The Evaluation of Osteoporosis:

Dual Energy X-ray Absorptiometry and Ultrasound in

Clinical Practice

Second Edition

The Evaluation of Osteoporosis:

Dual Energy X-ray Absorptiometry and Ultrasound in

Clinical Practice

Second Edition

GLEN M BLAKE PhD
Consultant Physicist and
Honorary Senior Lecturer
Guy's Hospital
London, UK

HEINZ W WAHNER MD FACP
Professor of Radiology and
Consultant Physician in Nuclear Medicine
The Mayo Clinic
Rochester
Minnesota, USA

IGNAC FOGELMAN MD FRCP
Professor of Nuclear Medicine and
Honorary Consultant Physician
Guy's Hospital
London, UK

MARTIN DUNITZ

© Martin Dunitz Ltd 1999

First published in the United Kingdom in 1999 by
Martin Dunitz Ltd
The Livery House
7–9 Pratt Street
London NW1 0AE

A CIP catalogue record for this book is available from the British Library

ISBN 1-85317-472-6

Distributed in the United States by:
Blackwell Science Inc.
Commerce Place, 350 Main Street
Malden, MA 02148, USA
Tel: 1–800–215–1000

Distributed in Canada by:
Login Brothers Book Company
324 Salteaux Crescent
Winnipeg, Manitoba, R3J 3T2
Canada
Tel: 204–224–4068

Distributed in Brazil by:
Ernesto Reichmann Distribuidora de Livros, Ltda
Rua Coronel Marques 335, Tatuape 03440–000
Sao Paulo,
Brazil

Composition by Wearset, Boldon, Tyne and Wear
Printed and bound in Great Britain by
Biddles Ltd, Guildford and King's Lynn

Contents

Guest Contributors

Carmelo A Formica PhD
Regional Bone Center
Helen Hayes Hospital
Route 9W, West Haverstraw
New York 10993-1195
USA

Didier Hans PhD
Osteoporosis and Arthritis Research Group
Department of Radiology
350 Parnassus Avenue, Suite 204
University of California
San Francisco
California 94117-1349
USA

H Theodore Harcke MD FACR
A.I. duPont Hospital for Children
Department of Medical Imaging
1600 Rockland Road
PO Box 269
Wilmington
Delaware 19899
USA

Miroslaw Jablonski MD PhD
Orthopaedic Department
Lubin Medical School
20–707 Lubin
Poland

Michael Jergas MD
Department of Radiology
Ruhr-University Bochum
St Josef-Hospital
Gudrunstr. 56
D-44791 Bochum
Germany

Colin G Miller PhD
Bona Fide Ltd
313 West Beltline Highway
Madison
Wisconsin 53713
USA

Christopher F Njeh PhD
Osteoporosis and Arthritis Research Group
Department of Radiology
350 Parnassus Avenue, Suite 204
University of California
San Francisco
California 94117-1349
USA

Jacqueline A Rea
Osteoporosis Research Unit
Guy's Hospital
London SE1 9RT
UK

John A Shepherd PhD
Hologic Inc
590 Lincoln Street
Waltham
Massachusetts 02154
USA

PREFACE TO THE SECOND EDITION

When writing the First Edition of this book in 1993, it was difficult to appreciate fully the growth and widespread acceptance of DXA that would occur within a few years. DXA measurements are no longer simply a research tool, but are generally recognised as being of immense clinical value and are considered a routine test.

To some extent the great increase in DXA use has followed on from intense interest and developments in the field of osteoporosis itself, with new and effective treatments becoming available, and with DXA studies now reimbursed in many countries. However, there have also been technical advances, with increased speed of examination the most noteworthy. The most dramatic development which has occurred in recent years, however, is the introduction of quantitative ultrasound for skeletal assessment, which has the obvious advantages of not using ionising radiation, being potentially portable and inexpensive. Clinical studies have shown that ultrasound measurements can evaluate risk of osteoporotic fracture as accurately as DXA, at least in the elderly population. In addition to conventional water based ultrasound systems for measuring the calcaneus, there are dry systems, imaging systems which improve accuracy for repositioning, systems that measure other skeletal sites, and recently semi-reflective systems that open up the tantalising possibility of obtaining ultrasound measurements in virtually any bone in the skeleton. Furthermore, since the FDA has recently approved the first bone ultrasound systems in the USA it is probable that ultrasound will be used extensively in clinical practice in the near future. We believe that the widespread use of ultrasound is inevitable and will eventually mean that effectively all women can have an assessment of osteoporotic fracture risk should they desire it. We are convinced that clinical ultrasound measurements of bone are here to stay and have therefore included it together with DXA in this comprehensive review of these techniques in the evaluation of osteoporosis.

ACKNOWLEDGEMENTS

I would like to thank Heinz Wahner and Ignac Fogelman for the help and encouragement they have given me in undertaking the task of producing a Second Edition of this book. Although much has changed in the technology and its applications over the past five years, the First Edition proved an excellent foundation on which to base an up-to-date account of the rationale and methodologies of bone densitometry. Secondly, I would like to thank all the guest contributors. The knowledge and expertise they have brought has added immensely to the overall scope and depth of the book.

I would especially like to thank the manufacturers and their representatives who have read and commented on sections of the manuscript and patiently answered my many requests for information. In particular, I would like to thank Jim Hanson (Lunar Corporation), Peter Steiger (Hologic Inc), Debbie Inskip (Aura Scientific), Joyce Paucek (Norland Medical Systems), John Aspinall (Norland Medical Systems), Tina Günther (Osteometer MediTech), Jean Luc Dumas (Diagnostic Medical Systems) and Nicole Hamilton (Schick Technologies Inc), all of whose assistance has been invaluable.

I would also like to thank the many colleagues at Guy's Hospital whose work and enthusiasm has provided a vital foundation for many chapters in this book. In particular, I would like to thank Rajesh Patel, Paul Ryan, Ruth Herd, Mandy Lewis, So-Jin Holohan, Jacqui Rea, Michelle Frost, Karen Knapp, Jane Parker, Anita Jefferies, Fiona Crane, Francesca Buxton, Matthew Sabin, Tania Jagathesan, Thesan Ramalingam, Ann-Marie Rees and Sanjiv Chhaya. Special thanks are due to Tanya Wheatley of Martin Dunitz Publishers for her tireless help and advice.

Finally, this book would not have been possible without long months of patient understanding on the part of my wife Chris.

Glen Blake

1

Metabolic Bone Disease and Osteoporosis: Relevant Information for Bone Mineral Measurements

CONTENTS • **Chapter overview** • **Introduction** • **Osteoporosis** • **Bone remodelling** • **Treatment** • **Clinical classification of osteoporosis** • **Contributions of bone mineral measurements to the understanding of metabolic bone disease**

CHAPTER OVERVIEW

This chapter reviews the different disease entities characterized by bone loss and defines the clinical terms used in dealing with patients affected by them. The diagnostic approach is briefly outlined to set the stage for discussing the role of bone mineral measurements in the diagnostic strategy and for making management decisions as described in later chapters. A brief description of the components of bone tissue is included. The latter is important for some techniques, such as quantitative computed tomography (QCT), but should cause little concern to the user of dual X-ray absorptiometry (DXA) procedures, except in very special circumstances.

INTRODUCTION

During the past 25 years, significant progress has been made in the development of techniques for measuring bone mass in vivo. A complex pattern of bone loss in health and disease has been revealed, and bone mineral measurements have come to be regarded as an essential tool for a rational approach to diagnosis and treatment of abnormal bone loss. Newer treatment regimens make it possible not only to decrease or stop bone loss, but in certain instances also to restore some bone to sites of frequent fracture[1,2] and thus reduce fracture risk.[3] Interest is now centred on how the results can be used effectively in the clinical work-up and management of patients suspected of having bone loss, and to identify patients who are likely to benefit from measures to reduce bone loss. A growing interest by pharmaceutical companies to develop more effective drugs to treat or prevent osteoporosis has resulted in multicentre studies of large populations based on bone density measurements. Increasingly, the focus of these studies is to demonstrate statistically significant reductions in fracture incidence.[3]

OSTEOPOROSIS

The term *osteoporosis* refers to a disease which is characterized by an absolute decrease in the amount of bone to a level below that required for mechanical support of normal activity and

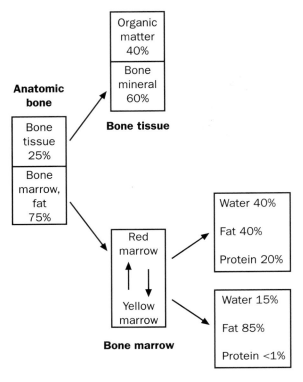

Figure 1.1 Composition of bone tissue. Values are approximate tissue compartments in axial skeletal bone and may vary widely with different skeletal sites.

tissue and 75% is bone marrow and fat. This proportion varies widely between different parts of the skeleton. Of the specific bone tissue, only 60% is bone mineral; 40% is organic matter, mainly collagen[4] (Figure 1.1).

Bone marrow consists of a stroma, myeloid tissue, fat cells, blood vessels, sinusoids and some lymphatic tissue. The yellow bone marrow contains mainly fat cells and the red marrow mainly erythropoietic tissue elements. There is no sharp demarcation between the two types of bone marrow. With advancing age, the proportion of red marrow decreases and is replaced with yellow marrow. At any age the proportion of yellow and red marrow varies with the skeletal site.

In osteoporosis, the anatomical bone volume (bone size) is unchanged, but the bone shows cortical thinning and porosis. Also, in the trabecular portion, the trabeculae are thinned and in certain regions have disappeared (Figure 1.2). Bone tissue constitutes less than the normal proportion of anatomical bone (Figure 1.1).

by the occurrence of skeletal fractures following minimal trauma. The distinction from age-related bone loss is only quantitative. The full aetiology of osteoporosis is not clearly understood and it is clearly a multifactorial disorder. Ageing, menopause, lifestyle, local factors regulating bone turnover, genetic factors and additional sporadic factors are considered to contribute to this bone loss. The current definition of osteoporosis is discussed and elaborated upon in Chapter 2.

The skeleton consists of cortical (70–80% by mass) and trabecular bone (20–30% by mass). In the normal axial skeleton approximately 25% of the anatomical bone volume is specific bone

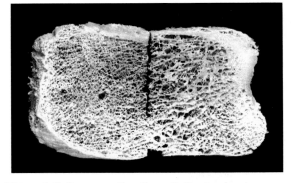

Figure 1.2 Cross-section through the trochanter region of a proximal femur, showing cortical and trabecular bone distribution. Normal (left) and osteoporotic (right) are compared. The cross-sectional area is the same on the two sides (From: Wahner HW. *Nuclear Medicine Annual* (Raven Press: New York, 1986), 195–226. Reproduced with permission from the author and publisher.)

The additional space is filled with fat. The ratio of specific bone tissue to bone marrow (fat or active marrow) is decreased. However, within the bone tissue, the ratio of mineral to organic matter remains unchanged. The chemical composition of the bone mineral in osteoporotic bone tissue is indistinguishable from that of normal bone.[5] If this were not the case, bone mineral results would be difficult to interpret in quantitative terms, because both chemical composition and mineral mass affect the measured X-ray attenuation.

In osteomalacia and rickets – another possible, although rare, cause of bone loss and fracture – the anatomical bone volume is also unchanged. In contrast to osteoporosis, the volume of bone tissue is normal or even increased. However, the bone tissue shows less than the normal mineral content and the organic matter is increased (uncalcified bone tissue). If both osteomalacia and osteoporosis are present, both mineral content and volume of bone tissue are decreased (Figure 1.3).

Analysis and quantification of the components of bone tissue as described above are only possible by bone histomorphometry performed on bone biopsy specimens. An understanding of the components of bone tissue is relevant to bone mineral analysis, especially when QCT is used, because these components of bone tissue have greatly differing attenuation properties at the X-ray energies used. When marrow fat and non-ossified bone tissue are present in abnormal amounts, this will falsely lower the measured bone density. This effect is negligible when DXA is used in patients who present for osteoporosis work-up. However, in severe osteomalacia in children bone mineral density (BMD) values may be falsely lower (by a few per cent) even with DXA due to the increase in organic matrix. The same may be true when marked bone marrow changes occur as a result of disease or treatment. Bone tissue components are summarized in Table 1.1. Bone loss constitutes a loss of bone mineral, which may be accompanied by a change of bone structure, and a change in the organic components in bone.

BONE REMODELLING

Throughout life, bone is remodelled by an orderly process of bone formation and resorption, which occurs in discrete foci throughout the skeleton called remodelling units. Each cycle consists of an activation process in which osteoclast precursor cells are activated, fuse and become multicellular osteoclasts that resorb bone, creating a tunnel in cortical bone or a lacuna on the surface of trabeculae. This period lasts 1–3 weeks. The osteoclasts disappear and are replaced by osteoblasts that fill in the tunnel, or lacuna. This period lasts 3–4 months. A rest period follows. The remodelling cycles are not synchronized. Resorption and formation are tightly coupled in young adulthood, so that the net balance of change in bone mass is zero. The rate of bone turnover is determined by the frequency of activation of new remodelling units. In age-dependent bone loss, there is an incomplete filling of normal size osteoclast resorption cavities, that is, a decrease in normal bone formation. This results in a thinning of trabeculae. In menopausal bone loss (high-turnover state), there is an increase in osteoclast numbers leading to the creation of an abnormally large resorption cavity. However, this is not accompanied by an increase in osteoblast activity, resulting in incomplete filling in of the cavity. This leads to a focal destruction of

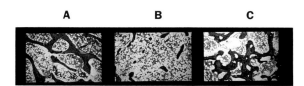

Figure 1.3 Iliac crest biopsies, Goldner's trichrome stain, 4-µm-thick sections; ×40. (A) General view of normal trabecular bone. (B) Osteoporosis; note the sparsity of trabecular bone and abundance of fat. (C) Osteomalacia; the increase in non-calcified osteoid (organic component of bone tissue) is apparent.

Table 1.1 Summary of gross anatomic and microscopic changes in bone with metabolic bone disease. (From: Wahner HW. *Nuclear Medicine Annual* (Raven Press: New York, 1986), 195–226. Reproduced with permission from the author and publisher.)

| | Gross anatomic bone composition | | | Chemical composition of bone tissue | | |
| | | | | Mineral phase | | |
Disease	Anatomic volume	Bone tissue (volume)	Bone marrow[a] (volume)	Ash weight	Ash composition	Organic phase
Osteoporosis	Normal	Decreased	Increased	Decreased	Normal	Decreased
Osteomalacia	Normal	Normal to increased	Normal to decreased	Decreased	Normal	Increased
Mixed osteomalacia and osteoporosis	Normal	Normal to decreased	Normal to increased	Decreased	Normal	Increased

[a] 'Marrow' is used here not to describe erythropoietic bone marrow but rather the fat and marrow that fill the spaces between the bone trabeculae.

trabeculae, which interrupts the normal structural integrity of the trabecular network.

TREATMENT

Drugs useful for treating osteoporosis decrease the abnormally increased rate of bone loss and may add bone to the skeleton. The mechanism can be explained using the concept of bone remodelling described above. The effect of drugs is not uniform throughout the skeleton and in particular may affect trabecular and cortical bone differently. Interestingly, some recent fracture prevention studies suggest that the increase in bone density during treatment can explain only 40% of the observed reduction in fracture incidence suggesting that other mechanisms are at work.[6] Presently used drugs can be classified as either anti-resorptive or formation-stimulating (Table 1.2).

CLINICAL CLASSIFICATION OF OSTEOPOROSIS

Osteoporosis can be classified into primary and secondary forms, depending on the presence or absence of other medical conditions. Such classifications are given in Tables 1.3 and 1.4. By far the most frequently encountered forms are Type I and Type II primary osteoporosis.

Clinical presentation

The clinical spectrum of osteoporosis has been extensively reviewed in several publications.[7-9] Only a short outline is given here.

The chief complaint of patients with spinal osteoporosis is acute or intermittent back pain following normal activity. The pain usually lasts a few days or weeks, and then subsides. Such episodes recur, and may result in chronic

Table 1.2 Drugs used in the treatment of osteoporosis.

Action	Drug	Remarks
Inhibition of bone resorption	Calcium	Minor retardation of bone loss and reduction of fractures in osteoporosis. Most widely prescribed drug.
	Oestrogen	Most effective in high-bone-turnover states. Retards bone loss, increases bone mass and reduces fractures. Side-effects.
	Bisphosphonates	Increase bone mass and reduce fractures by up to 50%. Convincing data regarding fracture efficiency.
	Selective oestrogen receptor modulators (SERMs)	Increase bone mass modestly without stimulating the endometrium. Possible protection against breast cancer and coronary artery disease.
	Calcitonin	Increases bone mass modestly and reduces fractures. Most effective in high-turnover states. Resistance in some patients.
	Vitamin D and compounds	Retard bone loss. Best if calcium absorption is impaired.
	Anabolic steroids	Some retardation of bone loss. Some are unsuitable for women.
Stimulation of bone formation	Sodium fluoride	Increases axial bone mass significantly. Cortical bone remains unchanged. Effect is dose dependent. At higher doses fracture risk is not affected despite higher bone mineral.
	Parathyroid hormone	Increases axial bone significantly with smaller effect on cortical bone. Possible fracture efficiency.

backache. These episodes are due to crush fractures of thoracic or lumbar vertebrae (Figure 1.4). As the disease progresses, loss of height, spinal deformity and fractures of hips, wrists and less frequently of other bones occur. The progression of the disease varies. Marked thoracic kyphosis and cervical lordosis can develop. Asymptomatic forms of the disease may occur where loss of height and deformity are the first clinical signs.

Table 1.3 Classification of osteoporosis. (From: Rubinstein E, Federman D, eds. *Scientific American Medicine*, Section 15, Subsection XI. Reproduced with permission. © 1988 Scientific American Inc. All rights reserved.)

Disorders of unknown cause in which osteoporosis is the major clinical abnormality

    Idiopathic osteoporosis: juvenile, adult
    Involutional osteoporosis

Disorders that contribute to osteoporosis in which the mechanism is partially understood
    Hypogonadism
    Hyperadrenocorticism: primary, iatrogenic
    Hyperthyroidism
    Intestinal malabsorption syndromes
    Scurvy
    Calcium deficiency
    Prolonged immobility
    Systemic mastocytosis
    Disorders caused by chronic heparin administration
    Disorders caused by chronic ingestion of anti-convulsant drugs
    Adult hypophosphatasia
    Disorders associated with other metabolic bone diseases: osteomalacia (of various causes),
        hyperparathyroidism

Heritable connective tissue disorders associated with osteoporosis
    Various forms of osteogenesis imperfecta
    Homocystinuria caused by cystathionine synthase deficiency
    Menkes' syndrome

Other systemic disorders or states associated with osteoporosis, possibly more frequently than accounted for by chance alone
    Rheumatoid arthritis
    Diabetes mellitus
    Chronic hepatic disease
    Alcoholism
    Down's syndrome
    Chronic pulmonary disease
    Waldenstrom's macroglobulinaemia
    Methotrexate-induced states

Impact on patient health

Osteoporosis is the leading cause of bone fractures in postmenopausal women and in the elderly population. In white women aged 65–84 years, 90% of fractures of the hip and spine, 70% of forearm fractures and 50% of fractures at other sites are caused by osteoporosis.[10] It is

Table 1.4 Classification of osteoporosis.

Classification		Clinical course	Diagnosis	Remarks
Primary osteoporosis (most frequent)	Involutional Type I	15–20 years, within menopause, women only	Vertebral crush fractures, high menopausal bone loss, bone turnover higher than 30%	Predominantly trabecular bone loss in axial skeleton
	Type II	Men or women over age 70	Vertebral crush fractures, hip and other fractures	Proportional loss of trabecular and cortical bone
(rare)	Idiopathic juvenile	Age 8–14, self-limited (2–4 years), both sexes	Fractures, low bone mass for age, normal laboratory	Normal growth, consider secondary forms
	Idiopathic young adult	Young adulthood, mild to severe (5–10 years), self-limited	Fractures, low bone mass, often hypercalcaemia, high- and low-bone-turnover forms	
Secondary osteoporosis	Endocrine, gastrointestinal, bone marrow disorders, connective tissue disorders, nutritional drugs	Associated with another disease, condition or drug	Underlying disease, low bone density, may present with fractures, pseudofracture	In general, partly reversible after treatment of primary disease

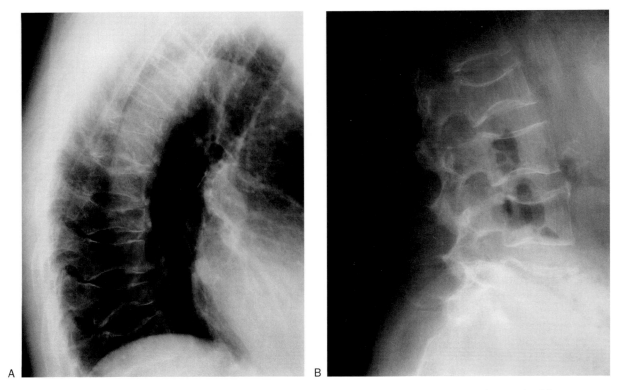

Figure 1.4 (A) Thoracic and (B) lumbar lateral spinal radiographs in a patient with multiple vertebral fractures.

estimated that in the USA in 1995 the total healthcare costs attributable to osteoporotic fractures exceeded $13 billion, of which two-thirds were due to hip fractures.[11] The consequences of the latter are particularly traumatic. The lifetime risk of hip fracture in women is as great as the risk of breast, endometrial and ovarian cancer combined. Half of all patients who survive a hip fracture are unable to walk unassisted and 25% are confined to nursing homes. In 12–20% of cases, the patient dies within 6 months.

The enormity of this health problem when set against the increasing population of elderly people in the western world is contrasted by our present therapeutic difficulties to significantly add bone and improve bone strength once it is lost. This has resulted in serious consideration of public health measures to prevent bone loss with guidelines for patients thought to be at risk of osteoporosis to undergo bone mineral measurements.

Diagnostic approach

The diagnostic approach to osteoporosis and bone loss includes a general examination, together with a radiograph (AP and lateral) of the thoracic and lumbar spine and of other sites with bone pain. Laboratory tests to evaluate endocrine, liver and renal function, calcium balance and absorption, and serum electrophoresis may be needed, depending on the degree of suspicion of secondary osteoporosis after a thorough clinical history and examination. Blood and urine tests that measure biochemical markers of bone turnover can be added. A bone density measurement should be obtained. With the widespread availability of DXA, spine and femur scans are generally performed. However, measurements of the peripheral skeleton are an acceptable alternative.[12]

With these tests, it should be possible to: (1) decide whether crush fractures or other signs of bone loss are present (radiograph); (2) judge the severity of bone loss (bone mineral measurements); and (3) exclude secondary causes of bone loss (laboratory tests).

For selection of the optimal treatment, it may be necessary to determine whether bone turnover is high or low, since treatments that depress bone resorption are most effective when used in high-turnover states. This historically was performed by iliac crest biopsy after double labelling with tetracycline, but biochemical markers such as alkaline phosphatase (bone isoenzyme), osteocalcin (Gla-protein), and urinary excretion of pyridinoline crosslinks and a number of other potential markers of bone turnover are being evaluated, and are likely to provide this information reliably in the future.[13] Repeated measurements of bone mineral are not sensitive enough to detect clinically significant rates of bone loss when performed within the short timespan of the weeks or months available for making the diagnosis.

Other potential indications for bone mineral measurements include screening for osteopenia, monitoring bone mass to assess efficacy of therapy and perhaps to identify 'fast bone losers' for more aggressive therapy. A detailed discussion of these indications is given in Chapter 16.

Evaluation of the skeletal radiograph is performed primarily to diagnose vertebral fracture, but is also of value to search for evidence of secondary causes and to establish a baseline for later measurements. Generalized osteopenia (picture frame appearance of end-plates, loss of horizontal trabeculae) and vertebral deformity (collapse, anterior wedging, ballooning, Schmorl's nodes) should be recorded. A detailed guide to the information obtainable from a review of skeletal radiographs in osteoporosis has been compiled by Eastell and Riggs.[14] Routine interpretation of radiographs usually identifies only advanced fractures. Guidelines are available on how to evaluate radiographs for vertebral fractures.[15] The subject of vertebral morphometry is discussed in Chapter 20.

CONTRIBUTIONS OF BONE MINERAL MEASUREMENTS TO THE UNDERSTANDING OF METABOLIC BONE DISEASE

Bone mineral determinations by X-ray absorptiometry measure the mass of bone mineral located in a region of interest defined on the two-dimensional projection image acquired by the scanning device. The results are expressed as the areal density, which is defined as the mass of bone mineral (or hydroxyapatite) per unit area of bone scanned. The information is different from that obtained using skeletal radiography, which evaluates the morphology of the skeleton with high image resolution, but is insensitive to changes in bone mineral mass.

Classification of bone diseases has historically been based on radiographic, biochemical and biopsy-related information, and bone mineral measurements cannot replace these tests for making a specific diagnosis such as osteomalacia. However, following the guidelines issued by the World Health Organization working group for the use of BMD in the diagnosis of osteoporosis (see Chapter 2), this condition is increasingly being diagnosed in this way and the clinical implications of this are further discussed in Chapter 16. Bone mineral measurements additionally allow: (1) estimation of whether bone mineral density or bone mineral mass are within a normal range and quantification of the degree of abnormality when present;

(2) use of these results to estimate the fracture risk; and (3) estimation of the rate of bone loss over a 1–2-year interval. This gives bone mineral measurements a front-line position in the diagnostic armament of the physician interested in bone disease.

REFERENCES

1. Liberman UA, Weiss SR, Bröll J et al. Effect of oral alendronate on bone mineral density and the incidence of fractures in postmenopausal osteoporosis. *N Engl J Med* (1995) **333**: 1437–43.
2. Herd RJM, Balena R, Blake GM et al. The prevention of early postmenopausal bone loss by cyclical etidronate therapy: a 2-year, double-blind, placebo-controlled study. *Am J Med* (1997) **103**: 92–9.
3. Black DM, Cummings SR, Karpf DB et al. Randomised trial of effect of alendronate on risk of fracture in women with existing vertebral fractures. *Lancet* (1996) **348**: 1535–41.
4. Nordin BEC, Crilly RG, Smith DA. Osteoporosis. In: Nordin B, ed. *Metabolic bone and stone disease*, 2nd edition (Churchill Livingstone: New York, 1984), 1–70.
5. Audran M, Basle MF, Galland F et al. X-ray microanalysis, ^{125}I single photon absorptiometry and histomorphometry of bone tissue in post menopausal osteoporosis. *Eur J Nucl Med* (1985) **11**(2/3): A24.
6. Cummings SR, Black DM, Vogt TM. Changes in BMD substantially underestimate the anti-fracture effects of alendronate and other anti-resorptive drugs. *J Bone Miner Res* (1996) **11**(suppl 1): S102.
7. Kanis JA. *Textbook of osteoporosis* (Blackwell Science: Oxford, 1996).
8. Marcus R, Feldman D, Kelsey J, eds. *Osteoporosis* (Academic Press: San Diego, 1996).
9. Meunier PJ, ed. *Osteoporosis: diagnosis and management* (Martin Dunitz: London, 1997).
10. Melton LJ, Thamer M, Ray NF et al. Fractures attributable to osteoporosis: report from the National Osteoporosis Foundation. *J Bone Miner Res* (1997) **12**: 16–23.
11. Ray NF, Chan JK, Thamer M, Melton LJ. Medical expenditures for the treatment of osteoporotic fractures in the United States in 1995: report from the National Osteoporosis Foundation. *J Bone Miner Res* (1997) **12**: 24–35.
12. Blake GM, Patel R, Fogelman I. Axial or peripheral bone density measurements? *J Clin Densitometry* (1998) **1**: 55–63.
13. Delmas PD. Biochemical markers for the assessment of bone turnover. In: Riggs BL, Melton LJ, eds. *Osteoporosis: etiology, diagnosis and management*, 2nd edition (Lippincott-Raven: Philadelphia, 1995), 319–33.
14. Eastell R, Riggs BL. Diagnostic evaluation of osteoporosis. In: Young WF, Klee GG, eds. *Endocrinology and metabolism clinics of North America* (WB Saunders: Philadelphia, 1988), 547–71.
15. Cummings SR, Melton LJ, Felsenberg D et al. Assessing vertebral fractures: report of the National Osteoporosis Foundation working group on vertebral fractures. *J Bone Miner Res* (1995) **10**: 518–23.

2

Bone Mass Measurements and Fracture Risk

Guest chapter by Michael Jergas

CHAPTER OVERVIEW

Over the last 20 years measurements of bone density have come to be recognized as an essential criterion for evaluating a patient's risk of osteoporotic fracture. More recently, ultrasound measurements of the calcaneus have been shown to have a predictive capability similar to conventional densitometry. This chapter reviews the evidence from epidemiological studies on which these conclusions are based. Although the differences in the ability of the various methodologies and measurement sites to predict fractures are marginal, it does seem that measurements at the site of fracture perform slightly better than measurements at other sites, especially for hip fractures. Although bone densitometry is well established, the concept of relying solely on a bone density threshold for making decisions on treatment does not do justice to the complexity of the disease. Clinical decisions should be based on a risk profile for each individual patient based on bone density and a full assessment of other risk factors. A brief review of the statistical methods used to interpret fracture studies is given in the Appendix to this chapter.

DEFINING OSTEOPOROSIS

The term osteoporosis is derived from the Greek language: *osteon* means bone, and *poros* is a small hole. Thus, the term *osteoporosis* is quite descriptive of the changes in bone tissue that can be observed in this generalized skeletal disease. Nevertheless, the definition of osteoporosis has changed through the times, mostly based on new evidence or new techniques that have become available for its diagnosis. Today, there is a tendency to define osteoporosis by means of quantitative determination of bone mineral density (BMD), or bone densitometry. Bone densitometry has played a major role as a means to measure objectively what radiologists subjectively describe as changes in the radiolucency of the skeleton on conventional radiographs. Today's importance of bone densitometry in the clinical diagnosis of osteoporosis is reflected in the definition of osteoporosis given by the Consensus Development Conference 1993, sponsored by the European Foundation for Osteoporosis and Bone Disease, the National Osteoporosis Foundation, and the National Institute of Arthritis and Musculoskeletal and Skin Disease: *Osteoporosis is a systemic skeletal disease characterized by low bone mass and microarchitectural deterioration of*

Table 2.1 Diagnostic categories for osteoporosis based on spinal bone density measurements as proposed by Kanis et al.[6]	
Category	*Definition by bone density*
Normal	A value for bone mineral density or bone mineral content that is not more than 1 SD below the young adult mean value.
Low bone mass (or osteopenia)	A value for bone mineral density or bone mineral content that lies between 1 and 2.5 SD below the young adult mean value.
Osteoporosis	A value for bone mineral density or bone mineral content that is more than 2.5 SD below the young adult mean value.
Severe osteoporosis (or established osteoporosis)	A value for bone mineral density or bone mineral content more than 2.5 SD below the young adult mean value in the presence of one or more fragility fractures.

SD, standard deviation.

bone tissue, with a consequent increase in bone fragility and susceptibility to fracture.[1]

The availability of a technique, i.e. bone densitometry in its various applications, clearly finds its expression in many definitions of osteoporosis that are entirely based on bone mass measurements. For example, Melton and Wahner proposed a definition of osteoporosis based on bone density.[2] The authors defined clinical osteoporosis as the presence of fractures resulting from minor trauma and simultaneous low bone density below a fracture threshold. The clinical consequence of such a finding would be to begin treatment for osteoporosis. The state of low bone density that is concurrent with a doubling or tripling of the risk for a fracture is defined as osteopenia, and represents an indication for starting prophylactic treatment. The World Health Organization (WHO) working group continued this approach in its definition of osteoporosis that was published in 1994.[3–5] In women, osteoporosis can be diagnosed if the value for BMD or bone mineral content (BMC) is 2.5 or more standard deviations (SD) below the mean value of a young reference population (T-score ≤ -2.5 SD). Kanis and co-workers commented on this definition and gave diagnostic categories that may be applied to white women (Table 2.1).[6]

Thus, the current diagnosis of osteoporosis relies mainly on bone mass measurements. The essential task of bone densitometry in a clinical setting is to identify patients at risk of osteoporotic fractures. Therefore, the association between bone mass and future fractures must be established, and various researchers have studied this association in a prospective fashion.

WHICH FRACTURES ARE OSTEOPOROTIC?

Fractures are the hallmark of osteoporosis, and often have a substantial impact on a patient's life. There is unanimous agreement that most fractures of the hip, wrist and vertebral body

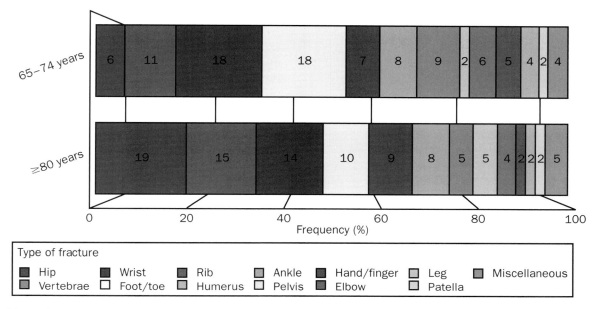

Figure 2.1 Frequency (in per cent) of fracture by type in white women aged 65–74 years and 80 years and older from the 'Study of Osteoporotic Fractures' 1986–92. (Data from Nevitt.[8])

without an adequate trauma may be attributed to osteoporosis.[7] In addition, there are a number of other fractures occurring in elderly people that may also be related to osteoporosis (Figure 2.1).[8] However, not all fractures in elderly people are associated with low bone density. In the setting of a large prospective study on the various aspects of osteoporosis in the ageing female population, the Study of Osteoporotic Fractures, Seeley et al. studied the relationship between bone mass and a variety of fractures.[9] The authors found that risks for fractures of the wrist, foot, humerus, hip, rib, toe, leg, pelvis, hand and clavicle were significantly related to reduced bone mass at the distal and mid-radius as well as the calcaneus (Figure 2.2). On the other hand, fractures of the ankle, elbow, finger and face were not associated with bone density at any measurement site. Thus, low bone density is associated with most types of fractures in elderly people. Few other studies offer such a detailed review of various fracture sites.

ASSOCIATION BETWEEN LOW BONE DENSITY AND FRACTURES

The first prospective study to evaluate the association between bone density and fractures was published as early as 1975. Smith and co-workers followed 278 women out of an initial study population of 571 white women aged 50 or above who had bone density measurements of the radius at baseline.[10] After a mean follow-up time of 1.7 years, 31 women had fractures. For both the distal and mid-radius, bone mass was inversely related to fracture incidence. A second study from the same group also used Singh's index of femoral trabecular pattern in addition to radius bone mass for fracture prediction in 106 white women, aged 70–95 years,

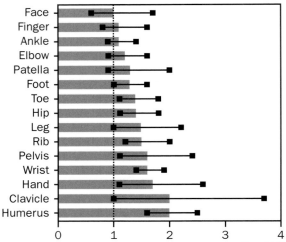

Hazard ratio per 1 SD decrease in proximal radius BMD

Figure 2.2 Age-adjusted hazard ratios (and 95% confidence intervals) of various fractures for a 1 standard deviation decrease in mid-radius bone density. (Data from Seeley et al.[9])

who were all nursing home residents.[11] Fractures occurred in 29 women after a mean follow-up period of 2.5 years. The authors again noted an association between bone mass at the radius and incident fractures, but did not find any correlation between the Singh index and subsequent fracture. The latter observation for the Singh index is probably due to the difficult assessment of this index.

Following these first prospective studies a number of researchers have studied the association between bone density and fracture risk. The Study of Osteoporotic Fractures (SOF) involved more than 9000 non-black women in four different regions of the USA and is probably the largest and most ambitious of a number of epidemiological studies. The different ways data are acquired and analysed can make it difficult to compare the results from the various studies. Often Cox's proportional hazards models or logistic regression analyses with a variety of predictors included in the models are

employed. There are also considerable differences in the populations studied as well as the length of the follow-up period. Table 2.2 lists some characteristics and results of prospective studies for prediction of osteoporotic fractures using bone densitometry. Risk ratios and odds ratios given in this table were taken directly from the respective publications.

Single photon (and X-ray) absorptiometry (SPA, SXA) as well as dual photon (and X-ray) absorptiometry (DPA, DXA) have been the most commonly used techniques to assess bone mass in the context of epidemiological studies. Almost all the measures derived from these techniques, BMC, BMD and bone mineral apparent density (BMAD), have been found to be associated with most types of fractures, especially in women (Table 2.2).[12–32] In a meta-analysis of prospective studies involving bone densitometry, Marshall and co-workers demonstrated that bone density measurements at the specific site of fracture tend to be slightly superior for predicting fractures at the respective site than measurements at other sites (Figure 2.3).[33] For example, a hip fracture is best predicted by hip bone density. However, while this seems to hold true for hip fractures, it is less obvious at other skeletal sites. For example, Black et al. found that measurements of the radius, calcaneus, hip and lumbar spine all provided similar predictive capability for a woman's subsequent risk of wrist fracture.[24] Overall, the different techniques and measurement sites do not differ substantially in their ability to predict future fracture, and the question whether one technique is significantly better than the others remains controversial.

There are few prospective data existing for quantitative computed tomography (QCT), even though this method has been applied widely in clinical practice since the early 1980s.[34] Ross and colleagues examined the vertebral fracture incidence in 380 women participating in a pharmaceutical trial, of whom 294 had an axial QCT measurement at baseline as well as DPA measurements of the spine and the femur.[17] Over an average 2.9 years follow-up time, 47 women experienced new vertebral fractures and 28 women had repeat fractures in

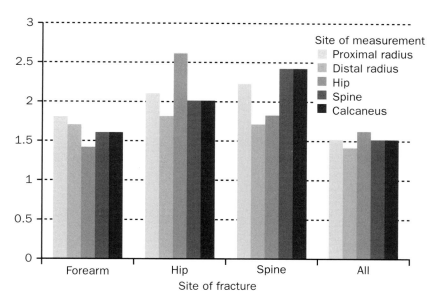

Figure 2.3 Relative risk of fracture for a 1 standard deviation (SD) decrease in bone density below aged-adjusted mean from the summary of a meta-analysis of prospective studies.[33] The results are given for various fracture sites as well as various sites of bone density measurements.

previously fractured vertebrae. For women with repeat fractures, rate ratios were higher for QCT measurements than for spinal or femoral DPA, while spinal and femoral DPA predicted new (incident) vertebral fractures somewhat better. There was also a strong association of incident vertebral fractures with prevalent fractures. The authors also found that the simultaneous use of two predictors (either two bone density measurements, or bone density and prevalent fracture) improved fracture prediction. The latter study is the only published prospective study including QCT measurements at baseline. However, there are many cross-sectional studies investigating the association between bone density and vertebral fracture, either for QCT alone or for QCT in comparison with other modalities. Most of these studies show a superior diagnostic capability for QCT with respect to discriminating patients with fractures from those without.[35–41] However, a recent cross-sectional study by Ito

and colleagues showed that QCT trabecular bone density was not superior to projectional bone density measurements of the calcaneus and the ultradistal forearm in the oldest study participants aged 70–79 years, while in younger participants QCT provided the best discrimination between fractured and non-fractured women.[42] This observation has to be confirmed in further studies.

Since there exist a large number of retrospective (or cross-sectional) studies of bone density measurements, an important question is whether cross-sectional study designs are valid for the evaluation of bone densitometry techniques and for the assessment of fracture risk. Stegman et al. compared prospective and retrospective study designs for assessing fracture risk within a 24-year cohort study.[26] The authors found that the estimates of relative risk of low-trauma fracture determined from a cohort study and the odds ratio determined from a nested case–control study within the

Table 2.2 Summary details from selected prospective studies of bone density and fracture risk. Odds or risk ratios were taken directly from the articles.

Study	Study population	Length of follow-up (years)	Site/type of fracture (number of patients)	Site/type of measurement	Model/adjustment	Odds/risk ratio
Melton III et al.[27]	304 women aged 30–94 years	7.8	Spine; mild to moderate trauma (n < 48)	BMD spine	Age-adjusted	2.2 (1.4–3.4)
				BMD femoral neck		2.0 (1.3–3.1)
				BMD trochanter		1.7 (1.1–2.6)
				BMD distal radius		1.6 (1.0–2.5)
				BMD mid-radius		2.5 (1.5–4.2)
			Proximal femur; mild to moderate trauma (n < 10)	BMD spine	Age-adjusted	2.3 (1.0–5.4)
				BMD femoral neck		2.8 (1.4–5.8)
				BMD trochanter		2.4 (1.1–5.2)
				BMD distal radius		3.1 (1.2–7.8)
				BMD mid-radius		1.5 (0.6–3.6)
			Distal forearm; mild to moderate trauma (n < 15)	BMD spine	Age-adjusted	1.4 (0.8–2.7)
				BMD femoral neck		1.5 (0.8–2.8)
				BMD trochanter		1.6 (0.9–2.8)
				BMD distal radius		2.3 (1.1–4.6)
				BMD mid-radius		1.5 (0.7–3.2)
			All sites; mild to moderate trauma (n < 125)	BMD spine	Age-adjusted	1.5 (1.1–2.0)
				BMD femoral neck		1.6 (1.2–2.2)
				BMD trochanter		1.5 (1.1–1.9)
				BMD distal radius		1.4 (1.0–1.9)
				BMD mid-radius		1.5 (1.1–2.1)
Stegman et al.[26]	131 Roman Catholic nuns	24	All sites (n < 31)	BMC radius	Adjusted for age and effective time postmenopausal	1.7 (1.1–2.6)[a] 1.9 (1.1–3.3)[b]

Table 2.2 Continued

Study	Study population	Length of follow-up (years)	Site/type of fracture (number of patients)	Site/type of measurement	Model/adjustment	Odds/risk ratio
Hui et al.[13]	386 free-living white women	6.7	Forearm (n = 7)	BMC radius	Age-adjusted	3.6 (1.9–6.8)
			All sites (n = 35)			2.6 (2.0–3.4)
	135 white women living in retirement home	5.5	Forearm (n = 10)			1.2 (0.7–2.2)
			Hip (n = 30)			1.9 (1.4–2.7)
			All sites (n = 54)			1.5 (1.2–2.0)
Hui et al.[14]	386 free-living white women	6.7	All sites (n = 35)	BMC radius	Unadjusted	3.1
				BMD radius		3.2
				BMAD radius		3.4
	135 white women living in retirement home	5.5	All sites (n = 54)	BMC radius		1.7
				BMD radius		1.7
				BMAD radius		1.6
Wasnich et al.[15]	699 Japanese-American women aged 43–80 years	3.6	Spine (n = 39)	BMD calcaneus	Age-adjusted; risks calculated for 2 SD difference	6.9 (4.3–10.6)
				BMD distal radius		5.7 (3.6–8.7)
				BMD spine		3.9 (2.4–6.2)
Ross et al.[16]	897 postmenopausal women	>4	Spine (n = 61)	BMD distal radius	Age-adjusted; risks calculated for 2 SD difference	3.6 (2.2–6.8)
				BMD prox. radius		4.0 (2.3–7.3)
				BMD calcaneus		5.8 (3.2–10.5)
				BMD spine		5.0 (2.8–9.1)

Table 2.2 Continued

Study	Study population	Length of follow-up (years)	Site/type of fracture (number of patients)	Site/type of measurement	Model/adjustment	Odds/risk ratio
Ross et al.[17]	380 women in clinical trial (294 with baseline QCT measurements)	2.9	All spine fractures; repeat and new (n = 57)	QCT spine	Age-adjusted; risks calculated for 2 SD difference	5.1 (2.8–9.1)
				BMD (DPA) spine		3.6 (2.0–6.6)
				BMD femoral neck		2.8 (1.4–5.6)
				BMD Ward's area		3.9 (2.0–7.3)
				BMD trochanter		4.8 (2.6–8.8)
			New spine fractures (n = 47)	QCT spine		4.8 (2.5–9.1)
				BMD (DPA) spine		5.8 (2.9–11.6)
				BMD femoral neck		5.2 (2.2–12.4)
				BMD Ward's area		3.8 (1.9–7.5)
				BMD trochanter		5.3 (2.7–10.3)
Gärdsell et al.[21]	1076 women	13	Distal radius (n = 66)	BMD distal radius	Age-adjusted	1.5
				BMD mid-radius		1.7
			Prox. humerus (n = 35)	BMD distal radius		1.9
				BMD mid-radius		1.7
			Hip, cervical (n = 28)	BMD distal radius		1.9
				BMD mid-radius		2.5
			Hip, trochanter (n = 17)	BMD distal radius		2.7
				BMD mid-radius		3.4
			All hip (n = 43)	BMD distal radius		2.5
				BMD mid-radius		3.2
			Spine (n = 70)	BMD distal radius		1.7
				BMD mid-radius		2.6
Gärdsell et al.[19]	654 men from various studies	11	Fragility fracture (n = 61)	BMD radius	Unadjusted; risk ratio for lowest vs. highest quintile	13

Table 2.2 Continued

Study	Study population	Length of follow-up (years)	Site/type of fracture (number of patients)	Site/type of measurement	Model/adjustment	Odds/risk ratio
Düppe et al.[22]	410 women aged 20–78 years at the time of measurement	20–25	Distal radius (n = 77)	BMD proximal radius	Age group 40–70 years at baseline measurement, age-adjusted relative risks At 25 years follow-up	1.3 (0.9–1.8)
			Spine (n = 63)			1.8 (1.2–2.6)
			All hip (n = 43)			1.7 (1.1–2.5)
			Hip, trochanter (n = 20)			2.1 (1.2–3.6)
			Hip, cervical (n = 23)			1.2 (0.7–2.1)
			All fragility fractures (n = 213)			1.3 (1.2–1.7)
			Distal radius		Age group 30–50 years at baseline measurement, age-adjusted relative risks at 25 years follow-up	1.7 (0.9–3.0)
			Spine			2.0 (0.9–4.6)
			All hip			1.4 (0.7–3.1)
			Hip, trochanter			
			Hip, cervical			1.1 (0.5–2.6)
			All fragility fractures			1.5 (1.0–2.4)
Cummings et al.[23]	8134 non-black women ≥65 years	1.8	Hip (n = 65)	BMD total femur	Age-adjusted	2.7 (2.0–3.6)
				BMD femoral neck		2.6 (1.9–3.6)
				BMD intertrochanter		2.5 (1.9–3.3)
				BMD trochanter		2.7 (2.0–3.6)
				BMD Ward's area		2.8 (2.1–3.6)
				BMD spine		1.6 (1.2–2.1)
				BMD distal radius		1.6 (1.2–2.1)
				BMD prox. radius		1.5 (1.2–1.9)
				BMD calcaneus		2.0 (1.5–2.7)

Table 2.2 Continued

Study	Study population	Length of follow-up (years)	Site/type of fracture (number of patients)	Site/type of measurement	Model/adjustment	Odds/risk ratio
Black et al.[24]	8134 non-black women ≥65 years	0.1–1.9 (0.7)	All sites (n = 191)	BMD total femur	Age-adjusted	1.4 (1.2–1.6)
				BMD femoral neck		1.4 (1.2–1.7)
				BMD intertrochanter		1.4 (1.2–1.7)
				BMD trochanter		1.4 (1.2–1.6)
				BMD Ward's area		1.4 (1.2–1.6)
				BMD spine		1.4 (1.2–1.6)
				BMD distal radius		1.5 (1.3–1.8)
				BMD prox. radius		1.4 (1.2–1.7)
				BMD calcaneus		1.3 (1.1–1.5)
			Wrist (n = 37)	BMD total femur	Age adjusted	1.5 (1.1–2.1)
				BMD femoral neck		1.7 (1.1–2.4)
				BMD intertrochanter		1.3 (0.9–1.9)
				BMD trochanter		1.5 (1.1–2.1)
				BMD Ward's area		1.4 (1.0–2.0)
				BMD spine		1.6 (1.1–2.3)
				BMD distal radius		1.8 (1.3–2.6)
				BMD prox. radius		1.6 (1.1–2.4)
				BMD calcaneus		1.8 (1.3–2.6)
Black et al.[25]	Random sample of 501 women from the 'Study of Osteoporotic Fractures'	3.7	Spine (n = 22)	BMD distal radius	Age-adjusted	1.8 (1.1–3.1)
				BMD prox. radius		1.6 (1.0–2.6)
				BMD calcaneus		2.7 (1.5–4.7)

Table 2.2 Continued

Study	Study population	Length of follow-up (years)	Site/type of fracture (number of patients)	Site/type of measurement	Model/adjustment	Odds/risk ratio
Seeley et al.[31]	9704 non-black women ≥65 years	5.9	Ankle (n = 191)	BMD distal radius	Age-adjusted	1.1 (1.0–1.3)
					Multivariable	1.2 (1.0–1.4)
			Foot (n = 204)		Age-adjusted	1.3 (1.1–1.5)
					Multivariable	1.3 (1.1–1.5)
Nguyen et al.[28]	1080 women ≥60 years	3.2	All atraumatic fractures (n = 192)	BMD femoral neck	Adjusted for quadriceps strength and body sway	2.4 (1.9–3.0)
	709 men ≥60 years	3.2	All atraumatic fractures (n = 89)	BMD femoral neck	Adjusted for quadriceps strength and body sway	2.0 (1.5–2.6)
Cheng et al.[29]	188 women aged 75 years, 133 women aged 80 years	29–34 months	Non-spine fractures in 17 75-year-olds, 10 80-year-olds	BMD calcaneus	75-year-olds	3.4 (1.4–8.1)
					80-year-olds	1.3 (0.2–5.9)
	103 men aged 75 years, 57 men aged 80 years		Non-spine fractures in 3 75-year-olds, 6 80-year-olds	BMD calcaneus	75- and 80-year-olds	3.6 (1.2–14.9)
Torgerson et al.[32]	1857 women aged 47–51 years	2	Self-reported non-spine and non-hip fractures (n = 44)	BMD spine	Unadjusted	1.9 (1.3–2.6)
				BMD femoral neck		1.1 (1.0–2.8)
				BMD Ward's area		1.4 (1.0–1.9)
				BMD trochanter		1.1 (0.8–1.5)
				BMD spine	Multivariate analysis	1.6 (1.2–2.3)

[a] Odds ratio for prospective study design; [b] odds ratio for retrospective study design.

BMC, bone mineral content; BMD, bone mineral density; BMAD, bone mineral apparent density.

For the study by Stegman et al. odds ratios are given for a prospective and a retrospective study design.[26]

For the study of Düppe et al. the number of fractures refers to the whole study population while the risk ratios apply to the respective subsets.[22]

cohort did not differ substantially. For each unit decrement in Z-score for forearm BMC, the adjusted relative risk ratio for the prospective study design was 1.67, while the odds ratio determined from the most recent BMC Z-score measurements was 1.87. Thus the measures from prospective and retrospective study designs are similar, and experience from several prospective and retrospective studies indicates that the results from these two types of studies may be comparable if carefully designed.[33] Nevertheless, further prospective studies are likely to be required, especially when new techniques are evaluated, or risk factors other than or in addition to bone density are assessed.

Based on results from some prospective studies, the value of bone densitometry for fracture prediction in very elderly patients has been questioned. In a prospective study by Gärdsell and co-workers, the authors found that BMC measured at the radius was associated with subsequent fractures in women aged 50–79 years, but fractures of the radius and the humerus as well as femoral neck fractures failed to show the same strong association with BMD in women aged 80 years and over as was found in the younger study population.[21] In the same study vertebral fractures showed a clear association with bone density at all ages. Similar results were reported by Hui et al. who studied elderly retirement home residents and a group of free-living women (Table 2.2).[13] Nevitt and colleagues studied the predictive value of bone mass in a larger group of women from the SOF study.[43] The authors found that for non-spine fractures, wrist and humerus fractures, a strong association with bone density existed. Fractures of the proximal femur were associated with bone density in all women. However, only trochanteric and not femoral neck fractures were associated with bone density in the oldest women (Figure 2.4). These results indicate that femoral neck fractures may be associated with factors other than bone density in elderly women and that efforts to maintain bone mass after age 80 may reduce the risk of trochanteric but not femoral neck fractures. Another important result from this study was that the excess risk of fracture of women with below-median bone density was greater in women aged 80 years and over compared with younger women. The latter study clearly demonstrates that bone density continues to be strongly associated with overall fracture risk in women aged 80 and over. Nevertheless, one must be aware that some limitations for bone densitometry in the prediction of certain types of fracture may exist in very elderly patients.

Looking at the average follow-up period in the various studies of bone densitometry, even in studies with follow-up periods of 20 years and more bone mass is significantly associated with incident fracture.[22,26] Figure 2.5 demonstrates the continuing association between baseline bone density and fracture risk over 25 years as reported by Düppe and colleagues.[22] The fact that bone density is a predictor of fractures over such a long period of time may be an argument for the importance of peak bone mass for future fracture. Hansen et al. found in a 12-year prospective study that radial bone density was associated with future Colles' fractures, but failed to predict vertebral fractures.[44] The authors found that an increased rate of bone loss existed in the patients who later suffered vertebral fractures. From these results the authors concluded that a baseline scan combined with a single estimation of bone loss may identify women at risk for developing osteoporotic fracture. Cheng and colleagues found in a 5-year prospective study that fracture occurrence was significantly associated with the initial bone mass measurement at the calcaneus.[30] The authors also noted that the change in BMD over that time period tended to relate to fracture occurrence in 75-year-old women while not being associated with fractures in 80-year-old women and in men. However, the results from this study in this respect are strongly limited by methodological issues. Both peak bone mass as well as bone loss resulting in low bone mass may be important predictors of future fractures. However, current evidence from other studies also suggests that the influence of initial bone mass on current bone mass and fracture risk is greater than that of bone loss in

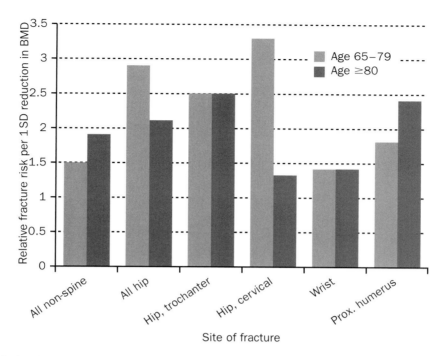

Figure 2.4 Relative risk of various fractures for a 1 standard deviation (SD) decrease in femoral neck bone densities in women aged 65–79 years and 80 years and over. Data are from a prospective study involving 8699 women who were followed for an average of 4.9 years.[43]

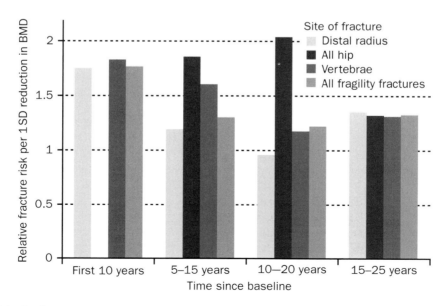

Figure 2.5 Risk of a fracture at various sites for a 1 standard deviation (SD) reduction in bone density at study baseline for subsequent 10-year periods (first 10 years, 5–15, 10–20, 15–25). All women were 50 years or older at study baseline. (Data from Düppe et al.[22])

women up to age 70 years.[13,20,21,45] It is estimated that 12 years after the menopause approximately 30% of the variance in density measurements may be explained on the basis of differential bone loss rates. Still, there is evidence that knowledge of bone loss improves the estimate of ultimate bone density.

DIAGNOSING OSTEOPOROSIS WITH QUANTITATIVE ULTRASOUND

Quantitative ultrasound (QUS) is one of the latest additions to the diagnostic toolbox of osteoporosis. This method, applied in the form of measurements of the speed of sound (SOS) and broadband ultrasound attenuation (BUA), has been used in industrial testing for a long time. The evolution in microelectronics made possible the easy application of QUS to the diagnosis of osteoporosis.

Quantitative ultrasound is a radiation-free method, and thus researchers as well as clinicians have embraced this technology enthusiastically as indicated by the large number of recently published studies. Also, QUS is not a simple measure of density, but rather a measure of other qualitative properties of bone. Clinical studies show that quantitative ultrasound measurements often correlate poorly with bone density at various sites. Several researchers have studied the association between quantitative ultrasonic measures and osteoporotic fractures, and some ongoing epidemiological studies on osteoporosis have included this method in their protocols. However, most results on this association are still derived from cross-sectional studies.

Table 2.3 lists the published prospective studies that focus on quantitative ultrasound measurements. The earliest such study was published in 1990 by Porter and colleagues.[46] The authors measured BUA in 1414 women aged 70 or above who were living in private or local authority homes for the elderly or in geriatric hospitals. Seventy-three women subsequently fractured a hip during the follow-up period of 2 years. Women with a low BUA, poor cognizance score and poor mobility had a higher incidence of fracture than those with a high BUA and good cognizance who were more mobile. These factors were partly independent. Heaney and colleagues reported on ultrasound transmission velocity measurements at the patella in 130 postmenopausal women who were free of vertebral fracture at baseline and were followed over 2 years.[47] Of these women, 19 developed fractures, and age-adjusted relative risk for the ultrasound measurement was 2.1. However, neither of these studies included bone density measurements for comparison.

Hans and co-workers studied the association between BUA, SOS, femoral neck BMD and hip fracture prospectively in 5662 women from the French EPIDOS study.[48] During the average follow-up period of 2 years, 115 new hip fractures occurred in the study population. The relative risks of hip fracture were 2.0 and 1.7 per 1 SD reduction in BUA and SOS respectively, compared to a relative risk of 1.9 per 1 SD reduction in femoral neck BMD. After inclusion of femoral neck density into a multivariate model the ultrasound variables remained predictive of hip fracture. Bauer and colleagues recently presented prospective data for the association between BUA, calcaneus BMD, femoral neck BMD and fracture risk in 6189 women from the SOF study.[49] The authors documented subsequent hip fractures and nonspine fractures during a mean follow-up of 2 years. Each 1 SD reduction in calcaneal BUA was associated with a doubling of the risk for hip fractures (relative risk (RR) = 2.0), which was similar to that for BMD measurements in the calcaneus (RR = 2.2) and the femoral neck (RR = 2.6). There was a stronger association between BUA and intertrochanteric fractures than between BUA and femoral neck fractures (RR = 3.3 versus RR = 1.3). Similar to the results from the EPIDOS study, Bauer et al. also found that BUA remained a significant predictor of hip fracture after adjustment for femoral neck BMD.

There are a number of retrospective studies worth mentioning since they represent further evidence of the diagnostic capability of quantitative ultrasound (Table 2.4). Bauer and coworkers studied BUA as well as bone density measurements of the hip, spine and the whole body in 442 women enrolling in a clinical trial.[50] After adjusting for age, weight and clinic, the relative risk for vertebral fracture was 1.8 (confidence interval (CI) 1.4–2.3) for each standard deviation reduction in BUA, while for each 1 SD reduction in bone density the relative risk was 1.7 at the femoral neck and 2.2 at the spine. Adjustment for spine, hip or whole body BMD did not significantly alter the association between BUA and vertebral fracture. Glüer and co-workers recently published a cross-sectional study of 4698 women from the Study of Osteoporotic Fractures population who had received BUA measurements at the heel as well as BMD measurements at the spine, hip and calcaneus.[51] In a multivariate logistic regression analysis, age, BUA and BMD of the calcaneus were independently associated with hip fractures, vertebral fractures at study baseline and recent vertebral fractures. The combination of femoral neck density and BUA showed only marginal improvement in the Receiver-Operating Characteristic (ROC) curve area. Further results from a number of retrospective studies are given in Table 2.4.[52–57]

OTHER PREDICTORS OF FRACTURE

The association between geometric properties of bone and biomechanical properties, such as the one between the cross-sectional area and the fracture load in vertebrae, or between the minimum moment of inertia, the cross-sectional area and forearm fracture force, is known from in vitro studies. An early technique for assessing skeletal status, the measurement of cortical thickness, represents a measurement of a geometric property of bone. Cortical thickness has been found to be related to age and bone density.[58–60] Several cross-sectional studies show an association between cortical thickness measures and prevalent fractures. A prospective nested case–control study for the prediction of hip fracture using metacarpal thickness was presented by Jergas and co-workers for the SOF study research group.[61] The combined cortical thickness and the cortical index provided a pre-

dictive capability (odds ratios between 1.7 and 2.2 per SD decrease) similar to that of bone density measurements at the calcaneus and the radius (odds ratios between 1.8 and 2.0).

Even though cortical thickness may be regarded as an architectural property of bone, it certainly reflects bone density too, and thus one would not necessarily expect cortical thickness to be predictive of only one particular type of fracture. However, there are architectural bone properties specific for a particular type of fracture. Hip axis length is the geometric measure that probably has received the most attention as indicated by the number of recent cross-sectional and prospective studies. It can be measured on radiographs and on DXA images, with the latter providing an automated and highly reproducible procedure.[62] Hip axis length is associated with hip fracture risk independent of age, height, weight and femoral bone density. In a prospective nested case–control study of 64 women with hip fracture and a random sample of 134 women from the SOF study, Faulkner and colleagues found that each standard deviation increase in hip axis length nearly doubled the risk of hip fracture (odds ratio 1.8; CI 1.3–2.5).[63] It is not associated with age, and is not predictive of fractures other than hip fractures.[64,65] Measuring a number of different geometric parameters from hip radiographs, Glüer et al. found that four measurements independently predicted hip fracture: reduced thickness of the femoral shaft cortex and of the femoral neck cortex; reduction in an index of tensile trabeculae; and a wider trochanteric region.[66] Two analyses by Nakamura et al.[67] and Cummings et al.[68] indicate that differences in geometric measures, including hip axis length, may explain differences in the rates of hip fracture between white, Asian and black women. Based on hip axis length, Cummings and colleagues estimated that Asians would have a 47% lower risk and blacks would have a 32% lower risk of hip fracture than whites because of their shorter hip axis.

Ross and colleagues measured vertebral depth from conventional radiographs in 804 women, of whom 100 developed new vertebral

Table 2.3 Summary details of prospective studies of quantitative ultrasound and fracture risk.

Study	Study population	Length of follow-up (years)	Site/type of fracture (number of patients)	Site/type of measurement	Model/adjustment	Odds/risk ratio
Porter et al.[46]	1414 women ⩾70 years	2	Hip (n = 73)	BUA calcaneus	Combinations with cognizance and mobility	Not given
Heaney et al[47]	130 postmenopausal women, no vertebral fracture	2	Spine (n = 19)	SOS patella	None	2.4 (1.3–4.3)
					Age-adjusted	2.1 (1.1–3.9)
Hans et al.[48]	5662 women ⩾75 years	2	Hip (n = 115)	BUA calcaneus	Unadjusted	2.1 (1.7–2.6)
				SOS calcaneus		1.9 (1.5–2.3)
				BMD femoral neck		2.1 (1.7–2.5)
				BUA calcaneus	Adjusted for age, weight and centre	2.0 (1.6–2.4)
				SOS calcaneus		1.7 (1.4–2.1)
				BMD femoral neck		1.9 (1.6–2.4)
				BUA calcaneus	Adjusted for age, weight and centre and including all BUA, SOS and femoral neck BMD in the model	1.7 (1.3–2.2)
				SOS calcaneus		1.1 (0.6–1.4)
				BMD femoral neck		1.8 (1.5–2.3)

Table 2.3 Continued

Study	Study population	Length of follow-up (years)	Site/type of fracture (number of patients)	Site/type of measurement	Model/adjustment	Odds/risk ratio
Bauer et al.[49]	6189 postmenopausal women ≥65 years	2	Any hip (n = 54)	BUA calcaneus	Adjusted for age and clinic	2.0 (1.5–2.7)
				BMD femoral neck		2.6 (1.9–3.8)
				BMD calcaneus		2.2 (1.9–3.3)
			Femoral neck (n = 26)	BUA calcaneus		1.3 (0.9–2.0)
				BMD femoral neck		2.0 (1.2–3.1)
				BMD calcaneus		1.4 (0.9–2.1)
			Trochanter (n = 28)	BUA calcaneus		3.3 (2.0–5.5)
				BMD femoral neck		3.9 (2.3–6.8)
				BMD calcaneus		3.4 (2.1–5.1)
			All non-spine (n = 350)	BUA calcaneus		1.3 (1.2–1.5)
				BMD femoral neck		1.3 (1.1–1.5)
				BMD calcaneus		1.4 (1.2–1.6)
			All hip (n = 54)	BUA calcaneus	Adjusted for age, clinic and femoral neck BMD	1.5 (1.0–2.1)
			Femoral neck (n = 26)			1.1 (0.7–1.6)
			Trochanter (n = 28)			2.4 (1.3–4.2)
			All non-spine (n = 350)			1.2 (1.1–1.4)
			Any hip (n = 54)		Adjusted for age, clinic and calcaneal BMD	1.3 (0.8–2.1)
			Femoral neck (n = 26)			1.1 (0.6–1.9)
			Trochanter (n = 28)			1.8 (0.9–3.7)
			All non-spine (n = 350)			1.1 (0.9–1.3)

BUA, broadband ultrasound attenuation; SOS, speed of sound; BMD, bone mineral density.

Table 2.4 Summary details of selected retrospective (cross-sectional) studies of quantitative ultrasound and fracture risk.

Study	Study population	Site/type of fracture (number of patients)	Site/type of measurement	Model/adjustment	Odds/risk ratio
Stegman et al.[56]	809 women ≥50 years	Low trauma fracture after age 40 (n = 204)	SOS patella BMD radius BMD ulna	Age-adjusted	1.5 (1.2–1.9) 1.6 (1.3–2.0) 1.8 (1.5–2.3)
		All fractures after age 40 (n = 314)	SOS patella BMD radius BMD ulna	Age-adjusted	1.2 (1.0–1.5) 1.5 (1.2–1.8) 1.6 (1.3–1.9)
	498 men ≥50 years	Low trauma fracture after age 40 (n = 44)	SOS patella	Age-adjusted	1.6 (1.1–2.3)
			BMD radius BMD ulna		1.7 (1.2–2.4) 1.9 (1.3–2.7)
		All fractures after age 40 (n = 163)	SOS patella BMD radius BMD ulna	Age-adjusted	1.7 (1.3–2.1) 1.5 (1.2–1.9) 1.5 (1.2–1.9)
Stegman et al.[57]	874 women ≥50 years	Spine (n = 201)	SOS patella	Age-adjusted	1.2 (1.0–1.5)
	522 men ≥50 years	Spine (n = 182)	SOS patella	Age and bone mass not significant in logistic regression model	1.3 (1.1–1.5)
Stewart et al.[52]	50 women with recent hip fracture, 50 age-matched controls	Hip (n = 50)	BUA calcaneus	Authors performed ROC analyses	No results given for logistic regression analyses

Table 2.4 Continued

Study	Study population	Site/type of fracture (number of patients)	Site/type of measurement	Model/adjustment	Odds/risk ratio
Bauer et al.[50]	442 women aged 55–80 enrolled in a clinical trial	Spine (n = 131)	BUA calcaneus	Unadjusted	1.6 (1.3–2.1)
			BUA calcaneus	Adjusted for age, weight and clinic	1.8 (1.4–2.3)
			BUA calcaneus	Adjusted for age, weight, clinic and femoral neck BMD	1.6 (1.2–2.1)
			BUA calcaneus	Adjusted for age, weight, clinic and spine BMD	1.5 (1.1–2.0)
			BUA calcaneus	Adjusted for age, weight, clinic and whole body BMD	1.6 (1.2–2.1)
			BMD femoral neck	Adjusted for age, weight and clinic	1.7 (1.3–2.1)
			BMD femoral neck	Adjusted for age, weight, clinic and BUA	1.5 (1.2–1.9)
			BMD spine	Adjusted for age, weight and clinic	2.2 (1.7–2.9)
			BMD spine	Adjusted for age, weight, clinic and BUA	2.0 (1.5–2.6)
			BMD whole body	Adjusted for age, weight and clinic	1.9 (1.5–2.3)
			BMD whole body	Adjusted for age, weight, clinic and BUA	1.5 (1.1–2.1)

Table 2.4 Continued

Study	Study population	Site/type of fracture (number of patients)	Site/type of measurement	Model/adjustment	Odds/risk ratio
Turner et al.[54]	Baseline measurements in 336 women ≥60 years enrolled in a clinical trial	Spine at baseline (n = 22) History of hip fracture after age 58 (n = 22)	BUA calcaneus SOS calcaneus BMD spine	Authors performed ROC analyses	No results given for logistic regression analyses
Schott et al.[53]	43 women with recent hip fracture and 86 age-matched controls	Hip (n = 43)	BUA calcaneus SOS calcaneus BMD femoral neck	Adjusted for height and weight	3.7 (2.0–6.6) 2.7 (1.7–4.5) 2.3 (1.4–3.7)
Gonnelli et al.[55]	304 Caucasian women	Spine (n = 225)	BUA calcaneus SOS calcaneus BMD spine	Unadjusted Adjusted for BMD Unadjusted Adjusted for BMD Unadjusted	3.1 2.0 4.6 2.3 6.5
Glüer et al.[51]	4698 women ≥65 years from the 'Study of Osteoporotic Fractures'	Spine at baseline (n = 812) Recent vertebral fractures (n = 168)	BUA calcaneus BMD spine BMD calcaneus BMD femoral neck BUA calcaneus BMD spine	Adjusted for age, centre and equipment	1.5 (1.4–1.6) 1.5 (1.4–1.6) 1.5 (1.4–1.6) 1.7 (1.5 –1.8) 1.7 (1.4–2.1) 1.9 (1.6–2.3)

Table 2.4 Continued

Study	Study population	Site/type of fracture (number of patients)	Site/type of measurement	Model/adjustment	Odds/risk ratio
		Hip (n = 106)	BMD calcaneus		1.8 (1.5–2.1)
			BMD femoral neck		2.0 (1.6–2.4)
			BUA calcaneus		1.9 (1.5–2.4)
			BMD spine		1.5 (1.2–1.9)
			BMD calcaneus		1.9 (1.5–2.4)
			BMD femoral neck		2.6 (2.0–3.4)
		All fractures (n = 1550)	BUA calcaneus		1.5 (1.4–1.6)
			BMD spine		1.4 (1.3–1.5)
			BMD calcaneus		1.5 (1.4–1.6)
			BMD femoral neck		1.6 (1.5–1.7)
	Subgroup of 1571 women	Vertebral fracture at study baseline (n = 259)	BUA calcaneus	Adjusted for age, centre and equipment	1.5 (1.3–1.7)
			SOS calcaneus		1.6 (1.3–1.9)
		Recent vertebral fractures (n = 43)	BUA calcaneus		2.3 (1.6–3.5)
			SOS calcaneus		2.3 (1.5 –3.5)
		Hip (n = 34)	BUA calcaneus		1.4 (1.0–2.1)
			SOS calcaneus		1.6 (1.0–2.4)
		All fractures (n = 477)	BUA calcaneus		1.4 (1.2–1.6)
			SOS calcaneus		1.4 (1.2–1.6)

BUA, broadband ultrasound attenuation, SOS, speed of sound, BMD, bone mineral density.

fractures on serial radiographs with the mean length of observation between radiographs of 8 years.[69] Vertebral depth was a consistent predictor of vertebral fracture incidents with an age-adjusted odds ratio of 1.23, and even improving when certain measures of bone density were included (odds ratio up to 1.45).

In many patients fractures are not just an expression of a traumatic event, but also of impaired skeletal status. Thus, one would expect that patients with fractures are at higher risk of suffering subsequent fractures and several authors have studied this association. For example, prevalent vertebral deformities are associated with subsequent vertebral deformities and also with non-spine fractures and vice versa.[16,17,19,25,70-73] The increased risk for subsequent fracture in patients with pre-existing fractures, in part independent of bone density, may be accounted for by the systemic effects of osteoporosis, or by shared risk factors for certain fractures. In a retrospective case–control study, Karlsson et al. found that even patients with non-osteoporotic fractures early in life may be at an increased risk for fragility fractures later in life.[74]

There is a long list of risk factors associated with osteoporotic fractures independent of bone density. In a large number of studies age is significantly associated with prevalent and incident fracture.[75] This association is independent of bone mass and most other measures. Thus, it must be concluded that additional factors that are reflected by age must play an important role in osteoporotic fracture. These factors may be related to bone quality, but also to other risk factors that are not yet accounted for. An extensive review of risk factors for hip fracture derived from the SOF study was published by Cummings and colleagues.[76] Aside from low calcaneal bone density, those women with an increased risk had maternal history of hip fracture, previous fractures of any type after age 50, were tall at age 25, rated their own health as fair to poor, had previous hyperthyroidism, had been treated with long-acting benzodiazepines or anti-convulsant drugs, ingested large amounts of caffeine, or spent 4 hours a day or less on their feet. Further findings associated with an increased risk of hip fracture were the inability to rise from a chair without using one's arm, poor depth perception, poor contrast sensitivity and tachycardia at rest. Thus, fracture risk in osteoporosis is multifactorial and knowledge of these risk factors must be taken into consideration for effective treatment of osteoporosis and prevention of its consequences.

DIAGNOSING OSTEOPOROSIS

The variety of risk factors for osteoporotic fracture may leave the reader with some doubt to what extent osteoporosis can be diagnosed at all. There is indeed some need for clarification about the role of bone density. What seems to be a relatively simple concept for diagnosing osteoporosis, the use of a threshold as proposed by the WHO working group,[3-6] needs some further thought. The use of a threshold for diagnosing osteoporosis is derived from the concept of a so-called fracture threshold. It is known from epidemiological studies that the rate of prevalent fractures increases substantially below a certain value. For clinical use, the fracture threshold is a relatively arbitrary level set at 2 SD below the mean of a young normal population. From a clinical perspective, this concept offers significant guidance for therapeutic and diagnostic procedures. On the other hand, the term fracture threshold in its literal sense may be misleading because of the substantial overlap between fracture and nonfracture patients. Speaking in terms of bone mass, an absolute discrimination between these groups is not possible. Furthermore, this discrimination is not the intent of bone mass measurements. Rather they should be used for an estimate of the risk of future fractures, and risk must be understood as a possibility of an untoward event (the fracture), not as absolute prediction. Osteoporosis should be understood as the lower part of a continuum of bone density, with the greatest risk among those people with the lowest absolute BMD values.[75,77]

Apart from these basic limitations in the concept of fracture threshold, there are practical considerations that make the use of a fracture threshold based on a T-score as proposed by the WHO working group quite controversial.[78] Probably the most important issue is the use of an appropriate reference database. Recent studies have shown that there may be limited agreement between a manufacturer's reference database and data derived from a study population. For example, mean values for femoral neck BMD from the NHANES III study population were approximately 3–5% lower than the manufacturer's reference values, and the standard deviations were 26–30% higher.[79] When comparing German normative data to a manufacturer's reference database, Lehmann et al. found good agreement for the female normative data.[80] However, data for the male reference population (30–39 years) were 7% lower

than the manufacturer's reference values. There are various reasons for such discrepancies, and the most obvious reasons lie in different sampling procedures of the various studies. Furthermore, across manufacturers comparable BMD values based on the recently proposed standardization conversions[81] can yield different T-score figures.[78]

T-score thresholds between different sites of BMD measurement, even within the same region, e.g. total hip, femoral neck and trochanter, will identify different proportions of patients and will create different risk groups (Figure 2.6).[78,82] This is even more so when one looks at multiple anatomic sites such as spine and hip, since densitometric results from different sites disagree in a significant proportion of patients. In a population-based study from

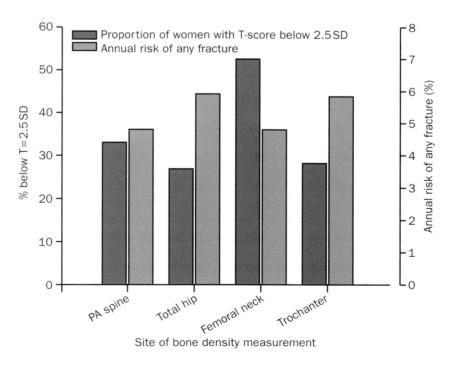

Figure 2.6 Using a T-score of 2.5 standard deviations (SD) as diagnostic threshold, different proportions of patients will be identified as being osteoporotic depending on the site or subregion measured. The use of such a threshold will also create different risk groups as indicated by the site-specific annual risk for any fracture. (Data from Black et al.[78])

Rochester, Minnesota, the proportion of women aged 80 years and older with a bone density more than 2 SD below the mean of young normal women is 48% when measured at the lumbar spine, 67% for either hip site, 68% for the mid-radius and rises to 84% for the combination of all measurements.[83]

Currently there is only limited existing data on whether a combination of multiple sites improves the diagnostic capability for fracture prediction as compared with measuring BMD at a single site. A prospective study of multiple site BMC measurements was presented by Wasnich and co-workers who reported that a combination of two sites strengthened the relationship to incident spinal fracture.[15] On the other hand, Black et al. found that a combination of femoral neck and lumbar spine BMD to identify elderly women at high risk for hip fracture was no better than using femoral neck BMD alone and adjusting the threshold.[84] Similarly, Genant and co-workers presented results for combinations of hip BMD and spinal, calcaneal or radius BMD for the prediction of hip fractures in 5568 women from the SOF study.[82] The authors found that when hip BMD was available, no additional information was gained from secondary measurements at the other sites. However, if BMD was low at the hip, low bone density at the calcaneus or the distal radius increased the risk of hip fracture. This result is in accordance with a cross-sectional study by Jergas et al. who found that a combination of spinal and femoral BMD did not improve the prediction of prevalent vertebral fracture.[85,86] It must be said, however, that even though adjusting thresholds for a single site measurement may identify a similar number of women at risk for fracture compared to multiple site measurements, it is of concern that a different group of women may be identified at risk. Therefore, although there may not be a compelling reason to perform routinely bone densitometry of both spine and hip in every patient, if there is evidence for artefacts that make BMD results of one site unreliable, e.g. anatomic variations, severe degenerative changes or fractures, measuring a second site may be useful for the assessment of a patient's bone mineral status. For general clinical practice, the interpretation and value of multiple site measurements are uncertain.

There is no question that in times of tight financial restraints the relative merits and imperfections of bone density measurements for the diagnosis of osteoporosis and estimate of future fracture risk must spark a controversial discussion.[87-90] Nevertheless, considering all the factors associated with fracture risk, bone densitometry still represents the most consistent predictive tool that is currently available. The predictive capability of bone density is comparable in its magnitude to that of blood pressure for stroke, and is better than that of serum cholesterol for coronary artery disease.[91,92] Despite this, there is still a wide overlap between those patients who will develop a fracture and those who will not. Therefore, rather than being considered a screening tool, the application of bone densitometry should remain confined to certain groups at risk of osteoporosis, and to those patients receiving drug therapy for osteoporosis.[93-96] The cost-effectiveness of therapeutic intervention based on densitometric results has been estimated to be comparable to the treatment of mild hypertension to prevent stroke.[97] Further studies of the cost-effectiveness of therapy are necessary in the light of emerging new therapeutic concepts in osteoporosis as well as the increased costs created by osteoporotic fractures. However, although cost-effectiveness is an important issue that has become increasingly relevant, it should not necessarily drive the provision of health care.

Several authors have developed models to estimate a woman's lifetime risk of suffering a hip fracture based on bone density and age.[98-100] The concept of lifetime risk appears to be very appealing for clinical use since it offers some advantages over the existing concept relying solely on bone density. Applying a nomogram to estimate directly a woman's hip fracture risk as proposed by Suman may facilitate the practical application of such a concept.[100] So far, this approach has only been proposed for prediction of hip fracture, and models for prediction of fractures at other sites still need to be developed. Also to be borne in mind is that low bone density is not the sole explanation for an increased risk of fracture. Other factors, such as an increased risk of falling and bone properties other than density are also of great importance. Concepts using current knowledge to determine a patient's risk of osteoporosis more exactly may finally replace the relatively simplistic approach of the T-score threshold. In any case, the treatment of a patient for osteoporosis does not depend solely on bone density, but on a range of clinical findings.[101]

SUMMARY AND CONCLUSIONS

Bone densitometry is an established tool for the diagnosis of osteoporosis, and bone mineral density is significantly associated with the risk of future fracture as shown in many prospective studies. This association is partly independent of age and other significant predictors of fracture such as falls, cognizance and mobility. The differences between the various densitometric techniques in predicting future osteoporotic fracture of any type are marginal. However, it seems that bone density measurements at the site of fracture do perform rather better than measurements at other sites. In general, retrospective and prospective study designs seem to deliver comparable results. There is currently no evidence that measuring a second site improves the diagnostic capability of bone densitometry. However, measuring a second site may identify a different group of patients at risk of osteoporosis.

From long-term prospective studies it can be concluded that peak bone density, and probably bone loss, are important predictors of subsequent fracture, and that fracture can be predicted from a single bone density measurement over a long period of time. Bone density also predicts fracture risk in the very elderly. However, some fractures, such as femoral neck fracture, may be more strongly influenced by other risk fractures in this age group.

Quantitative ultrasound has a predictive capability similar to bone densitometry even though it fails to show a close correlation to the quantitative measures of bone density. Results from the first prospective studies of QUS suggest that it may shortly be a viable alternative to bone density measurements as a screening tool. From the perspective that bone densitometry and quantitative ultrasound independently predict fractures, these measures actually seem complementary rather than competitive.

Simple geometric measures such as hip axis length and vertebral depth may also be derived from bone densitometry images and are predictive of hip fracture or vertebral fracture independently of bone density. In addition, prevalent fractures are strong predictors of future fracture and must be considered when therapeutic intervention is planned. Overall, there are various risk factors that contribute to the fragility of bone and the occurrence of osteoporotic fracture. The concept of using a threshold for bone density based on a comparison with young normals to define osteoporosis does not do justice to the complexity of the disease, even though bone density must currently be regarded as the most important contributor to osteoporotic fracture risk. Future concepts for determining a person's lifetime risk for fractures and making therapeutic decisions must be based on a risk profile of each individual consisting of bone mineral density, bone geometry, bone structure and a number of additional clinical risk factors.

APPENDIX: STATISTICAL ANALYSIS OF FRACTURE STUDIES

By Glen M Blake

As explained in this chapter, if bone densitometry or ultrasound techniques are to be proven as a reliable method of identifying patients at risk of osteoporotic fractures, it is essential to establish clearly the association between BMD or QUS measurements and future fractures. The most convincing way of doing this is through prospective epidemiological studies (often termed *cohort studies*) that quantify the association between bone density or ultrasound and fracture risk. However, when performing an initial evaluation of a new technique, a quick and simple approach is to perform a retrospective study (often termed a *case–control study*) by comparing measurements of patients known to have fractures (the cases) with individuals known to be free of fractures (the controls). Since few simple explanations exist of the principles behind the analysis of such studies, the following overview is intended for those without any knowledge of advanced statistics.

As an example, we shall consider the conduct and analysis of a prospective study such as the Study of Osteoporotic Fractures.[23] In such studies a large group of subjects representative of the at-risk population (usually elderly women) are enrolled for baseline BMD measurements and subsequent follow-up to record those individuals who suffer a fracture. It is generally found that the distribution of baseline BMD results approximates to a Gaussian curve (Figure 2.A1) that can be described by the mean and population standard deviation (SD). The mean and SD may be used to convert the individual BMD results into Z-score values:

Z-score =
(Measured BMD – Mean BMD)/Population SD

$$(A1)$$

Figure 2.A1 has been drawn with BMD values expressed in Z-score units on the horizontal axis. The Gaussian curve representing the distribution of the baseline data can then be written as:

$$N(Z) = \frac{N_0}{\sqrt{2\pi}} \exp(-Z^2/2) \qquad (A2)$$

where N_0 is the total number of subjects enrolled in the study and Z is the Z-score value.

Following recruitment, subjects are followed up and fracture data are collected over several years. Since lower BMD values are associated with higher fracture risk, a plot of the distribution of the baseline BMD values of fracture patients gives a second distribution curve with its peak shifted to the left (Figure 2.A1). Since the risk of a specific type of fracture is quite small (a few per cent or less), the curve for the fracture group in Figure 2.A1 has been multiplied by a factor of 100 to make it visible on the same vertical scale as the curve for the entire study population.

Mathematically, these studies are analysed using *linear logistic regression*[102,103] or *Cox proportional hazard*[103–105] models that express the dependence of fracture risk on BMD as an *odds ratio* or *risk ratio* respectively. The latter is the increased risk of fracture for each 1 SD decrease in BMD. The two types of model give very similar curves of fracture risk against BMD when the risk is small (see below). The most familiar type of statistical analysis is simple regression in which the best fitting straight line between two continuous variables, x and y, is written as:

$$y = \alpha + \beta x \qquad (A3)$$

The values of the two free coefficients, α and β, are determined using the principle of least squares. This type of analysis is often used in bone densitometry to find the relationship between BMD measurements at two different sites in the skeleton. However, examining the relationship between BMD and fracture risk is a more complex problem because one variable, fracture, is not continuous but is a *binary* quantity: i.e. each patient belongs to one of only two groups, fracture or non-fracture. In logistic regression a fit to the data is obtained by transforming the probability p that the patient will suffer a fracture using the logit

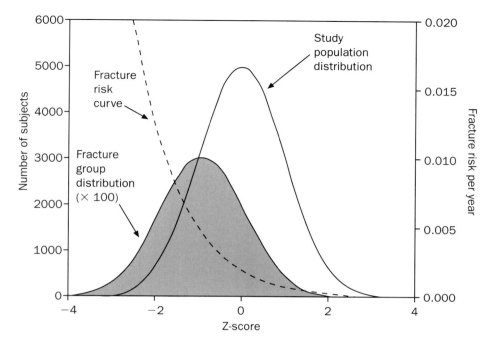

Figure 2.A1 Schematic illustration of the outcome and interpretation of a prospective epidemiological study to establish the relationship between bone density and fracture risk. Bone density is plotted on the horizontal axis in Z-score units. The three curves show: (1) the BMD distribution of the entire study population; (2) the BMD distribution of the fracture group (values ×100); and (3) (on the right-hand axis) the curve of fracture risk against Z-score inferred from statistical modelling. The latter is used to derive the risk ratio defined as the increased fracture risk for each 1 standard deviation (SD) decrease in BMD.

function and then expressing this as a linear function of BMD. If we continue to express BMD by the Z-score (equation A1) this can be written:

$$\mathrm{logit}(p) = \log(p/(1 - p)) = \alpha + \beta Z \quad \text{(A4)}$$

The advantage of the logit (or similar) function is that while the probability p can vary only between 0 and 1, $\mathrm{logit}(p)$ varies between $-\infty$ and $+\infty$ and can accommodate the full range of possible variation in the function on the right-hand side. The latter is often extended to construct a linear function of several relevant variables, e.g. age or BMD at other sites. Equation A4 can be rewritten to express p directly as a function of Z:

$$p = \exp(\alpha + \beta Z)/(1 + \exp(\alpha + \beta Z)) \quad \text{(A5)}$$

When equation A5 is used to plot fracture probability p as a function of BMD an S-shape curve (commonly called a sigmoid) is obtained (Figure 2.A2). The two free coefficients, α and β, are determined from optimizing the fit to the data. Further mathematical details can be found in the book by Collett.[102] As with simple regression (equation A3) or the Gaussian distribution (equation A2), the logistic function is a model chosen because it is found to fit the observations in a reasonably realistic manner.

If p_0 is the fracture risk of an individual with Z-score = 0, then the odds of this person experiencing a fracture are $p_0/(1 - p_0)$. Similarly, for an individual with $Z = -1$, the odds are

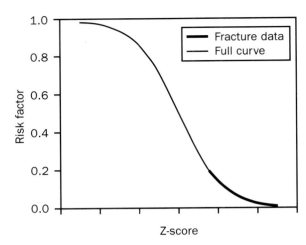

Figure 2.A2 Plot of the logit function used to relate fracture probability and bone density. In practice the full curve is often hypothetical since only data corresponding to low probability values are usually sampled in the application to fracture studies.

$p_{-1}/(1 - p_{-1})$. The *odds ratio* is defined as the ratio of the odds at $Z = -1$ to $Z = 0$:

$$\text{Odds ratio} = \frac{p_{-1}/(1 - p_{-1})}{p_0/(1 - p_0)} \quad (A6)$$

Substituting from equation A4 and reversing the sign of β so that a smaller (more negative) value of Z corresponds to higher fracture risk, then equation A6 reduces to:

$$\text{Odds ratio} = \exp\beta \quad (A7)$$

With the same proviso, when p is small, equation A5 becomes:

$$p \approx \exp(\alpha - \beta Z) = F_0 \exp(-\beta Z) \quad (A8)$$

where F_0 is the fracture risk at $Z = 0$. Hence, in the limit when p is small, the fracture prediction curve derived by logistic regression with odds ratio $\exp\beta$ approximates to the exponential curve derived from a Cox proportional hazards model in which risk increases with decreasing Z-score with a risk ratio $\exp\beta$. In this circumstance the distribution curve for the fracture group can be estimated by multiplying equation A2 by equation A8:

$$N_f(Z) = \frac{N_0 F_0}{\sqrt{2\pi}} \exp(-\beta Z - Z^2/2) \quad (A9)$$

Some rearranging of equation A9 gives the relationship:

$$N_f(Z) = \frac{N_0 F_0}{\sqrt{2\pi}} \exp(\beta^2/2) \exp(-(Z + \beta)^2/2) \quad (A10)$$

which means that the distribution curve of the fracture group (Figure 2.A1) is a Gaussian curve with the same standard deviation as the entire study population but with its peak shifted to the left by an amount β expressed in Z-score units. It is therefore possible to list the shift between the two peaks as a function of the risk ratio (Table 2.A1). Clearly, the larger the risk ratio, the wider the separation between the distribution curves for the fracture group and the entire study population, and the better the discrimination of the technique for identifying patients likely to have fractures.

A more intuitive way of presenting results of fracture studies is to divide the baseline BMD figures into four quartiles and plot the fracture risk for subjects in each quartile. If a technique has no predictive power (RR = 1.0) then 25% of all fracture cases will occur in each quartile. As the risk ratio becomes larger, however, a steadily higher percentage of fractures occurs in

Table 2.A1 Relationship between risk ratio and Z-score offset of fracture group.

Risk ratio	Z-score offset
1.0	0
1.5	0.41
2.0	0.69
2.5	0.92
3.0	1.10

Table 2.A2 Relationship between risk ratio and percentage of fractures expected in each quartile of the BMD range.

Risk ratio	1st quartile (%)	2nd quartile (%)	3rd quartile (%)	4th quartile (%)	*Ratio* 1st quartile:4th quartile
1.0	25	25	25	25	1.0
1.5	39	27	20	14	2.8
2.0	51	25	15	9	5.9
2.5	60	22	12	6	10.7
3.0	66	20	10	4	17.4

the lowest quartile and a dwindling percentage in the highest quartile. The exact percentages expected can be predicted using equation A10 and integral tables for the Gaussian distribution (Table 2.A2). For a risk ratio of 2.0 the model predicts that 51% of fractures occur in the lowest quartile and 9% in the highest. For a risk ratio of 3.0 the figures are 66% and 4% respectively. The figures in Table 2.A2 are intended to help readers interpret the clinical significance of the odds ratio and risk ratio figures presented in this chapter.

REFERENCES

1. Consensus Development Conference. Diagnosis, prophylaxis, and treatment of osteoporosis. *Am J Med* (1993) **94:** 646–50.
2. Melton LJ, Wahner HW. Defining osteoporosis. *Calcif Tissue Int* (1989) **45:** 263–4.
3. World Health Organization. WHO technical report series No. 843. Assessment of fracture risk and its application to screening for postmenopausal osteoporosis (WHO: Geneva, 1994).
4. Kanis JA, WHO Study Group. Assessment of fracture risk and its application to screening for postmenopausal osteoporosis: synopsis of a WHO report. *Osteoporos Int* (1994) **4:** 368–81.
5. Kanis JA, Devogelaer J-P, Gennari C. Practical guide for the use of bone mineral measurements in the assessment of treatment of osteoporosis: a position paper of the European foundation for osteoporosis and bone disease. *Osteoporos Int* (1996) **6:** 256–61.
6. Kanis JA, Melton LJ, Christiansen C et al. The diagnosis of osteoporosis. *J Bone Miner Res* (1994) **9:** 1137–41.
7. Melton LJ, Thamer M, Ray NF et al. Fractures attributable to osteoporosis: report from the National Osteoporosis Foundation. *J Bone Miner Res* (1997) **12:** 16–23.
8. Nevitt MC. Epidemiology of osteoporosis. *Rheum Dis Clin North Am* (1994) **20:** 535–59.
9. Seeley DG, Browner WS, Nevitt MC et al. Which fractures are associated with low appendicular bone mass in elderly women? *Ann Intern Med* (1991) **115:** 837–42.
10. Smith DM, Khairi MRA, Johnston CC. The loss of bone mineral with aging and its relationship to risk of fracture. *J Clin Invest* (1975) **56:** 311–18.
11. Khairi MRA, Cronin JH, Robb JA et al. Femoral trabecular-pattern index and bone mineral content measurement by photon absorption in senile osteoporosis. *J Bone Joint Surg* (1976) **58A:** 221–6.
12. Hui SL, Slemenda CW, Johnston CC. Age and

bone mass as predictors of fracture in a prospective study. *J Clin Invest* (1988) **81:** 1804–9.

13. Hui SL, Slemenda CW, Johnston CC. Baseline measurement of bone mass predicts fracture in white women. *Ann Intern Med* (1989) **111:** 355–61.

14. Hui SL, Slemenda CW, Carey MA et al. Choosing between predictors of fractures. *J Bone Miner Res* (1995) **10:** 1816–22.

15. Wasnich RD, Ross PD, Davis JW et al. A comparison of single and multi-site BMC measurements for assessment of spine fracture probability. *J Nucl Med* (1989) **30:** 1166–71.

16. Ross PD, Davis JW, Epstein RS et al. Pre-existing fractures and bone mass predict vertebral fracture incidence in women. *Ann Intern Med* (1991) **114:** 919–23.

17. Ross PD, Genant HK, Davis JW et al. Predicting vertebral fracture incidence from prevalent fractures and bone density among non-black, osteoporotic women. *Osteoporos Int* (1993) **3:** 120–6.

18. Gärdsell P, Johnell O, Nilsson BE. Predicting fractures in women by using forearm bone densitometry. *Calcif Tissue Int* (1989) **44:** 235–42.

19. Gärdsell P, Johnell O, Nilsson BE. The predictive value of forearm bone mineral content measurements in men. *Bone* (1990) **11:** 229–32.

20. Gärdsell P, Johnell O, Nilsson BE. The predictive value of bone loss for fragility fractures in women: a longitudinal study over 15 years. *Calcif Tissue Int* (1991) **49:** 90–4.

21. Gärdsell P, Johnell O, Nilsson BE et al. Predicting various fragility fractures in women by forearm bone densitometry: a follow-up study. *Calcif Tissue Int* (1993) **52:** 348–53.

22. Düppe H, Gärdsell P, Nilsson B et al. A single bone density measurement can predict fractures over 25 years. *Calcif Tissue Int* (1997) **60:** 171–4.

23. Cummings SR, Black DM, Nevitt MC et al. Bone density at various sites for prediction of hip fractures. *Lancet* (1993) **341:** 72–5.

24. Black D, Cummings SR, Genant HK et al. Axial and appendicular bone density predict fractures in older women. *J Bone Miner Res* (1992) **7:** 633–8.

25. Black D, Nevitt M, Palermo L et al. Prediction of new vertebral deformities. *J Bone Miner Res* (1993) **8**(suppl 1): S135.

26. Stegman MR, Recker RR, Davies KM et al. Fracture risk as determined by prospective and retrospective study designs. *Osteoporos Int* (1992) **2:** 290–7.

27. Melton LJ, Atkinson EJ, O'Fallon WM et al. Long-term fracture prediction by bone mineral assessed at different skeletal sites. *J Bone Miner Res* (1993) **8:** 1227–33.

28. Nguyen T, Sambrook P, Kelly P et al. Prediction of osteoporotic fractures by postural instability and bone density. *Br Med J* (1993) **307:** 1111–15.

29. Cheng S, Suominen H, Era P et al. Bone density of the calcaneus and fractures in 75- and 80-year-old men and women. *Osteoporos Int* (1994) **4:** 48–54.

30. Cheng S, Suominen H, Sakari-Rantala R et al. Calcaneal bone mineral density predicts fracture occurrence: a five-year follow-up study in elderly people. *J Bone Miner Res* (1997) **12:** 1075–82.

31. Seeley DG, Kelsey J, Jergas M et al. Predictors of ankle and foot fractures in older women. *J Bone Miner Res* (1996) **11:** 1347–55.

32. Torgerson DJ, Campbell MK, Thomas RE et al. Prediction of perimenopausal fracture by bone density and other risk factors. *J Bone Miner Res* (1996) **11:** 293–7.

33. Marshall D, Johnell O, Wedel H. Meta-analysis of how well measures of bone mineral density predict occurrence of osteoporotic fractures. *Br Med J* (1996) **312:** 1254–9.

34. Genant HK, Cann CE, Ettinger B et al. Quantitative computed tomography of vertebral spongiosa: a sensitive method for detecting early bone loss after oophorectomy. *Ann Intern Med* (1982) **97:** 699–705.

35. Cann CE, Genant HK, Kolb FO et al. Quantitative computed tomography for prediction of vertebral fracture risk. *Metab Bone Dis Relat Res* (1984) **5:** 1–7.

36. Reinbold WD, Genant HK, Reiser UJ et al. Bone mineral content in early-postmenopausal osteoporotic women and postmenopausal women: comparison of measurement methods. *Radiology* (1986) **160:** 469–78.

37. Nordin BEC, Wishart JM, Horowitz M et al. The relation between forearm and vertebral mineral density and fractures in postmenopausal women. *Bone Miner* (1988) **5:** 21–33.

38. Heuck A, Block J, Glüer CC et al. Mild versus definite osteoporosis: comparison of bone densitometry techniques using different statistical models. *J Bone Miner Res* (1989) **4:** 891–900.

39. van Berkum FNR, Birkenhäger JC, van Veen LCP et al. Noninvasive axial and peripheral assessment of bone mineral content: a compari-

son between osteoporotic women and normal subjects. *J Bone Miner Res* (1989) **5**: 679–85.

40. Pacifici R, Rupich R, Griffin M et al. Dual energy radiography versus quantitative computer tomography for the diagnosis of osteoporosis. *J Clin Endocrinol Metab* (1990) **70**: 705–10.

41. Guglielmi G, Grimston SK, Fischer KC et al. Osteoporosis: diagnosis with lateral and posteroanterior dual x-ray absorptiometry compared with quantitative CT. *Radiology* (1994) **192**: 845–50.

42. Ito M, Hayashi K, Ishida Y et al. Discrimination of spinal fracture with various bone mineral measurements. *Calcif Tissue Int* (1997) **60**: 11–15.

43. Nevitt M, Johnell O, Black DM et al. Bone mineral density predicts non-spine fractures in very elderly women. *Osteoporos Int* (1994) **4**: 325–31.

44. Hansen MA, Overgaard K, Riis BJ et al. Role of peak bone mass and bone loss in postmenopausal osteoporosis: 12 year study. *Br Med J* (1991) **303**: 961–4.

45. Hui SL, Slemenda CW, Johnston CC. The contribution of bone loss to postmenopausal osteoporosis. *Osteoporos Int* (1990) **1**: 30–4.

46. Porter R, Miller C, Grainger D et al. Prediction of hip fracture in elderly women: a prospective study. *Br Med J* (1990) **301**: 638–41.

47. Heaney RP, Avioli LV, Chesnut CH et al. Ultrasound velocity through bone predicts incident vertebral deformity. *J Bone Miner Res* (1995) **10**: 341–5.

48. Hans D, Dargent-Molina P, Schott AM et al. Ultrasonographic heel measurements to predict hip fracture in the elderly. *Lancet* (1996) **348**: 511–14.

49. Bauer DC, Glüer CC, Cauley JA et al. Bone ultrasound predicts fractures strongly and independently of densitometry in older women: a prospective study. *Arch Intern Med* (1997) **157**: 629–34.

50. Bauer DC, Glüer CC, Genant HK et al. Quantitative ultrasound and vertebral fracture in post menopausal women. *J Bone Miner Res* (1995) **10**: 353–8.

51. Glüer CC, Cummings SR, Bauer DC et al. Osteoporosis: association of recent fractures with quantitative ultrasound findings. *Radiology* (1996) **199**: 725–32.

52. Stewart A, Reid DM, Porter RW. Broadband ultrasound attenuation and dual energy x-ray absorptiometry in patients with hip fractures: which technique discriminates fracture risk? *Calcif Tissue Int* (1994) **54**: 466–9.

53. Schott AM, Weill-Engerer S, Hans D et al. Ultrasound discriminates patients with hip fracture equally well as dual energy x-ray absorptiometry and independently of bone mineral density. *J Bone Miner Res* (1995) **10**: 243–9.

54. Turner CH, Peacock M, Timmerman L et al. Calcaneal ultrasonic measurements discriminate hip fracture independently of bone mass. *Osteoporos Int* (1995) **5**: 130–5.

55. Gonnelli S, Cepollaro C, Agnusdei D et al. Diagnostic value of ultrasound analysis and bone densitometry as predictors of vertebral deformity in postmenopausal women. *Osteoporos Int* (1995) **5**: 413–18.

56. Stegman MR, Heaney RP, Recker RR. Comparison of speed of sound ultrasound with single photon absorptiometry for determining fracture odds ratios. *J Bone Miner Res* (1995) **10**: 346–52.

57. Stegman MR, Davies KM, Heaney RP et al. The association of patellar ultrasound transmissions and forearm densitometry with vertebral fracture, number and severity: the Saunders County bone quality study. *Osteoporos Int* (1996) **6**: 130–5.

58. Geusens P, Dequeker J, Verstraeten A et al. Age-, sex-, and menopause-related changes of vertebral and peripheral bone: population study using dual and single photon absorptiometry and radiogrammetry. *J Nucl Med* (1986) **27**: 1540–9.

59. Falch JA, Sandvik L. Perimenopausal appendicular bone loss: a 10-year prospective study. *Bone* (1990) **11**: 425–8.

60. Meema HE, Meindok H. Advantages of peripheral radiogrammetry over dual-photon absorptiometry of the spine in the assessment of prevalence of osteoporotic vertebral fractures in women. *J Bone Miner Res* (1992) **7**: 897–903.

61. Jergas M, San Valentin R, Black D et al. Radiogrammetry of the metacarpals predicts future hip fractures. *J Bone Miner Res* (1995) **10**(suppl 1): S371.

62. Faulkner KG, McClung M, Cummings SR. Automated evaluation of hip axis length for predicting hip fracture. *J Bone Miner Res* (1994) **9**: 1065–70.

63. Faulkner KG, Cummings SR, Glüer CC et al. Simple measurement of femoral geometry predicts hip fracture: the Study of Osteoporotic Fractures. *J Bone Miner Res* (1993) **8**: 1211–17.

64. Faulkner KG, Cummings SR, Nevitt M et al. Hip axis length and osteoporotic fractures. *J Bone Miner Res* (1995) **10**: 506–8.
65. Geusens P. Geometric characteristics of the proximal femur and hip fracture risk. *Osteoporos Int* (1996) **6**(suppl 3): S27–30.
66. Glüer CC, Cummings SR, Pressman A et al. Prediction of hip fractures from pelvic radiographs: the study of osteoporotic fractures. *J Bone Miner Res* (1994) **9**: 671–7.
67. Nakamura T, Turner CH, Yoshikawa T et al. Do variations of hip geometry explain differences in hip fracture risk between Japanese and white Americans? *J Bone Miner Res* (1994) **9**: 1071–6.
68. Cummings SR, Cauley JA, Palermo L et al. Racial differences in hip axis lengths might explain racial differences in rates of hip fractures. *Osteoporos Int* (1994) **4**: 226–9.
69. Ross PD, Huang C, Davis JW et al. Vertebral dimension measurements improve prediction of vertebral fracture incidence. *Bone* (1995) **16**: 257S–62S.
70. Wasnich RD, Davis JW, Ross PD. Spine fracture risk is predicted by non-spine fractures. *Osteoporos Int* (1994) **4**: 1–5.
71. Mallmin H, Ljunghall S, Persson I et al. Fracture of the distal forearm as a forecaster of subsequent hip fracture: a population based cohort study with 24 years of follow-up. *Calcif Tissue Int* (1993) **52**: 269–72.
72. Kotowicz MA, Melton LJ, Cooper C et al. Risk of hip fracture in women with vertebral fracture. *J Bone Miner Res* (1994) **9**: 599–605.
73. Burger H, van Daele PL, Algra D et al. Vertebral deformities as predictors of non-vertebral fractures. *Br Med J* (1994) **309**: 991–2.
74. Karlsson MK, Hasserius R, Obrant KJ. Individuals who sustain nonosteoporotic fractures continue to also sustain fragility fractures. *Calcif Tissue Int* (1993) **53**: 229–31.
75. Ross PD, Davis JW, Vogel JM et al. A critical review of bone mass and the risk of fractures in osteoporosis. *Calcif Tissue Int* (1990) **46**: 149–61.
76. Cummings SR, Nevitt MC, Browner WS et al. Risk factors for hip fractures in white women. *N Engl J Med* (1995) **332**: 767–73.
77. Wasnich R. Fracture prediction with bone mass measurements. In: Genant HK, ed. *Osteoporosis Update 1987* (Radiology Research and Education Foundation: San Francisco, 1987), 95–101.
78. Black DM, Palermo L, Genant HK et al. Four reasons to avoid the use of BMD T-scores in treatment decisions for osteoporosis. *J Bone Miner Res* (1996) **11**(suppl 1): S118.
79. Looker AC, Wahner HW, Dunn WL et al. Proximal femur bone mineral levels of US adults. *Osteoporos Int* (1995) **5**: 389–409.
80. Lehmann R, Wapniarz M, Randerath O et al. Dual-energy X-ray absorptiometry at the lumbar spine in German men and women: a cross-sectional study. *Calcif Tissue Int* (1995) **56**: 350–4.
81. Genant HK, Grampp S, Glüer CC et al. Universal standardization for dual x-ray absorptiometry: patient and phantom cross-calibration results. *J Bone Miner Res* (1994) **9**: 1503–14.
82. Genant HK, Lu Y, Mathur AK et al. Classification based on DXA measurements for assessing the risk of hip fractures. *J Bone Miner Res* (1996) **11**(suppl 1): S120.
83. Melton LJ, Chrischilles EA, Cooper C et al. How many women have osteoporosis? *J Bone Miner Res* (1992) **7**: 1005–10.
84. Black D, Bauer DC, Lu Y et al. Should BMD be measured at multiple sites to predict fracture risk in elderly women? *J Bone Miner Res* (1995) **10**(Suppl 1): S140.
85. Jergas M, Fuerst T, Grampp S et al. Assessment of spinal osteoporosis with dual x-ray absorptiometry of the spine and femur. *Radiology* (1995) **197**(suppl): 362.
86. Jergas M, Genant HK. Spinal and femoral DXA for the assessment of spinal osteoporosis. *Calcif Tissue Int* (1997) **61**: 351–7.
87. Sheldon TA, Raffle A, Watt I. Department of Health shoots itself in the hip. Why the report of the advisory groups undermines evidence based purchasing. *Br Med J* (1996) **312**: 296–7.
88. Barlow D, Cooper C, Reeve J et al. Department of Health is fair to patients with osteoporosis. *Br Med J* (1996) **312**: 297–8.
89. Lange S, Richter K, Köbberling J. Die Osteodensitometrie. In: Köhler W, Köpcke W, Naeve P, Weiss H, eds. *Biometrie*, Vol 3 (Lit Verlag: Münster, 1994).
90. Glüer CC. Osteoporosediagnostik – ein radiologisches Problem? *Fortschr Röntgenstr* (1996) **165**: 1–3.
91. Neaton JD, Wentworth D. Serum cholesterol, blood pressure, cigarette smoking and death from coronary artery disease: overall findings and differences by age for 316099 white men. *Arch Intern Med* (1992) **152**: 56–64.
92. Khaw K, Barrett-Connor E, Suarez L et al.

Predictors of stroke associated mortality in the elderly. *Stroke* (1984) **15:** 244–8.

93. Johnston CC, Melton LJ, Lindsay R et al. Clinical indications for bone mass measurements. *J Bone Miner Res* (1989) **4**(Suppl 2): 1–28.

94. Genant HK, Block JE, Steiger P et al. Appropriate use of bone densitometry. *Radiology* (1989) **170:** 817–22.

95. Jergas M, Genant HK. Current methods and recent advances in the diagnosis of osteoporosis. *Arthritis Rheum* (1993) **36:** 1649–62.

96. Compston JE, Cooper C, Kanis JA. Bone densitometry in clinical practice. *Br Med J* (1995) **310:** 1507–10.

97. Jönsson B, Christiansen C, Johnell O et al. Cost-effectiveness of fracture prevention in established osteoporosis. *Osteoporos Int* (1995) **5:** 136–42.

98. Melton LJ, Kan SH, Wahner HW et al. Lifetime fracture risk: and approach to hip fracture risk assessment based on bone mineral density and age. *J Clin Epidemiol* (1988) **41:** 985–94.

99. Black D, Cummings SR, Melton LJ. Appendicular bone mineral and a woman's lifetime risk of hip fracture. *J Bone Miner Res* (1992) **7:** 639–46.

100. Suman VJ, Atkinson EJ, Black DM et al. A nomogram for predicting lifetime hip fracture risk from radius bone mineral density and age. *Bone* (1993) **14:** 843–6.

101. Ettinger B, Miller P, McClung M. Use of bone densitometry results for decisions about therapy for osteoporosis. *Ann Intern Med* (1996) **125:** 623.

102. Collett D. *Modelling binary data* (Chapman & Hall: London, 1991).

103. Altman DG. *Practical statistics for medical research* (Chapman & Hall: London, 1991).

104. Cox DR. Regression models and life tables (with discussion). *J R Stat Soc* (1972) **B34:** 187–220.

105. Cox DR, Oakes D. *Analysis of survival data.* (Chapman & Hall: London, 1984).

3

Technical Principles of X-ray Absorptiometry

CHAPTER OVERVIEW

This chapter gives an introduction to the more widely used procedures available for the non-invasive measurement of bone density using the principles of X-ray absorptiometry. The principles behind the measurement of bone using quantitative ultrasound (QUS) techniques will be discussed in Chapter 6. The development of X-ray absorptiometry is outlined from both the technical and historical points of view. While the techniques of single-energy and dual-energy photon absorptiometry and quantitative computed tomography are considered in some detail, most emphasis is given to dual-energy X-ray absorptiometry (DXA). Since its introduction in 1987, DXA has been the technique most associated with the rapid growth in clinical applications of bone densitometry. Over this period, scans to measure bone density have become an essential part of the evaluation of patients at risk of osteoporosis. Recent technical developments such as fan-beam geometry and body composition analysis are also discussed. A detailed review of the commercially available DXA systems for measurements of the spine, femur and total body is given in Chapter 4. Commercial devices dedicated to measurements of the peripheral skeleton are described in Chapter 5. The mathematical background of

single photon, dual photon and dual-energy X-ray absorptiometry is explained in the Appendix to this chapter.

INTRODUCTION

A wide variety of methods for the non-invasive assessment of skeletal integrity based on the use of X- or γ-rays have been described (Table 3.1). While some involve subjective interpretation of radiographs, such as the assessment of the radiographic density of vertebrae or the evaluation of trabecular texture in the proximal femur (the Singh index), others involve sophisticated or expensive quantitative techniques such as high resolution CT imaging of trabecular microstructure or quantitative magnetic resonance imaging. A comprehensive and up-to-date review of current techniques for clinical investigation and research was published by Genant et al.[1] Some older techniques that have fallen into disuse in recent years are well described in a review by Tothill.[2]

In general, the techniques that have become most widely used are characterized by accurate and highly reproducible measurements, stable calibration and low radiation dose to the patient (Table 3.2). They include single photon

Table 3.1 Methods for the in vivo assessment of bone mineral and structure.

Subjective evaluation of radiographs
  Radiographic density of vertebrae
  Vertebral deformity
  Singh index

Quantitative evaluation of radiographs
  Radiogrammetry
  Radiographic absorptiometry
  Vertebral morphometry
  Fractal signature analysis

Methods based on absorptiometry
  Single photon and X-ray absorptiometry
  Dual photon and X-ray absorptiometry

Methods based on computed tomography
  Single-energy QCT
  Dual-energy QCT
  Peripheral QCT
  High-resolution pQCT

Non-imaging methods
  Compton scattering
  Total body neutron activation
  Part body neutron activation

Methods not using ionizing radiation
  Quantitative ultrasound
  Quantitative MRI
  High-resolution MRI

QCT, quantitative computed tomography; pQCT, peripheral quantitative computed tomography; MRI, magnetic resonance imaging.

(and X-ray) absorptiometry (SPA, SXA), dual photon (and X-ray) absorptiometry (DPA, DXA) and quantitative computed tomography (QCT). In recent years, DXA and QCT systems dedicated to measurements of the peripheral skeleton (pDXA, pQCT) have also become popular.

The most widely used types of bone densito-meter perform measurements at specific sites in the skeleton such as the spine, femur or forearm. Although osteoporosis is a systemic disease, the correlation coefficients between bone density values at different sites are typically around $r \approx 0.6$–0.7, and thus a bone density measurement at one site is far from being a perfect predictor of that at any other site. A detailed intercomparison of current techniques in a group of 124 healthy premenopausal, healthy postmenopausal and elderly osteoporotic women was published by Grampp et al.[3] From the point of view of cost, space requirements, radiation dose and the type of information provided, it is useful to divide X-ray absorptiometry equipment into those devices designed to measure axial and appendicular sites (spine and femur) and those designed to measure peripheral sites (forearm, hand and calcaneus). Equipment designed to measure the axial skeleton can often perform total body scans as well. Although whole body DXA studies give uniquely comprehensive information on total body bone density, bone mineral content and soft tissue composition, the spine and femur are widely regarded as the most important measurement regions because they are frequently sites of osteoporotic fractures that cause substantial impairment to quality of life, morbidity and mortality.

Most DXA, SXA and pDXA systems provide a two-dimensional projection image of the scan site (Figure 3.1). The principal information provided is the bone mineral density (BMD), defined as the integral mass of bone mineral in the measurement region of interest (ROI) divided by the projected area. The units of this type of BMD measurement are grams per square centimetre (g/cm^2). As well as BMD, figures are often provided for the bone mineral content (BMC) and projected area of the measurement ROI. In contrast, QCT and pQCT devices provide tomographic images that are slices through the chosen cross-section through the body (Figure 3.2). As a result, QCT measures true physical density in units of grams per cubic centimetre (g/cm^3) rather than the areal density measured by DXA.

Most of the other information on the com-

Table 3.2 The most widely used clinical methods for the assessment of skeletal status.

Technique	Measurement site	Precision error (%)	Effective dose (µSV)	Unit cost[a]
pDXA	Forearm	1	0.05	20–25 k
DXA	Spine	1	10	40–100 k
	Lat. spine	1.5	10	
	Femur	1.5	2	
	Total body	1	3	
QCT	Spine	2–4	100	350–500 k
pQCT	Forearm	1	1	40–80 k
QUS/BUA	Calcaneus	1–5	0	15–20 k
QUS/SOS	Calcaneus	0.3–1.0	0	
	Tibia	0.3	0	

[a] Pounds sterling (early 1998).
pDXA, peripheral dual X-ray absorptiometry; DXA, dual X-ray absorptiometry; QCT, quantitative computed tomography; pQCT, peripheral quantitative computed tomography; QUS, quantitative ultrasound; BUA, broadband ultrasound attenuation; SOS, speed of sound.

puter printout from a bone density scan is intended to provide an interpretation of the BMD result based on a comparison with a normal reference population matched for age, sex and ethnic origin. Usually the display includes a normal range plot in which the patient's BMD and age are plotted with respect to the reference population to provide a visual indication of the scan findings (Figure 3.1). To aid interpretation the report will also include T-score and Z-score values in which the BMD result is expressed as the difference from the mean BMD for young adult and age-matched normal populations respectively in units of the population standard deviation. T- and Z-scores are explained in more detail in Chapter 16. Finally, the patient's BMD result may also be expressed as a percentage of the mean value for the reference population. The mean used for this comparison can be either the young adult or the age-matched figure.

The purpose of all bone density measurements is to measure the quantity of the bone mineral phase with a stated chemical composition. Usually this is assumed to be hydroxyapatite $(Ca_{10}(PO_4)_6OH_2)$. Any variation in the chemical composition of the bone mineral phase can cause significant errors. However, in general, the qualitative changes in bone mineral composition, if present, are very small and need not be considered in bone mineral measurements. An interesting exception is the use of therapeutic agents based on strontium.[4] Because of the high atomic number ($Z = 38$ for strontium compared with $Z = 20$ for calcium), modification of the normal Sr/Ca composition of bone mineral (usually about 1×10^{-4} by weight) will cause a disproportionate change in BMD.

From studies over many years, the complex behaviour of bone mineral in the skeleton has gradually become understood. It appears that

k = 1.142   dθ = 43.8(0.928H) 5.981

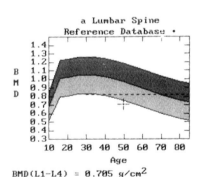

```
F0525960G    Sat 25.May.1996 11:05
Name:
Comment:
I.D.:                        Sex:     F
S.S.#:          - -     Ethnic:      C
ZIPCode:        Height: 162.30 cm
Operator:       Weight:  54.80 kg
BirthDate: 02.May.46    Age:    50
Physician:
Image not for diagnostic use

     TOTAL BMD CV FOR L1 - L4  1.0%

     C.F.   1.008     0.988    1.000

Region Est.Area  Est.BMC    BMD
         (cm2)   (grams)  (gms/cm2)
-------- ------- -------- ---------
   L1    12.11     7.34     0.606
   L2    13.08     8.99     0.687
   L3    14.94    11.15     0.746
   L4    17.92    13.47     0.751
TOTAL   58.05    40.94     0.705
```

·25.May.1996 11:07 [115 x 146]
Hologic QDR-4500A (S/N 45008)
Array Spine Medium V8.16a:3

HOLOGIC

A

a Lumbar Spine
Reference Database ·

B M D

BMD(L1-L4) = 0.705 g/cm²

Region	BMD	T(30.0)		Z	
L1	0.606	-2.90	66%	-2.26	71%
L2	0.687	-3.10	67%	-2.38	72%
L3	0.746	-3.07	69%	-2.31	75%
L4	0.751	-3.32	67%	-2.54	73%
L1-L4	0.705	-3.11	67%	-2.37	73%

· Age and sex matched
T = peak bone mass
Z = age matched   TK   04 Nov 91

```
F0525960G    Sat 25.May.1996 11:05
Name:
Comment:
I.D.:                        Sex:     F
S.S.#:          - -     Ethnic:      C
ZIPCode:        Height: 162.30 cm
Operator:       Weight:  54.80 kg
BirthDate: 02.May.46    Age:    50
Physician:
```

HOLOGIC

B

Figure 3.1 DXA scan of the lumbar spine: (A) scan image and BMD results; (B) scan interpretation with normal range plot, T-score and Z-score values, and BMD expressed as a percentage of the young adult and age-matched population means.

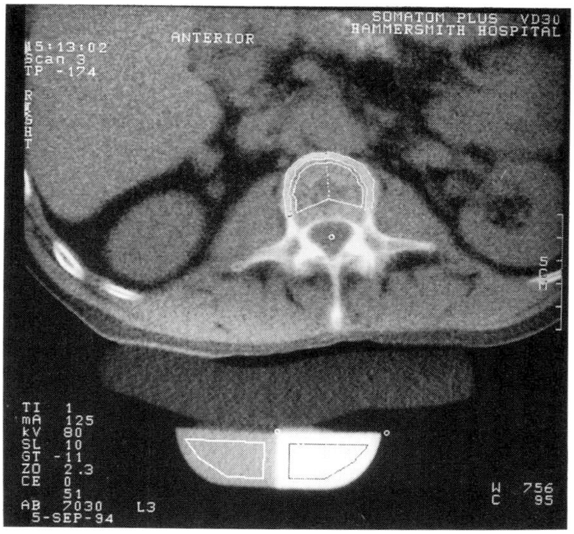

Figure 3.2 A QCT scan of a lumbar vertebra. BMD expressed in units of grams of hydroxyapatite per cubic centimetre can be measured separately in the trabecular bone and cortical shell of the vertebral body. The phantom below the patient serves to calibrate BMD in terms of the Hounsfield units of the CT image. (Courtesy of LM Banks.)

not only do cortical and trabecular bone respond differently to the effects of ageing, preventive treatment and different physical and hormonal stimuli, but also individual bones or even parts of a bone may vary in their degree of response. This explains why there is no single technique applicable to all questions regarding the mineral status of the skeleton raised in clinical and investigational medicine, and why selection of the appropriate site for a specific investigation is important if meaningful results are to be obtained.

GENERAL PRINCIPLES OF IN VIVO MEASUREMENTS WITH X- AND γ-RAYS

The various technical approaches to bone mineral measurements using X- and γ-radiation

have in common that they can be understood in terms of photon interactions with matter. The *photoelectric effect* and *Compton scattering* are the main processes. The photoelectric effect involves the complete absorption of the incident photon by an atom, while in Compton scattering the photon undergoes a collision with an atomic electron in which the photon is deflected and loses some of its energy in the process. Rayleigh scattering, involving the coherent scattering of an X-ray by all the electrons in an atom, may also be important at low photon energies.

Most bone densitometry techniques use the transmission of X- or γ-ray photons through the body. Methodologies such as SPA/SXA, DPA/DXA and QCT are based on making transmission measurements to record the attenuation of photons from an incident beam. At the relatively low photon energies used (30–140 keV), the photoelectric effect is the predominant mode of interaction in bone and Compton scattering in soft tissue. To ensure accurate measurements of the transmission factor it is important that those photons removed from the incident beam by scattering processes are prevented from reaching the detector. This requires the use of a narrow beam of radiation and efficient collimation of the detector.

The fraction of the incident radiation transmitted depends on: (1) the energy of the photons; (2) the elemental composition and physical density of the material through which they are travelling; and (3) the thickness of the material. The effect of the photon energy, composition and density of the material is described by the linear attenuation coefficient, μ. μ is defined as: *the fractional change in the intensity of the incident beam per unit thickness of the attenuating material* (Figure 3.3). If $I(x)$ is the intensity at position x and $I(x) - \delta I$ is the intensity at $x + \delta x$, then μ is defined by the equation:

$$\mu = \delta x \xrightarrow{\text{Limit}} 0 \; \frac{\delta I / I(x)}{\delta x} = \frac{1}{I} \frac{dI}{dx} \qquad (3.1)$$

Integration of equation 3.1 gives the exponential equation:

$$I(x) = I_0 \exp -\mu x \qquad (3.2)$$

Linear attenuation coefficient (μ)

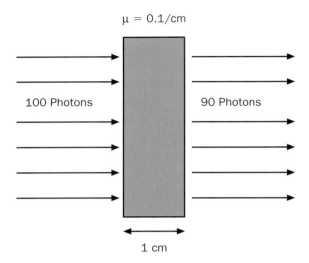

Figure 3.3 Definition of the linear attenuation coefficient. μ is the fractional change in X-ray beam intensity per unit thickness of the attenuating medium.

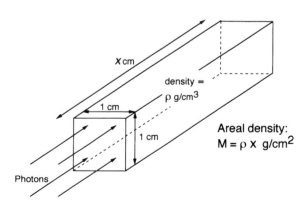

Figure 3.4 Definition of areal density. Areal density is the product of the physical density, ρ, and the total thickness of the attenuating material, x. In physical terms, ρx is the total mass in the column of unit cross-sectional area centred on the X-ray beam.

where I_0 is the incident intensity and $I(x)$ is the transmitted intensity for a slab of material of thickness x.

For the purposes of bone densitometry measurements it is helpful to consider not the linear attenuation coefficient, μ, but a closely related concept, the mass attenuation coefficient, μ_m. μ and μ_m are related by the physical density of the material, ρ.

$$\mu_m = \mu/\rho \qquad (3.3)$$

The advantage of the mass attenuation coefficient, μ_m, is that it depends solely on the energy of the incident photons and the atomic composition of the attenuating medium. The dependence on physical density is removed. This means that if, say, calcium atoms are present in a material, their contribution to μ_m depends solely on the fraction of all atoms that are calcium, and not on the physical state of the particular compound, crystalline state or mixture that is present.

If the mass attenuation coefficient is used instead of the linear attenuation coefficient, the exponential transmission equation, equation 3.2, can be written as:

$$I(x) = I_0 \exp{-\mu_m \rho x} \qquad (3.4)$$

Equation 3.4 is useful because of the product ρx in the exponential term. In physical terms, ρx is the total mass of material in a column of unit cross-sectional area centred on the X-ray beam (Figure 3.4). This quantity is just the local value of the areal density (units: g/cm^2), defined above as the integral mass of bone mineral at the measurement site divided by the projected area, that is routinely measured by SXA and DXA scans. Thus, equation 3.4 enables the combination of a measurement of the transmission factor $(I(x)/I_0)$ with knowledge of the mass attenuation coefficient to find the areal density, ρx. In practice, when making bone density measurements it is necessary to separate the contributions to the net attenuation of the X-ray beam by bone mineral and the overlying soft tissue. The methods of correcting for soft tissue in SPA/SXA and DPA/DXA scanning are explained in the Appendix to this chapter.

Quantitative computed tomography (QCT) studies differ from DXA because they provide quantitative information on bone density from cross-sectional rather than projectional images (Figure 3.2). Because the exact volume of bone tissue is known, true physical density (units: g/cm^3) rather than projectional areal density (units: g/cm^2) is measured. A CT scan provides an image that shows the value of the linear attenuation coefficient μ at each pixel in the image. Usually the μ values are given in Hounsfield units (HU), which are a linear rescaling of μ such that air takes the value HU = -1000 and water HU = 0. There is a linear correlation between HU numbers and bone mineral density that can be determined by including a calibration phantom in the scan. A detailed discussion of the current status of QCT can be found in a review by Genant et al.[1] Other technical details are given by Cann.[5] The chief limitation to the wider use of QCT is the high installation and running costs, so that an individual examination is expensive. Nevertheless, the possibility of carrying out what many people believe is the most relevant measurement of bone mineral, the true vertebral trabecular bone density, means that the technique continues to attract considerable attention.

A methodology widely studied in research laboratories is the Compton scattering technique.[6,7] In this method a narrow beam of photons interacts with bone by the incoherent (Compton) scattering process. The number of photons scattered from the bone sample is directly proportional to the density within this volume and is independent of the effective atomic number and the tissue surrounding the bone. Thus, like QCT, this technique can be used to study trabecular bone without interference from the surrounding cortex. Results are expressed in g/cm^3. To avoid difficulties of localization and multiple scattering, measurements in vivo are restricted to shallow and readily accessible sites such as the calcaneus and distal radius. Further details can be found in the review by Tothill.[2]

Neutron activation analysis is a method of studying body composition by irradiating the patient with neutrons. Many of the constituent elements become radioactive and can be quantified by their γ-ray emissions. After a short irradiation the patient is measured in a whole body counter in a low background environment. Its application to bone mineral measurements relies on the fact that 99% of calcium in the body is in the skeleton. The calcium radionuclide measured is ^{49}Ca, which has an 8.7-minute half-life and emits a 3.1-MeV γ-ray. Calcium-49 is formed by neutron capture by stable ^{48}Ca, which comprises 0.18% of natural calcium. Other gamma emissions give information on other elements in the body including nitrogen, sodium, phosphorus and chlorine. Potassium may be measured using the natural radionuclide ^{40}K. In vivo neutron activation analysis requires careful calibration and results in a fairly high radiation dose to the subject. During the 1970s and 1980s several facilities were operating in the USA and Europe, but the technique is used seldom now. Further details can be found in the review by Tothill.[2]

Techniques that avoid the use of X-rays are popular because they eliminate all concerns about radiation. The principles of quantitative ultrasound are discussed in Chapter 6. Another such methodology is quantitative magnetic resonance imaging (QMR). The technique is based on the application of a radiofrequency wave to excite hydrogen nuclei in a strong magnetic field and imaging the relaxation times of the processing protons. Bone tissue itself does not generate a signal, but the presence of the trabecular bone matrix modifies the signal from the adjacent marrow space. As with ultrasound, the method seems to be sensitive to a combination of bone density and bone microarchitecture. Further details can be found in the review by Genant et al.[1]

DESCRIPTION OF BONE DENSITOMETRY METHODS

This section discusses the historical development of bone densitometry methods and their evolution to the techniques that are most widely used today.

Single photon absorptiometry (SPA)

Photon absorptiometry was originally introduced by Cameron and Sorenson in 1963.[8] The original instruments used a radionuclide source emitting γ-rays with a single energy, either ¹²⁵I (28 keV) or ²⁴¹Am (60 keV), a feature that led to the name *single photon absorptiometry*. The underlying physics of these instruments limits them to measuring sites that can either be immersed in water or embedded in other materials with absorption properties equivalent to soft tissue. The first commercial SPA bone densitometers became available in the early 1970s. Measurement sites were assessed by scanning a single line either once or repeatedly and techniques were developed for measuring the mid- and distal radius, humerus, calcaneus and distal femur. Reproducible positioning of the scan imposed the biggest limitation on precision and in the radius it was usual for this to be based on manual location of a site one-third or one-half the length of the forearm where the bone is entirely cortical. Later SPA devices employed rectilinear scanning and performed a scout scan to find a location in the distal forearm with a predefined distance between the radius and ulna that could serve as an anatomical landmark called the *reference line* (Figure 3.5). Subsequently, techniques were developed to make measurements distally to the reference line where up to half the bone is trabecular.[9–11]

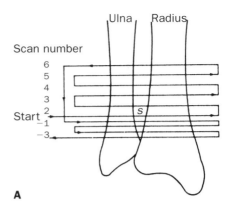

A

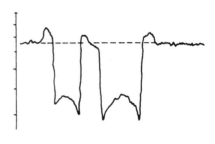

B

Figure 3.5 (A) Scan lines used in an SPA study of the forearm. The separation s determines the reference point for the BMD measurement. (B) Transmission plot across the wrist showing the soft tissue baseline. (Reproduced with permission from P Tothill.[2])

Single X-ray absorptiometry (SXA)

In recent years there has been continuing interest in small, low-cost devices dedicated to scanning the peripheral skeleton.[12] Such systems take up little space, are simple to operate and result in an exceptionally low radiation dose to the patient. Following the technical advances in DXA, an X-ray tube with a low-voltage generator (40 kV) has replace the radionuclide source in SPA devices resulting in the acronym *SXA* standing for *single X-ray absorptiometry*.[13,14] The use of an X-ray tube eliminates the need for frequent source replacement and recalibration,

which was a serious drawback of SPA using an ¹²⁵I radionuclide source. SXA devices still require the patient's forearm to be immersed in a waterbath to correct for the effects of soft tissue attenuation. However, in the latest development in forearm densitometry several manufacturers have introduced peripheral DXA (pDXA) devices based on similar principles to standard DXA equipment.[12] These dispense with the need for a water bath and allow the patient's forearm to be scanned in air resulting in a particularly compact and convenient device. Examination times have been reduced to 2–3 minutes for acquiring a projectional scan image of the distal forearm that allows the measurement of BMD at both trabecular and cortical sites. A more detailed discussion of these developments is given in Chapter 5.

Dual photon absorptiometry (DPA)

The substitution of a dual- for a single-energy source was an important advance in bone densitometry because it allowed the measurement of sites such as the lumbar spine and femur that cannot be surrounded with a bolus of constant soft tissue thickness. Although the first equipment for measuring bone mineral by this technique was constructed as early as 1965,[15] development was slow and a variety of research instruments were built by individual investigators with variations in design, choice of radionuclide sources and computer algorithms.[16–18] Initially, different source configurations were used depending on the measurement site: either ^{125}I and ^{241}Am (28 and 60 keV) or ^{241}Am and ^{137}Cs (60 and 662 keV). The radionuclide ^{153}Gd, which emits photons at two discrete energies (44 and 100 keV), became available in the early 1970s, and allowed the design of scanners measuring different sites of the skeleton with a single source. Furthermore, DPA systems for the first time had the capability of assessing total body bone mineral and body composition using a three compartment model of bone mass, lean mass and fat mass.[19] The widespread clinical use of DPA became possible in the early 1980s with the advent of the first commercial instruments produced by Novo and Lunar (Figure 3.6A).

While DPA brought significant improvements to the field of bone densitometry, there were numerous practical drawbacks. Scan times for high precision spine and femur scans could be as long as 20–40 minutes and the resolution was limited to 4–8 mm, giving poor quality images (Figure 3.6B). It is not physically possible to make a radionuclide source that is both small enough to limit loss of spatial resolution

by the penumbra effect and strong enough to give reasonable counting statistics in an acceptable scanning time. For these reasons, precision errors were as large as 1–2% in vitro and 2–4% in vivo. Moreover, ^{153}Gd has a relatively short half-life (T½ = 242 days) and the decreasing source strength with time required complicated corrections. The annual replacement of sources was costly and required recalibration of the system. The availability of ^{153}Gd sources was sometimes limited and could interrupt a continuous work schedule. Furthermore, in the USA the use of radioisotopes is strictly regulated by the Nuclear Regulatory Commission, which tended to restrict the use of this technique to established nuclear medicine laboratories.

Dual X-ray absorptiometry (DXA)

Dual X-ray absorptiometry overcame many of the shortcomings of DPA by replacing the radionuclide source with an X-ray tube. The technique had its origins in the method of X-ray spectrophotometry developed in the 1970s.[20,21] The introduction of an X-ray tube improved the performance of bone densitometers by combining higher photon flux with a smaller diameter source. The availability of an intense, narrow beam of radiation shortened scan times, enhanced image definition and improved precision.[22] These advantages were highlighted by Rutt and colleagues in a poster presented at the 1985 Annual Meeting of the American Society for Bone and Mineral Research.[23] From theoretical calculations they showed that replacement of the ^{153}Gd radionuclide source with an X-ray tube simultaneously improved image resolution from 2 mm to 1 mm, improved precision of the BMD measurements from 2% to 1% and shortened scan times from 20 minutes to 2 minutes. When the first commercial DXA scanner was introduced by Hologic in 1987 (Hologic Inc., Waltham, MA, USA),[24] DPA technology was immediately superseded.[25,26] As noted above, in recent years new X-ray devices for studying the peripheral skeleton have been

A

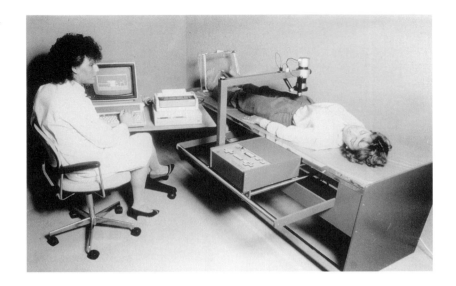

B

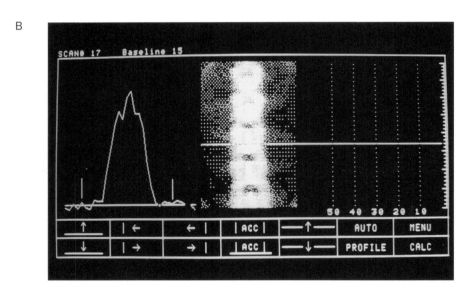

Figure 3.6 (A) A Novo BMC-LAB 22a DPA scanner as used in the mid-1980s. (B) A lumbar spine DPA scan being analysed on a Novo BMC-LAB 22a system.

introduced with similar improvements to SPA as DXA achieved for DPA.

Another significant advantage of DXA is the relative stability of calibration in clinical use.[27,28] DXA systems are factory calibrated and an analysis of records for 2700 DPX units manufactured by the Lunar Corporation (Madison, WI, USA) showed a coefficient of variation (CV) in system calibration of 0.5%.[29] With careful attention to the quality control procedures discussed in Chapter 9, this level of agreement should be maintained for the lifetime of the system.[30]

The replacement of a radioactive source by an X-ray tube requires the solution of several significant technical problems. A highly stable X-ray generator is essential. One advantage of a radionuclide source is that the rate of photon emission is constant and varies only due to statistical fluctuations (Poisson noise) and the slow decrease due to the half-life of the source. A constant source is necessary to ensure the fixed intensity of the incident beam. The advantages of higher photon flux are realized only to the extent that there is a corresponding reduction in the random fluctuations in X-ray output so they approach the theoretical limit set by Poisson noise.

A further advantage of a radionuclide source is its discrete line emissions. In contrast, X-ray tubes generate polyenergetic spectra and the effects of beam hardening are a potential source of error in DXA measurements. In beam hardening lower-energy photons are preferentially removed from the radiation beam compared with higher-energy photons, leading to a progressive shift in spectral distribution to higher effective photon energies with increasing body thickness. As a result the mass attenuation coefficients for bone and soft tissue change with body thickness and so vary between patients and sites within the body. Beam hardening can have two effects on BMD measurements: (1) for a particular true BMD, measured BMD may vary with body thickness; and (2) for a particular body thickness, BMD measurements may not lie on a truly linear scale.[31]

Quantitative computed tomography (QCT)

Quantitative computed tomography can determine the three-dimensional distribution of true volumetric bone density at any skeletal site.[1] However, because of the high responsiveness of spinal trabecular bone and its importance for vertebral strength, QCT is principally used to determine trabecular BMD in the vertebral body. In this application it is believed to be the technique with the highest diagnostic sensitiv-

ity to disease and age-related bone loss.[3] One advantage of QCT is that it can be performed on any commercial CT scanner with the use of specially designed calibration phantoms. More recent implementations of the technique have reduced the initially high radiation dose and improved the precision of the method by employing commercially available automated scanning and analysis software.[5,32] Nevertheless, the radiation dose is still significantly higher than DXA.[33]

QCT can be performed in single-energy (SEQCT) or dual-energy (DEQCT) modes, which differ in accuracy, precision and radiation dose.[34,35] The principal source of error for SEQCT measurements is variable marrow fat, which causes measurements to underestimate BMD and overestimate BMD loss. However, marrow fat increases with age and a correction reduces the BMD accuracy errors to levels that are small compared with the biological variation.[36] Although it is possible to improve accuracy by using DEQCT, this impairs precision and increases radiation dose.

Peripheral QCT (pQCT) measurement of the distal radius was one of the first bone densitometry techniques developed.[37] Originally an ^{125}I radionuclide source was used. However, in recent years commercial systems using X-ray tubes have been developed and the technique has gained wider acceptance.[38] Advantages of pQCT include the selective measurement of trabecular bone, low radiation dose and minimum impact of degenerative changes that can obscure DXA measurements of the spine. In addition, pQCT offers new possibilities that are only now being recognized in high resolution CT scans that allow the direct visualization of trabecular microstructure.[12] The radiation dose is small and structural parameters such as trabecular number and separation can be measured with high precision.[39] More details of pQCT instruments are given in Chapter 5.

Radiographic absorptiometry (RA)

The technique of radiographic absorptiometry involves measuring the optical density of bones

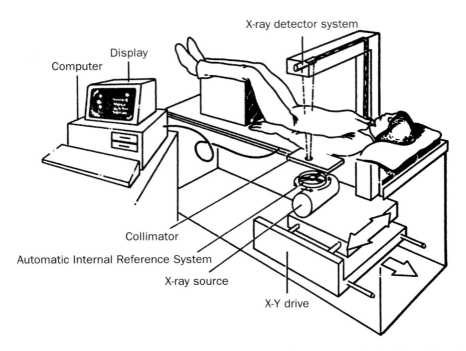

Figure 3.7 Components of a DXA scanner for scanning the spine, femur or total body. (Reproduced with permission from Hologic Inc.)

on X-ray film calibrated using a small reference wedge and is one of the oldest quantitative methods of evaluating bone mineral.[40] However, the simplicity belies the problems due to variation in kilovoltage, exposure, film characteristics, processing and soft tissue thickness.[2] The latter problem restricts the technique to peripheral sites, in particular the phalanges and metacarpal bones in the hand.

Recent improvements in technology have led to a revival in interest in RA. Exposed films can be mailed to central evaluation facilities provided that specific imaging and calibration protocols are followed.[41] In this form, RA does not require the purchase of any special purpose imaging equipment. Very recently, small dedicated systems for acquiring high resolution digital radiographic images of the hand have been developed. Like pDXA, these systems are particularly compact, deliver a very low radiation

dose and may be ideal for the physician's office. A more detailed discussion of these developments is given in Chapter 5.

TECHNICAL CONSIDERATIONS OF ABSORPTIOMETRY

Figure 3.7 shows the main components of an absorptiometry system. A radiation source, which can be either a radionuclide (for SPA or DPA) or an X-ray tube (for SXA or DXA), emits photons, which are collimated into a narrow pencil beam that can be turned on and off as required. The beam passes through the subject's bone and soft tissue and continues upward to enter a detector where the intensity of the transmitted radiation is registered. The source, collimator and detector are carefully aligned and mechanically connected by a scanning arm. As

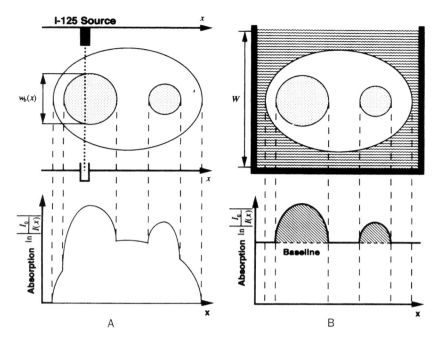

Figure 3.8 Principles of operation of an SPA/SXA device. (A) The top diagram shows a simulated forearm being scanned in air with the detector-source assembly. The curve below shows a tracing of the attenuated beam in air as the arm is scanned across its axis. (B) The same scan, but with the arm submerged in a water bath, which creates a constant thickness of soft-tissue-equivalent material around the bone. The effect is to create a fixed baseline against which the bone can be measured.

the arm moves across the subject's body a scan line is acquired representing the attenuation profile along a single projection. If the scanning arm performs a two-dimensional raster scan then a projectional image is acquired across the chosen scan field.

The basic principles of single photon (or X-ray) absorptiometry are illustrated in Figure 3.8A, which shows a simulated forearm being scanned in air. The attenuation through air alone is effectively zero, but starts to increase as the beam passes through the growing thickness of soft tissue. Where the beam path intersects the bone, the attenuation increases more rapidly. However, if the patient's forearm is first embedded in a constant thickness of a soft-tissue-equivalent material such as water, the

attenuation at points along the scan line not intersecting bone becomes constant (Figure 3.8B) and gives a reference baseline against which the additional attenuation caused by bone can be quantified. The incremental attenuation over and above the baseline gives a point-by-point profile of BMD along the scan line. Integrating this curve (the shaded area in Figure 3.8B) gives the total bone mineral content at the chosen projection. An example of a profile along an actual scan line is shown in Figure 3.5. Further mathematical details are given in the Appendix.

It is clear from Figure 3.8 that SPA/SXA can only work if soft tissue is composed of one homogeneous material of constant thickness. If this were not the case, an acceptable baseline could not be defined. The technique assumes that the muscle and other types of soft tissue at the measurement site can be closely simulated by water. However, this condition is not completely met. Fat surrounding the bone and subcutaneous fat both affect the uniform appearance of the baseline (Figure 3.5). A correction for this fat effect becomes necessary for certain measurement conditions.

In DPA/DXA, the requirement for a constant thickness of soft-tissue-equivalent material is eliminated by recording the attenuation profiles at two different photon energies. Because of the dependence of the attenuation coefficient on atomic number and photon energy (Figure 3.9), measurement of the transmission factors at two energies enables the areal densities (i.e. the mass per unit projected area) of two different types of tissue to be inferred. In DXA scans these are taken to be bone mineral (hydroxyapatite) and soft tissue respectively.

A simple explanation of the basic principle is shown in Figure 3.10. A DXA scan line records the attenuation profiles at two different photon energies, a high- and a low-energy profile. The low-energy profile shows somewhat higher attenuation than the high-energy profile for the soft tissue parts of the scan line, but markedly higher attenuation over bone due to the much larger attenuation coefficient of bone at lower photon energies (Figure 3.9). If the high-energy profile is multiplied by a suitable factor k (k is equal to the ratio of the soft tissue attenuation coefficients for the low- and high-energy beams), the two profiles become equal over the

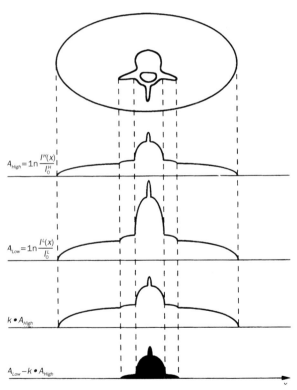

Figure 3.10 Principles of operation of a DPA/DXA device. The top two profiles show the attenuation curves for the high-energy and low-energy beams. The high-energy profile is multiplied by a factor k so that the soft tissue attenuation matches that in the low-energy profile. When the two profiles are subtracted the bone mineral distribution is left.

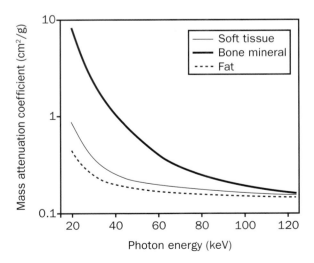

Figure 3.9 Variation of the mass attenuation coefficients for bone and soft tissue with photon energy.

soft tissue areas. Subtraction of the *k*-corrected high-energy profile from the low-energy profile gives a different profile that shows the point-by-point variation of BMD along the scan line. Further mathematical details are given in the Appendix.

When a DXA scan is acquired, the image is effectively a pixel-by-pixel map of BMD over the scan field. In practice, due to the variable composition of soft tissue from patient to patient and the effects of beam hardening on the polyenergetic X-ray spectrum, it is necessary to use the soft tissue regions adjacent to bone as a reference area of comparable thickness and composition. This serves as a baseline (an example is shown in the profile across the DPA scan in Figure 3.6B) and a line-by-line correction is applied to the BMD values. An edge detection algorithm is used to find the bone edges. The total projected area of bone is then derived by summing the pixels within the bone edges, and the reported value of BMD is calculated as the mean BMD over all the pixels identified as bone. Finally, bone mineral content (BMC) is derived by multiplying mean BMD by projected area:

$$BMC = BMD \times Area \qquad (3.5)$$

It is widely recognized that the accuracy of DXA scans is limited by the variations in soft tissue composition within the body. Because of its higher hydrogen content, the mass attenuation coefficient of fat is different from that of lean tissue. Differences in soft tissue composition in the path of the X-ray beam through bone compared with the adjacent soft tissue reference area will cause errors in the BMD measurements. These have been examined in a number of studies including theoretical studies based on the attenuation coefficients of hydroxyapatite, lean tissue and fat,[42] and studies using phantoms and cadavers.[43] Tothill used CT images to delineate the distribution of lean and fat tissue in transaxial scans through the lumbar vertebrae (Figure 3.11A) and hence estimated the effect on spine DXA scans.[44,45] For postero-anterior (PA) projection scans, errors of around 5% are found. However, for lateral spine scans larger and more variable effects are found.[45] In

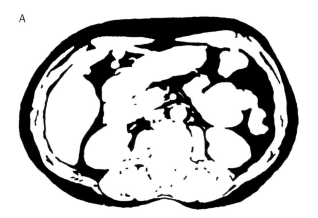

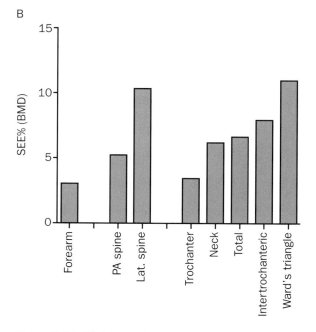

Figure 3.11 (A) Areas of adipose tissue in a CT image through the lumbar spine. (Reproduced with permission from P Tothill.[44]) (B) Random accuracy errors for BMD measurements in the spine, femur and distal forearm derived from linear regression analysis of in vivo and in vitro measurements in a cadaver study. (Adapted from Svendsen et al.[43])

a cadaver study, Svendsen et al. examined the effect of fat inhomogeneity on random accuracy errors for BMD measurements in the spine, femur and forearm.[43] The errors were smallest in the forearm, but within acceptable limits for

PA spine, femoral neck, trochanter and total hip BMD (Figure 3.11B).

DIFFERENT IMPLEMENTATIONS OF DUAL X-RAY ABSORPTIOMETRY

In DPA the required dual-energy spectrum is generated by the line emissions of the ^{153}Gd source (Figure 3.12A). In their original descrip-

tion of DXA, Rutt and colleagues suggested two ways of emulating the required spectrum with an X-ray tube:[23]

1) The use of constant-potential generator and a K-absorption edge filter (Figure 3.13) to split the polyenergetic X-ray spectrum (Figure 3.12B) into high- and low-energy components that mimic the emissions from ^{153}Gd (Figure 3.12C). K-edge filters made of the rare-earth metals cerium ($Z = 58$),

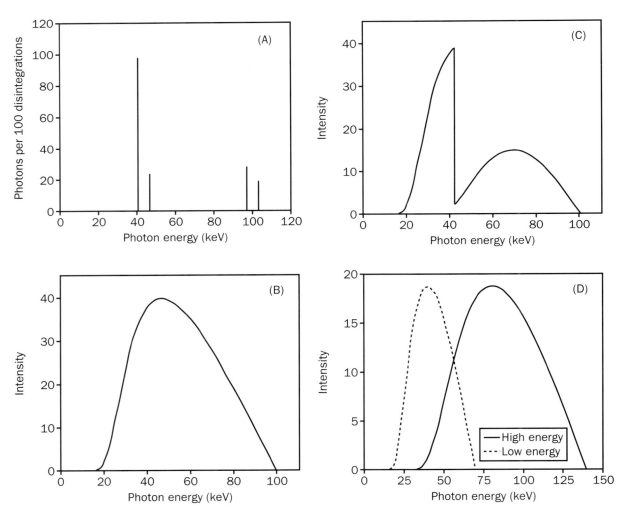

Figure 3.12 Energy spectra for different radiation sources used in DPA/DXA bone densitometers: (A) Spectrum for ^{153}Gd. There are two γ-ray emissions at around 100 keV and characteristic X-ray emissions at 41–48 keV. (B) Continuous spectrum from an X-ray tube. (C) Continuous X-ray spectrum modified by a K-edge filter. (D) High- and low-energy spectra from a kV switching system.

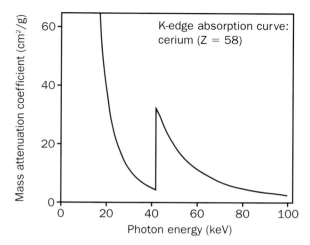

Figure 3.13 Variation of the mass attenuation coefficient with photon energy in cerium (Z = 58). The K-edge at 41 keV is the K-shell binding energy in cerium.

neodymium (Z = 60) and samarium (Z = 62) have been used for this purpose. In a DXA system using a K-edge filter, energy discriminating detectors able to sort each photon into the high- or low-energy channels are required. If errors are to be avoided careful attention must be paid to correcting the errors due to pulse pile-up at high count rates. This may limit the range of soft tissue thickness over which the equipment will function correctly.

2) In the second technique the high-voltage generator is switched between high and low kVp during alternate half-cycles of the mains supply. This technique leads to rather broader X-ray spectra (Figure 3.12D) and careful attention is required to correct for beam hardening. However, switched energy systems operate with a simple current-integrating detector with no need for energy discrimination. As a result the detectors are highly linear over a wide range of transmitted intensities.

The first commercially available DXA scanner was introduced by Hologic in 1987 and used the energy-switching principle.[25,26] Later implementations introduced by Lunar[46] and Norland (Norland Medical Systems Inc., Fort Atkinson, WI, USA) in 1988 and by Sopha (Sopha Medical, Buc, France) in 1989 used a constant-potential X-ray source combined with rare-earth filters. In 1997, a new DXA system was introduced by DMS (Diagnostic Medical Systems, Montpellier, France). Technical details of currently available systems are discussed in Chapter 4. The general principles of energy-switching and K-edge filter implementations are discussed in further detail below.

Energy switching

In energy-switching systems, the X-ray tube potential is rapidly switched between two different energies. In Hologic DXA scanners, which currently represent the only available implementation of this type, the X-ray potential is switched between 70 and 140 kVp during alternate half-cycles of the mains supply, resulting in 8.33 ms pulses in 60-Hz systems and 10 ms pulses in 50-Hz systems. To overcome the problems of beam hardening discussed above, Hologic systems are continuously calibrated by a rotating filter wheel that serves as an internal reference standard (Figure 3.14). The filter wheel is divided into three sectors containing respectively: (1) an open air gap; (2) an epoxy resin filter that is soft tissue equivalent; and (3) an epoxy resin filter containing hydroxyapatite that is bone equivalent. The latter has a BMD value of 1.0 g/cm^2. Each sector is itself divided in two for the high- and low-energy cycles. The former has a 3-mm brass filter that removes low-energy X-ray during the high-energy part of the cycle. Thus, each pixel in the scan image represents six transmission measurements that register the X-ray signal at high and low energies through the air gap, the soft tissue filter and the bone filter respectively (Figure 3.15). The differential attenuation through the two epoxy resin filters compared

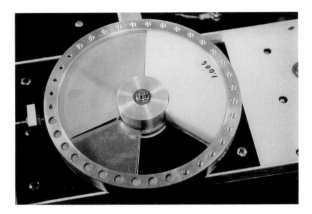

Figure 3.14 The calibration wheel used as the interval reference standard in Hologic DXA scanners. The different sectors in the wheel include bone- and soft-tissue-equivalent filters, together with an empty air sector. Each of these three sectors has a separate high- and low-energy segment with and without an additional brass filter. In the example shown, the BMD of the bone filter is 1.006 g/cm².

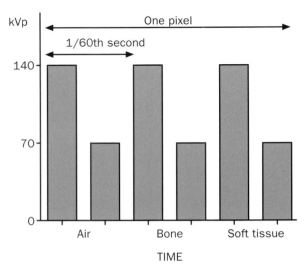

Figure 3.15 In Hologic DXA scanners, each pixel contains information at high and low kV through the air, bone and soft tissue sectors of the reference wheel. High and low kV measurements are made during alternate half-cycles of the mains supply. This is 60 Hz in the USA and 50 Hz in Europe.

with the air gap gives information from which the effective values of the mass attenuation coefficient for soft tissue and bone at high and low energies can be determined. Further information on this calculation is given in the Appendix.

The internal calibration wheel ensures that the system remains correctly calibrated irrespective of variations in soft tissue thickness from patient to patient or between scan sites. However, there remains a small residual linearity error because the calibration is only exactly correct for a BMD value equal to the BMD in the filter wheel (1.0 g/cm²) (Figure 3.16A). To correct the residual errors a linearity phantom is used consisting of an acrylic block with three slabs of bone-equivalent material with BMD values of 0.6, 1.0 and 1.6 g/cm² respectively. Using measurements of this phantom an algorithm is generated that corrects the measured bone densities to their true values. However,

this correction is only accurate for soft tissue thickness equivalent to the linearity phantom (16 cm). Small residual errors may still arise at other body thicknesses, in particular where total tissue thickness is small, as in scans of the forearm and hand (Figure 3.16B).

Unlike systems requiring energy discriminating detectors, kVp switching systems are not affected by pulse pile-up and cross-over. Instead, a current-integrating detector is used, which gives a wide dynamic range. This is particularly important for whole body scans, where the detector needs to register accurately both the unattenuated beam through air around the sides of the body as well as the highly attenuated beam through the thickest parts of the trunk. There is a similar advantage in performing scans of the forearm and hand.

In the latest Hologic systems using fan-beam technology, the energy switching is between 100 and 140 kVp instead of 70 and 140 kVp.

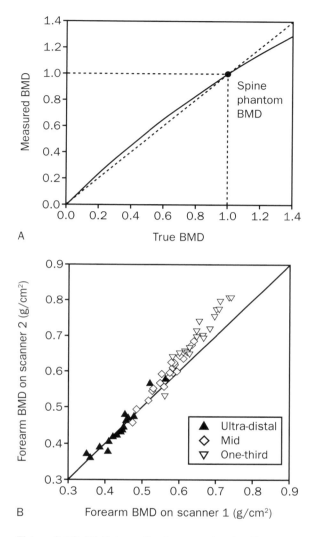

A

B

Figure 3.16 (A) Schematic diagram showing the effect of beam hardening on the bone density scale of a DXA densitometer. Unless a correction is made, measured and true BMD only agree at the calibration point. (B) Effect of an error in the beam hardening correction found during cross calibration of forearm BMD in two DXA densitometers. The differences are believed to have arisen during a software upgrade.

This change leads to somewhat improved performance of the system. To accommodate better the fan-beam geometry, the rotating filter wheel has been replaced by a rotating drum (Figure 3.17).

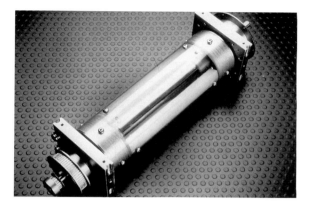

Figure 3.17 In the latest generation of Hologic fan-beam DXA scanners the internal reference wheel is replaced by a rotating drum.

Rare-earth filtered X-ray sources

An alternative method of implementing DXA uses a highly stable constant potential X-ray generator. The principle of operation is illustrated in Figure 3.18. In these systems, the X-ray beam is passed through a rare-earth filter with energy specific absorption characteristics (a K-edge) corresponding to the binding energy of the innermost atomic electrons (Figure 3.13). The K-edge filter divides the original X-ray spectrum into the high- and low-energy components shown in Figure 3.12C. The relatively narrow high- and low-energy components help reduce the problems caused by beam hardening.

K-edge filtered systems require pulse counting detectors with the associated problems of detector pile-up and energy cross-over (Figure 3.19). Detector pile-up results from the need to process each incoming X-ray photon individually so that the electronics can determine whether it should be assigned to the high- or low-energy channels. Incoming photons may be missed if they reach the detector while the electronics are still processing the previous pulse. This phenomenon is referred to as pulse pile-up. The detectors used in DXA are commonly based on sodium iodide scintillators coupled to photo-

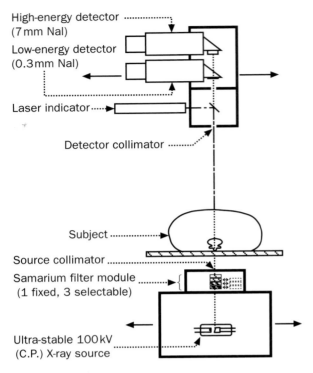

Figure 3.18 Principle of operation of a K-edge filter DXA system. Schematic drawing of a Norland XR-36 system. (Reproduced with permission from Norland Medical Systems Inc.)

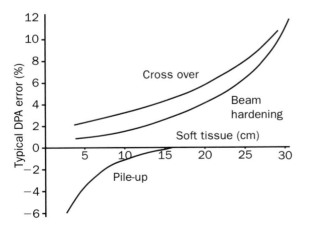

Figure 3.19 Effects of pulse pile-up, energy cross over and beam hardening on a pulse counting DXA system. (Reproduced with permission from Norland Medical Systems Inc.)

multiplier tubes. In such systems, up to 300 000 pulses per second can be processed without significant errors. To avoid this problem, tube current may need to be reduced in studies involving scanning thin body parts or air. Energy cross-over is another phenomenon that affects pulse counting detectors and is caused by high-energy photons erroneously being counted as low-energy photons. This phenomenon is corrected by subtracting a fraction of the high-energy counts from the low-energy channel. However, the fraction may vary with tissue thickness due to the effects of beam hardening and pulse pile-up (Figure 3.19).

BODY COMPOSITION MEASUREMENTS USING DXA

In addition to measuring bone mineral density and bone mineral content, the DXA technique has also been successfully applied to the measurement of body composition to determine the fat mass and lean mass components of the whole body. The physical basis of the measurement of body composition is that in those parts of the body where the X-ray beam does not intersect bone, the ratio of the attenuation values for the high- and low-energy beams is dependent on the composition of the material through which they pass and so the lean and fat mass can be separately evaluated. However, where bone is present, BMD and total soft tissue mass is determined instead. Over these latter sites lean and fat mass can be assigned based on interpolation from the composition of nearby soft tissue regions. By using known standards of various effective fat:lean ratios to calibrate the attenuation of the high- and low-energy beams, it is possible to measure the fat, lean and total masses as well as the BMC and BMD of the patient. Further details of this technique are given in Chapter 14.

FAN-BEAM DXA SYSTEMS

The first generation of DXA scanners used a pinhole collimator producing a pencil-beam of

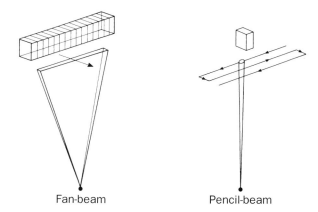

Figure 3.20 Comparison of the X-ray beam and detector geometry for a pencil-beam system with a single detector (right) and a fan-beam system with a multidetector array (left).

radiation coupled to a single detector in the scanning arm. Since then the most significant development in DXA technology has been the introduction of new systems that use a slit collimator to generate a fan-beam coupled to a linear array of detectors (Figure 3.20).[47,48] Fan-beam studies are acquired by the scanning arm performing a single sweep across the patient instead of the two-dimensional raster scan required by pencil-beam technology. As a result, scan times have been reduced from around 5–10 minutes for early generation pencil-beam scanners to 10–30 seconds for the latest fan-beam systems.

The short scan times for fan-beam DXA studies make these systems attractive to patient and technologist alike. However, there is clearly not a commensurate gain in patient throughput, since it is still necessary to inform the patient about the investigation, check for possible sources of technical artefacts such as belts, studs or buttons, position the patient for the scan and perform essential administrative tasks. In practice the introduction of fan-beam systems has decreased appointment times from perhaps one patient every 30 minutes to one every 15 minutes. However, this increase in patient throughput is probably the major advantage of fan-beam systems.

In the latest commercial DXA systems discussed in Chapter 4, the use of a fan-beam coupled to a solid-state detector constructed in the form of a multi-element linear array has significantly improved image resolution (Figure 3.21). This makes it easier to identify vertebral structure, together with artefacts such as degenerative disease, which can be a significant limitation in DXA studies of the lumbar spine. By supporting the source and detectors on a rotating C-arm, these systems enable lateral BMD scans of the spine to be acquired with the patient in the supine position. This type of study is discussed in Chapter 11. The advantage of reproducible positioning, short scan times and higher resolution images may enable useful clinical vertebral morphometry studies to be carried out on DXA systems to investigate vertebral fractures. This application is discussed in Chapter 20.

Alongside these advantages of fan-beam systems, it is important to recognize that an inevitable consequence of improved spatial resolution is slightly higher doses of radiation both to patients and to the staff operating equipment.[49,50] Radiation dose considerations are discussed further in Chapter 8.

APPENDIX: MATHEMATICAL BACKGROUND

X-ray absorptiometry scanners acquire data along an individual scan line (the x-direction) across the body, then increment axially (the y-direction), and repeat the process. The resulting raster scan results in the acquisition of a scan image composed of individual picture elements (pixels), each with a specific value of x and y. The mathematical algorithms outlined below illustrate how bone mineral density (BMD) is quantified pixel by pixel as a function of x and y.

During scan analysis, image processing algorithms identify anatomical landmarks, permit the definition of regions of interest (ROI) and then calculate the mean BMD in these regions expressed in units of g/cm^2. By multiplying the mean BMD by the projected area of the ROI (in cm^2), bone mineral content (BMC) is computed.

Interaction of photons with soft tissue and bone

When a beam passes through a substance at location (x,y) the radiation is attenuated by photon interactions with matter due to the photoelectric and Compton effects. The degree of attenuation depends on the energy of the photons, the atomic composition of the material and how thick the traversed section is. For a homogeneous material with mass attenuation coefficient μ (in cm^2/g), density ρ (in g/cm^3) and thickness w (in cm) at the point (x,y), the transmitted intensity I is related to the incident intensity I_0 according to the formula:

$$I = I_0 \exp{-\mu\rho w} \tag{A1}$$

In practice, there are often situations where the substance the beam is traversing is not homogeneous, but composed of layers of

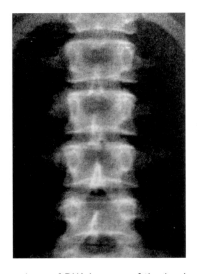
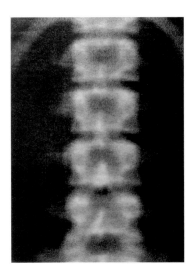

Figure 3.21 Comparison of DXA images of the lumbar spine obtained with a pencil-beam system (right) and a newer fan-beam system (left).

different materials each with its own mass attenuation coefficient, density and thickness. Assuming that the beam passes through N different materials, equation A1 can be rewritten as:

$$I = I_0 \exp[-\sum_{i=1}^{N} \mu_i \rho_i w_i] \qquad (A2)$$

Single photon (and X-ray) absorptiometry

In the case of SPA and SXA systems, the assumption is made that in equation A2 there are only two materials contributing to the attenuation, namely bone and soft tissue. Equation A2 therefore becomes:

$$I = I_0 \exp - (\mu_s \rho_s w_s + \mu_b \rho_b w_b) \qquad (A3)$$

where the subscripts s and b denote soft tissue and bone respectively. Taking the natural logarithm of equation A3 gives:

$$-\ln(I/I_0) = \mu_s \rho_s w_s + \mu_b \rho_b w_b \qquad (A4)$$

It is helpful to simplify equation A4 by writing J in place of the logarithmic transmission factor $-\ln(I/I_0)$ giving:

$$J = \mu_s \rho_s w_s + \mu_b \rho_b w_b \qquad (A5)$$

If the total thickness $W = w_s + w_b$ through soft tissue and bone is kept constant by placing the patient's forearm in a soft-tissue-equivalent medium such as water, then equation A5 can be rewritten as:

$$J = \mu_s \rho_s [W - w_b] + \mu_b \rho_b w_b \qquad (A6)$$

and the thickness of bone w_b at the point (x,y) can be computed:

$$w_b = \frac{J - \mu_s \rho_s W}{\mu_b \rho_b - \mu_s \rho_s} \qquad (A7)$$

The baseline transmission level in Figure 3.8B where the beam intersects only soft tissue and the bolus material is given by:

$$J_s = -\ln(I_s/I_0) = \mu_s \rho_s W \qquad (A8)$$

Substituting with J_s in equation A7 simplifies the equation to give:

$$w_b = \frac{J - J_s}{\mu_b \rho_b - \mu_s \rho_s} \qquad (A9)$$

The BMD at the point (x,y) in units of g/cm^2 is given by:

$$BMD = \rho_b w_b = \frac{\rho_b(J - J_s)}{\mu_b \rho_b - \mu_s \rho_s} \qquad (A10)$$

Dual photon (and X-ray) absorptiometry

For DPA and DXA systems it is helpful to replace the terms $\rho_s w_s$ and $\rho_b w_b$ in equation A3 with M_s and M_b to denote the areal densities of soft tissue and bone at the point (x,y) in units of g/cm^2. There are now two transmission equations, one for each photon energy. If primed variables denote the low-energy radiation beam and unprimed variables denote the high-energy beam, the two equations are:

low energy: $I' = I'_0 \exp^-(\mu'_s M_s + \mu'_b M_b) \quad$ (A11a)

high energy: $I = I_0 \exp^-(\mu_s M_s + \mu_b M_b) \quad$ (A11b)

As above, it is helpful to replace the logarithmic transmission factors with J giving the two equations:

$$J' = \mu'_s M_s + \mu'_b M_b \qquad (A12a)$$

$$J = \mu_s M_s + \mu_b M_b \qquad (A12b)$$

Provided the values of the four attenuation coefficients are known, equations A12a and A12b are two simultaneous equations that enable the areal densities of bone and soft tissue to be calculated from the transmission factors measured at the two photon energies. Solving the two equations we obtain:

$$M_b = \frac{J' - (\mu'_s/\mu_s)J}{\mu'_b - (\mu'_s/\mu_s)\mu_b.} \qquad (A13a)$$

$$M_s = \frac{(\mu'_b/\mu_b)J - J'}{(\mu'_b/\mu_b)\mu_s - \mu'_s} \qquad (A13b)$$

Equation A13a provides the basis for the determination of BMD in DPA and DXA. Its validity rests on the assumption that the attenuation coefficients for bone and soft tissue are exactly known at both energies. However, the composition of soft tissue varies from individual to individual due to the varying proportions of lean and adipose tissue so it may not be possible to use preset values of μ'_s and μ_s. For practical purposes, assume that the lean and fat are uniformly distributed throughout the subject's soft tissue. Define the 'R-factor' R_s as:

$$R_s = \mu'_s / \mu \qquad (A14)$$

Then equation A13a becomes:

$$M_b = \frac{J' - R_s J}{\mu'_b - R_s \mu_b} \qquad (A15)$$

Over the soft tissue part of the scan line where no bone is present then $M_b = 0$ and equation A15 can be solved for R_s in terms of the ratio of the logarithmic attenuation coefficients:

$$R_s = J'_s / J_s \qquad (A16)$$

where the subscript s denotes that the attenuation measurements are made over soft tissue.

In practice, the following iterative procedure can be used to make a line-by-line estimate of R_s and compute BMD:

1) Estimate R_s by an educated guess, for example by averaging J'/J for all points along the scan line.
2) Calculate BMD for each point using equation A15.
3) Separate the measured points into bone and soft tissue pixels by applying a threshold.
4) Recalculate R_s by averaging equation A16 over all pixels flagged as soft tissue.
5) Repeat steps 2–4 until R_s stops changing.
6) Smooth bone edges to eliminate isolated noise-generated bone points.
7) Display bone and soft tissue points for operator approval.
8) Determine regions of interest.
9) Determine the projected area of bone by counting all the pixels flagged as bone in each region of interest.
10) Determine mean BMD in each region of interest by averaging the BMD of all the individual bone pixels.
11) Calculate BMC as: BMC = BMD × Area.
12) Display the results and print the report.

The R_s value is related to the fat fraction and provides a basis for body composition measurements. The above method is only exact for uniform fat distribution. Unfortunately, fat tends to be concentrated in subcutaneous adipose tissue and in fat pockets in the abdomen. However, provided that the composition of the soft tissue baseline points along the scan line is representative of the soft tissue overlying bone, this method is still an excellent approximation.

Errors in the estimate of R_s result primarily in an accuracy error. Nevertheless, precision errors may be introduced if significant changes in body composition occur between consecutive measurements. Except for subjects with significant obesity, postero-anterior projection spine measurements are quite robust to variations in baseline. The same is true of femur scans provided that scan analysis is performed using vertical scan lines to reduce the effect of the pronounced gradient in soft tissue composition caused by subcutaneous fat on the lateral borders of the scan. The most serious effect is for lateral spine scans where soft tissue composition is especially sensitive to the choice of the reference baseline region.

The Hologic internal reference system

The approach outlined above yields accurate and precise results provided that the bone attenuation coefficients are stable and accurately known. However, with X-ray systems the effective values of μ'_b and μ_b vary with body thickness and composition due to the effects of beam hardening. Hologic densitometers employ an internal calibration wheel synchronized with the mains supply that continuously interposes known amounts of soft-tissue and bone-equivalent samples into the beam (Figure 3.13). Each pixel consists of six transmission measurements through the air, bone and soft tissue sectors of the calibration wheel at high and low X-ray energies. A logarithmic amplifier is used so that the output signal is proportional to the logarithmic transmission factor, J. Let J', J'_b and J'_s be the low-energy transmission factors for the air, bone and soft tissue sectors, and J, J_b

and J_s the corresponding high-energy factors. The increments in attenuation when the bone calibration filter rotates into the X-ray beam are given by:

$$\Delta J'_{cb} = J'_b - J' \qquad \text{(A17a)}$$

$$\Delta J_{cb} = J_b - J \qquad \text{(A17b)}$$

with similar equations for the soft tissue filter:

$$\Delta J'_{cs} = J'_s - J' \qquad \text{(A17c)}$$

$$\Delta J_{cs} = J_s - J \qquad \text{(A17d)}$$

Let M_{cb} and M_{cs} denote the areal densities of the bone mineral and soft-tissue-equivalent filters. The effective values of the four attenuation coefficients in equation A13a are given by:

$$\mu'_b = \Delta J'_{cb}/M_{cb} \qquad \text{(A18a)}$$

$$\mu_b = \Delta J_{cb}/M_{cb} \qquad \text{(A18b)}$$

$$\mu'_s = \Delta J'_{cs}/M_{cs} \qquad \text{(A18c)}$$

$$\mu_s = \Delta J_{cs}/M_{cs} \qquad \text{(A18d)}$$

Substitution of these attenuation coefficients into equation A13a gives the relationship:

$$M_b = \frac{(J' - (\Delta J'_{cs}/\Delta J_{cs})J)M_{cb}}{\Delta J'_{cb} - (\Delta J'_{cs}/\Delta J_{cs})\Delta J_{cb}} \qquad \text{(A19)}$$

Equation A19 can be simplified by writing:

$$k = \mu'_s/\mu_s = \Delta J'_{cs}/\Delta J_{cs} \qquad \text{(A20a)}$$

$$Q = J' - kJ \qquad \text{(A20b)}$$

$$d_0 = \Delta J'_{cb} - k\Delta J_{cb}, \qquad \text{(A20c)}$$

when we obtain:

$$M_b = (Q/d_0)M_{cb} \qquad \text{(A21)}$$

Because the R-factor in equation A14 is determined from the internal calibration wheel instead of the soft tissue points, the value of Q will be non-zero even for beam paths that do not pass through bone. However, in the case of spine and hip scans the variation in total tissue thickness along a scan line is relatively small. The quantity $(J' - kJ)$ corrects for these variations in soft tissue thickness and the value of Q for soft tissue pixels will therefore be constant. Bone and soft tissue pixels can be distinguished using thresholding and once bone pixels have

been identified, their Q values can be corrected by subtracting a baseline value Q_s equal to the average value for soft tissue pixels on that scan line. We therefore replace Q in equation A21 by $(Q - Q_s)$. The areal density M_{cb} is simply the bone density value of the calibration wheel, BMD_{cal}. Making these changes, the equation is finally obtained for the BMD value of the (x,y) pixel:

$$BMD = [(Q - Q_s)/d_0] BMD_{cal} \qquad \text{(A22)}$$

Values of k and d_0 are computed line by line by averaging over the soft tissue pixels in each scan line. Their global values are included on the scan printouts.

REFERENCES

1. Genant HK, Engelke K, Fuerst T et al. Noninvasive assessment of bone mineral and structure: state of the art. *J Bone Miner Res* (1996) **11:** 707–30.
2. Tothill P. Methods of bone mineral measurement. *Phys Med Biol* (1989) **34:** 543–72.
3. Grampp S, Genant HK, Mathur A et al. Comparisons of non-invasive bone mineral measurements in assessing age-related loss, fracture discrimination and diagnostic classification. *J Bone Miner Res* (1997) **12:** 697–711.
4. Meunier PJ, Slosman D, Delmas PD et al. Strontium ranelate as a treatment for vertebral osteoporosis. *J Bone Miner Res* (1997) **12**(suppl 1): S129.
5. Cann CE. Quantitative CT for determination of bone mineral density: a review. *Radiology* (1988) **166:** 509–22.
6. Webber CE, Kennett TJ. Bone density measured by photon scattering. I. A system for clinical use. *Phys Med Biol* (1976) **21:** 760–9.
7. Shukla SS, Leichter I, Karellas A et al. Trabecular bone mineral density measurement *in-vivo*: use of the ratio of coherent to Compton-scattered photons in the calcaneus. *Radiology* (1986) **158:** 695–7.
8. Cameron JR, Sorenson J. Measurement of bone mineral in-vivo: an improved method. *Science* (1963) **142:** 230–6.
9. Abwrey BJ, Jacobson PC, Grubb SA et al. Bone density in women: a modified procedure for

measurement of distal radius density. *J Orthop Res* (1984) **2**: 314–21.

10. Nilas L, Borg J, Gotfredsen A et al. Comparison of single and dual-photon absorptiometry in postmenopausal bone mineral loss. *J Nucl Med* (1985) **26**: 1257–62.

11. Wahner HW, Eastell R, Riggs BL. Bone mineral density of the radius: where do we stand? *J Nucl Med* (1985) **26**: 1339–41.

12. Glüer C-C, Jergas M, Hans D. Peripheral measurement techniques for the assessment of osteoporosis. *Semin Nucl Med* (1997) **27**: 229–47.

13. Kelly TL, Crane G, Baran DT. Single x-ray absorptiometry of the radius: precision, correlation and reference data. *Calcif Tissue Int* (1994) **54**: 212–18.

14. Borg J, Mollgaard A, Riis BJ. Single x-ray absorptiometry: performance characteristics and comparison with single photon absorptiometry. *Osteoporos Int* (1995) **5**: 377–81.

15. Reed GW. The assessment of bone mineralization from the relative transmission of ^{241}Am and ^{137}Cs radiations. *Phys Med Biol* (1966) **11**: 174.

16. Roos BO, Skoldborn H. Dual photon absorptiometry in lumbar vertebrae. I. Theory and method. *Acta Radiol Ther Phys Biol* (1974) **13**: 266–80.

17. Roos BO. Dual photon absorptiometry in lumbar vertebrae. II. Precision and reproducibility. *Acta Radiol Ther Phys Biol* (1975) **14**: 291–303.

18. Wilson CR, Madsen M. Dichromatic absorptiometry of vertebral bone mineral content. *Invest Radiol* (1977) **12**: 180–4.

19. Mazess RB, Peppler WW, Chesnut CH et al. Total body bone mineral and lean body mass by dual photon absorptiometry: comparison with total body calcium by neutron activation analysis. *Calcif Tissue Int* (1981) **33**: 361–3.

20. Jacobson B. X-ray spectrophometry in-vivo. *Am J Roentgenol* (1964) **91**: 202–10.

21. Gustavson L, Jacobson B, Kusoffsky L. X-ray spectrophometry for bone mineral determinations. *Med Biol Eng Comput* (1974) **12**: 113–18.

22. Sorenson JA, Duke PR, Smith SW. Simulation studies of dual-energy X-ray absorptiometry. *Med Phys* (1989) **16**: 75–80.

23. Rutt BK, Stebler BG, Cann CE. High speed, high precision dual photon absorptiometry. Poster presented at the Seventh Annual Meeting of the American Society for Bone and Mineral Research, Washington DC, 16 June 1985.

24. Stein JA, Lazewatsky JL, Hochberg AM. Dual energy x-ray bone densitometer incorporating an internal reference system. *Radiology* (1987) **165**(suppl): 313.

25. Wahner HW, Dunn WL, Brown ML et al. Comparison of dual energy X-ray absorptiometry and dual photon absorptiometry for bone mineral measurements of the lumbar spine. *Mayo Clinic Proc* (1988) **63**: 1075–84.

26. Cullum ID, Ell PJ, Ryder JP. X-ray dual photon absorptiometry: a new method for the measurement of bone density. *Br J Radiol* (1989) **62**: 587–92.

27. Orwoll ES, Oviatt SK. Longitudinal precision of dual energy X-ray absorptiometry in a multicenter study. *J Bone Miner Res* (1991) **6**: 191–7.

28. Glüer C-C, Faulkner KG, Estilo MJ. Quality assurance for bone densitometry research studies: concept and impact. *Osteoporos Int* (1993) **3**: 227–35.

29. Nord R, Mazess RB, Hanson JA. Inter-unit variation on 2700 DPX densitometers. *Osteoporos Int* (1997) **7**: 284.

30. Gaither KW, Faulkner KG, Ostrem EC et al. Variation in calibration amongst like-manufacturer DXA systems. *J Bone Miner Res* (1996) **11**(suppl 1): S119.

31. Blake GM, McKeeney DB, Chhaya SC et al. Dual energy x-ray absorptiometry: the effects of beam hardening on bone density measurements. *Med Phys* (1992) **19**: 459–65.

32. Steiger P, Block JE, Steiger S et al. Spinal bone mineral density by quantitative computed tomography: effect of region of interest, vertebral level, and technique. *Radiology* (1990) **175**: 537–43.

33. Kalender WA. Effective dose values in bone mineral measurements by photon absorptiometry and computed tomography. *Osteoporos Int* (1992) **2**: 82–7.

34. Genant HK, Boyd DP. Quantitative bone mineral analysis using dual energy computed tomography. *Invest Radiol* (1977) **12**: 545–51.

35. Glüer C-C, Reiser UJ, Davis CA et al. Vertebral mineral determination by quantitative computed tomography (QCT): accuracy of single and dual energy measurements. *J Comput Assist Tomogr* (1988) **12**: 242–58.

36. Glüer C-C, Genant HK. Impact of marrow fat on accuracy of quantitative CT. *J Comput Assist Tomogr* (1989) **13**: 1023–35.

37. Ruegsegger P, Elsasser V, Anliker M et al. Quantification of bone mineralization using computed tomography. *Radiology* (1976) **121**: 93–7.

38. Butz S, Wüster C, Scheidt-Nave C et al. Forearm

BMD as measured by peripheral quantitative computed tomography (pQCT) in a German reference population. *Osteoporos Int* (1994) **4:** 179–84.

39. Müller R, Hildebrand T, Häuselmann HJ et al. In vivo reproducibility of three-dimensional structural properties of non-invasive bone biopsies using 3D-pQCT. *J Bone Miner Res* (1996) **11:** 1745–50.

40. Mack PB, O'Brien AT, Smith JM et al. A method for estimating degree of mineralization of bones from tracings of roentgenograms. *Science* (1939) **89:** 467.

41. Cosman F, Herrington B, Himmelstein S et al. Radiographic absorptiometry: a simple method for determination of bone mass. *Osteoporos Int* (1991) **2:** 34–8.

42. Webber CE. The effect of fat on bone mineral measurements in normal subjects with recommended values of bone, muscle and fat attenuation coefficients. *Clin Phys Physiol Meas* (1987) **8:** 143–58.

43. Svendsen OL, Hassager C, Skodt V et al. Impact of soft tissue on in-vivo accuracy of bone mineral measurements in the spine, hip and forearm: a human cadaver study. *J Bone Miner Res* (1995) **10:** 868–73.

44. Tothill P, Pye DW, Teper J. The influence of extra-skeletal fat on the accuracy of dual photon absorptiometry of the spine. In: Ring EFJ, Evans WD, Dixon AS, eds. *Osteoporosis and bone mineral measurement* (IPSM Publications: York, 1989), 48–53.

45. Tothill P, Pye DW. Errors due to non-uniform distribution of fat in dual X-ray absorptiometry of the lumbar spine. *Br J Radiol* (1992) **65:** 807–13.

46. Mazess R, Collick B, Trempe J et al. Performance evaluation of a dual-energy x-ray bone densitometer. *Calcif Tissue Int* (1989) **44:** 228–32.

47. Blake GM, Parker JC, Buxton FMA et al. Dual X-ray absorptiometry: a comparison between fan beam and pencil beam scans. *Br J Radiol* (1993) **66:** 902–6.

48. Bouyoucef SE, Cullum ID, Ell PJ. Cross-calibration of a fan beam X-ray densitometer with a pencil beam system. *Br J Radiol* (1996) **69:** 522–31.

49. Patel R, Blake GM, Batchelor S et al. Occupational dose to the radiographer in dual X-ray absorptiometry: a comparison of pencil-beam and fan-beam systems. *Br J Radiol* (1996) **69:** 539–43.

50. Blake GM, Patel R, Lewis MK et al. New generation dual X-ray absorptiometry scanners increase dose to patients and staff. *J Bone Miner Res* (1996) **11**(suppl 1): S157.

4

Commercial Instruments for Spine, Femur and Total Body DXA

CHAPTER OVERVIEW

This chapter aims to familiarize the reader with the principal commercial dual-energy X-ray absorptiometry (DXA) instruments for bone densitometry investigations of the spine, femur and total body. Devices for X-ray absorptiometry studies of the peripheral skeleton (pDXA, pQCT, radiographic absorptiometry) are described in Chapter 5. As the year 2000 approaches, an important issue is the likely effect of the 'millennium bug' on the operation of bone densitometry systems. A discussion of this problem is given in the final section of this chapter. This chapter is based on information provided by the manufacturers and was current in early 1998.

INTRODUCTION

A list of the commercial instruments discussed in this chapter, with details of the manufacturers, including addresses, is given in Table 4.1. One of the most important distinctions between devices is in the scanning geometry. Instruments are conveniently classified into those that use pencil-beam (i.e. raster scan) geometry and those that use a fan-beam design.

The latter have the advantage of shorter scan times (5–30 seconds) and higher resolution images, and advanced systems such as the Lunar Expert-XL and Hologic QDR-4500A offer new research applications such as vertebral morphometry. However, pencil-beam systems are less expensive, radiation dose to patients and scatter dose to the technologist are lower[1,2] and, in response to the competition from fan-beam models, scan times as short as 1–2 minutes are now possible.

One of the most important aspects of fan-beam DXA systems is that they can be cross calibrated to reproduce with high precision the bone mineral density (BMD) measurements that would be obtained with a pencil-beam instrument.[3] However, because the apparent projected area depends on the height of the object above the scanning table, and because BMC is calculated from the equation:

$$BMC = BMD \times Area \qquad (4.1)$$

fan-beam instruments should not be relied upon to provide accurate measurements of BMC and projected area in the spine and femur.[4] In principle, a similar geometrical problem affects the measurement of BMC, lean tissue and adipose tissue mass in fan-beam total body studies.[5] However, improved

Table 4.1 DXA systems described in Chapter 4.

Manufacturer	Pencil-beam systems	Fan-beam systems
Diagnostic Medical Systems Parc de la Mediterannee, District de Montpellier, 34470 Perols, France	Challenger	
Hologic Inc. 590 Lincoln Street, Waltham, MA 02154, USA	QDR-4000	QDR-4500C QDR-4500W QDR-4500SL QDR-4500A
Lunar Corporation 313 West Beltline Highway, Madison, WI 53713, USA	DPX-MD (compact) DPX-MD (full-size) DPX-IQ (compact) DPX-IQ (full-size)	Expert-XL
Norland Medical Systems W6340 Hackbarth Road, Fort Atkinson, WI 53538, USA	XR-36 Eclipse	

algorithms based on the known scan geometry and use of the high-energy X-ray transmission factor to measure body thickness, now permit accurate whole body mass measurements even with fan-beam instruments.[6] The principal attraction of fan-beam systems for total body applications is the shorter scan times (3 minutes instead of 15 minutes) coupled with the higher resolution images.

Many clinicians and technologists find fan-beam DXA systems attractive because of the short scan times and the ability to investigate more patients in a working day (or equivalently, to complete a given case load in less time). However, pencil-beam systems remain of interest for those with lighter patient loads or for whom cost is a primary consideration.

When evaluating the relative merits of fan-beam instruments, it is notable that there is little evidence that the technical advance that they undoubtedly represent has resulted in any appreciable improvement in one of the benchmark indices of system performance, the precision of BMD measurements. However, fan-beam systems deliver comparable precision with shorter scan times. Also, other improvements mean that results are less operator dependent than with older pencil-beam designs. The newer fan-beam systems have been designed with the clinical user in mind and offer improvements in patient positioning, scan localization and software features that make it easier for the operator to maintain optimum precision.

It is often forgotten that one of the significant advances in bone densitometry that occurred when DXA technology replaced dual photon absorptiometry (DPA) was the improved software applications made possible by the rapid evolution of personal computers. The specification of the PC continues to improve making scan analysis faster and providing greater on-line storage of patient data. PCs now also offer new options such as networking, Windows-based applications, on-line manuals and teaching information on CD-ROM, and remote service diagnostics. Purchasers of a DXA scanner for the first time will certainly wish to scrutinize the software for their individual preferences just as closely as the function and performance of the bone densitometer. Purchasers of replacement equipment or those adding a second densitometer will probably be more concerned about issues such as cross calibration to ensure continuity of the BMD scale, and backward compatibility to ensure that old studies can be recovered and reanalysed if necessary.

The following review of commercial systems deals first with the pencil-beam systems before describing fan-beam instruments.

COMMERCIAL PENCIL-BEAM DXA SYSTEMS

The Hologic QDR-4000

Hologic produced the first commercially available DXA instrument, the QDR-1000, in 1987.[7,8] In the first systems, PA lumbar spine and proximal femur scans with scan times of 6–8 minutes were the only applications offered. Later developments included distal forearm, decubitus lateral scans of the lumbar spine, paediatric, orthopaedic and small-animal software. Scan times were halved by adding an option to change the sampling frequency in the axial direction from 10 lines/cm to 5 lines/cm with little detriment to precision.

Another significant development was the QDR-1000W system in which the table-top was modified for performing whole body scans for total body BMD and body composition studies.

The integrating detector used on QDR series densitometers results in a wide dynamic range and this is beneficial for total body and forearm applications where a significant fraction of the scan area is through air and, in the case of total body scans, there is a wide range of tissue thicknesses.

In the latest evolution, Hologic now offers the QDR-4000 pencil-beam system (Figure 4.1). The QDR-4000 features improvements in styling, an upgraded computer system (Pentium 300 MMX or better), improved data archiving facilities (now a 1 GB JAZ drive), CD-ROM capability and software using Windows 95.

The QDR-4000 has an X-ray tube with a tungsten stationary anode target and a high-voltage generator that switches between 70 and 140 kVp for alternate half-cycles of the mains supply. The effective photon energies are approximately 43 keV and 110 keV respectively, although these figures will vary by a few keV depending on tissue thickness in the scan field. X-ray output is highly stable and for tissue thickness greater than a few centimetres noise characteristics approach the limits set by Poisson noise (Chhaya SC, Blake GM, unpublished data). The single radiation detector is a cadmium tungstate scintillator coupled to a photomultiplier tube. The system is calibrated by a rotating reference wheel that generates the high- and low-energy attenuation coefficients for each scan line and corrects for beam hardening due to variation in tissue thickness. One advantage of the internal calibration system is that the scanner calibration is very robust in the event of replacement of the X-ray tube or HV generator circuit board, either of which may cause small changes in the effective photon energy.

Quality control measurements are performed by scanning the Hologic anthropomorphic spine phantom which is made of hydroxyapatite and moulded from a cadaver lumbar spine. The simulated L1–L4 vertebrae are encased in a block of tissue-simulating epoxy resin. The spine phantom is scanned daily and the results added to a database so that sudden shifts or long-term trends in calibration can be

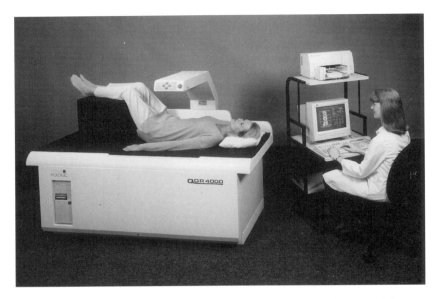

Figure 4.1 The Hologic QDR-4000 pencil-beam DXA scanner performs spine, femur and forearm scans. (Reproduced with permission from Hologic Inc., Waltham, MA, USA.)

detected. The software will not allow patient scanning until the daily system check has been performed. Daily scanning of the phantom does not modify system calibration but provides an independent check on continuity. In the event of a serious system failure, the spine phantom can be used to reset the calibration with a high degree of accuracy.

The QDR-4000 is intended as a basic clinical system with software and internal calibration that makes it compatible with both the earlier Hologic pencil-beam models and the company's more advanced fan-beam systems. Further details of scan modes and system performance are given in Table 4.2.

The Lunar DPX series

The Lunar DPX scanner[9] was first produced in 1988 to an initial design based on theoretical studies by Sorenson[10] to optimize dose efficiency. Over a 10-year period the basic configu-

ration has been developed to produce a family of instruments with a wide variety of capabilities and to date over 5000 units have been sold world-wide. At the time of writing the basic model is the DPX-MD (Figure 4.2), which is available in either a compact (scanning table length 1.8 m) or full-size version (scanning table length 2.4 m). The compact model is offered as a basic clinical system for bone densitometry of the PA spine and femur with scan times of 4–5 minutes. Optional software is available for forearm, decubitus lateral spine, prosthetic implant, paediatric and small-animal applications. The full-size version is intended for users wishing to perform total body scans in addition to the spine, femur and other specialist applications mentioned above. Whole body scans for total body BMD and body composition take 10 minutes. Acquisition times for spine and femur scans are the same as for the compact model.

The DPX-MD was introduced to give an easy upgrade path to the top-of-the-range DPX model, the DPX-IQ (Figure 4.3). The latter offers

Table 4.2 The Hologic QDR-4000.

X-ray generator	70 and 140 kVp (switched kV)
Applications (and scan times)	PA spine (2.5, 5 min) Femur (3.5, 7 min) Forearm (5 min)
Calibration	Internal calibration wheel
Quality control	Daily scan of Hologic spine phantom
Entrance surface dose	30 µGy (fast mode)
Effective dose	0.3 µSv (fast mode PA spine)
Computer	Pentium 300 or higher Windows 95

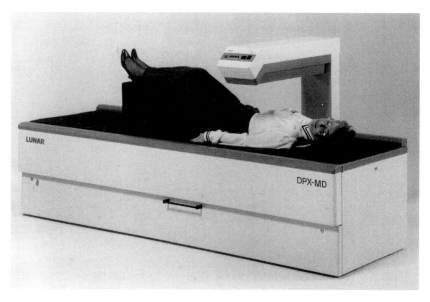

Figure 4.2 The DPX-MD pencil-beam scanner is the basic DXA system offered by Lunar. (Reproduced with permission from Lunar Corp., Madison, WI, USA.)

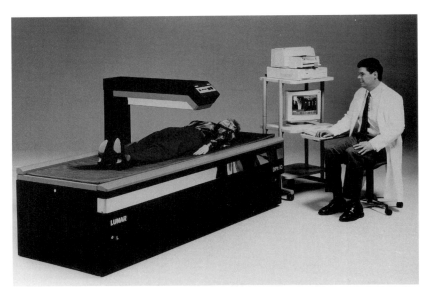

Figure 4.3 The DPX-IQ pencil-beam scanner is the top-of-the-range DPX model. (Reproduced with permission from Lunar Corp., Madison, WI, USA.)

improvements in scan speed, image resolution, image display and the computer system. Like the DPX-MD, the DPX-IQ is available in either compact or full-size versions, with the latter offering the additional option of total body scanning. Scan times are shortened to 1 minute for a spine scan and 2 minutes for a femur scan. These scan speeds are made possible by a combination of higher tube current (3 mA instead of 0.75 mA) and a system of dynamic turning that shortens the step reversals of the scanning arm during execution of the raster scan. Image quality is enhanced by improvements in image resolution and display. A PC with a Pentium 300 MHz processor (or higher) allows the use of Windows 95-based software, a CD-ROM manual, networking to an analysis workstation, and a DICOM print option that allows printing to radiology laser film systems.

The option of networking to a second PC (IQ:NET) is offered as standard on the DPX-IQ,

but an upgradable extra on the DPX-MD. It has the advantage that scan analysis and printing as well as entry of biographical information for the next patient can be performed at the workstation PC while the acquisition PC performs the current scan. Time can be saved by undertaking these tasks in parallel.

All DPX models are based on a constant potential X-ray generator with a cerium (Z = 58) K-edge filter and a single sodium iodide scintillation detector. The stationary anode X-ray tube is operated at 76 kV and with the K-edge filter generates effective photon energies of 38 and 70 keV. The X-ray generator is highly stable with fluctuations restricted to less than ±0.05%. Pulse counting is used at the detector and pulse height analysis is used to discriminate between high- and low-energy photons. The DPX-MD uses a current setting of 0.75 mA for the 4-minute scan time spine and femur modes. The higher 3 mA current setting

Table 4.3 The Lunar DPX-MD and DPX-IQ.

X-ray generator	76 kV constant potential (cerium K-edge filter)
Applications (and scan times)	PA spine (1, 4 min) Femur (2, 4 min) Whole body (4, 10 min) Forearm (2 min)
Calibration	Daily scan of Lunar block phantom
Quality control	Lunar aluminium phantom
Entrance surface dose	10 µGy (0.75-mA scan)
Effective dose	0.1 µSv (0.75-mA PA spine)
Computer	Pentium 300 or higher Windows 95 or Windows NT

used in the DPX-IQ fast scan modes offers better precision and shorter scan times. A 2-minute interval between scans to avoid overheating has been removed with the most recent software upgrade. All DPX scanners use a system of intelligent scan positioning (SmartScan) in which acquisition starts with a full-width scan window and then automatically centres on the spine or femur. Scan time is shortened by restricting the amount of soft tissue included to just the area required for the soft tissue baseline. However, perhaps the most striking aspect of the DPX is the achievement of good precision with an exceedingly low radiation dose to the patient and corresponding minimal scatter dose hazard to the technologist.[1,2]

Daily quality control scans on DPX scanners are performed using the Lunar block phantom. However, because these scans serve to calibrate the system, additional regular quality control scans of another phantom such as the Lunar four-step aluminium spine phantom are strongly recommended (see Chapter 9) to provide an independent check on the continuity of calibration. In certain situations the detection of instrumental drift, as well as recalibration following a serious system failure, may depend on diligent performance of scans of the aluminium spine phantom, ideally at least once a week.

Further details of DPX instruments are given in Table 4.3.

The Norland XR-36 and Eclipse

Norland Medical Systems was the first company to produce a commercial bone mineral device, an SPA densitometer, and today specializes in instruments for peripheral densitometry and research. However, the company still manufactures two full-size DXA systems for spine, femur and total body studies, the XR-36 and the Eclipse.

The Norland XR-36 (Figure 4.4) is capable of

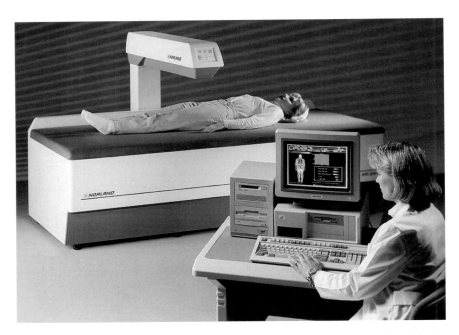

Figure 4.4 The Norland XR-36 pencil-beam DXA scanner will perform spine, femur and total body scans. (Reproduced with permission from Norland Medical Systems, Fort Atkinson, WI, USA.)

performing total body scans as well as PA spine, femur, forearm and decubitus lateral spine studies. A stationary anode X-ray tube is operated at a constant potential of 100 kV and a stabilized 1.3-mA anode current. K-edge filtration is employed using a variable thickness samarium filter ($Z = 62$, K-edge $= 46.8$ keV). The scanner is unique in that, prior to performing the BMD scan, the system measures the patient's thickness with a short pulse of radiation and then automatically chooses the most appropriate K-edge filter thickness from a range of selectable filters based on the patient's size. This feature allows scanning of a wide range of patient thicknesses, optimizing accuracy and precision over the broadest range of patient sizes while minimizing radiation dose. A dual sodium iodide scintillation detector system is used to detect high- and low-energy photons, which are separated by physical filtration

(see Chapter 3, Figure 3.18). The first sodium iodide crystal is very thin and detects the low-energy photons, filtering them from the beam. The second, thicker crystal detects the remaining high-energy photons. The system of dynamic filtration automatically adjusts the X-ray beam intensity pixel by pixel to match varying body thicknesses by switching the samarium filters in and out of the beam and ensuring that each scan pixel receives the proper exposure regardless of tissue thickness.

The Norland Eclipse (Figure 4.5) is a compact version of the XR-36 system, in which the scanning table is shortened from 2.4 m to 1.8 m. It employs the same system of dynamic filtration for automatic exposure control as the XR-36 and the same scanning applications are offered with the exception of total body scans. In both the XR-36 and Eclipse, a QuickScan mode optimizes the raster scan enabling spine, femur and

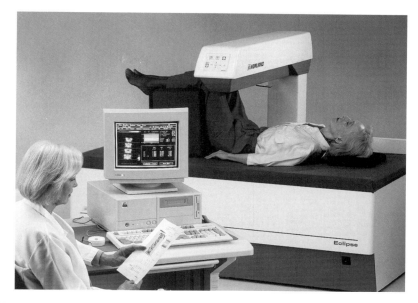

Figure 4.5 The Norland Eclipse pencil-beam DXA scanner is a smaller version of the XR-36 and will perform spine, femur and forearm scans. (Reproduced with permission from Norland Medical Systems, Fort Atkinson, WI, USA.)

forearm studies to be acquired with scan times of 2–3 minutes.

Both Norland systems include a 77-step double step-wedge calibration phantom made from aluminium and acrylic which is designed to cover the full range of bone density and soft tissue thickness found in adults and children. Calibration scans are used to derive a fourth-order polynomial function that enables measurements of logarithmic transmission in the high- and low-energy beams to be converted into BMD results. This system eliminates the pulse pile-up, energy cross over and beam-hardening corrections otherwise necessary for X-ray absorptiometry measurements. A scan of the calibration phantom is performed automatically as part of the daily quality assurance. Following this an automatic scan is performed of the Norland spine phantom made from hydroxyapatite and tissue-equivalent epoxy resin. The entire quality assurance procedure takes 15 minutes.

Further details of the XR-36 and Eclipse instruments are given in Table 4.4.

The DMS Challenger

In late 1997, Diagnostic Medical Systems, manufacturer of the UBIS-5000 imaging ultrasound scanner, announced a new range of DXA systems. The DMS Challenger (Figure 4.6) is a pencil-beam DXA system for scanning the spine, proximal femur and distal forearm. A stationary anode X-ray tube is operated at a constant potential of 86 kV and a stabilized 0.8-mA anode current. K-edge filtration is employed using a samarium filter delivering a dual-energy beam with effective photon energies of 35 and 75 keV. The scanner has an auto-

Table 4.4 The Norland XR-36 and Eclipse.

X-ray generator	100 kV constant potential (samarium K-edge filter)
Applications (and scan times)	PA spine (2 min) Femur (3 min) Whole body (5 min) Forearm (3 min)
Calibration	Norland 77-step aluminium and acrylic step-wedge phantom
Quality control	Norland spine phantom
Entrance surface dose	20 μGy (2 min QuickScan)
Effective dose	0.2 μSv (QuickScan PA spine)
Computer	Pentium 300 or higher

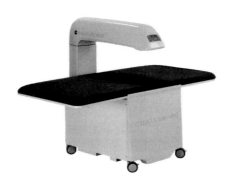

Figure 4.6 The DMS Challenger is a compact, transportable DXA system for scanning the spine, femur and forearm. (Reproduced with permission from Diagnostic Medical Systems, Perols, France.)

matic calibration that is performed before each examination. In addition, weekly quality control scans are performed using calibrated phantoms of the spine and forearm. Measurement sites in the femur are the femoral neck, the greater trochanter and Ward's triangle. Measurement sites in the forearm are the ultra-distal, distal and mid-radius. Vertebral examination is performed between L2 and L4. The bone mineral content (BMC), bone mineral density (BMD), bone homogenicity index (BHI) and projected area are given as examination results. Reference curves are provided for each of the above anatomical locations in order to generate T-score and Z-score values as diagnostic values. Compared with other DXA systems, Challenger is compact (the 1.9-m-long scanning table folds away to 0.8 m for storage) and is mounted on castor wheels for easy transport.

Table 4.5 The DMS Challenger.	
X-ray generator	86 kV constant potential (samarium K-edge filter)
Applications (and scan times)	PA spine (3, 6 min) Femur (3, 6 min) Forearm (2, 4 min)
Calibration	Internal calibration
Quality control	Spine, hip and forearm phantoms
Entrance surface dose	<7 µGy
Effective dose	
Computer	Pentium 300 or higher

Further details of the Challenger system are given in Table 4.5.

COMMERCIAL FAN-BEAM DXA SYSTEMS

Hologic fan-beam systems

Hologic was the first company to introduce a commercial fan-beam system with the QDR-2000 in 1991. The device had a linear array of 32 cadmium tungstate scintillation detectors and could be operated in either pencil-beam or fan-beam modes to perform PA spine, femur, forearm and total body scans. In addition, the scanning arm could be rotated through 90° so that a PA projection scan of the spine could be followed by a lateral projection fan-beam scan with the patient remaining in the supine position. In pencil-beam mode the scans emulated the QDR-1000. In fan-beam mode scan times for the spine and femur were 1–2 minutes depending on the scan speed chosen. The use of cross-calibration factors ensured that BMD results agreed closely with those of

pencil-beam scans.[3] However, comparison of fan-beam and pencil-beam measurements of BMC and the projected area showed a somewhat greater scatter[4] because of the effects of X-ray beam geometry, as discussed earlier.

The QDR-2000 was the first DXA system to offer the vertebral morphometry application described in Chapter 20. Subsequently, a modified system was produced, the QDR-2000*plus*, which enhanced image quality for lateral imaging of the spine by reducing focal spot size, incorporating an anti-scatter plate and providing both single-energy and dual-energy images to optimize placement of the vertebral height markers.

In 1995 the QDR-2000 and QDR-2000*plus* were replaced by a new range of fan-beam systems, the QDR-4500 series.

The Hologic QDR-4500 Acclaim series

The QDR-4500 Acclaim product line (Figure 4.7) is a modular family of DXA bone densitometers with a wide range of capabilities to meet

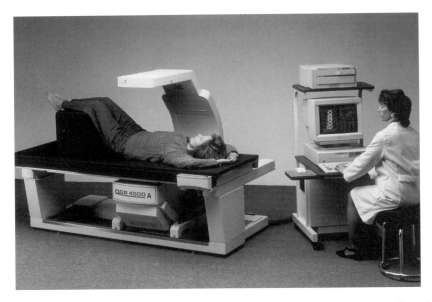

Figure 4.7 The Hologic QDR-4500 Acclaim fan-beam DXA scanner. The different models will perform either just spine and femur scans or additional applications such as total body, supine-lateral and vertebral morphometry. (Reproduced with permission from Hologic Inc., Waltham, MA, USA.)

the requirements of the clinical user. All QDR-4500 models operate only in fan-beam mode, since this scan mode is now well proven for accurate and precise measurements of BMD. The fan-beam geometry was designed to emulate the QDR-2000. The X-ray generator switches between 100 and 140 kVp and utilizes a rotating calibration drum instead of the internal reference wheel used in the QDR-1000 and QDR-2000. The advantage of the latter change is that the system is very quiet in operation and very compact compared with the QDR-2000. The scintillation detectors in earlier Hologic models have been replaced by a high-density linear array of 216 solid state detectors.

The basic model in the series is the QDR-4500C, which is intended for users who require a basic clinical system for scans of the spine, femur and forearm. Scan times are 30 seconds for the fast-array mode, which is suit-able for most routine clinical applications. Slower scan modes (1 minute, 2 minutes) are also available and can be selected for unusual patients or special applications. Bouyoucef et al.[11] demonstrated the equivalence in calibration of the three QDR-4500 scan modes with each other and with pencil-beam scans on a QDR-1000W system. All QDR-4500 systems have a scout scan (turbo) mode intended to aid patient repositioning from the PC console. This latter mode is used during most procedures and helps to ensure optimal positioning of the patient. There is also a high-speed (7-second) single-energy mode for acquiring decubitus lateral scans of the thoracic and lumbar spine for the evaluation of vertebral deformity. All QDR-4500 systems have been designed to aid use in the clinical setting with features such as an adjustable scanning table for loading and unloading the patient.

Table 4.6 The Hologic QDR-4500 Acclaim.

X-ray generator	100 and 140 kVp (switched kV)
Applications (and scan times)	PA spine (10, 30, 60 sec)
	Femur (10, 30, 60 sec)
	Whole body (3 min)
	Lateral spine (120 sec)
	Forearm (30 sec)
	Morphometry (10 sec, 10 min)
Calibration	Internal calibration drum
Quality control	Daily scan of Hologic spine phantom
Entrance surface dose	150 µGy (fast mode)
Effective dose	3 µSv (fast mode PA spine)
	3 µSv (total body)
Computer	Pentium 300 or higher
	Windows 95

Patel et al.[12] evaluated the turbo mode (10-second scan time) for BMD studies and found that although image quality is poorer than for other modes, turbo scans are acceptable for many bone densitometry applications provided small adjustments are made to the relevant cross-calibration factors to ensure complete consistency with the 30-second scan mode.

Other units in the product line include the QDR-4500W, which adds the facility to perform whole body scans, the QDR-4500SL, which incorporates a rotating C-arm so that supine lateral BMD scans of the lumbar spine can be performed and the QDR-4500A, which adds the supine lateral vertebral morphometry application. Other special applications include software for paediatric, orthopaedic and small-animal studies.

System quality control of QDR-4500 systems is based on daily scans of the Hologic spine phantom as described earlier. Further technical details are given in Table 4.6.

The Lunar Expert-XL

The Expert-XL (Figure 4.8)[13] is the first fan-beam densitometer manufactured by Lunar Corporation. Unlike previous DXA systems, spine and hip BMD scans are performed with the X-ray tube above and the detector array underneath the patient, an arrangement that minimizes the geometrical distortion caused by the fan-beam geometry. A rotating anode tube is used, which operates at a constant potential of 134 kV. The detectors are a high-density solid-state linear array of scintillators and photodiodes with 288 elements at each of two photon energies. The basic principle is K-edge filtration with a tantalum filter ($Z = 73$), although compared with conventional DXA more emphasis is placed on generating the dual-energy signal at the detectors. A rotating C-arm allows lateral images for vertebral morphometry, and a motorized table-top that changes the height of the object gives flexibility

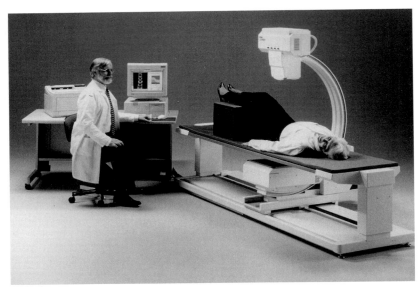

Figure 4.8 The Lunar Expert-XL fan-beam DXA scanner will perform spine, femur, total body and vertebral morphometry studies. (Reproduced with permission from Lunar Corp., Madison, WI, USA.)

in varying the magnification factor and image resolution.

Perhaps the most significant feature of the Lunar Expert is the high resolution image which is significantly improved compared with first generation DXA systems. This is essential for vertebral morphometry and other research applications, and assists in the detection of osteophytes, sclerosis and vertebral compression fractures that cause inaccuracies in routine bone mineral measurements in the lumbar spine. However, it should be noted that higher image resolution is always obtained at the price of using more radiation. Comparison with the Lunar DPX suggests that patient dose from the Expert is significantly above the minimum required for high precision densitometry of the spine and femur.[2] As a consequence of this, and dependent on workload, precautions for the radiation protection of the technologist may be necessary. A helpful booklet produced by Lunar gives detailed information on this aspect of installing and operating the Expert-XL.[14] The relatively high radiation output from the Expert is, however, advantageous for vertebral morphometry studies in that it allows high quality lateral images of the spine to be obtained at a fraction of the dose of conventional radiography.

Daily quality control on the Expert-XL consists of a scan of the Lunar block phantom and checks on the C-arm and motorized scanning table. The system has an internal hydroxyapatite calibration and regular quality control scans of the Lunar aluminium spine phantom are recommended. Further technical details are given in Table 4.7.

THE MILLENNIUM BUG

With the approach of the year 2000, all centres operating bone densitometry equipment should

Table 4.7 The Lunar Expert-XL.	
X-ray generator	134 kV constant potential (tantalum K-edge filter)
Applications (and scan times)	PA spine (6, 12 sec) Femur (6, 12 sec) Whole body (4 min) Forearm (10 sec) Morphometry (40 sec)
Calibration	Internal hydroxyapatite calibration
Quality control	Daily scan of Lunar block phantom Lunar aluminium phantom
Entrance surface dose	530 µGy (12 sec scan)
Effective dose	20 µSv (12 sec spine scan)
Computer	Pentium 300 or higher Windows 95

be aware of the potential failure of systems that may occur after 1 January 2000. All commercial DXA instruments use date information to calculate patients' ages for plotting BMD with respect to the reference population. The same information is needed for calculations of the rate of change of BMD with time in patients having follow-up studies.

There are two potential problems that may affect the proper operation of systems. First, manufacturers' software algorithms might not calculate ages correctly when the patient's date of birth and scan date span the millennium. Secondly, IBM clones will fail to function after 1 January 2000 if the year date stored in the system is a shortened two-digit number (i.e. '98 for 1998) rather than the full four-digit number.

The principal manufacturers (Lunar, Hologic and Norland) were approached for statements on how the millennium bug would affect instruments. All gave assurances that either current versions of system software or new versions about to be released are year-2000 compliant. All users of equipment should therefore approach their service centres to ensure that they have the latest millennium-proof version of software loaded on their systems.

Less is known about the function of PCs. Newer systems (486 microprocessors and above) supplied by reputable manufacturers should operate correctly. However, given the complexity of the problem it is difficult to give absolute assurances. Manufacturers stated that their policies were to work only with suppliers of PCs who guaranteed their equipment to be year-2000 proof. However, it seems likely that some older IBM clones will fail and need replacing. For specific advice, users should approach their service centres. Given the relatively modest cost of PCs, it would be better to plan to replace older computer equipment now rather than risk a disabling failure.

REFERENCES

1. Patel R, Blake GM, Batchelor S et al. Occupational dose to the radiographer in dual X-ray absorptiometry: a comparison of pencil-beam and fan-beam systems. *Br J Radiol* (1996) **69:** 539–43.
2. Blake GM, Patel R, Lewis MK et al. New generation dual X-ray absorptiometry scanners increase radiation dose to patients and staff. *J Bone Miner Res* (1996) **11**(suppl 1): S157.
3. Faulkner KG, Glüer C-C, Estillo M et al. Cross-calibration of DXA equipment: upgrading from a QDR-1000/W to a QDR-2000. *Calcif Tissue Int* (1993) **52:** 79–84.
4. Blake GM, Parker JC, Buxton FMA et al. Dual X-ray absorptiometry: a comparison between fan-beam and pencil-beam scans. *Br J Radiol* (1993) **66:** 902–6.
5. Fuerst T, Genant HK. Evaluation of body composition and total bone mass with the Hologic QDR-4500. *Osteoporos Int* (1996) **6**(suppl 1): 203.
6. Kelly TL, Shepherd JA, Steiger P, Stein JA. Accurate body composition assessment using fan-beam DXA: technical and practical considerations. *J Bone Miner Res* (1997) **12**(suppl 1): S269.
7. Wahner HW, Dunn WL, Brown ML et al. Comparison of dual-energy X-ray absorptiometry and dual photon absorptiometry for bone mineral measurements of the lumbar spine. *Mayo Clin Proc* (1988) **63:** 1075–84.
8. Cullum ID, Ell PJ, Ryder JP. X-ray dual photon absorptiometry: a new method for the measurement of bone density. *Br J Radiol* (1989) **62:** 587–92.
9. Mazess R, Collick B, Trempe J et al. Performance evaluation of a dual-energy X-ray bone densitometer. *Calcif Tissue Int* (1989) **44:** 228–32.
10. Sorenson JA, Duke PR, Smith SW. Simulation studies of dual-energy X-ray absorptiometry. *Med Phys* (1989) **16:** 75–80.
11. Bouyoucef SE, Cullum ID, Ell PJ. Cross-calibration of a fan-beam X-ray densitometer with a pencil beam system. *Br J Radiol* (1996) **69:** 522–31.
12. Patel R, Seah M, Blake GM et al. Concordance and precision of dual X-ray absorptiometry with a 10 s scan. *Br J Radiol* (1996) **69:** 816–20.
13. Lang T, Takada M, Gee R et al. A preliminary evaluation of the Lunar Expert-XL for bone densitometry and vertebral morphometry. *J Bone Miner Res* (1997) **12:** 136–43.
14. Lunar Expert-XL. Radiation safety information. Madison, WI: Lunar Corporation.

5

Commercial Instruments for X-ray Absorptiometry of the Peripheral Skeleton

CONTENTS • Chapter overview • Introduction • Commercial peripheral DXA systems
• Commercial peripheral QCT systems • Radiographic absorptiometry

CHAPTER OVERVIEW

This chapter describes the commercially available X-ray absorptiometry devices for studies of the peripheral skeleton. The various technologies may be divided conveniently into peripheral dual-energy X-ray absorptiometry (DXA) systems, peripheral quantitative computed tomography (QCT) systems, and methods for performing radiographic absorptiometry. For users requiring compact, low-cost equipment for studying the peripheral skeleton, the alternative to X-ray technology is quantitative ultrasound (QUS). While this chapter describes the X-ray systems, commercial QUS devices are described in Chapter 7. The chapter is based on information provided by the manufacturers and was current in early 1998.

INTRODUCTION

Although the first commercially available bone densitometers used the technology of single photon absorptiometry (SPA) for studies of the peripheral skeleton, interest in recent years has centred mainly on conventional DXA measurements of the spine and femur. However, in most countries there are inadequate resources to meet demand and DXA scans are not available to all patients who might benefit. Furthermore, conventional DXA scanning is perceived as costly, not least because of the need to refer patients to hospital-based facilities. Thus, despite the widespread popularity of bone mineral density (BMD) studies of the spine and femur, there has been a recent revival of interest in small, low-cost, X-ray absorptiometry devices dedicated to scanning the peripheral skeleton. As a result, a wide variety of innovative equipment has become available in the past few years.

Until recently much commercial instrumentation for the assessment of the peripheral skeleton was based on the technique of single X-ray absorptiometry (SXA), the technological successor of SPA. In the past 2 or 3 years, however, manufacturers have generally replaced SXA systems with peripheral DXA (pDXA) devices. Several studies have examined the relationship between pDXA measurements and SXA in the forearm.[1-5] Peripheral DXA is methodologically equivalent to conventional DXA with the use of a second photon energy to correct for varying soft tissue thickness, which eliminates the need for placing the patient's arm in a water bath. As discussed in Chapter 2, BMD measurements at forearm sites are well proven in predicting fracture risk. However, it should be noted that for the prediction of hip fracture risk, measurements in the proximal femur are generally believed to provide the optimal assessment.[6] Also, amongst measurement sites in the peripheral skeleton, there is considerable evidence that the calcaneus may be more predictive than the forearm.[6,7] Longitudinal studies conducted during clinical trials have generally suggested that the forearm is not a particularly sensitive site for monitoring response to treatment.[8,9] However, it should be noted that recently a new region of interest localized within the ultra-distal forearm has been reported to show percentage BMD changes as large as those in the axial skeleton during clinical trials of hormone replacement therapy (HRT) and bisphosphonates.[10]

Peripheral QCT (pQCT) of the radius was one of the first densitometric techniques developed.[11] In recent years the availability of lower-cost commercial instruments has stimulated wider interest in the technique and a number of studies have reported on the accuracy, precision and diagnostic sensitivity of the technology.[12,13] One reason for the interest in pQCT is the ability of the technique to provide assessments that go beyond the basic BMD result. Because of the complete information on the distribution of bone mineral within the tomographic slice images, pQCT makes it possible to calculate biomechanical parameters descriptive of bone strength such as the cross-sectional moment of interia and strength–strain index (SSI)[14–17] which allow a more accurate assessment of bending strength. High-resolution pQCT studies also allow the imaging of trabecular microstructure and the direct visualization of osteoporotic changes.[18] Parameters such as bone volume, trabecular number, trabecular thickness and trabecular separation can be derived and show good agreement with histological sections.[19] The technique may in future allow the routine non-invasive assessment of three-dimensional trabecular microstructure.[20]

In radiographic absorptiometry (RA), BMD in the hand is assessed using a radiograph calibrated with an aluminium wedge. The technique was first described 60 years ago,[21] but its application was limited by factors such as voltage setting, exposure time, film quality and film

processing, which affected the apparent density of bones on a standard X-ray film. However, advances in the ability to capture and digitize high-resolution radiographic images, and computerized techniques for image analysis that can correct for variations in radiographic exposure and tissue thickness, have resulted in greatly enhanced precision relative to older, less sophisticated implementations of RA.[22–25] As currently practised, radiographs are acquired using standardized protocols and mailed to a central reading facility for analysis. In the most recent development the X-ray film has been eliminated by devices designed to acquire a direct digital radiographic image of the hand.[26] The direct digital approach preserves the high-resolution image and precision of the film technique while enabling bone density analysis to be performed on site. Among other developments, the method has also been adapted to give high-resolution DXA images of the hand.[27]

A list of the commercial instruments discussed in this chapter with full details of the manufacturers is given in Table 5.1. Peripheral DXA devices for studying the forearm and calcaneus will be discussed first, followed by pQCT and methods for performing RA.

COMMERCIAL PERIPHERAL DXA SYSTEMS

The Norland pDEXA system

The Norland pDEXA system (Figure 5.1) is a compact table-top device that performs dual-energy absorptiometry scans at distal and proximal (one-third) sites in the radius and ulna. The X-ray tube operates at a constant potential of 60 kV and is used in conjunction with a tin (Z = 50) K-edge filter to provide effective photon energies of 28 and 48 keV. There are dual solid-state detectors of cadmium-telluride (or zinc cadmium-telluride) mounted side by side which monitor the high- and low-energy signals. System calibration is analogous to the Norland XR-36 with a 16-step-wedge phantom of aluminium and acrylic used to calibrate

Table 5.1 Peripheral X-ray absorptiometry systems described in Chapter 5.		
Manufacturer	*System*	*Technology*

CompuMed
  1230 Roscrans Avenue
  Manhattan Beach
  CA 90266, USA
	OsteoGram	RA

Lunar Corporation
  313 West Beltline Highway
  Madison, WI 53713, USA
	PIXI	pDXA

Medilink
  80 Rue de l'Hortus
  34280 Carnon,
  France
	Osteoview	pDXA

Nederburgh BV
  Amersfoortseweg 32
  3751 LK Bunschoten
  The Netherlands
	OsteoScan	pDXA

Norland Medical Systems
  W6340 Hackbarth Road
  Fort Atkinson
  WI 53538, USA
	pDEXA
	Apollo
	XCT-2000
	XCT-3000
		pDXA
		pDXA
		pQCT
		pQCT

Osteometer MediTech A/S
  1, Kogle Alle
  DK-2970 Hoersholm
  Denmark
	DTX-200	pDXA

Scanco Medical AG
  Avenring 6–8
  CH-8303 Bassersdorf
  Switzerland
	Densiscan-1000	pQCT

Schick Technologies Inc.
  31-00 47th Avenue
  Long Island City
  NY 11101, USA
	AccuDEXA	pDXA

pDXA, peripheral dual X-ray absorptiometry; pQCT, peripheral quantitative computed tomography; RA, radiographic absorptiometry.

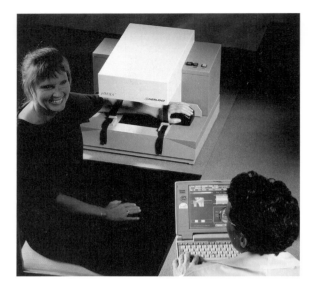

Figure 5.1 The Norland pDEXA forearm DXA scanner. (Reproduced with permission from Norland Medical Systems, Fort Atkinson, WI, USA.)

Table 5.2 The Norland pDEXA.

X-ray generator	60 kV constant potential (tin K-edge filter)
Applications	Distal radius and ulna One-third radius and ulna One-third radius
Calibration	Norland 16-step aluminium and acrylic step-wedge phantom
Quality control	Hydroxyapatite forearm phantom
Dimensions	52 cm (L) × 43 cm (W) × 43 cm (H)
Weight	27 kg

BMD in terms of a polynomial function of the high- and low-energy logarithmic attenuations. System quality control is based on regular scanning of the step-wedge phantom together with daily scans of an anatomically correct forearm phantom made of hydroxyapatite and soft-tissue-equivalent epoxy resin.

For in vivo studies, total scan time is around 5 minutes. A scout scan is first performed, which identifies a reference line located at the proximal edge of the ulna end-plate. Scans are then performed of a 10-mm-wide strip proximal to the reference line (referred to as the distal region on the scan report) corresponding to the area of minimal BMD. This is followed by a second 10-mm strip located in cortical bone at the one-third site. The latter is located from information on forearm length entered during scan set-up. The report sheet (Figure 5.2) provides information on BMD, BMC, T-score and Z-score at the two measurement sites. A large multicentre study in the USA to obtain reference data has recently been described.[28] Further

details of the Norland pDEXA device are given in Table 5.2.

The Osteometer DTX-200

The Osteometer DTX-200 (Figure 5.3). is a compact system mounted on castor wheels that performs dual-energy X-ray absorptiometry scans of the distal radius and ulna. It has replaced an earlier generation SXA device, the DTX-100.[1] While the DTX-200 is similar in outward appearance to the DTX-100, it has dispensed with the need to perform scans with the patient's forearm immersed in a water bath.

The DTX-200 X-ray tube operates at a constant potential of 55 kV and a tube current of 0.3 mA. A tin K-edge filter provides a dual-energy source. The detector is a sandwich of two scintillation crystals and two photodiodes, the first scintillator detecting predominantly the low-energy X-rays, while the remaining signal

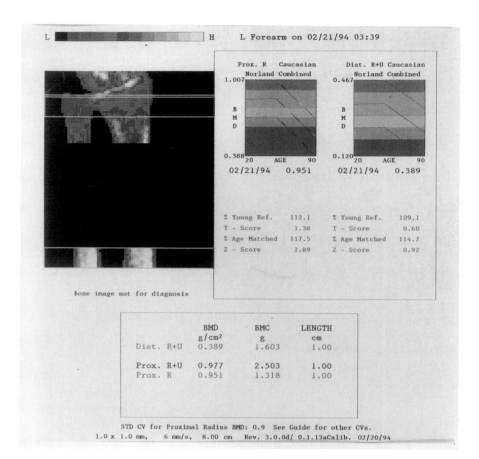

Figure 5.2 Scan report sheet for the Norland pDEXA scanner. (Reproduced with permission from Norland Medical Systems, Fort Atkinson, WI, USA.)

is detected in the second scintillator. There is an in-line calibration system which measures an aluminium calibrator with a BMD equivalence of $0.63 \, \text{g/cm}^2$ once per scan line. This latter measurement is performed at the lower end of each scan line, while at the upper end a lead filter monitors the dark current in the photodiodes. Daily quality control scans are performed using an aluminium and lucite forearm phantom.

Total scan time for an in vivo forearm scan using the standard speed mode is 4.5 minutes. After scan acquisition is completed, the system software automatically identifies a reference line at the point where the separation of the radius and ulna is exactly 8 mm. Bone density is measured in a region of interest (ROI) referred to as the distal ROI and defined as the 24-mm-long section of bone immediately proximal to the 8-mm reference line. This site consists of approximately 87% cortical bone and 13% trabecular bone. In a recent development, a new ROI (nROI) has been added based on the area distal to the reference line but excluding the end-plates and the projection of the cortical shell of the radius and ulna. This latter site comprises 65% trabecular and 35% cortical bone. Clinical trial studies of HRT and bisphos-

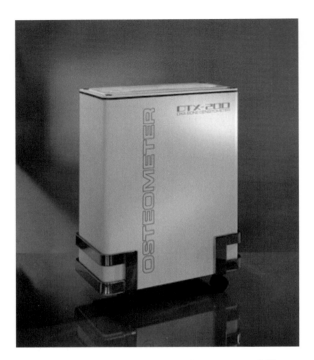

Table 5.3 The Osteometer DTX-200.

X-ray generator	55 kV constant potential (tin K-edge filter)
Applications	Distal radius and ulna Ultradistal radius and ulna (nROI) One-quarter distal radius and ulna
Calibration	Internal calibration
Quality control	Aluminium forearm phantom
Dimensions	59 cm (L) × 29 cm (W) × 78 cm (H)
Weight	33 kg

Figure 5.3 The Osteometer DTX-200 forearm DXA scanner. (Reproduced with permission from Osteometer MediTech, Hoersholm, Denmark.)

phonates show that this region provides a sensitive site for monitoring response to treatment.[10]

The scan report sheet (Figure 5.4) provides information on BMD, BMC (bone mineral content) and the projected area for the distal and nROI sites with T-score and Z-score figures for distal BMC and BMD. Further details of the DTX-200 are given in Table 5.3.

The Nederburgh OsteoScan

The Nederburgh OsteoScan (Figure 5.5) is a compact dual-energy X-ray absorptiometry system that performs measurements at the ultra- and mid-distal (one-third) radius sites. The X-ray tube operates at a constant potential of 60 kV and a tube current of 0.5 mA. A tin

K-edge filter provides a dual-energy source with effective photon energies of 27 and 52 keV. The system is calibrated by orthogonal soft tissue and bone-equivalent wedges that are sampled at 2800 points to provide accurate and linear BMD measurements over the entire range of possible bone and soft tissue combinations.

Total scan time is 3 minutes and results in separate images of the ultra- and mid-distal radius. The system software then automatically identifies the proximal point of the radius endplate and sets the ultra-distal ROI as the 15-mm-wide strip immediately proximal to the reference point (Figure 5.6). The mid-distal ROI is a 10-mm strip measured at the one-third radius site. The scan report sheet provides information on BMD, BMC, T-score and Z-score for the two measurement sites. An optional additional software package further analyses the BMD image at the mid-distal site to measure cortical wall thickness, the wall to lumen ratio, volumetric bone density and the

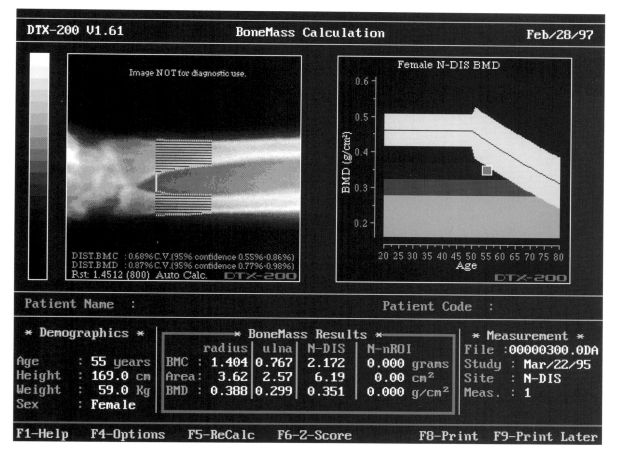

Figure 5.4 Scan report sheet for the Osteometer DTX-200. (Reproduced with permission from Osteometer MediTech, Hoersholm, Denmark.)

breaking-bending resistance index (BBRI), which is a function of the moment of inertia and maximum diameter of the bone. These supplementary morphometric and mechanical parameters are offered on the premise that fractures have a mechanical cause and fracture risk may be better assessed by evaluations that include information on mechanical properties.

Further details of the OsteoScan are given in Table 5.4.

The Medilink Osteoview

The Medilink Osteoview (Figure 5.7) is a new DXA forearm densitometer announced in late 1997 that performs measurements at the distal radius and ulna, the proximal radius and ulna, and the ultra-distal, distal and mid-radius. The X-ray tube operates at a constant potential of 75 kV and in conjunction with a cerium ($Z = 58$) K-edge filter provides effective photon energies of 30 and 70 keV. An automatic internal calibration system and phantom are

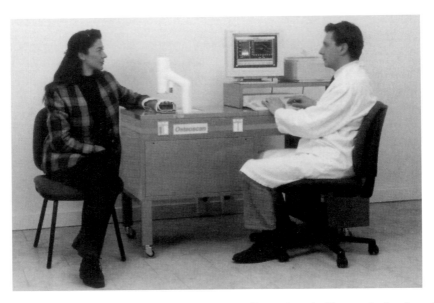

Figure 5.5 The Nederburgh OsteoScan forearm DXA scanner. (Reproduced with permission from Nederburgh BV, Bunschoten, The Netherlands.)

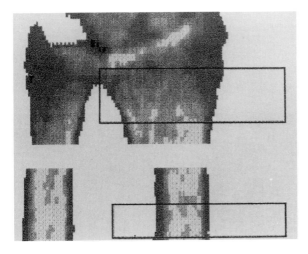

Figure 5.6 Scan image from the Nederburgh OsteoScan. (Reproduced with permission from Nederburgh BV, Bunschoten, The Netherlands.)

Table 5.4 The Nederburgh OsteoScan.	
X-ray generator	60 kV constant potential (tin K-edge filter)
Applications	Ultra-distal radius One-third radius
Calibration	Dual-wedge phantom
Quality control	Aluminium forearm phantom
Dimensions	58 cm (L) × 50 cm (W) × 116 cm (H)
Weight	80 kg

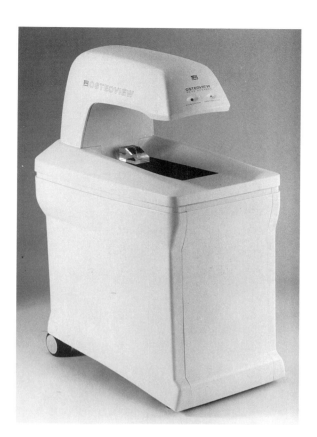

Table 5.5 The Medilink Osteoview.

X-ray generator	75 kV constant potential (cerium K-edge filter)
Applications	Distal radius and ulna Ultra-distal radius and ulna Proximal radius and ulna Ultra-distal and distal radius Proximal radius
Calibration	Automatic calibration system
Quality control	Forearm phantom
Dimensions	80 cm (L) $\times$ 50 cm (W) $\times$ 130 cm (H)
Weight	70 kg

Figure 5.7 The Medilink Osteoview forearm DXA scanner. (Reproduced with permission from Medilink, Carnon, France.)

provided. The scan time for in vivo studies is 2 minutes. The report sheet (Figure 5.8) provides information on projected area, BMC, BMD and bone homogenicity index (BHI) at each measurement site. Reference curves are provided for each ROI, and T-score and Z-score results are given. The system is mounted on castor wheels for easy transport. Further details of the Medilink Osteoview device are given in Table 5.5.

The Lunar PIXI

The Lunar PIXI (Figure 5.9) is a novel, ultra-compact, dual-energy absorptiometry system designed to measure the calcaneus and the distal forearm.[29] Unlike conventional pDXA devices such as the Norland pDEXA and Osteometer DTX-200, which perform pencil-beam rectilinear scans of the forearm, the PIXI system uses cone-beam geometry and a charge-coupled device (CCD) area detector coupled to a 80 mm by 100 mm scintillation screen. Low-energy (55 kV) and high-energy (80 kV) images, each of approximately 1 second duration, are acquired in quick succession. The entire acquisition cycle takes approximately 5 seconds. It is important that the patient does not move during this time. A complete study including acquisition, scan analysis and report printout can be completed in 2 minutes, making this one of the quickest devices presently available.

The PIXI system may be placed on the floor with a heel support to perform studies of the calcaneus. Unlike water-based or contact ultrasound systems, it is not necessary for the

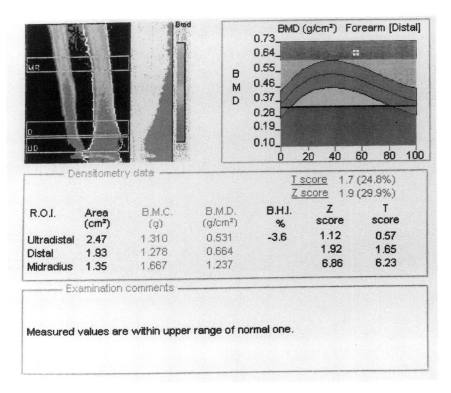

Figure 5.8 Scan report sheet from the Medilink Osteoview. (Reproduced with permission from Medilink, Carnon, France.)

patient to remove hosiery or socks before the scan is performed. As discussed in Chapter 2, prospective epidemiological studies based on SPA have consistently shown the calcaneus to be one of the best sites for predicting fracture risk.[6,7] However, it should be noted that as a measurement site it is also particularly sensitive to the amount and type of exercise taken by the patient. As an alternative, the PIXI device can be placed on a table-top for measuring distal forearm BMD. At both sites the scan analysis programme places regions of interest whose size and location are automatically fitted to individual anatomical landmarks. The scan report sheet provides information on BMD and T-score at the measurement site.

Daily quality control scans are performed using aluminium and lucite phantoms of the calcaneus and distal forearm. During image acquisition, part of the CCD detector is used to acquire an air baseline (for normalizing the attenuation image) together with a soft-tissue- and bone-equivalent block phantom (for internal calibration). The 512×512 detector gives a pixel size of 0.2 mm enabling additional applications where high resolution is an advantage, for example imaging of the hand or small animals. Further details of the PIXI system are given in Table 5.6.

The Norland Apollo

The Norland Apollo (Figure 5.10) is a new DXA system that measures BMD in the calcaneus. The Apollo was developed from the

OsteoAnalyzer system, an instrument that used to be manufactured by Dove Medical Systems until production and distribution was taken over by Norland Medical Systems.

The OsteoAnalyzer was one of the earliest developed commercial SPA systems. It was designed to measure either the forearm or the calcaneus[5] and was used for several of the most influential studies of the relationship between bone mineral measurements and fracture risk.[6,7] Subsequently the ^{125}I radionuclide source was replaced by an X-ray tube and the system was sold as an SXA device for measuring the calcaneus. In its latest evolution as the Norland Apollo, the system is a DXA device optimized for performing rapid BMD measurements of the calcaneus. The X-ray tube operates at 60 kV$_\mathrm{p}$ and is used in conjunction with a tin K-edge filter to provide effective photon energies of 28 and 48 keV. To perform a scan, the patient's heel is placed in a moulded V-shaped support to ensure correct positioning. During the measurement the system performs a series of 15 scan lines across the calcaneus with a total scan time of 15 seconds. The system then automatically selects the optimum site for the BMD measurement. The entire examination takes less than 2 minutes. Calibration and daily quality control studies are undertaken using internal phantoms.

Further details of the Apollo system are given in table 5.7

The Schick AccuDEXA

The Schick AccuDEXA (Figure 5.11) is an innovative and ultra-compact table-top device designed to measure BMD and BMC in the phalanges of the middle finger.[27] The system is manufactured by Schick Technologies Inc., and is available either through Schick or a number of licensed distributors in the USA and elsewhere. The AccuDEXA device can be viewed as either an extension of DXA technology to measure BMD in the hand, or as a development of radiographic absorptiometry that makes digitized X-ray images of the phalanges available for immediate BMD analysis. Hence this section

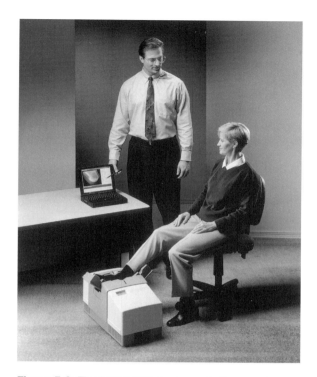

Figure 5.9 The Lunar PIXI dual-energy X-ray system can image the calcaneus and the forearm. (Reproduced with permission from Lunar Corp., Madison, WI, USA.)

Table 5.6 The Lunar PIXI.	
X-ray generator	55 kV and 80 kV
Applications	Calcaneus
	Distal forearm
	Hand
	Small animal
Calibration	Internal calibration
Quality control	Aluminium phantoms
Dimensions	63 cm (L) × 30 cm (W) × 33 cm (H)
Weight	29 kg

Table 5.7 The Norland Apollo.	
X-ray generator	60 kV constant potential (tin K-edge filter)
Applications	Calcaneus
Calibration	Internal calibration
Quality control	Internal phantom
Dimensions	52 cm (L) × 52 cm (W) × 50 cm (H)
Weight	33 kg

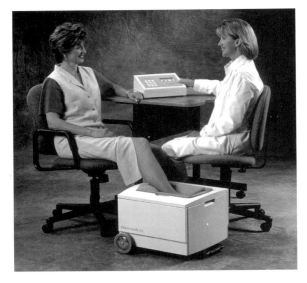

Figure 5.10 The Norland Apollo dual-energy X-ray system images the calcaneus. (Reproduced with permission from Norland Medical Systems, Fort Atkinson, WI, USA.)

should be read in conjunction with the later description of radiographic absorptiometry in this chapter.

During scan acquisition the patient places their non-dominant hand within the unit which houses a finger placement plate with a guide for the patient's middle finger and a spring-loaded lever to hold the finger in place during the examination. The principle used is cone-beam DXA, with an area detector that acquires high-energy (70 kV) and low-energy (50 kV) images within a 5-second period. Reference wedges serve as internal calibration and enable the device to compute phalangeal BMC and BMD. The effective dose to the patient is extremely low (estimated at 0.0003 μSv) and the box-shaped geometry of the device provides effective shielding from scattered radiation.

A separate PC is not required to operate the system. To perform an examination, the operator enters the patient information on a touch-sensitive LCD screen. After instructing the patient on the positioning of his or her hand, the operator can verify the correct placement of the finger through a viewing window. After completion of the acquisition cycle, the image is displayed for the operator to verify before BMD is calculated and displayed. Recently completed studies with AccuDEXA in the USA have provided reference data, and studies of ashed bone have verified the accuracy of the BMC measurements. Studies ongoing at the time of writing include assessments of fracture prediction and the ability to monitor response to treatment. Further details of the system are given in Table 5.8.

COMMERCIAL PERIPHERAL QCT SYSTEMS

The Norland–Stratec XCT-2000 and XCT-3000

The peripheral DXA instruments described thus far generate projectional images that mea-

Table 5.8 The Schick AccuDEXA.	
X-ray generator	50 kV and 70 kV
Applications	Phalanges of middle finger
Calibration	Internal calibration
Quality control	
Dimensions	38 cm (L) × 36 cm (W) × 36 cm (H)
Weight	26 kg

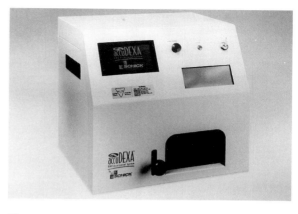

Figure 5.11 The Schick AccuDEXA DXA system measures BMD and BMC in the phalanges of the middle finger. (Reproduced with permission from Schick Technologies Inc., Long Island City, NY, USA.)

sure integral bone. With such systems the cortical and trabecular compartments cannot be measured separately. However, a German company, Stratec Medizintechnik (Pforzheim, Germany), has developed a series of scanners that use the principles of quantitative computed tomography to determine the volumetric BMD of trabecular and cortical bone in the distal radius. The technique is usually known as peripheral QCT (pQCT). Stratec systems are now sold world-wide in a joint marketing operation with Norland Medical Systems. Unlike DXA technology, the three-dimensional information in pQCT images allows the separation of cortical and trabecular elements and the quantification of geometrical parameters related to bending strength[14–17] that supplement the conventional assessments based on bone density.

The basic pQCT system offered for clinical use is the XCT-2000 (Figure 5.12). This is a table-top evolution of the earlier XCT-960 model, of which many clinical studies have been reported in the literature.[12–17] The X-ray tube is operated at 59 kVp with an effective photon energy of around 37 keV. Before scan acquisition the length of the patient's forearm is first measured. A planar scout scan taking 1 minute is then performed and used to identify

the proximal point of the radius endplate. The CT measurment site is then set at 4% of the forearm length measurement (approximately 10 mm) proximal to the reference point. The CT acquisition takes a further 1 minute and uses a translate-rotate principle with a set of 12 semiconductor detectors. The time for a complete examination including scout scan, CT slice generation, scan analysis and printed report is approximately 8 minutes. During scan analysis the cortical and subcortical regions are identified and a measurement of trabecular bone made in the radial spongiosa. This latter region is identified as the inner subregion with a cross-sectional area of 45% of the total cross section. The scan report provides figures for total BMD (cortical, subcortical and trabecular) and trabecular BMD alone. Reference ranges for a Northern European population are provided. After the BMD report the Stress Strain Index (SSI) based on the cross sectional moment of inertia can be printed out to give a measure of the mechanical strength of the bone. In the 4% plane, the measurement of cortical BMD is limited by the partial volume effect. However, cortical bone can be measured at a position

15% of ulna length proximal to the radial end-plate.

A larger free-standing model, the XCT-3000, is also available and is designed for studies of the femur, tibia and jaw-bone. There is also a range of specialized high-resolution systems for animal research that vary in gantry diameter and voxel size. Radiation doses from the animal systems are higher and therefore these devices cannot be used for human investigations. However, studies of biomechanical parameters and trabecular microarchitecture based on animal studies are being extended to humans measured with clinical systems.[30]

Further details of the XCT-2000 system are given in Table 5.9.

The Scanco Medical Densiscan-1000

The Scanco Densiscan-1000 is a high-resolution pQCT system that allows direct visualization of trabecular bone microstructure. The radiation dose is small, and structural parameters such as trabecular separation and number can be measured with precision errors of less than 0.5%.[20] Comparison with histological sections showed agreement within ±10%, except for trabecular thickness, which is more difficult to measure.[19] Further information about the system can be found in the review article by Glüer et al.[18]

RADIOGRAPHIC ABSORPTIOMETRY

The time-honoured technique of radiographic absorptiometry[21] assumes a proportionality between BMD and the optical density of

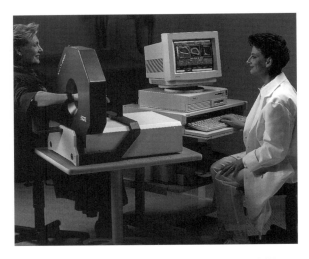

Figure 5.12 The Norland–Stratec XCT-2000 pQCT scanner. (Reproduced with permission from Norland Medical Systems, Fort Atkinson, WI, USA.)

Table 5.9 The Norland–Stratec XCT-2000.	
X-ray generator	59 kV
Applications	Distal forearm, tibia
Calibration	European forearm phantom
Quality control	Hydroxyapatite cone phantom
Dimensions	93 cm (L) × 55 cm (W) × 62 cm (H)
Weight	45 kg

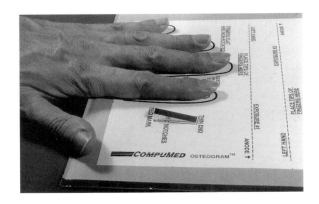

Figure 5.13 In radiographic absorptiometry, an X-ray of the hand is calibrated with a small aluminium wedge.

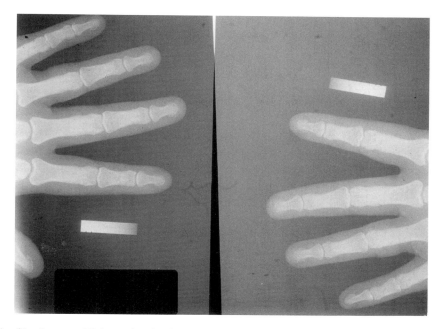

Figure 5.14 The film from an RA investigation is digitized to measure BMD in the phalanges.

conventional radiographs so that a wedge of aluminium or hydroxyapatite can be used to calibrate the film. Typically, this method is applied to the metacarpals or phalanges of the hand where the thickness of overlying tissue is small. Originally the calibration and evaluation of each radiograph were performed manually making the technique labour intensive and highly operator dependent.[25] However, recently the procedure has attracted renewed interest as special protocols and central evaluation laboratories have made the technique widely available as a simple screening method for the primary care physician.[22,25] Improvements in obtaining radiographs under standard conditions and computer-assisted optical density calculations from X-rays allow bone mineral measurements on the fingers with a precision of 2% and an accuracy of 6%, figures that are comparable with other bone mineral measurement techniques.

In the OsteoGram technique (CompuMed) two radiographs of the non-dominant hand are taken consecutively at 50 and 60 kVp (300 mA) with non-screened film. An aluminium reference standard is simultaneously exposed (Figure 5.13). The exposed films are then mailed to a central facility for processing and analysis. During film analysis the radiograph is digitized and calibrated using the image of the aluminium wedge (Figure 5.14). The area and mineral content of the middle phalanges are determined. Results from the three phalanges are averaged, and mineral mass, length, area, volume, area density and volume density of composite bone are calculated, as well as densities of compact and trabecular bone. As a quality control check, the two films are analysed separately, and results have to be within 2%. An example of results from a longitudinal RA study is shown in Figure 5.15. Other variants of updated RA techniques include Osteoradiometer (NIM, Verona, Italy) and Bonalyzer (Teijin, Tokyo, Japan).[25]

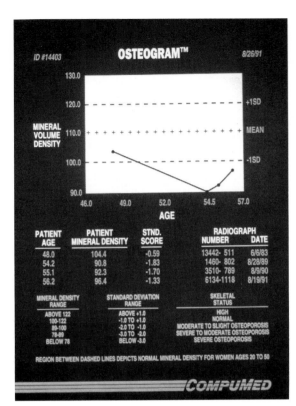

Figure 5.15 Report sheet for a longitudinal study performed using radiographic absorptiometry.

In a recent development from CompuMed, the X-ray film has been eliminated in a device designed to acquire a direct digital radiographic image of the hand, thus enabling the bone density analysis to be performed on site. A prototype device has been described based on a CCD detector which is optically coupled to an X-ray phosphor.[26] Single-energy images are acquired at 60 kVp with an image area of 6 × 6 cm and a pixel resolution of 0.11 mm.

In a parallel development, Schick Technologies have developed the AccuDEXA device described earlier in this chapter, which extends the technique of dual-energy X-ray absorptiometry to measurements in the hand.[27]

REFERENCES

1. Nelson D, Feingold M, Mascha E et al. Comparison of single-photon and dual-energy x-ray absorptiometry of the radius. *Bone Miner* (1992) **18:** 77–83.
2. LeBoff MS, El-Hajj A, Fuleihan G et al. Dual-energy x-ray absorptiometry of the forearm: reproducibility and correlation with single photon absorptiometry. *J Bone Miner Res* (1992) **7:** 841–6.
3. Faulkner KG, McClung MR, Schmeer MS et al. Densitometry of the radius using single and dual-energy absorptiometry. *Calcif Tissue Int* (1994) **54:** 208–11.
4. Fuerst T, Hottya GA, Blunt BA et al. Comparison of single and dual x-ray absorptiometry for measuring forearm BMD: the Osteometer DTX forearm densitometers. *J Bone Miner Res* (1997) **12**(suppl 1): S377.
5. Wasnich R, Ross P, Vogel J. Comparison of pDEXA and SXA BMD of the radius. *J Bone Miner Res* (1997) **12**(suppl 1): S378.
6. Cummings SR, Black DM, Nevitt MC et al. Bone density at various sites for prediction of hip fractures. *Lancet* (1993) **341:** 72–5.
7. Wasnich RD, Ross PD, Heilbrun LK, Vogel JM. Selection of the optimal site for fracture risk prediction. *Clin Orthop* (1987) **216:** 262–9.
8. Liberman UA, Weiss SR, Bröll J et al. Effect of oral alendronate on bone mineral density and the incidence of fractures in postmenopausal osteoporosis. *N Engl J Med* (1995) **333:** 1437–43.
9. Faulkner KG, McClung MR, Ravn P et al. Monitoring skeletal response to therapy in early postmenopausal women: which bone to measure? *J Bone Miner Res* (1996) **11**(suppl 1): S96.
10. Christiansen C, Ravn P, Alexandersen P, Mollgaard A. A new region of interest (nROI) in the forearm for monitoring the effect of therapy. *J Bone Miner Res* (1997) **12**(suppl 1): S480.
11. Rüegsegger P, Elsasser U, Anliker M et al. Quantification of bone mineralization using computed tomography. *Radiology* (1976) **121:** 93–7.
12. Grampp S, Lang P, Jergas M et al. Assessment of skeletal status by peripheral quantitative computed tomography of the forearm: short-term precision in vivo and comparison to dual x-ray absorptiometry. *J Bone Miner Res* (1995) **10:** 1566–76.
13. Takada M, Engelke K, Hagiwara S et al. Accuracy and precision study in vitro for peripheral quantitative computed tomography. *Osteoporos Int* (1996) **6:** 207–11.

14. Louis O, Willnecker J, Soykens S et al. Cortical thickness assessed by peripheral quantitative computed tomography: accuracy evaluated on radius specimens. *Osteoporos Int* (1995) **5:** 446–9.

15. Louis O, Boulpaep F, Willnecker J et al. Cortical mineral content of the radius assessed by peripheral QCT predicts compressive strength on biomechanical testing. *Bone* (1995) **16:** 375–9.

16. Augat P, Reeb H, Claes LE. Prediction of fracture load at different skeletal sites by geometric properties of the cortical shell. *J Bone Miner Res* (1996) **11:** 1356–63.

17. Ferretti JL, Capozza RF, Salica D et al. Noninvasive estimation of bending or torsion strength of the human radius by peripheral quantitative computed tomography (pQCT). *J Bone Miner Res* (1995) **10**(suppl 1): S372.

18. Glüer C-C, Jergas M, Hans D. Peripheral measurement techniques for the assessment of osteoporosis. *Semin Nucl Med* (1997) **27:** 229–47.

19. Müller R, Hahn M, Vogel M et al. Morphometric analysis of noninvasively assessed bone biopsies: comparison of high-resolution computed tomography and histologic sections. *Bone* (1996) **18:** 215–20.

20. Müller R, Hildebrand T, Häuselmann HJ, Rüegsegger P. In vivo reproducibility of three-dimensional structural properties of noninvasive bone biopsies using 3D-pQCT. *J Bone Miner Res* (1996) **11:** 1745–50.

21. Mack PB, O'Brien AT, Smith JM, Bauman AW. A method for estimating degree of mineralization of bones from tracings of roentgenograms. *Science* (1939) **89:** 467.

22. Cosman F, Herrington B, Himmelstein S, Lindsay R. Radiographic absorptiometry: a simple method for determination of bone mass. *Osteoporos Int* (1991) **2:** 34–8.

23. Yang S-O, Hagwara S, Engelke K et al. Radiographic absorptiometry for bone mineral measurement of the phalanges: precision and accuracy study. *Radiology* (1994) **192:** 857–9.

24. Kleerekoper M, Nelson DA, Flynn MJ et al. Comparison of radiographic absorptiometry with dual-energy X-ray absorptiometry and quantitative computed tomography in older white and black women. *J Bone Miner Res* (1994) **9:** 1745–9.

25. Yates AJ, Ross PD, Lydick E, Epstein RS. Radiographic absorptiometry in the diagnosis of osteoporosis. *Am J Med* (1995) **98**(suppl 2A): 415–75.

26. Sechopoulos I, Levis I, Karellas A et al. A new method for high resolution digital radiographic absorptiometry. *J Bone Miner Res* (1997) **12**(suppl 1): S267.

27. Bouxsein ML, Michaeli DA, Plass DB et al. Precision and accuracy of computed digital absorptiometry for assessment of bone density of the hand. *Osteoporos Int* (1997) **7:** 444–9.

28. Miller PD, Paucek JM, Harrold LM. Normative forearm data for ambulatory female adults using a new DXA device. *J Bone Miner Res* (1997) **12**(suppl 1): S258.

29. Borg J, Mazess R, Hanson J. Peripheral instantaneous x-ray imager: the PIXI bone densitometer. *J Bone Miner Res* (1997) **12**(suppl 1): S376.

30. Ferretti JL. Perspectives of pQCT technology associated to biochemical studies in skeletal research employing rat models. *Bone* (1995) **17:** 353S–64S.

6

Technical Principles of Ultrasound

CHAPTER OVERVIEW

This chapter provides an introduction to the technical principles behind quantitative ultrasound measurements in bone. The emphasis is on water-based and contact ultrasound systems that make transmission measurements through the calcaneus, since these are the best established in terms of proven ability to predict fracture risk. However, attention is also given to newer 'semi-reflection' devices designed to measure the speed of sound along a fixed longitudinal section of bone. While the present chapter explains the principles behind the measurement of broadband ultrasonic attenuation and speed of sound, Chapter 7 gives a comprehensive review of the commercial ultrasound systems currently available. The potential of bone ultrasound technology as a clinical tool was first demonstrated in 1984 by Chris Langton. For most of the intervening years ultrasound has been a research tool, either studied in comparison with X-ray absorptiometry, or investigated in its own right for fracture prediction or in in vitro studies of the relationship with bone architecture. However, the recent approval by the Food and Drug Administration (FDA) of the first commercial ultrasound system means that the technology is set to enter a new phase of rapid expansion as it enters routine clinical use.

INTRODUCTION

Interest in the use of ultrasonic measurements in bone as a clinical tool to investigate skeletal status developed following the pioneering report of Langton and colleagues[1] that a measurement of broadband ultrasonic attenuation (BUA) in the calcaneus could discriminate between elderly women who had sustained a recent hip fracture and healthy elderly women with no history of fracture. Over the past decade, many studies have examined the use of bone ultrasound for the investigation of osteoporosis. Comprehensive and up-to-date reviews of the technology and its clinical applications have been published by Njeh et al.[2] and Gregg et al.[3] Genant et al.[4] proposed that the acronym QUS should be used as a generic term to describe quantitative ultrasound measurements of bone, similar to the use of the acronyms SXA, DXA and QCT to describe the various types of X-ray absorptiometry measurements. There is now a widespread consensus that QUS has a proven role in the assessment of fracture risk, especially in elderly women.[5] In the USA, the FDA has approved for the first time the use of a commercial ultrasound device for routine investigations, and this will undoubtedly lead to a rapid expansion in the clinical applications of QUS technology.

The clinical value of bone ultrasound is established best for water-based systems that measure the calcaneus.[5] The calcaneus was chosen as the measurement site because it is easily accessible, has a high percentage of trabecular bone and is weight bearing, with a pattern of loss in osteoporosis similar to the spine.[6] Another advantage of the calcaneus is that, as described in Chapter 2, the ability of measurements at this site to predict fractures is well established from earlier studies using single photon absorptiometry. Following Langton's report describing the measurement of BUA, commercial ultrasound devices have been developed that are also capable of measuring the speed of sound (SOS) in the calcaneus.[7,8] Several manufacturers have since developed new ultrasound systems able to make SOS measurements at other sites in the skeleton.[9–11]

Although many cross-sectional studies have confirmed the original observation that BUA measurements can discriminate patients with osteoporotic fractures retrospectively, prospective fracture studies are the most convincing way of establishing the clinical value of QUS. The first such study was reported in 1990 by Porter et al.[12] using the prototype ultrasound system developed by Langton and colleagues to measure BUA in 1414 institutionalized elderly women in Hull and Doncaster, UK. In combination with cognizance and mobility ratings, BUA was significantly related to the incidence of hip fracture. More recently, Hans and colleagues[13] reported the results of the French EPIDOS study in which 5662 women aged 75 years or over were measured with the Achilles system (Lunar Corp., Madison, WI, USA). During 2 years of follow-up, 115 hip fractures were recorded. The increased risk of fracture for each 1 standard deviation (SD) decrease in the QUS and DXA measurements was 2.0 for BUA, 1.7 for SOS and 1.9 for femoral neck bone mineral density (BMD) (Figure 6.1A). Further analysis of the data showed that the QUS and femoral neck BMD measurements were significant and independent predictors of hip fracture risk.

A similar study to EPIDOS based on subjects enrolled in the USA in the Study of Osteoporotic Fractures (SOF) was published by Bauer et al.[14] Measurements were made on 6189 women aged 65 or over using the UBA575 system (Walker Sonix Inc., Worcester, MA, USA). Fifty-four hip fractures were recorded during a 2-year follow-up period. The conclusions were similar to those of Hans et al.[13] Each 1 SD reduction led to an increased risk of hip fracture of 2.0 for BUA, 2.2 for calcaneal BMD and 2.6 for femoral neck BMD (Figure 6.1B). As well as analysing data in terms of risk ratios, results from fracture studies are also conveniently presented by giving the hip fracture risk in each of the four quartiles of the QUS and BMD variables (Figure 6.1C). In Bauer's study, 50% of hip fractures occurred in subjects in the lowest quartile of BUA and 63% in the lowest quartile of femoral neck BMD. Other prospective and case–control studies of QUS measurements and fracture risk are discussed in Chapter 2.

The attraction of QUS devices is that they do not use ionizing radiation and are cheaper and more portable than conventional bone densitometers that scan the spine and femur. Although at the time of writing DXA is the more widely accepted procedure, there is growing acceptance that a QUS scan is an effective substitute for a BMD measurement in the calcaneus[15] and may be a more suitable technology for assessing fracture risk in large populations than conventional DXA bone densitometry.[5]

BASIC PRINCIPLES OF ULTRASOUND

Sound can be defined as a longitudinal compression wave in which the particles in the medium execute an oscillatory motion parallel to the direction in which the sound wave is travelling. This manifests itself as a sinusoidal variation in *strain* (defined as the fractional change in length, $\Delta l/l$), and a consequent variation in the *pressure*, Δp. In the elastic region of the stress–strain curve (Figure 6.2), the ratio of $(\Delta p/(\Delta l/l))$ is constant and for a solid material

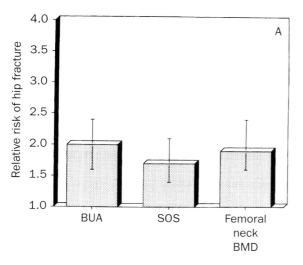

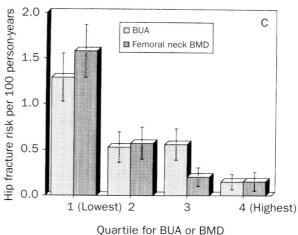

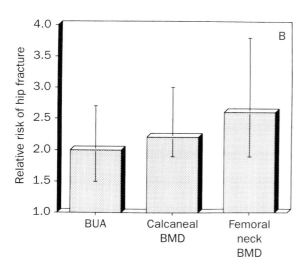

Figure 6.1 Relative risk for hip fracture found in two prospective studies of quantitative ultrasound. Results are expressed as the increased risk of fracture for each standard deviation decrease in the QUS or BMD parameter. Error bars show the 95% confidence intervals. (A) Results from the EPIDOS study for BUA, SOS and femoral neck BMD. BUA and SOS measurements were performed using the Lunar Achilles system. (Data from Hans et al.[13]) (B) Results from the SOF study for BUA, calcaneal BMD and femoral neck BMD. BUA measurements were performed using the Walker Sonix UBA575 system. (Date from Bauer et al.[14]) (C) As an alternative to relative risk, results may be presented as the fracture risk for subjects in each quartile of BUA or BMD. (Data from Bauer et al.[14])

is called Young's elastic modulus, E. For a homogeneous solid medium the speed of sound for longitudinal waves is given by:[16]

$$c_{\text{long}} = \sqrt{\left(\frac{E(1 - \sigma)}{\rho(1 + \sigma)(1 - 2\sigma)} \right)} \quad (6.1)$$

where ρ is the density of the material and σ is the ratio of transverse to longitudinal strain

(Poisson's ratio). Since σ is small (typically 0.1–0.4 for bone[17,18]), equation 6.1 is often approximated to:

$$c_{\text{bar}} = \sqrt{(E/\rho)} \quad (6.2)$$

which is the equation for the SOS of a longitudinal wave in a bar whose cross-section is smaller than the wavelength. Longitudinal sound waves can travel through a gas, liquid or

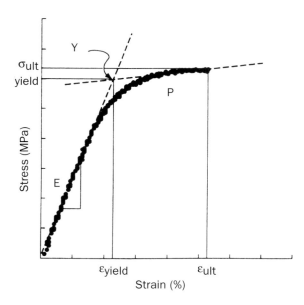

Figure 6.2 A stress–strain curve from a study of the breaking strength of tibial bone. The slope of the stress–strain curve in the elastic region defines Young's elastic modulus, *E*. (Reproduced with permission from SC Lee.[40])

solid medium. However, in solids it is also possible to generate transverse (or shear) waves in which particles in the medium execute an oscillatory motion at right angles to the direction of propagation of the wave. The speed of propagation of shear waves is given by:[16]

$$c_{\text{shear}} = \sqrt{\left(\frac{E}{2\rho(1+\sigma)}\right)} \quad (6.3)$$

and is typically around half the figure for longitudinal waves.

The human ear is sensitive to sound waves with frequencies between 20 Hz and 15 kHz. Frequencies above 20 kHz are generally referred to as *ultrasound*. Ultrasound is widely used in radiology with applications that include medical imaging and Doppler ultrasound measurements of blood flow.[19] For these applications, frequencies in the range 2–10 MHz are often used. However, because of the high

attenuation of ultrasound in cancellous bone, rather lower frequencies in the range 0.1–1 MHz are used for QUS studies.

Ultrasonic transducers

To transmit and receive signals at the high frequencies required, medical ultrasound systems use the *piezoelectric effect*. The term is derived from the classical Greek *piezo* meaning press. This is a property shared by many dielectric materials in which the application of a mechanical stress induces an electric field that can be detected by electrodes placed across the two ends of the transducer. The effect is caused by the relative movement of positive and negative charges in a crystal when it is compressed or stretched. Conversely, when an electric field is applied, a change in physical dimensions occurs. Piezoelectric transducers can therefore convert an electrical signal into a sound wave and vice versa. Suitable materials should ideally have both a large *receiving constant* (the voltage induced by a given applied pressure) and a large *transmitting constant* (the strain induced by a given applied voltage). Transducers for medical applications are often made from ceramic compounds of lead–zirconate–titanate (PZT).

Sound intensity and the measurement of attenuation

As with many physiological stimuli, human observers grade sounds into equal steps of perceived intensity on a logarithmic scale. Similarly, when sound is amplified or attenuated in stages, the different steps combine together multiplicatively. Sound intensity is therefore conveniently measured on a logarithmic scale in units called decibels (dB). In physical terms, the intensity of sound is defined as the rate of flow of energy through unit cross-sectional area (units: watts/m²). A tenfold step in intensity corresponds to a change of 10 dB, a 100-fold step to 20 dB, a 1000-fold step to 30 dB, and so on. If sound signals with two intensities,

I_1 and I_2 are expressed in decibels as dB_1 and dB_2 respectively, their difference is given by:

$$\text{Difference in sound intensity} = dB_1 - dB_2$$

$$= 10 \log_{10}(I_1/I_2) \text{ dB} \qquad (6.4)$$

In practice, sound level is often measured on the basis of the sound pressure amplitude, p. Because intensity is related to the square of the pressure amplitude, equation 6.4 can also be written:

$$dB_1 - dB_2 = 20 \log_{10}(p_1/p_2) \text{ dB} \qquad (6.5)$$

When an ultrasound signal is detected by a piezoelectric transducer, the voltage V induced is proportional to p. Hence, the difference in sound intensity expressed in decibels is related to the voltage amplitude by the equation:

$$dB_1 - dB_2 = 20 \log_{10}(V_1/V_2) \text{ dB} \qquad (6.6)$$

Sound levels experienced in everyday life are also measured on an absolute scale using decibels. A jet aircraft at close quarters registers around 140 dB, a normal conversation 70 dB and a ticking watch 20 dB.

Reflection and transmission of sound waves at boundaries

When a sound wave passes from one material to another reflection and transmission will occur at the boundary (Figure 6.3). In general, the transmitted sound will be refracted at the boundary because of the different values of the speed of sound in the two media. The intensities of the reflected (I_r) and transmitted (I_t) signals are related to the intensity of the incident wave (I_i) by the values of the *acoustic impedance* (Z) in the two media. Acoustic impedance is the product of the density and the speed of sound in a medium, i.e. $Z = \rho c$. If two adjacent materials have equal values of Z, then there is no reflected wave. However, for the general situation where there is an acoustic mismatch across the boundary, the following relationships hold:[20]

$$\frac{I_r}{I_i} = \left(\frac{Z_2\cos\theta_i - Z_1\cos\theta_t}{Z_2\cos\theta_i + Z_1\cos\theta_t} \right)^2 \qquad (6.7)$$

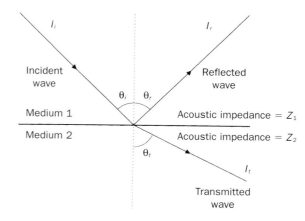

Figure 6.3 Transmission and reflection of a sound wave at the boundary between two materials.

and:

$$\frac{I_t}{I_i} = \frac{4Z_1Z_2\cos\theta_i\cos\theta_t}{(Z_2\cos\theta_i + Z_1\cos\theta_t)^2} \qquad (6.8)$$

where Z_1 and Z_2 are the acoustic impedances in the two media and θ_i and θ_t are the angles of incidence and refraction (Figure 6.3). In calcaneal ultrasound systems the sound transmitted from soft tissue to bone in the heel is approximately normally incident on the boundary so that $\theta_i = \theta_t = 0$. In this circumstance, equations 6.7 and 6.8 simplify to:

$$\frac{I_r}{I_i} = \left(\frac{Z_2 - Z_1}{Z_2 + Z_1} \right)^2 \qquad (6.9)$$

and:

$$\frac{I_t}{I_i} = \frac{4Z_1Z_2}{(Z_2 + Z_1)^2} \qquad (6.10)$$

From equations 6.9 and 6.10 it is evident that at the boundary between air and tissue the large change in density means that sound energy is virtually totally reflected. From this, the importance of achieving good acoustic contact across the gap between the ultrasound transducer and the skin can be appreciated, and in QUS studies this is done using either water in the wet systems or ultrasound gel in contact systems. A full explanation of the reflection and transmission of sound at a boundary is complicated because in general an incident longitudinal wave will generate both longitudinal and transverse reflected and transmitted waves.[16]

The ultrasound beam from a circular transducer

QUS systems generally measure BUA using large aperture piezoelectric transducers with a diameter significantly greater than the wavelength of the sound. For a speed of sound of 1500 m/s and a frequency range 0.2–0.6 MHz (the range often used for BUA measurements), wavelength varies from 7.5 mm down to 2.5 mm. Large diameter transducers (typically 20 mm) reduce the spread of the ultrasound beam caused by diffraction and hence enhance the signal at the receiving transducer.

The size and shape of the beam can be calculated using Huygen's principle in which each point on the surface of the transducer acts as a source of wavelets whose effect is summed to find the beam profile in front of the transducer.[20] Interference between wavelets leads to the characteristic diffraction pattern of the beam. Let the radius of the transducer be a and the wavelength of the sound λ. The space in front of the transducer is divided into two zones (Figure 6.4):

1) The 'near-field' zone lies at distances closer than a^2/λ to the transducer face. Here, phase differences between wavelets from different points of the transducer exceed 2π and they interfere constructively or cancel each other out. The diffraction pattern is a complicated set of concentric rings in which the sound pressure amplitude is alternately at a maximum or at zero and whose pattern varies rapidly with distance from the transducer face.

2) The 'far-field' zone lies at distances beyond a^2/λ. Here, phase differences are smaller and wavelets add constructively to create a conical-shaped primary beam whose dia-

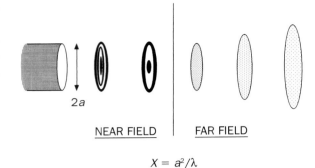

$$X = a^2/\lambda$$

Figure 6.4 The size and shape of the ultrasound beam are determined by the interference of wavelets from each point of the transducer. In the near field the beam is a complicated pattern of rings and nulls. At distances greater than a^2/λ the beam is conical with a diameter at distance x of $1.22 \times \lambda/a$ (a is the radius of the transducer).

meter at distance x is given by the equation $d = 1.22 \times \lambda/a$. Outside the primary beam the wavelets cancel and apart from some weak sidelobes sound intensity is zero.

For 20 mm-diameter transducers and wavelengths from 7.5 mm to 2.5 mm, the transition between the two zones lies at distances varying from 13 mm to 40 mm. It is clear that when measuring BUA the exact volume of bone interrogated by the ultrasound beam varies significantly with frequency.

The frequency content of a sound pulse

A sound wave represented by a continuous sine wave has a frequency content with a single value (Figure 6.5A). However, in practice sound signals that quickly fade away (Figure 6.5B) or consist of a single narrow pulse (Figure 6.5C) are often encountered. The frequency content of such signals can be found using Fourier analysis:[21]

$$A(f) = \int_{-\infty}^{\infty} F(t) \exp(-2\pi i f t) \, dt \qquad (6.11)$$

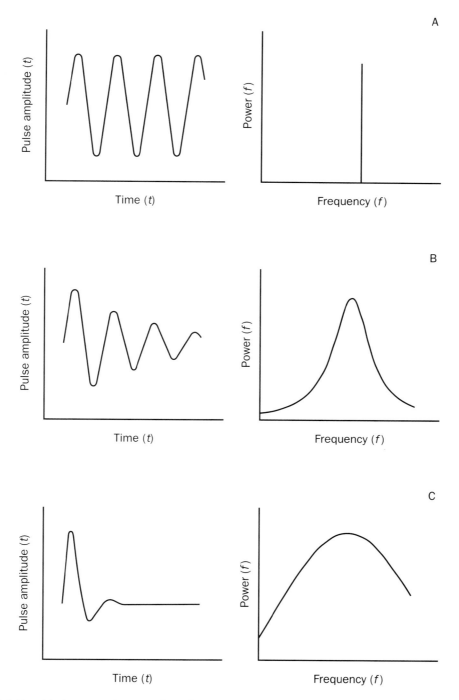

Figure 6.5 Relationship between the wave form for a sound pulse in the time domain (left-hand figures) and the corresponding power spectrum in the frequency domain (right-hand figures). (A) A signal represented by a continuous sine wave has a frequency content with a single value. (B) A sound pulse with the form of a damped sine wave contains a range of frequencies centred on the frequency of the underlying sine wave. (C) A narrow pulse contains a broad range of frequencies.

$A(f)$, the Fourier transform of the signal, is useful because it gives the decomposition of the sound pulse $F(t)$ into its constituent frequencies. Since $A(f)$ is a complex number, it contains information on both the amplitude and the phase as a function of frequency. Computing $A(f)$ from $F(t)$ is a standard procedure performed in signal analysis and image processing.[21] One advantage of dividing a signal into its component frequencies is that it makes it easier to calculate the effect of filters that act to transmit or block the signal selectively at different frequencies. The analysis of a sound pulse transmitted through the heel is in effect investigating the properties of the calcaneus as a filter. Often it is required to know the intensity present at different frequencies. The power spectrum, $P(f)$, is the product of $A(f)$ and its complex conjugate. As shown in Figure 6.5A–C, the narrower the sound pulse the broader the frequency distribution. In general, a pulse of width τ seconds will contain significant power at frequencies up to $1/\tau$ Hz. Thus, a pulse of 1 μs duration contains frequencies up to 1 MHz. In principle an infinitely narrow pulse contains equal power over an infinitely wide range of frequencies.

BROADBAND ULTRASONIC ATTENUATION

The measurement of BUA

When an ultrasound beam is transmitted through tissue some of the energy is lost as the beam becomes attenuated. Let $A(f)$ be the signal amplitude at frequency f determined from Fourier analysis of the sound pulse. In general, $A(f)$ decreases with increasing thickness of the attenuating material according to the exponential relationship:[2,22]

$$A_x(f) = A_0(f) \exp{-\mu(f)x} \qquad (6.12)$$

where $A_0(f)$ is the amplitude of the incident signal, $A_x(f)$ the amplitude after traversing thickness x, and $\mu(f)$ (units: cm^{-1}) is the frequency-dependent attenuation coefficient. In ultrasound studies it is conventional to define

the attenuation coefficient in relationship to the signal amplitude (i.e. the sound pressure) rather than the intensity.[22] Substitution into equation 6.5 leads to the relationship:

$$\text{Change in sound intensity} = dB_0 - dB_x$$
$$= 8.686\,\mu(f)x\ \text{dB} \qquad (6.13)$$

where the factor $8.686 = 20\log_{10}(e)$. It is convenient to change the attenuation coefficient into units of dB/cm by multiplying $\mu(f)$ by this factor. Equation 6.13 then becomes:

$$dB_0 - dB_x = \mu_{\mathrm{dB}}(f)x\ \text{dB} \qquad (6.14)$$

Equation 6.14 shows that the attenuation expressed in decibels increases linearly with thickness, x.

In the original ultrasound system developed by Langton, the patient's foot was placed between transmitting and receiving transducers in a small tank containing degassed water and a surfactant. The principles behind the measurement of BUA are explained in Figures 6.6A–C. After carefully positioning the heel, a frequency analyser was used to measure the spectrum of the transmitted signal from a short (0.5 μs) duration pulse (Figure 6.6A). The product of the attenuation coefficient $\mu_{\mathrm{dB}}(f)$ and the bone thickness x were measured using the substitution method in which the power spectrum of the transmitted signal is compared with and without the patient's heel in place (Figure 6.6B). In this way the effect of pulse shape, beam profile, transducer efficiency and attenuation in the water tank are properly corrected. When the signal attenuation due to the heel is plotted against frequency, a linear relationship is found (Figure 6.6C). The slope of the graph has units of dB/MHz and is referred to as broadband ultrasonic attenuation (BUA). For further mathematical details of the measurement refer to the review article by Njeh et al.[2]

The commercial QUS systems that were developed from Langton's prototype, which include the Walker Sonix, CUBA and Sahara instruments, all measure BUA from the slope of the regression line between 0.2 MHz and 0.6 MHz (Figure 6.7). Langton's studies showed that measurements over this frequency range gave good discrimination between normal

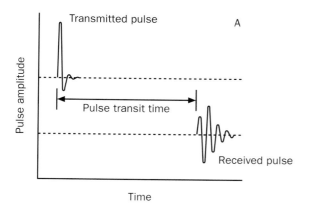

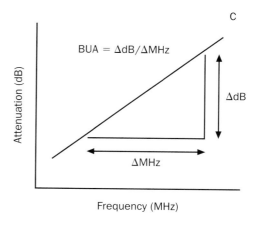

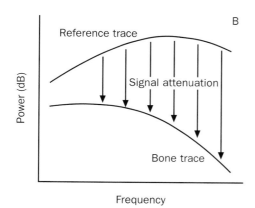

Figure 6.6 The physical principles behind the measurement of BUA. (A) The received pulse is digitized and Fourier analysis used to determine the power spectrum. The pulse transit time between the start of the transmitted pulse and the start of the received pulse is used for the SOS measurement. (B) In the substitution method, the power spectrum of the sound pulse transmitted through the patient's heel is compared with the reference trace determined from the signal transmitted through the water without the patient's foot. The difference between the bone trace and the reference trace is the attenuation due to the patient's heel. (C) When the attenuation through the patient's heel is plotted against frequency, a linear relationship is found for frequencies below 1 MHz. BUA is defined as the slope of the regression line and is measured in units of dB/MHz.

subjects and patients who had suffered a hip fracture.

Should BUA be normalized for bone width?

Clinical ultrasound systems generally do not determine the calcaneal thickness x, and therefore measure the product $\mu_{dB}(f)x$ rather than $\mu_{dB}(f)$. In principle, normalizing attenuation for bone size should result in a parameter that is more indicative of the true status of the calcaneus since the incidental factor of bone thickness at the measurement site is removed. The difference between normalized BUA (nBUA: units dB/MHz per cm) and non-normalized BUA (units: dB/MHz) is analogous to the difference between a true volumetric measurement of bone density (units: g/cm^3) as measured by a QCT scan and the areal density (units: g/cm^2) measured in conventional X-ray absorptiometry.

One commercial system, the UBA575+, does routinely measure calcaneal thickness. However, the measurement is performed to determine the true speed of sound in bone

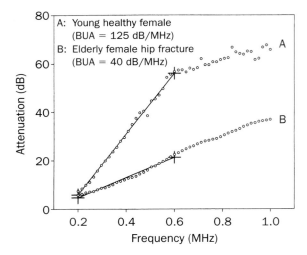

Figure 6.7 Measurement of BUA in: (A) a healthy young female subject; (B) an elderly patient after a hip fracture. BUA was measured from the slope of the linear regression line between 200 and 600 kHz. (Data courtesy of C Langton.[1])

rather than normalized BUA. Bone width is measured using the pulse–echo technique in which each transducer emits a pulse and the reflected signal from the soft tissue to bone interface is recorded (Figure 6.8). However, while the lateral face of the calcaneus is smooth, flat and approximately normal to the propagating signal, the medial surface is curved, which may make detection of the reflected signal more difficult.

The effect of normalizing BUA for bone thickness has been investigated mainly in in vitro studies. Using measurements of bovine trabecular bone on a UBA575 system, Wu et al.[23] concluded that BUA results depended on thickness in a complex, non-linear fashion, and that simple normalization is not appropriate. However, Langton,[1] Njeh[2] and Serpe and Rho[24] all report a linear relationship between BUA and sample thickness. Figure 6.9 shows the distribution of calcaneal bone width measured in 558 women aged 18–82 years scanned in the Guy's Hospital Osteoporosis Unit, London using a UBA575+ system. Mean calcaneal width was 30.1 mm, the population SD was 3.2 mm and the precision determined from duplicate measurements was 1.1 mm. The mean and SD agree well with data reported by Wu et al. from measurements of radiographs and CT scans.[23] The latter authors found only a weak correlation between BUA and bone size in in vivo studies and concluded that, with the exception of children, the effect of bone size on BUA used in the clinical setting is small.

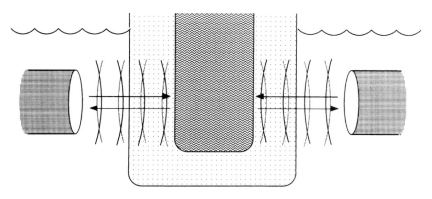

Figure 6.8 Measurement of bone width in the calcaneus using the pulse–echo technique as performed by the Walker Sonix UBA575+ system.

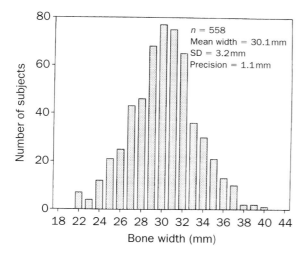

Figure 6.9 Distribution of bone width in the calcaneus in 558 women aged 18–82 years measured with a Walker Sonix UBA575+ system. Mean bone width was 30.1 mm, the population SD was 3.2 mm and the precision determined from duplicate measurements was 1.1 mm. (Data courtesy of Ms M Frost, Guy's Hospital Osteoporosis Unit, London.)

CUBA device, the CUBA Clinical, is available commercially (McCue Ultrasonics, Winchester, UK), and recently the UBA575 has been replaced by a new dry system, the Sahara (Hologic Inc., Waltham, MA, USA). Both these devices are exceptionally light and portable and clinical studies show their performance approximates to that of the water-based systems.[26,27] In contact systems, the substitution method of determining BUA is not directly applicable. Hence, the amplitude trace used to normalize the patient trace in Figure 6.6B must be measured using a phantom and stored in the system software.

In each of the four devices mentioned above, a foot support is used to position the patient's heel between fixed transducers. Thus, the measurement site cannot readily be adapted to different sizes and shapes of the calcaneus. The exact anatomical location of the BUA measurement varies from patient to patient, and in some individuals might even lie partly outside bone. However, two water-based systems, the UBIS-5000 (DMS, Montpellier, France)[28] and the DTU-one (Osteometer, Roedovre, Denmark) produce BUA images by performing a raster scan of the calcaneus (Figure 6.10) thus allowing a more consistent placement of the measurement site. At the present time it is too early to tell whether this gives a significant improvement in diagnostic accuracy.

Wet, dry and imaging systems for measuring BUA

To date, the large majority of clinical studies of BUA have been performed on either the Walker Sonix UBA575 or Lunar Achilles systems. Both these devices use a water bath to achieve acoustic coupling between the ultrasound transducers and the subject's heel. However, for a light and truly portable device there is an advantage in using a dry contact system in which the transducers are coupled directly to the heel using silicone pads and ultrasound gel. The first such system, the Contact Ultrasonic Bone Analyser (CUBA), was described by Langton et al.[25] An upgraded

The effect of phase cancellation on BUA measurements

As discussed above in 'The ultrasound beam from a circular transducer' section, conventional QUS systems use large aperture piezoelectric transducers with diameters significantly larger than the wavelength of the sound. This has the advantage of limiting the spread of the ultrasound beam by diffraction, but may create problems in the measurement of BUA.

Sound waves propagating through a homogeneous medium arrive at different points on

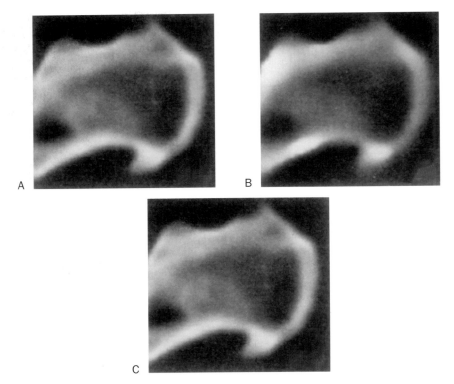

Figure 6.10 Comparison between QUS and BMD images of a human calcaneus obtained in an in vitro study: (A) normalized broadband ultrasonic attenuation; (B) ultrasound bone velocity; (C) bone mineral density. QUS images were obtained using an imaging ultrasound system and the BMD image using QCT. (Reproduced with permission from P Laugier.[15])

the face of the receiving transducer exactly in phase (Figure 6.11A), and so give rise to the maximum response in the detector. However, because cancellous bone is a heterogeneous medium, in practice there may be phase differences along different pathways through bone (Figure 6.11B). Since a piezoelectric transducer responds to the average pressure over its surface, signals that are out of phase will interfere, leading to an underestimate of the true intensity of ultrasound and therefore an overestimate of attenuation. The effect is greater at higher frequencies, thereby tending artificially to increase BUA.

Petley et al.[29] investigated this effect in 10 normal volunteers and showed that it caused BUA to be overestimated by between 15 and 57 dB/MHz. It may also be a contributing factor to the often quoted problem of the poor precision of QUS scans, since it would enhance the sensitivity of BUA measurements to small changes in the position of the measurement site. Njeh et al. showed that the frequency dependence of phase cancellation may assist in its detection by causing significant scatter in the linear plot of attenuation against frequency.[30] Also, it is possible that the effect is beneficial in that it may enhance the differences in BUA between normal and osteoporotic.

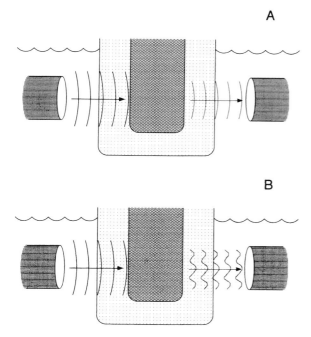

A

B

Figure 6.11 Schematic illustration of the effects of phase cancellation in the measurement of BUA. (A) In a uniform medium sound waves arrive at all points of the receiving transducer in phase; (B) inhomogeneities cause phase fluctuations in the wavefront leading to partial cancellation at the detector.[29]

SPEED OF SOUND MEASUREMENTS IN THE CALCANEUS

Commercial QUS systems for measuring BUA in the calcaneus also produce a measurement of the SOS by dividing the propagation distance by the pulse transit time (Figure 6.6A). As with normalized BUA, an accurate determination of the true velocity of sound in bone requires a measurement of bone thickness. However, as mentioned above, the UBA575+ is the only commercial device that makes this measurement. As emphasized above in relation to BUA measurements, cancellous bone is not a homogeneous medium, and therefore the equations

for the speed of sound given above (equations 6.1–6.3) are only approximations. Several in vitro studies have examined the relationship between Young's modulus E and the apparent density ρ, finding equations of the form:

$$E = k\rho^n \qquad (6.15)$$

where K is a constant and n the power function. The results give values for n in the range 2–3[31,32] and explain the observation that SOS values are larger for higher densities.

SOS measurements in wet systems

In general, those QUS systems that use a water bath to couple the ultrasound transducers to the patient's heel simply measure the average SOS through water, soft tissue and bone, a quantity usually referred to as the *time of flight velocity*.[33] Time of flight velocity (V_{tof}) is conveniently measured using the substitution method.[2] If x_{trans} is the separation of the two transducers, V_{water} is the SOS in water, and Δt the decrease in the propagation time of the sound pulse between the transducers when the patient's heel is placed in the sound path, then it is readily shown that:[2]

$$V_{tof} = \frac{V_{water}x_{trans}}{x_{trans} - (\Delta t V_{water})} \qquad (6.16)$$

To find the true velocity of sound in bone (bone velocity, V_{bone}) it is necessary to know the transducer separation x_{trans} and the bone thickness at the measurement site, x_{bone} (Figure 6.12A). It is assumed that the velocity of sound in soft tissue is the same as in the water. By summing the time it takes the sound pulse to travel through the water and the bone, the following relationship between V_{tof} and V_{bone} is found:

$$\frac{x_{trans}}{V_{tof}} = \frac{(x_{trans} - x_{bone})}{V_{water}} + \frac{x_{bone}}{V_{bone}} \qquad (6.17)$$

Equation 6.17 can be simplified by writing $\alpha = x_{bone}/x_{trans}$ when we obtain:

$$\frac{1}{V_{tof}} = \frac{(1 - \alpha)}{V_{water}} + \frac{\alpha}{V_{bone}} \qquad (6.18)$$

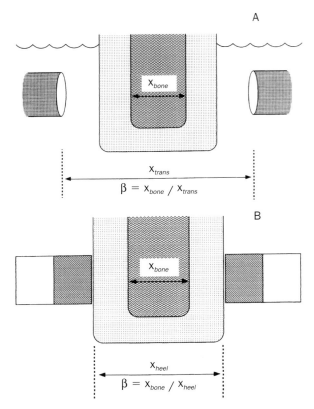

Figure 6.12 (A) Measurement of SOS using a water bath ultrasound system. Time of flight velocity (V_{tof}) is the mean speed of sound through water, soft tissue and bone. Determination of the true speed of sound in bone (V_{bone}) requires the measurement of bone width in the calcaneus (x_{bone}). The relationship between V_{bone} and V_{tof} is a function of α, the ratio of bone width to transducer separation.
(B) Measurement of SOS using a contact ultrasound system. Heel velocity (V_{heel}) is the mean speed of sound through soft tissue and bone. The relationship between V_{bone} and V_{heel} is a function of β, the ratio of bone width to heel width.

It can be seen from equation 6.18 that the relationship between V_{tof} and V_{bone} depends on α and, to the extent that there is a narrow range of bone thickness values in the measured population (Figure 6.9), then V_{tof} is a reasonable substitute for V_{bone}. This is confirmed by scatter plots of V_{bone} against V_{tof} from measurements on the UBA575+ system (Figure 6.13A). Values for V_{bone} span the range 1450–1900 m/s and include the SOS in water ($V_{water} \approx 1485$ m/s) when equation 6.18 has the solution $V_{tof} = V_{bone} = V_{water}$. This has the useful practical consequence that V_{tof} and V_{bone} are especially tightly correlated in the lower part of the range of bone velocity values that is important for identifying patients with osteoporosis.

In the Lunar Achilles system, velocity is measured using the substitution method described above (equation 6.16). However, the transit time is measured from the zero-crossing point of the first negative slope of the received signal trace instead of the first point of detection of a positive signal (Figure 6.6A). The Achilles SOS parameter is an estimate of V_{bone} calculated on the assumption that all subjects have a bone thickness of 40 mm.[2]

SOS measurements in dry systems

In contact systems such as the CUBA Clinical and Sahara, the transducers are coupled to the patient's heel using soft pads. Unlike the water-based systems, transducer separation is not fixed but depends on the heel thickness, x_{heel}. The velocity measurement obtained by dividing transducer separation by pulse transit time is the average SOS through soft tissue and bone (Figure 6.12B). Miller et al.[33] called this velocity parameter the *heel velocity* (V_{heel}), although it is sometimes also called *limb velocity*.[2] The relationship between heel velocity and bone velocity can be calculated in a similar manner to that between time of flight velocity and bone velocity by summing the time it takes the sound pulse to travel through the soft tissue and bone:

$$\frac{x_{heel}}{V_{heel}} = \frac{(x_{heel} - x_{bone})}{V_{soft}} + \frac{x_{bone}}{V_{bone}} \quad (6.19)$$

where V_{soft} is the SOS in soft tissue. Equation 6.19 can be simplified by writing $\beta = x_{bone}/x_{heel}$ when we obtain:

$$\frac{1}{V_{heel}} = \frac{(1 - \beta)}{V_{soft}} + \frac{\beta}{V_{bone}} \quad (6.20)$$

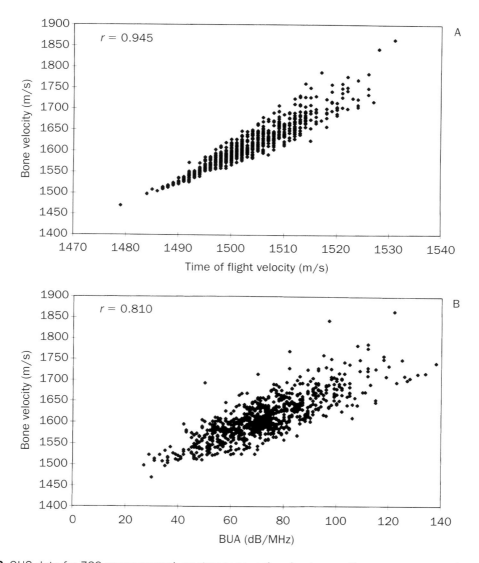

Figure 6.13 QUS data for 739 young normal, postmenopausal and osteoporotic women measured on a Walker Sonix UBA575+ system. (Data courtesy of Ms M Frost, Guy's Hospital Osteoporosis Unit, London.) (A) Plot of bone velocity (V_{bone}) against time of flight velocity (V_{tof}). The high correlation reflects the narrow dispersion in bone width shown in Figure 6.9. Note that the distribution converges at the point $V_{bone} = V_{tof} = 1485$ m/s where both velocity parameters equal the SOS in water. (B) Plot of bone velocity against

The relationship between V_{heel} and V_{bone} was investigated by Miller and colleagues[33] using a CUBA Research system. Based on measurements in 200 young normal, postmenopausal and osteoporotic women, they showed that the narrow dispersion in β led to a close correlation between V_{heel} and V_{bone} similar to that for V_{tof} and V_{bone} shown in Figure 6.13A. Hence, there is no clinical advantage in making the extra measurement of soft tissue thickness required to determine bone velocity. Miller also concluded that for longitudinal studies there was definitely no advantage in measuring V_{bone} since the additional measurement errors involved detract from rather than enhance the clinically useful precision.

COMBINATIONS OF BUA AND SOS IN THE CALCANEUS

Commercial QUS systems measuring the calcaneus generally produce both a BUA and an SOS measurement. Scatter plots show that the two parameters are reasonably well correlated (Figure 6.13B). This suggests that combining the BUA and SOS values to produce a single new QUS parameter might reduce random measurement errors and improve precision and diagnostic accuracy.

The first such parameter, introduced on the Lunar Achilles system, was called 'Stiffness'. Stiffness is derived by first expressing the BUA and SOS values on a sliding percentage scale such that healthy young adults have average values of 100% and elderly osteoporotic subjects around 60%. The algorithms used for converting BUA and SOS into percentages of the expected young normal (%YN) values are:

$$\text{BUA:} \quad \%YN_{BUA} = \frac{(BUA - 50)}{75} \times 100\% \quad (6.21a)$$

$$\text{SOS:} \quad \%YN_{SOS} = \frac{(SOS - 1380)}{180} \times 100\% \quad (6.21b)$$

Stiffness is then calculated as the arithmetic mean of the two %YN values:

$$\text{Stiffness} = \frac{\%YN_{BUA} + \%YN_{SOS}}{2} \quad (6.21c)$$

Substituting from equations 6.21a and 6.21b into equation 6.21c gives a direct relationship between Stiffness and BUA and SOS:

$$\text{Stiffness} = 0.667 \times BUA + 0.278 \times SOS - 417 \quad (6.21d)$$

The Achilles Stiffness parameter has no independent physical meaning and is not related to the mechanical stiffness of the bone. The advantages in its use relate to the smoothing entailed in the averaging of the BUA and SOS contributions in Equation 6.21c and the faster convergence of measurments to a stable value when the patient's foot is placed in the waterbath than for BUA or SOS alone. Also, by combining the results in a single index, scan interpretation may be made easier for clinicians unfamiliar with the physical basis of quantitative ultrasound measurements.

The other commercial system to offer a combined QUS parameter is the Sahara. In this case a slightly different algorithm is used, which gives equal weighting to BUA and SOS. The new parameter is referred to as the quantitative ultrasound index (QUI):

$$QUI = 0.41 \times (BUA + SOS) - 571 \quad (6.22)$$

QUI has been shown to correlate reasonably accurately ($r = 0.85$) with BMD measurements in the calcaneus and the Sahara scan report provides the user with an estimated BMD value. In this context, the BMD estimate is probably best regarded as a substitute for fracture probability. In future, longer-term data from studies such as EPIDOS and SOF[13,14] might enable ultrasound findings to be reported directly in terms of fracture risk.

SOS MEASUREMENTS AT OTHER SKELETAL SITES

Recently, new ultrasound systems have been developed that measure SOS in an entirely different way from the heel transmission systems described above. Instead of measuring the velocity of ultrasound waves transmitted across bone, the new instruments are designed to measure SOS in a fixed longitudinal section of bone, usually parallel to the long axis. In this way the effect of the uncertainties caused by varying bone and soft tissue thickness in calcaneus measurements is removed. The technique is sometimes referred to as *semi-reflection* to distinguish it from the conventional transmission method.

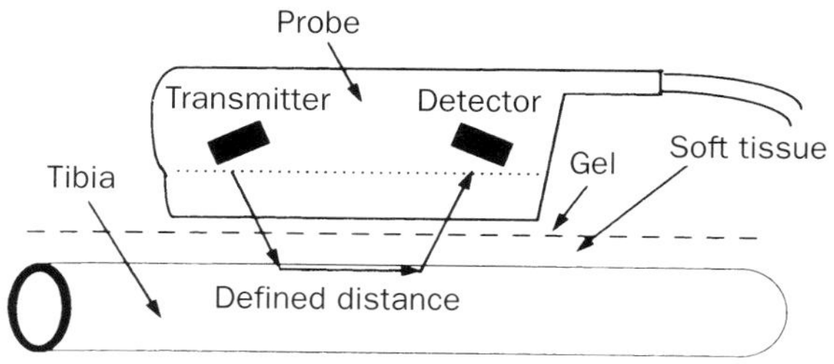

Figure 6.14 Schematic illustration of the technique for the measurement of tibial SOS using the semi-reflection method. The SOS is measured along a fixed longitudinal section of bone. (Reproduced with permission from A Foldes.[34])

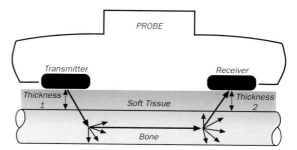

Figure 6.15 Physical principles of the Omnisense bone ultrasound system. Piezoelectric transducers at either end of a small hand held probe measure the thickness and speed of sound in the soft tissue overlying bone. Proprietary algorithms use a measurement of the shortest sound propagation time to infer the SOS in bone.

The first of these devices, the Soundscan 2000 (Myriad Ultrasound Systems, Rehovot, Israel), measures SOS in the cortical layer of the mid-tibia.[9,34] The tibia was chosen because of its long, straight smooth surface and the thin and fairly constant layer of overlying soft tissue. A single hand-held probe is used, which measures the transit time of a 250-kHz pulse along a defined 50-mm distance. Because the SOS is much higher in cortical bone than in soft tissue (4000 m/s versus 1500 m/s), the transmitted sound wave is strongly refracted (Figure 6.14). The probe houses a proprietary array of ultrasound transducers designed to reduce the effect of soft tissue on the velocity measurement. The probe is moved back and forth across the tibial surface and a minimum of 150–200 velocity readings are recorded. The final SOS result is the average of the five highest readings.

Recently, a new semi-reflection system has been developed, the Omnisense (Sunlight Ultrasound Technologies, Rehovot, Israel).[11] This device has a smaller and more sophisticated probe that can correct for larger and more variable thicknesses of soft tissue. As a result, the Omnisense system can perform SOS measurements at a large number of different sites in the skeleton and is the first ultrasound instrument capable of measurements in the spine and proximal femur. While the exact algorithms used are proprietary, it seems likely that they are based on using Fermat's principle to identify the sound path with the shortest propaga-

tion time between the transmitter and detector (Figure 6.15).

DOES ULTRASOUND PROVIDE DIFFERENT INFORMATION FROM DENSITOMETRY?

A widely cited advantage of QUS technology is that it gives different information from X-ray absorptiometry that is more related to bone quality than bone density. The high attenuation found in the measurement of BUA in cancellous bone is largely caused by the scattering of sound waves by the large numbers of trabeculae. Hence, BUA is believed to be related to structural factors such as porosity, connectivity and trabecular thickness. In contrast, equation 6.2 shows that the information over and above density provided by an SOS measurement is the elastic modulus.

The most convincing evidence that BUA values relate to bone structure is provided by in vitro studies comparing measurements of cubes of cancellous bone along different orthogonal axes. Since the BMD of a cube of bone should be independent of the axis studied, any variation in ultrasound properties suggests a significant structural component. A variation of BUA with orientation was reported by Nicholson et

A

$y = -2.3095 + 0.067563x \quad r = 0.86856$

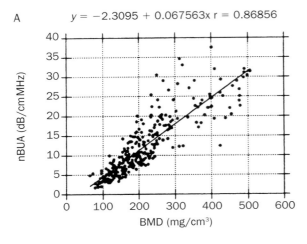

B

$y = 1452.8 + 0.30995x \quad r = 0.94035$

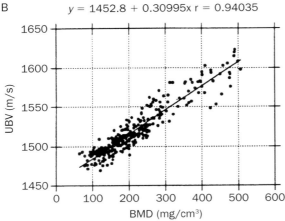

Figure 6.16 Relationship between bone mineral density (BMD) and: (A) normalized broadband ultrasonic attenuation (nBUA); (B) ultrasonic bone velocity (UBV). QUS parameters were obtained using an imaging ultrasound system and BMD using QCT. (Reproduced with permission from P Laugier.[15])

al.[35] in measurements of human vertebrae. Glüer et al.[36] measured cubes of bovine bone, which they radiographed and scored for trabecular alignment. Large differences along the three axes were found, with BUA values highest when the sound waves propagated parallel to the principal axis of the trabeculae. Hans et al.[37] and Glüer et al.[38] studied the relationship between BUA and histomorphometric parame-

ters representing the microarchitecture of bone. In a study of bovine trabecular bone, Glüer et al.[38] were able to demonstrate a significant association between structural parameters and BUA independent of BMD. However, in a study of human bone, Hans et al.[37] failed to show any significant correlation between ultrasonic parameters and bone microarchitecture. One problem may be that many of the important histomorphometric parameters such as porosity and trabecular thickness are themselves strongly correlated with BMD. In contrast to bone microarchitecture, in vitro studies have been quite successful in demonstrating a significant relationship between SOS measurements and the mechanical properties of bone (Figure 6.2).[39,40]

It is often argued that the relatively poor correlation between ultrasound parameters and BMD measurements in the calcaneus itself constitutes evidence that QUS studies are measuring different properties of bone.[41] However, this overlooks the many difficulties of the comparison such as ensuring that QUS and BMD measurements are made at exactly the same site in the calcaneus, the fact that the volume of bone measured by ultrasound is ill-defined because of the spreading of the sound beam by diffraction, and the phase cancellation effects described by Petley.[29] In this context, it is worth noting that the advent of imaging ultrasound has allowed more careful mapping of BUA, SOS and BMD in the calcaneus (Figure 6.10) and resulted in considerably higher correlations than previously reported. Laugier et al. found correlation coefficients of $r = 0.94$ between SOS and BMD and $r = 0.87$ between nBUA and BMD (Figure 6.16).[15] As used in current practice, QUS scans are often regarded as a convenient substitute for a BMD measurement in the calcaneus. However, it should not be forgotten that certain collagen diseases may modify the relationship between ultrasound and densitometric measurements found in normal subjects.[42] This, and many other aspects of quantitative bone ultrasound, require further research if the physical basis and clinical interpretation of QUS measurements are to be understood better.[5]

REFERENCES

1. Langton CM, Palmer SB, Porter RW. The measurement of broadband ultrasonic attenuation in cancellous bone. *Eng Med* (1984) **13**: 89–91.
2. Njeh CF, Boivin CM, Langton CM. The role of ultrasound in the assessment of osteoporosis: a review. *Osteoporos Int* (1997) **7**: 7–22.
3. Gregg EW, Kriska AM, Salamone LM et al. The epidemiology of quantitative ultrasound: a review of the relationships with bone mass, osteoporosis and fracture risk. *Osteoporos Int* (1997) **7**: 89–99.
4. Genant HK, Glüer C-C, Faulkner KG et al. Acronyms in bone densitometry [letter]. *J Bone Miner Res* (1992) **7**: 1239.
5. Glüer C-C. Quantitative ultrasound techniques for the assessment of osteoporosis – expert agreement on current status. *J Bone Miner Res* (1997) **12**: 1280–8.
6. Vogel JM, Wasnich RD, Ross PD. The clinical relevance of calcaneus bone mineral measurements: a review. *Bone Miner* (1988) **5**: 35–58.
7. Waud CE, Lew R, Baran DT. The relationship between ultrasound and densitometric measurements of bone mass in the calcaneus in women. *Calcif Tissue Int* (1992) **51**: 415–18.
8. Lees B, Stevenson JC. Preliminary evaluation of a new ultrasound bone densitometer. *Calcif Tissue Int* (1993) **53**: 149–52.
9. Orgee JM, Foster H, McCloskey EV et al. A precise method for the assessment of tibial ultrasound velocity. *Osteoporos Int* (1996) **6**: 1–7.
10. Ventura V, Mauloni M, Mura M et al. Ultrasound velocity changes at the proximal phalanges of the hand in pre-, peri- and postmenopausal women. *Osteoporos Int* (1996) **6**: 368–75.
11. Hans D, Weiss M, Fuerst T et al. A new reflection quantitative ultrasound system: preliminary results of multi site bone measurements. *Osteoporos Int* (1997) **7**: 300.
12. Porter RW, Miller CG, Grainger D et al. Prediction of hip fracture in elderly women: a prospective study. *Br Med J* (1990) **301**: 638–41.
13. Hans D, Dargent-Molina P, Schott AM et al. Ultrasonographic heel measurements to predict hip fracture in elderly women: the EPIDOS prospective study. *Lancet* (1996) **348**: 511–14.
14. Bauer DC, Glüer C-C, Cauley JA et al. Broadband ultrasonic attenuation predicts fractures strongly and independently of densitometry in older women. *Arch Intern Med* (1997) **157**: 629–34.
15. Laugier P, Droin P, Laval-Jeantet AM et al. In-vitro assessment of the relationship between acoustic properties and bone mass density of the calcaneus by comparison of ultrasound parametric imaging and quantitative computed tomography. *Bone* (1997) **20**: 157–65.
16. Gooberman GL. *Ultrasonics: theory and application* (English Universities Press: London, 1968), 1–9.
17. Reilly DT, Burstein AH. The elastic and ultimate properties of compact bone tissue. *J Biomech* (1975) **8**: 393–405.
18. Yahia LH, Drouin G, Duval P. A methodology for mechanical measurement of technical constants of trabecular bone. *Eng Med* (1988) **17**: 169–73.
19. Goldberg BB, Wells PNT. *Ultrasonics in clinical diagnosis*, 3rd edition (Churchill Livingstone: Edinburgh, 1983).
20. Woodcock JP. *Ultrasonics* (Adam Hilger: Bristol, 1979), 5.
21. Herman GT. *Image reconstruction from projections* (Springer-Verlag: New York, 1979).
22. Bhatia AB. *Ultrasonic absorption: an introduction to the theory of sound absorption in gases, liquids and solids* (Clarendon Press: Oxford, 1967), 5.
23. Wu CY, Glüer C-C, Jergas M et al. The impact of bone size on broadband ultrasound attenuation. *Bone* (1995) **16**: 137–41.
24. Serpe LJ, Rho J. Broadband ultrasonic attenuation dependence on bone width in vitro. *Phys Med Biol* (1996) **41**: 197–202.
25. Langton CM, Ali AV, Riggs CM et al. A contact method for the assessment of ultrasonic velocity and broadband ultrasonic attenuation in cortical and cancellous bone. *Clin Phys Physiol Meas* (1990) **11**: 243–9.
26. von Stetten E, Wilson K, Steiger P et al. In-vivo comparison of two calcaneal ultrasound scanners: the Sahara clinical bone sonometer and the Walker–Sonix UBA-575+. *J Bone Miner Res* (1996) **11**(suppl 1): S244.
27. Frost ML, Blake GM, Fogelman I. Evaluation of a new heel ultrasound system: the Sahara clinical bone sonometer. *Osteoporos Int* (1997) **7**: 303.
28. Laugier P, Fournier B, Berger G. Ultrasound parametric imaging of the calcaneus: in-vivo results with a new device. *Calcif Tissue Int* (1996) **58**: 326–31.
29. Petley GW, Robins PA, Aindow JD. Broadband ultrasonic attenuation: are current measurement techniques inherently inaccurate? *Br J Radiol* (1995) **68**: 1212–14.
30. Njeh CF, Hans D, Fuerst T et al. Trace analysis as

a form of quality assurance in QUS assessment of bone. *J Bone Miner Res* (1997) **12**(suppl 1): S261.

31. Gibson LJ. The mechanical behaviour of cancellous bone. *J Biomech* (1985) **18**: 317–28.

32. Turner CH, Cowin SC, Rho JY et al. The fabric dependence of the orthotropic elastic constants of cancellous bone. *J Biomech* (1990) **23**: 549–61.

33. Miller CG, Herd RJM, Ramalingam T et al. Ultrasonic velocity measurements through the calcaneus: which velocity should be measured? *Osteoporos Int* (1993) **3**: 31–5.

34. Foldes AJ, Rimon A, Keinan DD et al. Quantitative ultrasound of the tibia: a novel approach for assessment of bone status. *Bone* (1995) **17**: 363–7.

35. Nicholson PH, Haddaway MJ, Davie MW. The dependence of ultrasonic properties on orientation in human vertebral bone. *Phys Med Biol* (1994) **39**: 1013–24.

36. Glüer C-C, Wu CY, Genant HK. Broadband ultrasonic attenuation signals depend on trabecular orientation: an in-vitro study. *Osteoporos Int* (1993) **3**: 185–91.

37. Hans D, Arlot ME, Schott AM et al. Do ultrasound measurements on the *os calcis* reflect more the bone microarchitecture than the bone mass: a two dimensional histomorphometric study. *Bone* (1995) **16**: 295–300.

38. Glüer C-C, Wu CY, Jergas M et al. Three quantitative ultrasound parameters reflect bone structure. *Calcif Tissue Int* (1994) **55**: 46–52.

39. Bouxsein ML, Radloff SE. Quantitative ultrasound of the calcaneus reflects the mechanical properties of calcaneal trabecular bone. *J Bone Miner Res* (1997) **12**: 839–46.

40. Lee SC, Coan BS, Bouxsein ML. Tibial ultrasound velocity measured in situ predicts the material properties of tibial cortical bone. *Bone* (1997) **21**: 119–25.

41. Glüer C-C, Vahlensieck M, Faulkner KG et al. Site-matched calcaneal measurements of broadband ultrasound attenuation and single X-ray absorptiometry: do they measure different skeletal properties. *J Bone Miner Res* (1992) **7**: 1071–9.

42. Cheng S, Tylavsky FA, Rho J et al. Do collagen abnormalities affect ultrasound assessment? *J Bone Miner Res* (1997) **12**(suppl 1): S175.

7

Commercial Ultrasound Instruments

Guest chapter by Christopher F Njeh and Didier Hans

CHAPTER OVERVIEW

Since the pioneering work of Langton et al.[1] in 1984, many clinical quantitative ultrasound machines have been developed. The objective of this chapter is to give a broad review of the current commercially available quantitative ultrasound (QUS) systems. While some QUS devices such as the Walker Sonix UBA575 are no longer available, they will be discussed since they provide background for current systems and also because most of the early reported studies were carried out using these systems. The chapter starts by introducing the various anatomical sites currently measured by QUS. The systems will be described in alphabetical order, with system specifications provided by the manufacturers. The last sections will deal with QUS quality assurance and cross-calibration issues.

INTRODUCTION

Clinical QUS systems first became available in early 1990, and there are currently a multitude of different machines on the market. These include, in alphabetical order: Achilles+ (Lunar; Madison, WI, USA); AOS100 (Aloka, Japan); CUBA Clinical (McCue; Winchester, England, UK); DBM Sonic (IGEA; Carpi, Italy); DTU-one (Osteometer MediTech A/S;

Hoersholm, Denmark); Omnisense (Sunlight; Rehovot, Israel); Paris (Norland, Fort Atkinson, WI, USA); Sahara (Hologic; Waltham, MA, USA); SoundScan 2000 (Myriad; Rehovot, Israel); and UBIS-3000 (DMS; Montpellier, France). Continual improvements are being made by either enhancing hardware performance or optimizing analysis algorithms. The examination requires less time and there is ongoing effort to improve reproducibility of broadband ultrasonic attenuation (BUA). In general terms, commercial QUS devices show a greater technological diversity than bone densitometry equipment. Though based on similar principles, the instruments listed above have significant differences, particularly in their calibration methods, site of measurement (mainly at calcaneus, phalanges or tibia), analysis software and scanner design. They also vary in precision, the mode of data acquisition (fixed single point or imaging), coupling (water or gel), velocity definition (bone velocity, limb velocity and time of flight) and transit time measurement. These differences, combined with the fact that no absolute standard exists for ultrasound measurement, cause the readings obtained on the different instrumentation to vary dramatically. As a consequence, results obtained on a validated device cannot be directly translated into performance statements of other technologically different QUS devices and thus are not directly comparable. Different

QUS devices have been developed to measure various anatomical sites (Table 7.1).

Calcaneus

The calcaneus is the most popular measurement site for several reasons. The calcaneus is 90% cancellous bone, which, due to its high surface:volume ratio, has a higher metabolic turnover rate than cortical bone. Hence, cancellous bone will manifest bone metabolic changes before cortical bone.[2] The calcaneus is also easily accessible, and the medio-lateral surfaces are fairly flat and parallel, thus reducing repositioning errors. The choice of the calcaneus as the test site has been supported by Wasnich et al.[3] and Black et al.,[4] who reported that the calcaneus appeared to be the optimal bone mineral density (BMD) measurement site for routine screening of perimenopausal women to predict the risk of any type of osteoporotic fracture.

Finger phalanges

The measurement site is the distal metaphysis of the first phalanx of the last four fingers. The medio-lateral surfaces are approximately parallel thus reducing ultrasound scattering. In the metaphysis, both cortical and trabecular bone are present. Both types of bone tissue are extremely sensitive to age-related bone resorption. Cortical bone usually becomes more porous with advancing age. In addition, the cortices of long bone become thinner because the rate of endosteal resorption exceeds the rate of periosteal formation of bone. Taken together, the age-related losses of cortical and cancellous bone substantially increase the fragility of bone. In one study, the phalanges of elderly women had the highest deviation from peak adult bone mass compared with other techniques such as spine dual X-ray absorptiometry (DXA), spine quantitative computed tomography (QCT), femoral neck DXA and forearm DXA.[5] They are, therefore, appropriate to evaluate the risk of fracture.

Tibia

The mid-tibia has been chosen because of its long, straight and smooth surface. Also, the overlying soft tissue is very thin thereby minimizing errors in speed of sound (SOS) measurement. Since 80% of the skeleton is cortical, and osteoporotic fracture may also involve cortical bone, it might be of clinical interest to measure a cortical bone such as the tibia. In addition, cortical bone loss may play an important role in determining whole bone strength. Measurement at this site is usually longitudinal ultrasound velocity along the antero-medial cortical border of mid-tibia, thereby taking advantage of a site that is easily accessible in most individuals.

Other sites

Measurement sites have been restricted to peripheral skeleton due to the highly attenuating nature of ultrasound. However, with the advent of semi-reflection techniques, the accessible sites now include many others such as the femur, posterior process of the spine, radius and ulna.

CLINICAL QUANTITATIVE ULTRASOUND BONE MEASUREMENT SYSTEMS

These systems measure either ultrasound velocity, attenuation or both. Most manufacturers have quoted precision values for the parameters measured. This is usually quoted as the coefficient of variation (CV) from repeated measurements. A brief description will be given of the commercial systems mentioned above according to the site measured.

Calcaneal wet QUS systems

UBA575 (Walker Sonix, USA)
This was the first commercial system for the assessment of bone status (Figure 7.1). Based on the initial work of Langton et al.,[1] Walker Sonix

Device	Manufacturer	Anatomical site	Coupling medium	Parameter	Precision CV^a (%)	CV^b (%)	Comments
Table 7.1 Commercially available QUS devices for bone assessment.							
Achilles	Lunar	Calcaneus	Water	BUA	0.8–2.5	1.6	
				SOS	0.2–0.4	0.2	TOF velocity
				Stiffness	1.0–2.0	2.13	
AOS	Aloka	Calcaneus	Gel	SOS	0.3–0.4	0.15	Limb velocity
				TI	0.76–1.53	0.97	
				OSI	1.21–1.85	1.25	
CUBA Clinical	McCue	Calcaneus	Gel	BUA	1.5–4.0	3.4	Limb velocity
				SOS	0.2–0.6	0.30	
DBM Sonic 1200	IGEA	Phalanges	Gel	Ad-SOS	0.5–1.0	1.1	Amplitude-dependent velocity
DTU-one	Osteometer	Calcaneus	Water	BUA	1–1.4	N/A	Imaging system, TOF velocity
				SOS	0.1–0.2		
Omnisense	Sunlight	Multisite	Gel	SOS	0.2–1.0	1.0	Semi-reflection
Paris	Norland	Calcaneus	Gel	BUA	1.8	N/A	Limb velocity
				SOS	0.4		
				Soundness			
Sahara	Hologic	Calcaneus	Gel	BUA	0.8–2.5	3.68	Limb velocity
				SOS	0.2–0.4	0.2	
				QUI	1.0–2.0	2.4	
				Est. BMD	2.5	N/A	
SoundScan	Myriad	Mid-tibia	Gel	SOS	0.2–1.0	N/A	Semi reflection
UBIS 5000	DMS	Calcaneus	Water	BUA	0.8–2.5	1.82	Imaging system, phase velocity, fully automatic, ROI
				SOS	0.2–0.4	0.24	
				BUB			
UBA575+	Walker Sonix	Calcaneus	Water	BUA	2.0–5.0	5.2	No longer in production; two velocity results are given: bone velocity and TOF
				SOS	0.2–0.6	0.1	

^{a}CV, % coefficient of variation reported in the literature.
^{b}CV, short-term precision measurement on elderly and osteoporotic women by the authors.
N/A = not available.
TOF = time of flight

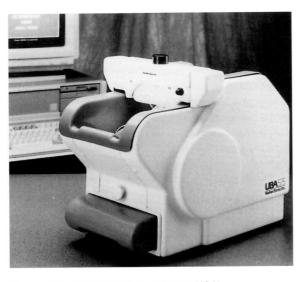

Figure 7.1 UBA575 (Walker Sonix, USA).

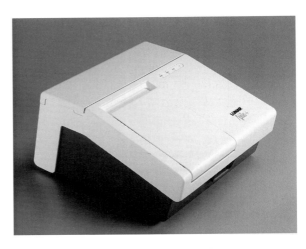

Figure 7.2 Achilles+ (Lunar Corp., USA).

Inc. developed a prototype instrument UBA1001. This system had a variable frequency tone burst generator producing a sequence of short bursts of single frequency ultrasound rather than a single broadband pulse. The frequency range of 200–1000 kHz was produced in 28 kHz steps. The UBA1001 provided only BUA measurements carried out in a room temperature water bath between two fixed 25-mm diameter transducers, both resonant at 1 MHz.[6]

The UBA575 model introduced the refinements of rectilinear scanning of the transducers and a pneumatic foot restraint to improve reproducibility. The rectilinear scan was made of nine points in a 3 × 3 grid in a 22 × 22-mm region. The transducers were changed to 18-mm diameter with a 500-kHz resonant (nominal) frequency and signal amplitudes registered at 12 equally spaced intervals between 200 and 600 kHz.

A reference trace is obtained with degassed water, then the subject's heel is immersed and allowed to stabilize for approximately 3 minutes. The calculation of BUA at each point is as previously described, the final result being obtained via a nine-point averaging sequence. The UBA575 has recently been upgraded to the UBA575+ with the capability of measuring time of flight (TOF) velocity by the substitution method. A pulse–echo technique is used to measure the width of the calcaneus[7] and this information is used to estimate the true bone velocity. BUA is now calculated using a fast Fourier transform method (FFT) rather than the tone–burst technique. This system is no longer commercially available.

Achilles+ (Lunar Corp., USA)

The Achilles+ (Figure 7.2) uses a high-precision, heated water bath with pre-measured surfactant maintained at a constant 37°C, since both velocity and BUA are temperature dependent.[8,9] It has two tanks: the reservoir to feed the bath and the drain. The filling and draining of the water bath are fully automated and each measurement is carried out in fresh water. Two single element-unfocused 25-mm diameter transducers are mounted coaxially at a fixed separation of approximately 95 mm.[10]

Data are collected in the time domain, thus enabling both velocity and BUA to be measured. Velocity is calculated using the TOF substitution method,[11] with the transit time measured from the zero-crossing point of the first negative slope of the received signal trace. An assumption that all subjects have the same heel width of 40 mm is used in the velocity calculation. This means that the SOS measurement approximates to an estimate of limb velocity. An FFT algorithm is used to calculate the amplitude spectrum. BUA is then calculated by the same substitution method described by Langton et al.,[1] but it is not normalized for heel width.

Lunar has introduced an index called 'Stiffness' (not related to mechanical stiffness), defined as a combination of normalized velocity and BUA: Stiffness = 0.67*BUA + 0.28*SOS − 420. Stiffness is claimed to improve the standardized coefficient of variation of velocity or BUA alone.[12]

To help standardize the measurement position, special shims that elevate the heel according to foot size are now available. Paediatric positioners are also available with adaptors to cone down the diameter of the transducers.

The Achilles is supplied with two quality assurance phantoms: a water reference insert and a calibration standard. The water reference insert is used when the Achilles is collecting water reference data and the standard is used in daily system checks. The expected values are BUA: ~75 dB/MHz and velocity: ~1600 m/s. The acceptable range for these values is unique to each scanner.

Normative data collected for a European population are available. Additionally, specific reference data are available for Japanese, French and German populations. Detailed system specifications are presented in Table 7.2.

UBIS-5000 (Diagnostic Medical Systems (DMS), SA, France)

The UBIS (Ultrasound Bone Imaging Scanner) instruments are water-based systems which measure both BUA and SOS.[13] They use a technologically different approach by generating a BUA image of the calcaneus and also using phase velocity in calculating SOS (Figure 7.3). An upgraded model introduced in 1998, the UBIS-5000, also measures a new parameter, broadband ultrasound backscatter (BUB). The

UBIS systems obtain ultrsound images in transmission mode by using a pair of single-element-focused, 29-mm diameter broadband transducers immersed in a water bath at 30°C. The transducers are co-axially and confocally aligned with a separation of 110 mm. The

Table 7.2 Technical specifications for the Achilles.

Clinical

	Precision (CV%)	Annual change	
		%/year	units/year
BUA	1.7	0.7	0.5 dB/MHz
Velocity	0.3	0.07	1.1 m/s
Stiffness	1.7	0.9	0.9

Transducer

Diameter	25 mm
Central frequency	0.5 MHz
Frequency range	0.230 MHz bandwidth (FWHM)
Frequency used to calculate BUA	Proprietary
Mode	Unfocused

Data acquisition

Scan time	2 minutes
Scan area	Fixed point
Computer requirement	486 Dx50 processor

Physical dimension of scanner

Weight	20 kg
Length	33 cm
Width	51 cm
Height	65 cm

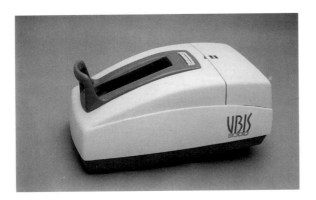

Figure 7.3 UBIS-5000 (Diagnostic Medical Systems (DMS), SA, France).

examination and restrain the heel from moving from side to side during the examination. The new UBIS-5000 model has an improved water management system with automatic filling and draining using self-contained reservoirs and a temperature controlled waterbath maintained at 30°C. The UBIS systems feature a unique electronic internal calibration and quality control with display of results. There is no manipulation of a phantom involved and therefore it is supposed that this procedure will provide long-

ultrasound beam scans both the x and y directions in 1-mm steps until the entire calcaneus is imaged. The scan area is typically 60×60 mm (maximum 85×85 mm). A value of BUA is obtained for each position and images of it are then processed. Then a small circular region of interest (ROI) of approximately 1 cm² based on the lowest attenuation is selected in the middle of the posterior part of the calcaneus.[14] The advantage of the image is that it allows the evaluation of standardized regions of interest (automatic regions of interest have been included in the software) in all patients; and the analysis of exactly the same volume of bone in repeated examinations of the same patient. The image also makes it possible for measurement artefacts to be identified and avoided.

The UBIS-5000 system also measures phase velocity throughout the scanned region. Because phase velocity is highly dependent on frequency, the UBIS-3000 manufacturers defined ultrasound bone velocity (UBV) as the average value of phase velocity in the frequency range 200–600 kHz. The reported UBV is the average UBV in the ROI.[13]

The operator, with the help of the on-screen display, could adjust the calcaneus using the built-in mechanical system so that the foot is always held at an adequate angle. A strap is provided to maintain the leg in position during

Table 7.3 Technical specifications for the UBIS-5000.

Clinical		Precision (CV%)	Annual change	
			%/year	units/year
BUA		0.5	0.64	0.84 dB/MHz
Velocity		0.25	0.046	0.7 m/s

Transducer	
Diameter	29 mm
Central frequency	0.5 MHz
Frequency range	0.1–0.9 MHz
Frequency used to calculate BUA	0.2–0.6 MHz
Mode	Focused

Data acquisition	
Scan time	2 minutes
Scan area	60×60 mm
Computer requirement	486 DX4-100/1.2 GB

Physical dimension of scanner	
Weight	27 kg
Length	75 cm
Width	42 cm
Height	39 cm

term stability of calibration. Before each examination, UBIS makes two measurements: a water reference and a test using the two internal phantoms in order to check that the system is operating correctly.

Normative data are available for European and Asian populations aged 20–80 years. Detailed system specifications are presented in Table 7.3.

DTU-one (Osteometer MediTech A/S, Denmark)

This is also a water-based imaging system similar to the UBIS-3000 described above (Figure 7.4A and B). Both SOS and BUA images are obtained in transmission mode by using a pair of focused 20-mm diameter broadband transducers immersed in a water bath at room temperature. High resolution images (0.6 mm) are acquired on the calcaneus, the maximum scanning area being 60 × 80 mm. A region of interest (ROI) is defined in the posterior part of the calcaneus as an area with a local minimum attenuation.[15] The ability to identify precisely a well defined area of the calcaneus ensures that the same area of the bone is assessed at repeated measurement. This is supposed to make the measurements independent of overall heel size and positioning of the foot.

TOF velocity is calculated using an assumed fixed heel thickness. A daily quality assurance phantom is also provided. Detailed system specifications are presented in Table 7.4.

Calcaneal dry QUS systems

AOS-100 (Aloka Co. Ltd, Japan)

AOS-100 (Acoustic Osteo Screener) (Figure 7.5) uses gel as a form of coupling (dry system), measures SOS and transmission index (TI) and generates an index called osteo sono-assessment index (OSI). The 25-mm diameter broadband ultrasound transducers are manually positioned over the calcaneus in direct contact with the patient's skin. The transducers are encased in a rubber material that is soft enough to adapt to the shape of the calcaneus. The time of ultrasound propagation through the heel

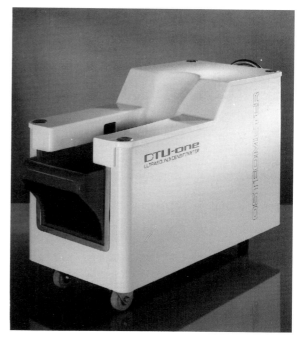

A

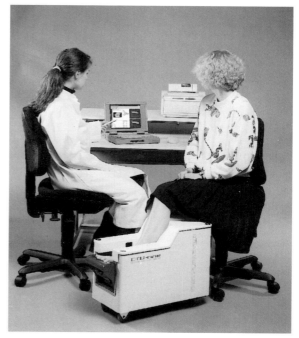

B

Figure 7.4 DTU-one (Osteometer MediTech A/S, Denmark).

Table 7.4 Technical specifications for the DTU-one.

Clinical			
	Precision (CV%)	Annual change	
		%/year	units/year
BUA	1.2		
Velocity	0.16		

Transducer	
Diameter	20 mm
Central frequency	0.5 MHz
Frequency range	200–800 kHz
Frequency used to calculate BUA	300–650 kHz
Mode	Focused

Data acquisition	
Scan time	3 minutes
Scan area	60 × 80 mm
Computer requirement	75 MHz Pentium

Physical dimension of scanner	
Weight	22 kg
Length	53 cm
Width	28 cm
Height	44 cm

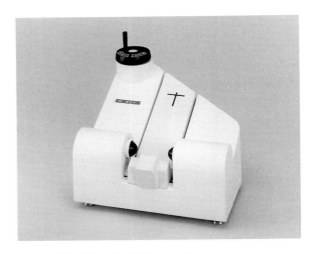

Figure 7.5 AOS-100 (Aloka Co. Ltd, Japan).

(transit time) is automatically measured from the start of the transmitted wave to the start of the leading edge of the received pulse. The heel width is also automatically measured and the velocity thus calculated by dividing the heel width by the transit time.

The TI is a value related to the frequency-dependent attenuation when ultrasound is transmitted through the bone. The received waveform is displayed in the time domain and TI is defined as the half-width of the first maximum value of the received waveform. The OSI is then calculated as: $OSI = TI*SOS^2$.

Two standard types of foot adapters are available. A large type is for a foot of 25 cm or more, while the medium type is for a foot of 22 cm to less than 25 cm. The adapters are an attempt to measure the same location on varying foot sizes. Detailed system specifications are presented in Table 7.5.

CUBA Clinical (McCue plc, UK)
A detailed description of this dry system's mode of operation is given by Langton et al.[16] Two 19-mm diameter broadband ultrasound transducers are positioned by spring action over the calcaneus with a constant pressure in direct contact with the patient's skin. The clinical version has coupling silicone pads which assist in accommodating various heel shapes (Figure 7.6). To improve precision, an iterative algorithm ensures consistency of coupling and positioning by requiring the complete removal of the heel from the system, recoupling and repositioning.

Table 7.5 Technical specifications for the AOS-100.			
Clinical			
	Precision (CV%)	Annual change	
		%/year	units/year
SOS	0.1		
TI	0.95		
OSI	1.9		
Transducer			
Diameter	25 mm		
Central frequency	0.5 MHz		
Frequency range			
Frequency used to calculate BUA	N/A		
Mode	Unfocused		
Data acquisition			
Scan time	2 seconds		
Scan area	Fixed point		
Computer requirement			
Physical dimension of scanner			
Weight	38 kg		
Length	38 cm		
Width	38 cm		
Height	30 cm		

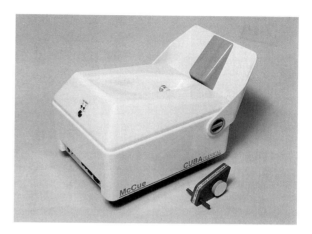

Figure 7.6 CUBA Clinical (McCue plc, UK).

The time of ultrasound propagation through the heel (transit time) is automatically measured from the start of the transmitted wave to the start of the leading edge of the received pulse. Heel width is also automatically measured and the velocity calculated by dividing the heel width by the transit time.

BUA is calculated via an FFT algorithm. The calculated amplitude spectrum for a patient's heel is compared with a reference spectrum stored within the system (see Chapter 6). BUA values are not normalized for heel thickness in the clinical system. There is a CUBA Research version that allows the user to normalize BUA for heel thickness and permits varying transducer arrangements and frequency ranges.

The CUBA Clinical has incorporated an electronic phantom.[17] This is a two-stage active low-pass filter, which provides two levels of BUA (~40–~80 dB/MHz) simulation within the dynamic working range. A water-filled phantom is also provided, which is used to couple the transducers and allows the electronic phantom to be used for all calibration and quality assurance check procedures. Detailed system specifications are presented in Table 7.6.

Sahara (Hologic Inc., USA)
The Sahara is a dry and contact heel ultrasound system, developed to emulate the wet Walker Sonix system. Two single-element, 19-mm diameter broadband ultrasound transducers are mounted on a motorized caliper mechanism, and are coupled to the heel via soft elastomer pads and a coupling gel. The pads

Table 7.6 Technical specifications for the CUBA Clinical.

Clinical			
	Precision (CV%)	Annual change	
		%/year	units/year
BUA	2.5	0.8	
Velocity	0.5		
Transducer			
Diameter	19 mm		
Central frequency	1 MHz		
Frequency range	0.2–1 MHz		
Frequency used to calculate BUA	0.2–0.6 MHz		
Mode	Unfocused		
Data acquisition			
Scan time	2 minutes		
Scan area	Fixed point		
Computer requirement	40 MB hard drive; 4 MB RAM		
Physical dimension of scanner			
Weight	10 kg		
Length	45.4 cm		
Width	35.4 cm		
Height	25.8 cm		

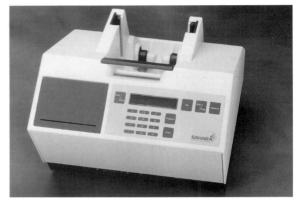

A

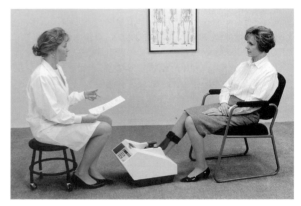

B

Figure 7.7 Sahara (Hologic Inc., USA).

(shaped to improve contact with the calcaneus) are placed in direct contact with the patient's skin (Figure 7.7A and B), and position encoders mechanically measure the width of the heel.

BUA is measured as previously described and SOS is determined by comparing the transit time to the mechanically measured heel width. The Sahara system linearly combines BUA and SOS values, with equal weighting into a single parameter called quantitative ultrasound index (QUI). QUI has a young adult value of about 100. This is analogous to Stiffness used by Achilles (Lunar). The QUI parameter is highly correlated to heel BMD results obtained by DXA, and thus the estimated heel BMD is obtained from the QUI by linear rescaling. Estimated heel BMD results are reported by Sahara in g/cm^2.

Two configurations are available, namely the 'clinical' and 'advanced clinical' models. The standard clinical model is a self-contained unit with LCD display and internal printer that produces hard copy output with SOS, BUA and QUI values. The advanced clinical model includes an external computer with a database for storage of patient information and measurement results.

A rigid foot positioning device is provided to insure reproducibility of leg and foot position during data acquisition. Detailed system specifications are presented in Table 7.7.

Paris (Norland Medical Systems, USA)

The Paris (Figure 7.8) is the most recent commercial calcaneal ultrasound scanner and this review is based on the initial information released by the manufacturer at the time of the first announcement of the system in late 1997.

The Norland Paris is a development of the Concordant, a dry QUS system initially manufactured in Canada and chosen for CaMos

Table 7.7 Technical specifications for the Sahara.

Clinical

	Precision		Annual change	
	$CV\%^a$	SCV^b	%/year	units/year
BUA	3.5	(3.5)	1.0	0.75 dB/MHz
Velocity	0.22	(2.3)	0.09	1.45 m/s
QUI	2.1	(2.5)	0.92	0.90 (QUI)
Est. heel BMD	2.4	(2.4)	1.0	0.0057 g/cm²

Transducer

Diameter	19 mm
Central frequency	0.6 MHz
Frequency range	0.1–1.0 MHz
Frequency used to calculate BUA	0.2–0.6 MHz
Mode	Unfocused

Data acquisition

Scan time	10 seconds
Scan area	Fixed point
Computer requirement	Optional

Physical dimension of scanner

Weight	10 kg
Length	36 cm
Width	43 cm
Height	30 cm

[a] CV in % of young adult value.
[b] SCV, (precision error)/(annual change).

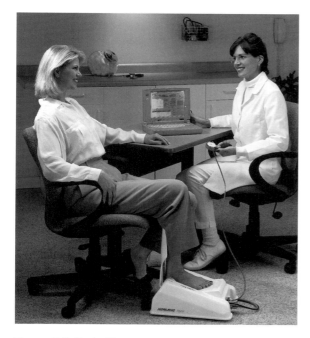

Figure 7.8 Paris (Norland Medical Systems, USA).

(Canadian Multicentre Osteoporosis Study), a study of the prevalence and incidence of osteoporosis in Canada conducted nationwide in 10 000 subjects aged 25 years and over, which commenced in 1996. The Concordant was chosen for the CaMos study because of its portability, ease of use, speed and stability.

The Paris is a dry system with pads coupled to the patient's heel using gel. However, to incorporate some of the advantages of water-based ultrasound systems, the contact pads are inflated by a small pressurized reservoir of air-free water, which forms the main coupling medium between the transducers and the heel.

Measurements are made of BUA and limb velocity (called VOS), and the two measures are combined to give a quantity called Soundness, an index of bone fragility similar in concept to Stiffness on the Lunar Achilles and QUI on the Hologic Sahara. A probe monitors ambient temperature with an accuracy of $\pm 0.1°C$ and allows corrections to be made for the temperature variation of the SOS in water. The weight is 4 kg, making the system light and portable. Population reference values for Caucasian male and female subjects are available from the CaMos study. Further technical information is given in Table 7.8.

Finger QUS systems

DBM Sonic 1200 (IGEA srl, Italy)
This system uses fixed point transmission technique to measure amplitude-dependent ultrasound velocity through the proximal phalanges of the last four fingers of the hand[18] (Figure 7.9). Two 16-mm diameter, 1.25 MHz transducers are assembled on a high precision caliper (± 0.02 mm) that measures the distance between the probes. The probes are positioned on the medio-lateral surfaces of the distal metaphysis of the phalanx using the phalanx head as reference point. Coupling is achieved by using standard ultrasound gel. The TOF is defined as the time from emitted pulse to received signal that is above a predetermined amplitude value. When a normal bone is tested, the amplitude of the first signal received is above the predetermined threshold, but for osteoporotic bone, significant attenuation occurs and the amplitude of the first signal is not enough to trigger the reading. The velocity thus measured is amplitude related, hence amplitude-dependent SOS

(Ad-SOS). This enables the differences in SOS measured between normal and osteoporotic bone to be magnified. The positioning of the probes is slightly adjusted until the optimum signal (defined in terms of number of peaks and the amplitude of the peaks) is recorded on the screen. Measurements are carried out on each

Table 7.8 Technical specifications for the Paris.

Clinical			
		Precision (CV%)	Annual change
			%/year units/year
BUA		1.8	
Velocity		0.4	
Soundness			

Transducer	
Diameter	23 mm
Central frequency	0.5 MHz
Frequency range	
Frequency used to calculate BUA	
Mode	Unfocused

Data acquisition	
Scan time	2 seconds
Scan area	Fixed point
Computer requirement	Pentium

Physical dimension of scanner	
Weight	4 kg
Length	36 cm
Width	29 cm
Height	13 cm

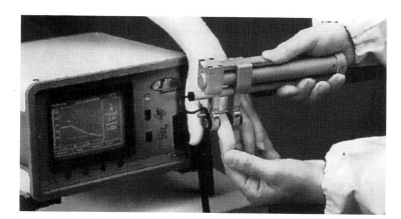

Figure 7.9 DBM Sonic 1200 (IGEA srl, Italy).

of the four phalanges and the results averaged. The proximal phalanges were chosen because of their cortical and cancellous bone composition and because of the high degree of bone turnover occurring at the metaphiseal level.

The manufacturers are also working on improving the system's diagnostic sensitivity by analysing the pattern of the received signal and by generating what is termed 'ultrasound bone profile score (UBPS)' based on the fuzzy logic approach. This grades the transmitted ultrasound signal by combining a number of parameters affected by the status of the bone. These include: number of peaks, relative amplitudes of peaks, peak regression and the trend of velocities in the four fingers. A Plexiglas phantom is provided for daily check system stability. The Ad-SOS reading should be 2760 ± 20 m/s; the exact values vary from system to system. Detailed system specifications are presented in Table 7.9.

Tibial QUS systems

SoundScan (Myriad Ultrasound Systems Ltd, Israel)
This system is the first instrument designed to measure longitudinal transmission of an acoustic pulse along the cortical layer of bone.

A proprietary multi-element ultrasound probe measures velocity along a defined and fixed longitudinal distance of the cortical layer of the mid-tibia, parallel to its long axis (Figure 7.10). The mid-tibia was chosen because of its long, straight and smooth surface. This site is defined as the mid-point between the distal apex of the medial malleolus and the distal aspect of the patella. The transducers are coupled to the anterior surface of the tibia through standard ultrasound gel. The transit time of a 250-kHz pulse along a defined 50-mm distance is measured. A single-unit, ultrasound probe houses all the components together with a proprietary array of ultrasound transducers designed to eliminate the effect of soft tissue on velocity. The measurement is performed by placing the probe at the mid-tibial plane parallel to the longitudinal axis of the bone. Then, the probe is moved back and forth across the tibia surface and a minimum of 150–200 discrete velocity readings are recorded. The resultant velocity is a computed average of the five highest readings.[19]

The SoundScan family consists of the SoundScan 2000, designed for the multi-user, research environment and the SoundScan Compact, a portable, lightweight instrument for the individual practitioner. A phantom is supplied for daily check of system stability and the

Table 7.9 Technical specifications for the DBM-Sonic.

Clinical

	Precision (CV%)	Annual change	
		%/year	units/year
Velocity	0.53	0.47	

Transducer

Diameter	12 mm
Central frequency	1.25 MHz
Frequency range	N/A
Frequency used to calculate BUA	N/A
Mode	Unfocused

Data acquisition

Scan time	5–10 minutes
Scan area	Fixed point
Computer requirement	Optional

Physical dimension of scanner

Weight	6.5 kg
Length	26 cm
Width	15 cm
Height	38 cm

Table 7.10 Technical specifications for the SoundScan.

Clinical

	Precision (CV%)	Annual change	
		%/year	units/year
Velocity	0.3–0.4	0.14–0.24	5.4–9.4 m/s

Transducer

Diameter	20 mm
Central frequency	0.25 MHz
Frequency range	0.25–1 MHz
Frequency used to calculate BUA	N/A
Mode	Unfocused

Data acquisition

Scan time	2 minutes
Scan area	12.5 cm^2
Computer requirement	486 DX2-66, 1.2 MB hard drive

Physical dimension of scanner

Weight	4.4 kg
Length	32 cm
Width	36 cm
Height	15 cm

velocity reading should be within 3940 ± 10 m/s. Normative data are available for the female and male Caucasian population as well as the paediatric population. Detailed system specifications are presented in Table 7.10.

Multi-site QUS systems

Omnisense (Sunlight Ultrasound Technologies Ltd, Israel)

To date, QUS using the transmission technique has been limited to peripheral sites because of the high attenuating nature of bone and the varying degree of soft tissue. Sunlight has

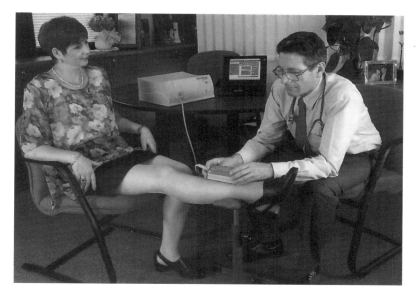

Figure 7.10 SoundScan Compact (Myriad Ultrasound Systems Ltd, Israel).

developed a system to measure velocity based on semi-reflection. The Omnisense prototype is, in fact, a multi-site bone assessment device, capable of measuring SOS at almost any skeletal site, including spine (posterior spinous process and arch), radius, phalanx, calcaneus, iliac crest and many other bones. Femoral neck and greater trochanter capability is currently under development (Figure 7.11).

The Omnisense consists of a desktop unit and a family of up to five proprietary probes designed for different skeletal sites. Bone SOS measurements are based on a complex proprietary ultrasound measurement sequence which compensates for the actual soft tissue characteristics (i.e. velocity and thickness) at the skeletal site measured. Fermat's principle is used to identify the sound path at the critical angle of refraction at which the propagation time between transmitter and detector is a minimum. Since the soft tissue characteristics are measured at different points along the bone surface, one does not have to assume the constancy of the surrounding soft tissue. The sequence is executed by several transducers (transmitter/receiver) packed tightly in each probe. The bone velocity obtained will reflect either cortical or trabecular bone depending on cortex thickness at the skeletal site being measured.

The Omnisense is designed for small clinics and primary care providers, as well as large

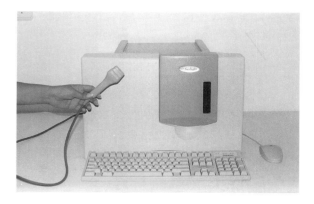

Figure 7.11 Omnisense (Sunlight Ultrasound Technologies Ltd, Israel).

clinics and hospitals. Preliminary data gathered for these first generation devices demonstrate good fracture discrimination for individual sites as well as for a combination of sites.[20–22] Detailed system specifications are presented in Table 7.11.

Miscellaneous

There are other ultrasound systems developed and locally distributed such as in Canada, Italy, Germany and France. However, detailed information is not yet available. In addition, it is expected that more commercial ultrasound systems will become available in the near future.

CROSS CALIBRATION

Table 7.11 Technical specifications for the Omnisense.		
Clinical		
	Precision (CV%)	*Annual change*
		%/year *units/year*
Velocity[a]	0.24–1.2	0.18–0.3 5–10 m/s
Transducer		
Diameter	Variable	
Central frequency	0.5 MHz	
Frequency range	N/A	
Frequency used to calculate BUA	N/A	
Mode	Unfocused	
Data acquisition		
Scan time	1 minute per site	
Scan area	Vary with site	
Computer requirement	Included with the system	
Physical dimension of scanner		
Weight	15 kg	
Length	44 cm	
Width	47 cm	
Height		

[a]These values vary depending on the site measured.

The scientific community has not yet seriously addressed the issue of cross calibration for different QUS devices. In many situations, the differences between different QUS devices are not important. For example, in a clinic with only one machine on which all patients are measured, the relative differences between manufacturers are not important. As long as the scanner used is stable, the analysis technique is consistent and patients are not scanned on any other systems, any observed changes in ultrasound parameter over time can be assumed to be real and not due to machine artefact. However, investigators often do not have the luxury of using only a single machine for the duration of a study. Also, many older QUS devices will be replaced in the coming years, and a hospital or clinic may choose to switch to another manufacturer's system. In either case, the continued monitoring of bone status in patients would be complicated by this change in equipment.

In clinical drug trials using ultrasonic information, multiple centres are typically used in order to enroll the number of patients needed to establish the efficacy of a particular pharmaceutical. More often than not, the centres enrolled will be equipped with a variety of different scanners. Due to differences in ultrasound values, direct comparisons of centres with different equipment cannot be made without performing cross calibration measurements. The determination of a 'true' ultrasound parameter becomes arbitrary at this point, as no ultrasound standard has yet been established.

Simple comparisons of patient ultrasound values with established normals are also complicated by the disparate results obtained on different scanners. Evaluations can only be performed properly by using normative data obtained on the same type of system, otherwise the comparisons will be invalid. By quantifying the differences between manufacturers, a set of universal normative data would be possible, compiled from the normative data results of all the manufacturers. The establishment of a single normative data set would unify the diagnostic results obtained on the various systems.

As ultrasound systems become widely used both for diagnosis and drug trials, the question of how to compare results from different machines arises. As described in the preceding sections, clinical systems have differences in the diameter of transducer used, the frequency range and the method of measuring velocity, resulting in a disparity in the results obtained and a difference in the dynamic range of values.

Causes of variation

1) Differences in transducer diameter resulting in unequal amounts of calcaneus being interrogated by the ultrasound wave.
2) The use of focused and unfocused transducers.
3) Physically, there are differences in the area of the calcaneus measured by the different systems, and it is known that the calcaneus is very heterogeneous.
4) The definition of transit time results in significant differences in calculated velocities. Nicholson et al.[23] found that zero-crossing used by Achilles resulted in the lowest velocity compared to first deviation from zero used by CUBA Clinical.
5) The definition of velocity also adds another complexity – bone velocity, limb velocity and time of flight velocity.[11]
6) Use of fixed or assumed fixed heel width in velocity calculation.
7) Different algorithm for calculating BUA resulting in systematic differences in BUA between manufacturers. For example, the Achilles and DTU-one have a range of BUA

values significantly narrower than the Sahara and CUBA.

There is a need to identify accurately the sources and magnitude of all the variations so that accurate cross calibration can be achieved and measurements interchanged between machines.

Glüer et al.[24] carried out a study on a group of 30 women using both the Walker Sonix UBA575 and the Lunar Achilles. They reported that the BUA readings obtained on the two machines differed substantially, and the correlation between the UBA575 BUA and the Achilles BUA was markedly lower than correlations between bone densitometers measuring the same site. Therefore, BUA results cannot accurately be extrapolated from one device to another. No large comparative assessment of velocity has been reported for these clinical systems. Strelitzki et al.[25] have also addressed this problem using phantoms on three different manufacturers' systems. They found intra- and intermanufacturer variation in measured values.

QUALITY CONTROL (QC) IN THE USE OF QUS

It is very important to apply a stringent QC programme when using QUS in bone status assessment. This is partly because changes in SOS and BUA due to disease or treatment are relatively small. Therefore, measurements of bone status changes have to be very precise because procedural errors, malfunctioning equipment or erroneous data analysis may cause substantial interference, even if the data are erroneous by only a few percentage points. The QC protocols should be designed to ascertain that the equipment is functioning properly. Machine differences and lack of an absolute ultrasound bone phantom or of universally accepted cross-calibration procedures result in BUA and/or SOS variations when measuring the same subject on different systems.

The degree of complexity of the QC programme will depend on whether it is for an individual site or for a multicentre clinical trial.

At an individual site, for example, two types of testing could be carried out: acceptance testing and routine testing.

Acceptance testing includes accuracy, in vivo and in vitro precision and power output measurement. In vivo measurement should cover a wide age and body status range. This is because precision has been reported to vary between normal and osteoporotic subjects.

Routine testing includes regular measurement of a QC phantom to detect any drift in the machine and periodic graphical analysis of QC data. Ultrasound bone phantoms are not yet available but most manufacturers will provide system-specific ones. However, these system-specific phantoms are not anthropomorphic and their daily changes may not reflect what might happen in vivo.

Another aspect of QC is operator training. Indeed, positioning error is one of the major sources of imprecision in QUS.[26] It is the main source of error that depends on the working procedures of technicians.

PRECISION

Before discussing this issue, it is important for readers to understand some fundamental concepts, which will allow them to form their own opinions concerning precision. Most instrument performance evaluations have focused on reproducibility of measurement results and on assessing variations in measurement results in response to age, disease and treatment. The results and the interpretation of these comparisons have been complicated due to differences in the technology used, the variability of the parameters measured, the site and the system. Consequently, simple comparison of precision is inadequate because a technique with poor precision but ability to demonstrate larger changes over time is preferable to a competing 'high-precision' approach.[27,28] In the past, people used to report reproducibility as the coefficient of variation (CV), defined by reporting the precision error as a percentage of the mean measured value. The CVs generally quoted in the literature are presented in Table

7.1, while the manufacturers' quoted CVs are presented in Tables 7.2–7.11. However, the limitation of using the CV as a reliable figure of merit is its failure to take into account the possible range of values of BUA and velocity in clinical studies. To overcome these hurdles, proposals have been made to standardize the precision error of ultrasound measurement.[29,30] So far, several standardized coefficient of variation (SCV) definitions have been proposed, for example, dividing precision errors by one of the following factors: (1) the difference between healthy and osteoporotic individuals; (2) rates of changes due to disease or treatment; (3) the natural variability of healthy individuals; and (4) normal annual rates of skeletal changes. Other more sophisticated approaches for expressing diagnostic sensitivity have been suggested.[31,32] For example, Miller et al.[29] based their approach to standardized precision errors on the ratio of per cent precision and per cent range of results (5th to 95th percentile). There is a consensus that the methods of assessing longitudinal sensitivity require standardization, but there is disagreement about the preferred approach. As long as there is no consensus on the standard method, employing one of the simpler approaches for standardization may be recommended; for example, dividing the precision error by the age-related change typical for that subject group. If this statistic is not available, a crude estimate could be obtained by dividing the precision error by the standard deviation of the subjects of the study. The smaller the resulting ratios, the better the longitudinal sensitivity.

Factors affecting precision

In vivo precision is affected by soft tissue, heel thickness, coupling and repositioning error. Using the Walker Sonix UBA1001, Evans et al.[26] carried out an extensive study of the factors that might affect precision. These included: immersion time of the foot in the water bath, water depth, water temperature, concentration of detergents and various rotations of the foot. They found that foot positioning was the major cause of measurement imprecision in BUA. This is due to the spatial variation of BUA in the calcaneus. They proposed that the optimum measuring temperature of the water bath was $32 \pm 2°C$ since they demonstrated a decrease in BUA with temperatures above 34°C. The thickness of the overlying soft tissue has been reported, using the Achilles system, to affect only velocity and not BUA.[33] It might be expected that for the UBA575+, where soft tissue corrections are made and true bone velocity is measured, the effect will be negligible.

REFERENCES

1. Langton CM, Palmer SB, Porter RW. The measurement of broadband ultrasonic attenuation in cancellous bone. *Eng Med* (1984) **13:** 89–91.

2. Vogel JM, Wasnich RD, Ross PD. The clinical relevance of calcaneus bone mineral measurements: a review. *Bone Miner* (1988) **5:** 35–58.

3. Wasnich RD, Ross PD, Heilbrun LK, Vogel JM. Selection of the optimal skeletal site for fracture risk prediction. *Clin Orthop* (1987) **216:** 262–9.

4. Black DM, Cummings SR, Genant HK et al. Axial and appendicular bone density predict fractures in older women. *J Bone Miner Res* (1992) **7:** 633–8.

5. Kleerekoper M, Nelson DA, Flynn MJ et al. Comparison of radiographic absorptiometry with dual-energy x-ray absorptiometry and quantitative computed tomography in normal older white and black women. *J Bone Miner Res* (1994) **9:** 1745–9.

6. Truscott JG, Simpson M, Stewart SP et al. Bone ultrasonic attenuation in women: reproducibility, normal variation and comparison with photon absorptiometry. *Clin Phys Physiol Meas* (1992) **13:** 29–36.

7. Waud CE, Lew R, Baran DT. The relationship between ultrasound and densitometric measurements of bone mass at the calcaneus in women. *Calcif Tissue Int* (1992) **51:** 415–18.

8. Evans JA, Tavakoli MB. Temperature and direction dependence of the attenuation and velocity of ultrasound in cancellous and cortical bone. In: Ring EFG, Bhalla AK eds. *Current research in osteoporosis and bone measurement II.* (British Institute of Radiology: London, 1992) 43.

9. Njeh CF. The dependence of ultrasound velocity and attenuation on material properties of cancellous bone [PhD]. (Sheffield Hallam University: Sheffield, UK, 1995).

10. Zagzebski JA, Rossman PJ, Mesina C et al. Ultrasound transmission measurements through the os calcis. *Calcif Tissue Int* (1991) **49:** 107–11.

11. Njeh CF, Boivin CM, Langton CM. The role of ultrasound in the assessment of osteoporosis: a review. *Osteoporos Int* (1997) **7:** 7–22.

12. Lees B, Stevenson JC. Preliminary evaluation of a new ultrasound bone densitometer. *Calcif Tissue Int* (1993) **53:** 149–52.

13. Laugier P, Droin P, Laval-Jeantet AM, Berger G. In vitro assessment of the relationship between acoustic properties and bone mass density of the calcaneus by comparison of ultrasound parametric imaging and quantitative computed tomography. *Bone* (1997) **20:** 157–65.

14. Laugier P, Giat P, Berger G. Broadband ultrasonic attenuation imaging: a new imaging technique of the os calcis. *Calcif Tissue Int* (1994) **54:** 83–6.

15. Jorgensen HL, Hassager C. Improved reproducibility of broadband ultrasound attenuation of the os calcis by using specific region of interest. *Bone* (1997) **21:** 109–12.

16. Langton CM, Ali AV, Riggs CM et al. A contact method for the assessment of ultrasonic velocity and broadband attenuation in cortical and cancellous bone. *Clin Phys Physiol Meas* (1990) **11:** 243–9.

17. Langton CM. Development of an electronic phantom for calibration, cross-correlation and quality assurance of broadband ultrasound attenuation measurement in the calcaneus [abstract]. *Osteoporos Int* (1997) **7:** 309.

18. Cadossi R, Cane V. Pathways of transmission of ultrasound energy through the distal metaphysis of the second phalanx of pigs: an in vitro study. *Osteoporos Int* (1996) **6:** 196–206.

19. Orgee JM, Foster H, McCloskey EV et al. A precise method for the assessment of tibial ultrasound velocity. *Osteoporos Int* (1996) **6:** 1–7.

20. Hans D, Barkmann R, Kantorovich E et al. Discrimination of hip fractures by quantitative ultrasound at multiple measurement sites. *J Bone Miner Res* (1997) **12:** S383.

21. Barkmann R, Hans D, Kantorovich E et al. Discrimination of forearm fractures by quantitative ultrasound at multiple measurement sites. *J Bone Miner Res* (1997) **12:** S385.

22. Hans D, Weiss M, Fuerst T et al. A new reflection quantitative ultrasound system: preliminary

results of multisite bone measurments. *Osteoporos Int* (1997) **7**: 300.

23. Nicholson PHF, Lowet G, Langton CM et al. A comparison of time-domain and frequency-domain approaches to ultrasonic velocity measurement in trabecular bone. *Phys Med Biol* (1996) **41**: 2421–35.

24. Glüer CC, Wu CW, Genant HK. Disparity of different BUA approaches. *Calcif Tissue Int* (1993) **52**: S171.

25. Strelitzki R, Clarke AJ, Evans JA. The measurement of the velocity of ultrasound in fixed trabecular bone using broadband pulses and single-frequency tone bursts. *Phys Med Biol* (1996) **41**: 743–53.

26. Evans WD, Jones EA, Owen GM. Factors affecting the in vivo precision of broad-band ultrasonic attenuation. *Phys Med Biol* (1995) **40**: 137–51.

27. Genant HK, Engelke K, Fuerst T et al. Noninvasive assessment of bone mineral and structure: state of the art. *J Bone Miner Res* (1996) **11**: 707–30.

28. Genant HK, Block JE, Steiger P et al. Appropriate use of bone densitometry. *Radiology* (1989) **170**: 817–22.

29. Miller CG, Herd RJ, Ramalingam T et al. Ultrasonic velocity measurements through the calcaneus: which velocity should be measured? *Osteoporos Int* (1993) **3**: 31–5.

30. Moris M, Peretz A, Tjeka R et al. Quantitative ultrasound bone measurements: normal values and comparison with bone mineral density by dual X-ray absorptiometry. *Calcif Tissue Int* (1995) **57**: 6–10.

31. Davis JW, Ross PD, Wasnich RD et al. Long-term precision of bone loss rate measurements among postmenopausal women. *Calcif Tissue Int* (1991) **48**: 311–18.

32. Glüer CC, Blunt B, Engelke K et al. 'Characteristic follow-up time' – a new concept for standardized characterization of a technique's ability to monitor longitudinal changes. *Bone Miner* (1994) **25**(suppl 2): S40.

33. Kotzki PO, Buyck D, Hans D et al. Influence of fat on ultrasound measurements of the os calcis. *Calcif Tissue Int* (1994) **54**: 91–5.

8

Assessment of Instrument Performance: Precision, Installation of New Equipment and Radiation Dose

CHAPTER OVERVIEW

This chapter discusses three aspects of instrument performance that are important in the evaluation of bone densitometry equipment. The first of these is *measurement precision*, which is frequently used to characterize the ability of a device to monitor significant change in the skeleton. Precision, usually expressed as the coefficient of variation (CV) of repeated measurements, is the most widely quoted index used in the evaluation of instrument performance. Probably the majority of published clinical studies include some assessment of precision. However, despite the popularity of the concept, the best way to express precision is still the subject of controversy. The limitation of quoting precision using the CV is that it takes no account of the relative magnitude of the changes associated with ageing, established osteoporosis or response to treatment. To allow for the size of likely changes, and thus derive an index that gives a truer reflection of an instrument's clinical potential, many authors have proposed substituting CV with the standardized coefficient of variation (SCV), in

which reproducibility is normalized to some measure of the range of clinical values. As yet, however, there is no generally agreed definition of SCV.

The second section of this chapter discusses the *installation of a new DXA system*, including advice on radiation safety requirements. Although bone densitometry equipment is robust and will generally function well for many years, some research studies may continue for 5 years or longer. On this timescale it is inevitable that many centres will feel the need to replace equipment, often to expand facilities or to take advantage of advances in technology. In such circumstances it is important to ensure the continuity (or at least the traceability) of the bone mineral density (BMD) measurement scale. A discussion is given of the cross calibration of new dual-energy X-ray absorptiometry (DXA) systems to ensure agreement with the older systems being replaced.

The final aspect of equipment performance discussed in this chapter is *radiation dose*. The exceptionally low dose to patients and technologists from DXA investigations has undoubtedly been a major factor in the widespread acceptance and rapid expansion of the technology. Detailed assessments of patient dose are required for submissions to local ethics committees for research projects, and a knowledge of radiation dose can be useful for reassuring anxious patients. The introduction of fan-beam DXA systems has tended to increase radiation levels, and has required a re-evaluation of the radiation protection of technologists.

ACCURACY AND PRECISION

This review of the evaluation of equipment performance begins with a discussion of the methods used to assess the accuracy and precision of bone densitometry investigations.

The accuracy errors of a test reflect the degree to which the measured results deviate from true values. In the case of bone mineral measurements it is generally accepted that true bone mineral content (BMC) is obtained by defatting bone and ashing under standard conditions (600°C for 24 hours) in a muffle furnace. To find true BMD, it is also necessary to radiograph specimens to measure the projected area. Despite the obvious importance of validating the accuracy of bone densitometry techniques, only a few studies of dual photon absorptiometry (DPA) or DXA have addressed this issue.[1-8] Comparisons of in situ BMD measurements in cadavers with results of ashing show differences between 0% and 15%. These may be explained by factors such as errors caused by soft tissue composition, the fat content of bone and errors in the measurement of the projected area inherent in different edge-detection algorithms.

In general, small accuracy errors are of little clinical significance provided they remain constant. Precision errors reflect the reproducibility of a diagnostic technique and in practice often have greater clinical relevance than accuracy errors. A knowledge of precision errors is important for two reasons. First, results are interpreted against the relevant reference range and if the population standard deviation is relatively narrow as, for example, for some speed of sound (SOS) measurements, a technique with

extremely poor precision may actually lead to the misinterpretation of results. More frequently, however, precision errors are important because it is necessary to decide whether a follow-up scan shows evidence of significant change.

Short-term precision

All studies of new instrumentation or new applications should include an assessment of short-term precision. This entails performing a number of repeated measurements on a representative set of individuals to characterize the reproducibility of the technique. Generally, for studies of short-term precision the repeated measurements on each individual subject are performed either on the same day or extending over a time period of no more than 2 weeks. Over such a short time period no true change in BMD is expected (Figure 8.1A). If the repeated measurements on each subject are performed immediately following each other, then it is important that the patient should stand up and be repositioned between measurements if the effects of both instrumental and positioning errors are to be properly assessed. For any one individual, the repeated measurements may be used to calculate the mean and standard deviation (SD):

$$\bar{x}_j = \Sigma_i x_{ij}/m \qquad (8.1)$$

$$\mathrm{VAR}(x_j) = \Sigma_i(x_{ij} - \bar{x}_j)^2/(m - 1) \qquad (8.2)$$

$$\mathrm{SD}(x_j) = \sqrt{\mathrm{VAR}(x_j)} \qquad (8.3)$$

where x_{ij} is the ith measurement on the jth subject, $\bar{x}_j$ is the mean, $\mathrm{VAR}(x_j)$ the variance and $\mathrm{SD}(x_j)$ the SD for the jth subject, and m is the number of measurements for each subject. Note in equation 8.2 that the sum of squares term is divided by $(m - 1)$, not by m. On some pocket calculators and computer programs the user is given the option of calculating SD by dividing by either m or $(m - 1)$. However, $(m - 1)$ should be used in circumstances where the mean is not known to start with, but has to be

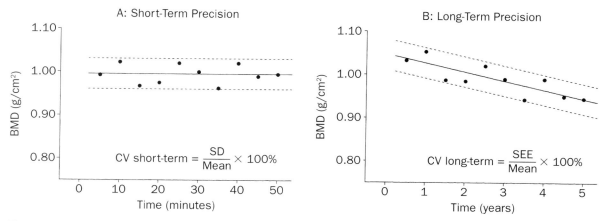

Figure 8.1 (A) Definition of short-term precision. Over short time periods no real change in BMD is expected. Precision is expressed as the coefficient of variation by writing the standard deviation (SD) as a percentage of the mean. (B) Definition of long-term precision. Over long time periods real changes in BMD are likely. If the secular change is linear with time then the random measurement errors are expressed by the standard error of the estimate (SEE) derived from linear regression analysis. Precision is expressed as the coefficient of variation by writing the SEE as a percentage of the mean.

calculated from the same data set as the SD (i.e. as in equations 8.1 and 8.2).

For many purposes the absolute error expressed by the SD is the most satisfactory way of expressing the short-term precision. However, given the widely differing numerical values of BMD or quantitative ultrasound (QUS) parameters, it is a popular convention to express precision data as the relative error (or CV) by dividing the SD by the mean:

$$CV(x_j) = (SD(x_j)/\bar{x}_j) \cdot 100\% \qquad (8.4)$$

which gives a more intuitive presentation of the precision error. Thus, when expressed as the SD, the precision for a DXA measurement of spine BMD and a ultrasound measurement of SOS might be 0.01 g/cm² and 16 m/s respectively. However, when expressed as the CV, both measurements have a precision of 1%.

It is frequently necessary to combine precision data obtained from a number of subjects. In this case the precision error is calculated by first finding the mean and variance of the

repeated measurements on each subject using equations 8.1 and 8.2, and then averaging the individual means and variances for all the subjects studied:

$$\bar{x} = \Sigma_j \bar{x}_j / n \qquad (8.5)$$

$$\overline{VAR(x)} = \Sigma_j VAR(x_j)/n \qquad (8.6)$$

where n is the number of subjects studied. A statistically unbiased estimate of the true precision error is obtained by finding the root mean square (RMS) SD calculated from the square root of the mean variance:

$$RMS\ SD(x) = \sqrt{\overline{VAR(x)}} \qquad (8.7)$$

The most widely adopted convention for calculating the coefficient of variation for data from a group of subjects is to divide the RMS SD by the mean of all subjects and express the result as a percentage:

$$CV(x) = (RMS\ SD(x)/\bar{x}) \cdot 100\% \qquad (8.8)$$

One of the most frequently adopted study

designs is to perform duplicate measurements on each subject ($m = 2$). In this instance the SD for each subject is conveniently calculated by dividing the difference, d, between the two measurements by $\sqrt{2}$. Hence, for the special case of duplicate measurements:

$$SD(x_j) = d_j/\sqrt{2} \text{ where} \tag{8.9}$$

$$d_j = (x_{1j} - x_{2j}) \tag{8.10}$$

The mean is found by adding all the results together and dividing by the total number of measurements, i.e. $2n$:

$$\bar{x} = \Sigma_j(x_{1j} + x_{2j})/2n \tag{8.11}$$

The coefficient of variation is then calculated from the equation:

$$CV(x) = \frac{\sqrt{(\Sigma_j d_j^2/2n)}}{\bar{x}} \cdot 100 \tag{8.12}$$

Some authors choose to combine the precision data from different subjects by taking the arithmetic mean rather than the RMS of the individual SD. However, this approach is unsatisfactory because it leads to a systematic underestimation of the true Gaussian error, σ, by a factor that varies with the number of repeated measurements per subject, m. These factors were calculated by Glüer et al.[9] and are listed in Table 8.1.

It is often not appreciated that, because the evaluation of precision involves determining an SD, the random statistical errors are inherently large unless the study design includes a sufficiently large number of repeated measurements. If (as above) the design involves m repeated measurements made on each of n subjects, there will be a total of $n \cdot m$ measurements. However, since it is necessary to calculate the mean BMD of each subject, there are only $n \cdot (m - 1)$ independent measurements from which to evaluate precision. This number is the *degrees of freedom* (df), and is an essential item of information for evaluating the statistical weight of a study.

The statistical errors in estimates of the coefficient of variation are dominated by errors in determining the RMS SD. This latter has two components, the first arising from the size of

Table 8.1 Determination of precision by combining data from repeated measurements on a number of different subjects. The table shows the ratio of the calculated precision error to the true Gaussian error when precision is calculated as: (1) the simple average; (2) the root mean square (RMS) average. (Data from Glüer et al.[9])

Number of repeat measurements per subject	Ratio to true Gaussian error	
	Simple average	RMS average
2	0.798	1.00
3	0.866	1.00
4	0.921	1.00
6	0.952	1.00
12	0.978	1.00

the available data set (given by df), and the second from any true (i.e. non-statistical) differences between subjects in their individual SD. The combined error cannot be smaller than the figure determined by the finite data set available. This latter can be calculated from tables of the chi-squared distribution given the number of degrees of freedom entering into the estimate of the RMS SD. Factors for multiplying the RMS SD to derive the lower (2.5%) and upper (97.5%) confidence limits are shown plotted as a function of df in Figure 8.2, and selected figures are tabulated in Table 8.2. As an example, if four repeated measurements are made on each of 10 subjects, df = 30, i.e. there are three independent measurements on each subject contributing to the estimation of the RMS SD. In this example the resulting 2.5% and 97.5% confidence limits are obtained by multiplying the RMS SD by 0.80 and 1.34 respec-

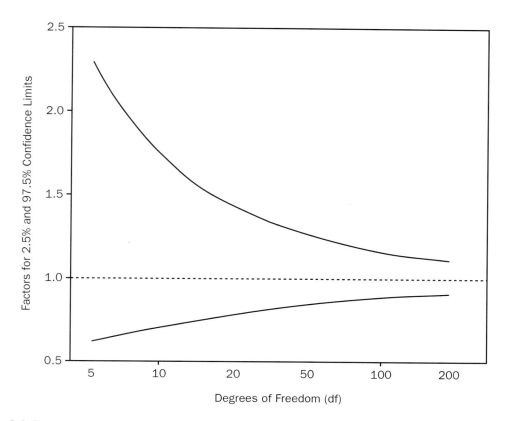

Figure 8.2 The statistical errors in a precision study cannot be smaller than the component arising from the finite data set available. This limit can be calculated from the chi-squared distribution. In this figure the 2.5% and 97.5% confidence limits are plotted as a function of the number of degrees of freedom (df) for a measured coefficient of variation of 1%. For a study with m measurements performed on each of n subjects: df $= n \times (m - 1)$ (after Glüer et al.[9]).

tively. However, it is important to realize that the true errors may be even larger if real differences in precision exist between subjects. The evaluation of this is a complex problem and the interested reader is referred to the article by Glüer et al.[9]

When performing a precision study it is important that the measurements are made on a well defined patient group, i.e. young normal subjects, healthy postmenopausal women or osteoporotic patients. In general with DXA or QUS equipment, the CV is expected to differ between these groups. The issue of real differ-

ences in precision between subjects within such general groups is more difficult to assess because it is unusual for studies to include a sufficient number of repeated measurements on each subject to characterize properly such differences. In the author's experience, obesity can be an important factor in influencing the precision of DXA studies, and care is needed if data from patients with body mass index (BMI) > 30 kg/m² are included because of the effects of excessive attenuation of the radiation and increased heterogeneity of soft tissue composition. For QUS studies, where there is no

Table 8.2 2.5% to 97.5% confidence limits derived from the chi-squared distribution for the estimation of errors in precision studies. Upper and lower error limits are calculated by multiplying the measured precision by the listed factors for the relevant degrees of freedom.[a]

Degrees of freedom	Lower limit	Upper limit
10	0.70	1.75
20	0.77	1.44
30	0.80	1.34
50	0.84	1.24
100	0.88	1.16
200	0.91	1.11

[a]The true errors will be larger if there are real differences in precision between individual subjects.

Table 8.3 Recommendations for conducting precision studies. (From Glüer et al.[9])

Precision errors of individual subjects should be based on standard deviations (for short-term precision) or standard errors of the estimate (for long-term precision) using formulae with correctly calculated degrees of freedom.

For short-term precision measurements, the subjects should be repositioned between measurements.

Averaging of precision errors of several individuals should be based on root mean square (RMS) averages.

The subject group on which the precision estimates are obtained should be clearly characterized (e.g. by giving the mean and SD of age and BMD).

Sufficient data should be obtained to provide at least 30 degrees of freedom for the calculation of precision (i.e. 30 subjects with two measurements each, or 15 with three measurements, or 10 with four measurements, etc.).

radiation safety issue, is it easier to perform the large numbers of measurements on each subject required to evaluate individual precision. When this is done, surprisingly large differences in the CVs of different individual subjects are found, which probably reflect the degree of inhomogeneity of the calcaneus at the measurement site. In this circumstance the finite data set errors shown in Figure 8.2 and Table 8.2 may significantly underestimate the true errors. To avoid selection bias, it is important that precision studies should include measurements spread over a large number of representative subjects.

A summary of advice for performing precision studies is listed in Table 8.3.

Long-term precision

It is important to recognize that precision errors may depend on the time interval between repeated measurements.[9] When new equipment or new applications are evaluated, often only the short-term precision errors are assessed from repeated measurements performed either in a single session or at most over a period of a few weeks. Frequently such studies are likely to reflect optimal conditions unlikely to be realized in routine practice. Although short-term precision studies are relatively easy to perform, it is often more relevant to the interpretation of clinical data to know the long-term precision error defined by the random measurement errors over time periods of months or years.

Generally, long-term precision errors are expected to be larger than short-term errors because they reflect additional sources of random variations such as small drifts in instrument calibration, changes in a patient's weight and soft tissue composition, and variations in patient positioning and other differences in technique for performing and analysing scans that arise over time or between different personnel performing a test.

Because long-term precision errors are measured over time periods in which true changes in BMD may occur, the calculation of long-term precision requires a different mathematical approach from that for short-term precision. Because of these changes, use of the SD (Figure 8.1A) would result in overestimation of the true precision errors. Instead, it is often assumed that many subjects will experience a long-term secular decrease of bone mass with ageing (Figure 8.1B). A parameter that correctly quantifies sources of variability other than a true linear change is the standard error of the estimate (SEE), which can be calculated from linear regression analysis. When repeated measurements are made of the same patient over a long period of time, the SEE quantifies the variability about the regression line. Thus, SEE rather than SD should be taken as the estimate of the long-term precision error. As with short-term precision, results form different individuals can be combined to find the average SEE:

$$\text{RMS SEE}(x) = \sqrt{(\Sigma_j \text{SEE}(x_j)^2/n)} \quad (8.13)$$

and the long-term precision expressed as the coefficient of variation by dividing the RMS SEE by the mean for all subjects and expressing the results as a percentage:

$$\text{CV}(x) = (\text{RMS SEE}(x)/\bar{x}) \cdot 100\% \quad (8.14)$$

The considerations for estimation of the statistical errors in the determination of precision are similar to those for the short-term precision discussed above. However, since linear regression analysis involves the fitting of two free parameters (the slope and intercept) to each patient's data, if m measurements are performed on each of n subjects the total number of degrees of freedom will be df $= n \cdot (m - 2)$.

It is important to be aware that this definition of long-term precision based on the SEE might still include variability because of non-linear changes in bone density. It may not be appropriate therefore in patients who have recently commenced or discontinued treatment for osteoporosis, or women in the first few years after the menopause. However, the data can be examined for systematic deviations from linearity by expressing each measurement in each patient as the residual from the regression line and plotting the trend of the mean of the n residuals at each of the m time points. Statistical analysis for significant deviations from linearity can be performed using analysis of variance.

The interpretation of follow-up scans

In many osteoporosis centres, patients attending outpatient clinics or recommended to take preventive treatment may have one or more follow-up scans. Verifying response to medication is widely believed to have a beneficial function in encouraging compliance with treatment. However, realistic figures for the long-term precision error are essential for the proper evaluation of follow-up scans since they enable a set of clear rules to be drawn up for determining whether the measured changes in BMD indicate a statistically significant response to treatment, or whether BMD is unchanged, or perhaps continuing to fall significantly.

In calculating the smallest detectable change in BMD it is necessary to allow not just for the precision error, but also the statistical significance and power required, since these must be chosen to reflect the importance attached to avoiding a false negative (a type II error) as well as a false positive finding (a type I error).

If CV is the coefficient of variation of the long-term precision error then, because both measurements are affected by precision errors, a 1 SD difference between the initial baseline and a follow-up investigation will be $\sqrt{2}\text{CV}\%$.

The statistical significance of a measured percentage change in BMD of Δ BMD% is therefore:

$$Z_\alpha + Z_\beta = \Delta \text{ BMD}\%/\sqrt{2}\text{CV} \qquad (8.15)$$

where α is the significance level for a type I, and β is the power for a type II error. If a 10% significance level is chosen ($Z_\alpha = 1.28$) and 80% power ($Z_\beta = 0.84$), then equation 8.15 becomes:

$$\Delta \text{ BMD}\% = 3\text{CV} \qquad (8.16)$$

Equation 8.16 defines a figure for the smallest change in BMD that must occur before the clinician can determine with 10% significance and 80% power that a patient's BMD result has shown a statistically significant response to treatment.

In Figure 8.3, results for the smallest detectable change in PA spine and femoral neck BMD are shown superimposed on the results for the mean change in BMD with time

reported by Liberman et al. in postmenopausal osteoporotic women (PA spine T-score < −2.5) treated daily with 10 mg alendronate or placebo.[10] Figures for the long-term precision of 1.5% for PA spine BMD and 2.5% for femoral neck BMD are assumed,[11] giving figures for the smallest measurable change of 4.5% and 7.5% respectively. The increase of 4.5% required for detecting a significant change in the spine was on average reached after 6 months of treatment (Figure 8.3A), while the mean change in femoral neck BMD did not approach the required figure of 7.5%, even after 3 years of treatment (Figure 8.3B).

Choice of measurement site for follow-up scans

It is clear from Figure 8.3 that the choice of the

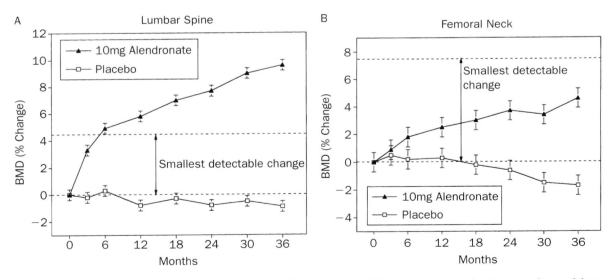

Figure 8.3 Mean (± SE) changes in BMD from baseline in women with postmenopausal osteoporosis receiving placebo or 10 mg alendronate daily for 3 years. (A) PA lumbar spine (L1–L4) BMD; (B) femoral neck BMD. In each plot, the smallest detectable change is plotted assuming a long-term precision error of 1.5% for PA spine BMD and 2.5% for femoral neck BMD (alendronate data from Liberman et al.[10]).

optimum site for performing follow-up scans depends on both the magnitude of the response to treatment and the precision of the measurements. It follows that the ratio of treatment effect over precision is a useful index for comparing the merits of different techniques and measurement sites. The exact numerical results for this ratio depend, however, on the type of treatment and the study population (i.e. elderly osteoporotic versus early postmenopausal women), and so generally can only be applied in the context of a single large study in which data from multiple measurement sites or technologies are available from patient follow-up. Nevertheless, useful comparisons can be made between, for example, spine and femur BMD, PA and lateral spine DXA, comparison between femur sites, or peripheral and axial measurements.

The recently completed multicentre clinical trials of alendronate give an opportunity to make such comparisons. Faulkner et al.[12] have presented data from the EPIC study, an evaluation of the use of low-dose alendronate to prevent bone loss in early postmenopausal women. DXA BMD measurements were available for PA and decubitus lateral spine, four sites in the femur, the total body and two forearm sites. The study findings are summarized in Figure 8.4A, which shows the total treatment effect (defined as the difference between the baseline to 2-year changes in the alendronate-treated and placebo groups) for the different measurement sites. When the total treatment effect is divided by the precision error, the PA spine is shown to be the optimum measurement site for monitoring longitudinal change (Figure 8.4B). Although lateral spine BMD shows a larger treatment effect

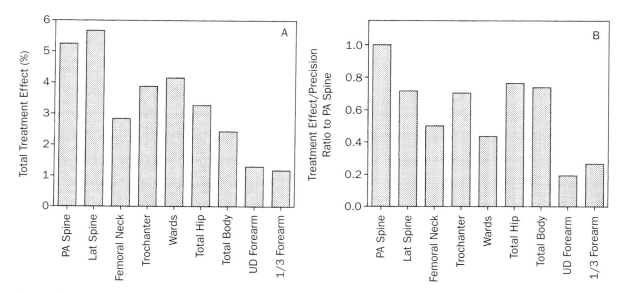

Figure 8.4 Comparison of BMD measurements at nine different skeletal sites in early postmenopausal women receiving placebo or 5 mg alendronate daily. (A) Total treatment effect, defined as the difference in the mean changes in BMD from baseline between the alendronate and placebo groups at 2 years; (B) sensitivity of the different scan sites for monitoring longitudinal change obtained by dividing the total treatment effect by the long-term precision. Results are shown normalized to PA spine BMD (data from Faulkner et al.[12]).

(Figure 8.4A), this is outweighed by the poorer precision for lateral measurements. In the femur, the trochanter and total hip are the best sites. Interestingly, the EPIC study data suggest that the forearm is a relatively poor site for longitudinal studies (Figure 8.4B). However, Christiansen et al. reported much better results for forearm BMD measurements from data collected during four clinical trials (including one study using alendronate) by using a new region of interest with a high percentage of trabecular bone.[13]

Herd reported a similar trial to the EPIC study using cyclical etidronate therapy to prevent early postmenopausal bone loss,[14] although in a smaller group of patients. This study gave an opportunity to compare supine lateral projection scans of the lumbar spine with the conventional PA projections.[15] The results (Figure 8.5) confirm Faulkner's conclusion that although lateral spine BMD shows a larger response to treatment, this advantage is cancelled by the poorer precision. Preston[16] analysed data for the femur sites from Herd's etidronate study, including the new central hip site proposed by Takada et al.,[17] and confirmed that the trochanter and total hip were the optimum sites in the femur.

Standardized coefficient of variation (SCV)

Short-term precision expressed by the coefficient of variation is the index most fre-

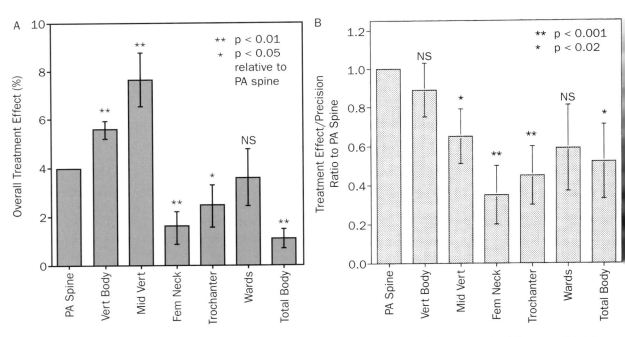

Figure 8.5 Comparison of BMD measurements for the PA spine, supine lateral spine, proximal femur and total body in early postmenopausal women receiving placebo or cyclical etidronate therapy. (A) Total treatment effect, defined as the difference in the mean changes in BMD from baseline between the etidronate and placebo groups at 2 years; (B) sensitivity of the different scan sites for monitoring longitudinal change obtained by dividing the total treatment effect by the long-term precision. Results are shown normalized to PA spine BMD (data from Blake et al.[15]).

quently used to measure the clinical perfor-mance of instrumentation. The discussion above has emphasized some of the limitations of short-term CV as an index of performance, including the fact that: (1) short-term precision studies are often conducted in idealized con-ditions that may underestimate the true errors that arise in studies conducted over several years; and (2) in longitudinal studies it is important to consider the magnitude of the response to treatment as well as the precision errors.

There is, however, another problem inherent in the definition of precision as the SD error normalized to the bone density parameter (equation 8.4). This practice overlooks the sig-nificance of the ratio of the SD error to the range of values arising in clinical measurements in limiting the diagnostic sensitivity of equip-ment. Thus, a parameter such as ultrasound velocity with a relatively narrow range of val-ues requires a corresponding improvement in measurement precision if it is to provide as pre-cise an index of skeletal status. Thus, the stan-dardized coefficient of variation (SCV) defined as:

$$SCV = (RMS\,SD/clinical\,range) \cdot 100\% \quad (8.17)$$

gives a more realistic indication of the true clin-ical sensitivity of measurements than conven-tional short-term precision measured by the CV.

Different authors have adopted different choices for the definition of *clinical range* in equation 8.17. Thus, Miller et al. used the dif-ference between the 5th and 95th centiles in a large group of pre- and postmenopausal women to compare different operational defini-tions of the ultrasound velocity parameter.[18] Another definition of clinical range might be the difference between the mean values in young normal subjects and patients with estab-lished osteoporosis. These definitions, however, restrict the evaluation of SCV to particular groups of patients studied at multiple measure-ment sites or by several technologies. A defini-tion of clinical range with more general applicability is the population SD of young nor-mal subjects used in the measurement of the T-score parameter:

$$T\text{-score precision} = (RMS\,SD/young\,adult\,SD) \quad (8.18)$$

An advantage of equation 8.18 is that it gives a figure for short-term precision expressed in T-score units. This is a useful concept because it gives a direct indication of the resolution with which the measurements can categorize patients in the context of the WHO criteria for the definition of osteoporosis.[19] The evaluation of T-score precision requires the determination of two different SD measurements and, as emphasized in Table 8.2, it is important to obtain large data sets if statistical errors are to be minimized and meaningful comparisons made between different types of measurement.

Other authors have preferred to generalize the concept of precision by normalizing the RMS error of repeated measurements to the average *rate of change* of the chosen variable in untreated women.[20,21] Such a ratio has units of time, and indicates the interval between succes-sive measurements required for statistically sig-nificant changes to be detected. For example, Glüer et al.[20] defined the characteristic follow-up time (CFT) by the equation:

$$CFT = 3\,SEE/r \quad (8.19)$$

where SEE is the standard error of the estimate derived from linear regression analysis as explained above, and r is the rate of change. The origin of the factor 3 in equation 8.19 is the same as that in equation 8.16. Before such con-cepts can become more widely used, greater consensus is needed on the operational defini-tion of rate of change, for example from cross-sectional or longitudinal studies, and over what age range of subjects.

Concepts such as SCV, T-score precision and CFT are particularly useful for the objective evaluation of the wide variety of commercial QUS systems now available. These may rely on different or incompatible definitions of the speed of sound (SOS) and broadband ultrasonic attenuation (BUA) variables that can signifi-cantly influence the numerical value of the coefficient of variation, and so mask the true clinically useful precision. The interested reader is referred to Table 17.1 in Chapter 17 where some numerical examples are given.

INSTALLATION OF A NEW DXA SCANNER

One of the convenient aspects of modern DXA instruments is that they are calibrated in the factory and supplied with a factory calibrated phantom (a spine phantom for devices such as the Lunar DPX (Lunar Corp., Madison, WI, USA) and Hologic QDR-4500 (Hologic Inc., Waltham, MA, USA), a forearm phantom for devices such as the Norland pDEXA (Norland Medical Systems, Fort Atkinson, WI, USA) and Osteometer DTX-200 (Osteometer Meditech, Hoersholm, Denmark)) with a stated BMD value printed on the side. This phantom therefore serves as a secondary standard with its calibration derived directly from the primary standard kept in the factory, and can be used to check the accuracy of the scanner calibration throughout its operational life. At installation, the manufacturer's engineer will perform a series of scans with the phantom to ensure that the instrument is correctly set up. Regular scans of the phantom as part of the system quality control will then serve to check against any drift on the BMD scale.

Interunit variation after installation

Results of the factory calibration of 2700 DPX units supplied by Lunar Corporation were described by Nord.[22] Measurements of a spine phantom containing actual vertebrae embedded in lucite gave a CV of 0.5%. Measurements of the aluminium spine phantom supplied with all Lunar DPX densitometers similarly gave a CV of 0.5%. However, measurements with the European Spine Phantom (ESP) gave 1.8%. This poor result was explained by difficulties the design of the ESP phantom poses for edge-detection algorithms.[23] Users of DXA equipment are strongly advised to base their quality control programmes on the phantom supplied by the manufacturer and not to try to substitute

or recalibrate with other phantoms. Strict adherence to the manufacturer's protocols is the only guarantee that the BMD calibration can be maintained in the event of a serious system failure.

A better idea of the variation in calibration amongst DXA systems in the period following installation is obtained from data acquired by quality assurance centres monitoring DXA clinical trials, who send phantoms around the world for measurement on a large number of instruments. Gaither et al. reported data from the Oregon Osteoporosis Center on 61 Hologic QDR and 67 Lunar DPX densitometers using a Hologic spine phantom (Figure 8.6).[24] There were 94 out of 128 (71%) calibrated within 0.5% of the mean BMD for their manufacturer group, 116 (91%) within 1% and 125 (98%) within 1.5%. Three units showed deviations of 2.5%. Such large errors are likely to be caused by changes since installation and should be readily identified by the users of these systems if the manufacturer's recommendations on quality control are adhered to (see Chapter 9).

Radiation safety checks at installation

In the United Kingdom it is mandatory to inform the local radiation protection adviser of all new medical equipment delivering ionizing radiation. Before installation, advice should be sought on the siting of equipment, the possible provision of shielding and the writing of local rules on radiation safety. Afterwards, measurements should be made of the environmental dose arising from scattered radiation (to protect the operator) and entrance surface dose (to protect the patient). Typical results are described later in this chapter. In general, with pencil-beam DXA systems such as the Lunar DPX, Norland XR-36 and Hologic QDR-1000, radiation hazards are extremely small. However, more care may be necessary with some fan-beam systems. If the operator's desk is closer than 2–3 metres from the patient, then it may be necessary to provide shielding against scattered radiation. Because of the low levels of radiation involved, writing local rules is straightforward.

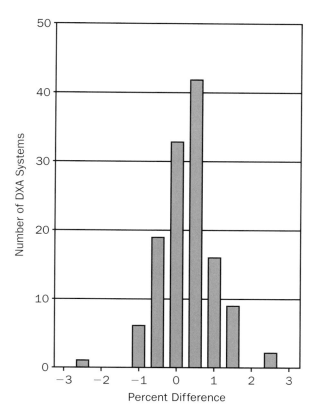

Figure 8.6 Results for intramanufacturer variation in calibration as assessed by scanning a single spine phantom on 128 DXA systems (61 Hologic QDR-series, 67 Lunar DPX-series). Of the 128 systems studied, 91 (71%) were calibrated within ±0.5% of the mean BMD for their manufacturer group, and 116 (91%) within ±1%. For three systems (2%) the differences were as large as 2.5% (data from Gaither et al.[24]).

Table 8.4 Some radiation protection requirements for bone densitometry.
When planning a new installation, the radiation protection adviser should be consulted.
Staff planning to operate equipment should attend a POPUMET course.
When not in use, equipment producing X-rays should be protected against misuse by switching off, locking and placing the key in a secure place.
Operators should never expose themselves to the primary X-ray beam.
During a scan, only the patient should be within the controlled area limit.[a]
The PC monitor and the operator's desk should be placed well outside the controlled area limit.[a] For pencil-beam axial DXA systems this means at least 1 metre away, and for fan-beam systems at least 3 metres away. If this is not possible a radiation barrier should be installed.

[a]The controlled area is the region within which the time-averaged dose rate exceeds 7.5 µSv/hour.

Some points that should be included are listed in Table 8.4. Note that in the United Kingdom all staff operating medical equipment delivering ionizing radiation should attend a POPUMET course.[25]

Cross calibration between densitometers

For users of DXA equipment who are installing a second scanner or replacing an old densitometer with a new unit, it is important to consider the agreement between the BMD measurements on the two instruments.[26] This is especially important for the conduct of clinical trials and other longitudinal studies. Some trials may last for 5 years or longer, and it is likely that over such a time period many centres will find a need to replace a DXA system, whether due to ageing equipment or to take advantage of advances in technology.

It is widely recognized that, due to differences in technology, edge-detection algorithms, scan analysis software and calibration, the replacement of a DXA system with an instrument from a different manufacturer is likely to cause serious difficulties for the interpretation of longitudinal studies.[27] However, when upgrading a scanner with a new model from the same manufacturer it should be possible, using suitable phantoms, to ensure consistency of the in vivo BMD calibration with only small residual errors. The agreement can be improved if at installation the new densitometer is set up and calibrated to agree with the old instrument using the manufacturer's spine phantom supplied with the old unit. The old spine phantom should then be kept and used for the subsequent daily quality control scans on the new scanner.

The question arises as to whether cross calibration using phantoms is sufficient, or whether additional in vivo data are required to verify the accuracy of the phantom cross calibration. Undoubtedly, if equipment behaved ideally and there were no human errors, then phantom studies might be acceptable. However, it is the incidence of unexpected findings during in vivo cross-calibration studies that suggests the importance of considering a human study whenever DXA scanners are replaced. An example was shown in Chapter 3 (Figure 3.16B) in which an in vivo cross-calibration study between two pencil-beam DXA systems showed a non-linear relationship between BMD measurements in the distal forearm. In contrast, there was close agreement between lumbar spine and femoral neck BMD between the two systems, a result that strongly suggests that the difference in forearm BMD was software related and probably due to differences in the forearm beam-hardening correction on the two instruments.

Another example of a difference in vivo not predicted by phantom measurements is shown in Figure 8.7. In this study, measurements of the Hologic spine phantom on two fan-beam DXA systems suggested that their BMD calibrations agreed to 0.2 ± 0.1%, while in vivo data on 46 female subjects showed a difference of 2.7 ± 0.3%.[28] In this instance, the error was believed to have originated in a service visit that resulted in a misalignment of the collima-

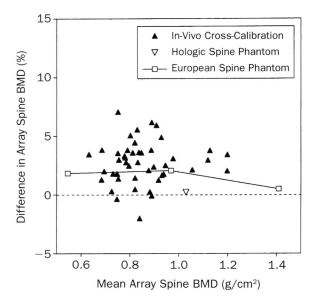

Figure 8.7 Results from phantom and in vivo cross calibrations of a Hologic QDR-2000*plus* and a Hologic QDR-2000. The difference in the fan-beam PA spine BMD measured on the two systems (expressed as a percentage) is plotted against the mean BMD. Data are shown for 46 postmenopausal women. Also shown are data points for the Hologic spine phantom and the three vertebrae of the European Spine Phantom (ESP). Mean percentage differences (and SEM) were: (A) in vivo spine data: +2.9 (0.2)%; (B) Hologic phantom: +0.2 (0.1)%; (C) ESP phantom at 1.0 g/cm² : +2.1 (0.3)%.

tor slit and multidetector array in one of the instruments. Experiences such as these last two examples suggest that in vivo cross-calibration studies are an essential precaution and should be regarded as the final safeguard for the continuity of BMD calibration.

The analysis of in vivo cross-calibration data

If in vivo cross-calibration studies are to be performed in an adequate fashion, careful planning is required. Since the study entails increased radiation dose, local ethics approval and informed consent from patients are required. Ideally, if space allows the two scanners should be operated side by side during the study so that subjects can be scanned on the two systems on the same day. This saves patients the need for an extra visit as well as causing minimal interruption to a busy appointments programme as both systems can be operated simultaneously.

In general, a study of around 50–100 subjects is required if the BMD calibrations are to be compared with a 95% confidence error of $\pm 0.5\%$. Around 20–25 subjects are probably the smallest worth-while study size, since the 95% error will increase to $\pm 1\%$.[28] It is important to include patients with a wide range of BMD values if the best data are to be obtained. All scans should be analysed using the standard protocols recommended by the manufacturer with identical regions of interest. This latter protocol is facilitated by performing the analysis using the scan comparison facility in which the two scans are displayed on the screen side by side so that the regions can be correctly placed. This may not be possible if fan-beam images are being compared with pencil beam. In this case anatomically identical ROIs must be superimposed by eye as accurately as possible.

Since it is likely that a new DXA system will have updated software, the possibility of software-related differences should be considered by analysing scans performed on the old unit on the new system to differentiate between the effects of the hardware and software changes.

Cross-calibration data are analysed using linear regression analysis[29] with BMD measurements on the old unit plotted on the horizontal axis and the new system on the vertical axis for each scan site. In this way equations are derived so that measurements on the old unit can be converted to agree with the new system. The statistical error in the intercept of each regression line is evaluated and, if the 95% confidence limits include zero, the regression analysis is repeated with the intercept forced through the origin. A data analysis package with this latter option is available on the widely used Microsoft Excel spreadsheet. Finally, the slope and 95% confidence limits of the regression line through the origin for each scan site should be examined to determine whether it is statistically significantly different from unity. If the slope is significantly different from unity, then BMD results on the old scanner should be multiplied by this factor to put them on a consistent BMD scale with the new system.

If the opposite correction is required, i.e. a factor to multiply the measurements on the new unit to make them agree with the old, then the axes should be reversed, i.e. the BMD measurements on the new unit plotted on the horizontal axis and the old system on the vertical axis. This latter is required if the calibration file on the new system is to be edited to force agreement with the in vivo BMD calibration of the old scanner. This latter step is used, for example, by manufacturers to ensure continuity of BMD calibration on successive generations of equipment, in particular to obtain exact agreement between fan-beam and pencil-beam instruments.

Results of an in vivo cross-calibration study between a Hologic QDR-4500 and an QDR-2000*plus* are shown in Figure 8.8.[30] In this study, linear regression analysis gave an intercept that was not significantly different from zero at every BMD site analysed (Table 8.5). While most published cross-calibration studies include data for spine and femoral neck BMD, much less information is available for the other sites in the hip, the forearm and total body BMD. This is unfortunate, since data for the other femur sites have assumed greater importance since the recommendation of the International Committee for Standards in Bone Measurement that femur BMD should be standardized and interpreted using the total hip site.[31] With the widespread use of the NHANES III reference data for femur BMD,[31–33] continuity of the BMD scale at the total hip site has assumed particular importance.

One of the most frequently performed upgrades of DXA scanning equipment in recent years has been the replacement of QDR-1000 units by QDR-4500. Results of some in vivo

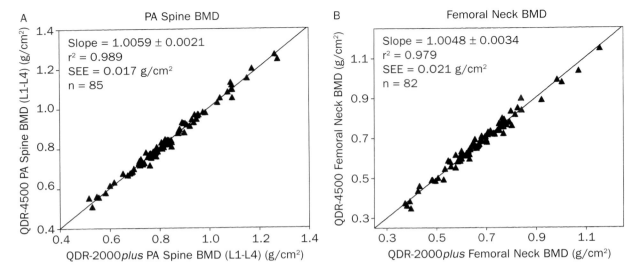

Figure 8.8 Scatter plots of: (A) PA spine BMD; (B) femoral neck BMD measured on QDR-4500 and QDR-2000*plus* DXA bone densitometers. The subjects were 85 postmenopausal women. Also shown on the plots are the results of linear regression analysis with the line forced through the origin (data from Blake et al.[30]).

Table 8.5 Results of linear regression analysis of an in vivo cross-calibration study between a Hologic QDR-4500 and a QDR-2000*plus*.[30]

BMD site	n	r^2	Intercept	Slope (and standard error)	SEE (g/cm^2)
PA spine	85	0.989	NS	1.0059 (0.0021); $p < 0.01$	0.017
Femoral neck	82	0.979	NS	1.0048 (0.0034); NS	0.021
Trochanter	82	0.979	NS	1.0280 (0.0034); $p < 0.001$	0.018
Intertrochanter	82	0.980	NS	1.0304 (0.0030); $p < 0.001$	0.024
Total hip	82	0.988	NS	1.0276 (0.0023); $p < 0.001$	0.016
Ward's triangle	82	0.969	NS	0.9953 (0.0067); NS	0.033

n, number of subjects; NS, not significant; SEE, standard error of the estimate.

Table 8.6 Results of some in vivo cross-calibration studies between Hologic QDR-4500 and QDR-1000 DXA systems. (Data from refs 51 and 52 and unpublished analyses by the author.)

Centre	n	PA spine BMD slope (and SE)	Femoral neck BMD slope (and SE)
Centre A	154	0.994 (0.002)	0.995 (0.003)
Centre B	104	1.004 (0.002)	0.996 (0.003)
Centre C	60	0.980 (0.004)	1.012 (0.005)
Centre D	54	1.004 (0.003)	–
Centre E	105	0.984 (0.002)	1.006 (0.004)
Centre F	104	0.987 (0.002)	1.009 (0.006)
Mean		0.992 (0.010)	1.004 (0.008)

n, number of subjects.

cross-calibration studies known to the author are listed in Table 8.6.

RADIATION DOSE IN DXA

Studies of radiation exposure to patients from DXA scans have confirmed that dose levels are small compared with many other radiological investigations involving ionizing radiation.[34-45] However, clinicians requesting and technologists performing scans should be aware that any exposure to ionizing radiation carries a risk. With diagnostic procedures this is always very small, and especially for bone densitometry studies where radiation levels are often so low that, for example, the scatter dose to the operator from some pencil-beam systems can be difficult to detect and quantify accurately.[43]

The hazards involved are carcinogenesis (the induction of cancer by exposure to radiation), and in men or women with child bearing potential, genetic injury to future children.[46] Both these hazards are examples of the *stochastic* effects of radiation. This means that in each individual undergoing a radiological investigation there is a small chance (with a risk proportional to the dose) that the radiation exposure will cause a cancer. A familiar analogy would be the risk of death in an aeroplane accident. One person might make many hundreds of transcontinental flights without mishap, while a victim of a crash might be making his or her first flight. Despite such examples, people generally understand that the risk of death in an accident increases in proportion to the number of flights made. Unlike aeroplane flights, however, it has not proved easy to quantify the risks of radiation because cancer is a relatively common disease with many other causes unrelated to radiation. Except in a few special circumstances, such as studies of the survivors of the Japanese atomic bombings,[46] these other cancers totally mask the small effects of radiation.

Some risks in life comparable to having a DXA study are listed in Table 8.7

Table 8.7 Some activities carrying a risk of death comparable to receiving an effective dose of 1 μSv from a DXA scan. (Data from Pochin.[49,50])

Exposure to natural background radiation for 4 hours

Smoking one-tenth of a cigarette

Travelling 3 miles by car

Travelling 15 miles in an aeroplane

Rock climbing for 5 seconds

Canoeing for 20 seconds

Working in a factory for half a day

Being a woman aged 30 for 60 minutes

Being a woman aged 40 for 20 minutes

Being a woman aged 50 for 8 minutes

Being a woman aged 60 for 3 minutes

Being a woman aged 70 for 1 minute

Units of radiation dose

Accurate measurements of radiation dose are all made with the help of *ionization chambers*. These measure the amount of electric charge released in a given volume of air when the chamber is placed in the radiation beam. The intensity of an X-ray beam measured in this way is called *exposure*, and is measured in units called *roentgens* (symbol, R). Manufacturers' specification sheets for DXA systems often give figures for the X-ray beam expressed in milliroentgens (mR). This is a simple measurement to make because it only involves performing scans of the ionization chamber in air. However, it is important that a large mass of tissue-equivalent material is placed behind the chamber to generate *backscatter*, otherwise the measurement does not reflect the true dose in vivo.

Measurements of exposure express the effects of the radiation on air. To find the radiation dose to the human body, it is necessary to relate this to the effects in tissue. The first step in doing this is to convert the measurement of exposure in air into the *absorbed dose* in soft tissue. Absorbed dose expresses the radiation dose in tissue in terms of the energy absorbed from the X-ray beam per unit mass of tissue. The concept here is that the energy absorbed from the radiation beam damages the tissue and, on the molecular scale, results in broken atomic bonds and direct damage to biologically important molecules such as DNA. The unit of absorbed dose is the *gray* (symbol, Gy), and 1 Gy is an absorbed dose of 1 joule/kilogram. One gray is a large dose of radiation, and in diagnostic radiology absorbed dose is usually expressed in milligray (mGy). With DXA systems, dose is often so low that a more convenient unit is the microgray (μGy). Because the air in an ionization chamber is so similar in its average atomic number to soft tissue, measurements of exposure in air expressed in mR are readily converted into absorbed dose in soft tissue expressed in μGy with a factor that varies only slightly with photon energy. For lean tissue and X-rays generated at 100 kVp, the conversion factor is 9.2 μGy/mR.[37]

An important quantity usually expressed as absorbed dose is the *entrance surface dose*. This is the absorbed dose to the skin at the point where the X-ray beam enters the patient's body. Some figures for entrance surface dose for widely used DXA systems are listed in Table 8.8. As the X-ray beam passes through the patient's body the radiation is attenuated due to the absorption and scattering of photons. Internal organs therefore receive progressively lower doses the more shielded they are by overlying tissues. A plot of absorbed dose as a function of tissue depth is called a *depth dose curve* (Figure 8.9).

Because absorbed dose measures the energy transferred by the radiation to the tissue, it is not the most appropriate way of expressing the biological effects of the radiation such as the risks of cancer induction. The biological harm is instead expressed as the *dose equivalent* (DE). Dose equivalent is derived from absorbed dose

Table 8.8 Measurements of entrance surface dose (ESD) for some DXA systems.[a]

DXA system	Scan mode	ESD (µGy)
Lunar DPX	0.75 mA medium	10
Hologic QDR-1000	Quick mode (4 min)	30
Hologic QDR-1000	Performance mode (8 min)	60
Hologic QDR-4500	Fast mode (30 sec)	150
Hologic QDR-4500	Medium mode (60 sec)	300
Lunar Expert-XL	2 mA fast (12 sec)	320
Lunar Expert-XL	5 mA fast (12 sec)	800

[a]Measurements made by the author using an MDH-1015 ionization chamber (MDH Industries, Monrovia, CA, USA) and a tissue-equivalent phantom to provide backscatter.

by multiplying by the *quality factor* of the radiation:

$$\frac{\text{Dose}}{\text{equivalent}} = \text{absorbed dose} \times \text{quality factor}$$

The quality factor (QF) is a measure of the relative ability of the ionizing radiation to do biological damage. For the various different types of ionizing radiations (alpha-, beta-, gamma-rays and neutrons), it is always measured relative to X-rays. Thus, for X-rays, QF = 1.0 by definition, and the dose equivalent is always numerically equal to the absorbed dose. Nevertheless, the distinction is still made to show that the concept of the quality factor has been taken into account. To differentiate between measurements of dose equivalent and those of absorbed dose, the former are quoted

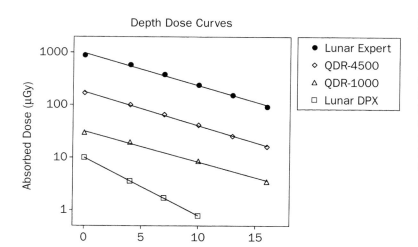

Figure 8.9 Depth dose curves measured for PA spine BMD scans on four DXA bone densitometers: Lunar DPX: 0.75 mA medium mode; QDR-1000: Quick scan mode; QDR-4500: fast scan mode; Expert-XL: 5 mA fast mode. Measurements were made using an MDH-1015 180-cm³ ionization chamber (MDH Industries, Monrovia, CA, USA) and a tissue-equivalent phantom.[37]

in units of *sieverts* (symbol, Sv). As with the gray, 1 sievert is a relatively large dose. Hence, in diagnostic radiology, dose equivalent is usually expressed in millisievert (mSv). For DXA scans, dose is often so low that a more convenient unit is the microsievert (μSv).

The final step in the derivation of radiation dose is to convert the dose equivalent figures for each organ into the *effective dose*. This is done by multiplying the dose equivalent for each organ by a weighting factor proportional to the sensitivity of that organ to the stochastic effects of radiation, and summing over all the organs exposed:

$$\text{Effective dose} = \Sigma_j \text{DE}_j \cdot w_j \qquad (8.20)$$

where DE_j and w_j are the dose equivalent and weighting factor respectively for the *j*th organ. The advantage of the concept of effective dose is that it summarizes the radiation risks from any radiological investigation in a single figure and thus the radiation hazard to the patient from a DXA scan can be compared directly with a chest X-ray, a CT scan of the abdomen, a radionuclide bone scan, or any other investigation that uses ionizing radiation. The weighting factors w_j are chosen so that their sum is unity, i.e.:

$$\Sigma_j w_j = 1 \qquad (8.21)$$

From this it can be seen from equation 8.20 that, were every organ in the body to be exposed to the same uniform dose, the effective dose would equal this uniform dose. Thus, effective dose can be defined as *the uniform dose to the whole body that carries the same stochastic risks to the patient as the given radiological investigation.*

The above scheme for calculating effective dose was established by the International Commission on Radiological Protection (ICRP) and is explained in greater detail in ICRP Publication 60.[46] The list of tissue weighting factors derived by the ICRP is summarized in Table 8.9. These weighting factors replace an earlier set published in 1977[47] and are based on updated information about cancer induction by radiation. Calculations using the old 1977

Table 8.9 Tissue weighting factors from ICRP-60 (1990).[46]

Tissue type	Weighting factor
Ovaries	0.20
Bone marrow (red)	0.12
Colon	0.12
Lung	0.12
Stomach	0.12
Bladder	0.05
Breast	0.05
Liver	0.05
Oesophagus	0.05
Thyroid	0.05
Skin	0.01
Bone surfaces	0.01
Remainder	0.05[a]

[a]The following 10 tissues are included in the remainder with weighting factors of 0.005 each: adrenal, brain, upper large intestine, small intestine, kidney, muscle, pancreas, spleen, thymus and uterus.

weighting factors are distinguished by using the term *effective dose equivalent* instead of *effective dose.*

Patient doses from DXA

Effective dose is the preferred method of specifying patient dose from DXA investigations because it relates directly to the total radiation risk involved. A number of studies have published figures for Hologic[34-38] and Lunar[39-43] DXA systems and results are summarized in Tables 8.10–8.12. Dose findings for vertebral morphometry studies using DXA systems are summarized in Table 20.6 in Chapter 20. The

Table 8.10 Effective doses for DXA studies on a Hologic QDR-1000 and a QDR-4500. Scan times are given in brackets. (Data from Lewis et al.[37,44])

Scan mode	QDR-1000	QDR-4500
PA spine (L1–L4)	0.5 µSv (8 min)	2.0 µSv (30 sec)
Proximal femur		
excluding ovaries[a]	0.1 µSv (6 min)	0.6 µSv (30 sec)
including ovaries	1.4 µSv (6 min)	5.4 µSv (30 sec)
Total body		
excluding ovaries[a]	3.6 µSv (16 min)	2.6 µSv (3 min)
including ovaries	4.6 µSv (16 min)	3.4 µSv (3 min)
Forearm	0.07 µSv (6 min)	0.05 µSv (30 sec)

[a]Dose excluding ovaries applies to postmenopausal women.

Table 8.11 Effective doses for DXA studies on a Lunar DPX-L and an Expert-XL. Scan times are given in brackets. (Data for spine and femur from Njeh et al.[39] Total body dose for Expert-XL calculated by author using method of Lewis et al.[37])

Scan mode	DPX-L	Expert-XL
PA spine (L1–L4)	0.21 µSv (5 min)	75 mSv (12 sec)
Proximal femur		
excluding ovaries[a]	0.08 µSv (5 min)	18 µSv (12 sec)
including ovaries	0.15 µSv (5 min)	45 µSv (12 sec)
Total body		
excluding ovaries[a]	–	41 µSv (4 min)
including ovaries	–	54 µSv (4 min)

[a]Dose excluding ovaries applies to postmenopausal women.

Table 8.12 Effective doses for paediatric mode studies on a Lunar DPX-L. Scan times are given in brackets. (Data from Njeh et al.[43])

Scan mode	Child aged 5 years	Child aged 10 years
PA spine	0.28 µSv (5 min)	0.20 µSv (5 min)
Total body	0.03 µSv (9 min)	0.02 µSv (12 min)

most commonly adopted approach to estimating dose is to scan an anthropomorphic phantom containing thermoluminescent (TLD) dosimeters. However, TLD is not a particularly sensitive technique, and because of the low dose from DXA investigations, especially with pencil-beam systems, a large number of repeated scans may be required to achieve a detectable signal.

There is general agreement that patient dose for a spine and femur DXA examination on a pencil-beam system is exceptionally low, around 1 µSv or less. Dose from the Lunar DPX system is lower than for the Hologic QDR-1000, as is evident from the lower depth dose values in Figure 8.9. To translate this dose into a figure for the actual risk of inducing cancer, the estimate for the total lifetime risk for a 30-year-old adult from 1 µSv of 0.6×10^{-7} can be used,[46] equivalent to odds of 16 million to one. As discussed earlier, some examples of comparable risks from other activities are listed in Table 8.7. Because of the long latent period for many radiation-induced cancers (up to 30 years), the risks to older patients who are the majority of referrals for bone densitometry investigations are significantly lower. Correspondingly, the risks to children will be larger. Njeh et al. studied the effective dose to 5- and 10-year-old children scanned using the paediatric mode on the Lunar DPX-L system (Table 8.12).[43] Results were only marginally greater than the dose of

0.2 µSv found for adult scans.[39] However, care is needed when using adult modes to scan children because the relatively wider scan fields and smaller tissue depths will result in significantly higher effective doses.

Rather higher doses have been reported for DXA investigations on fan-beam systems[37,39–41,44] and may relate to the improvement in image resolution. Again, the differences are evident in the depth dose curves shown in Figure 8.9. Doses for the Hologic QDR-4500 are around 10 times greater than for the QDR-1000, and for the Lunar Expert-XL are around 100 times greater than for the DPX. Some reports for the Expert-XL suggest doses of around 70 µSv for a 5-mA fast mode AP spine scan,[39,40] which is equivalent to around four chest X-rays. However, this figure can be significantly reduced by use of shorter scan times or lower tube current.

Patient dose from DXA scans of the peripheral skeleton is exceptionally low. Lewis et al. reported an effective dose of 0.07 µSv for a forearm scan on a Hologic QDR-1000,[37] and unpublished studies by the author have found similar figures for forearm studies on the Norland pDEXA and Osteometer DTX-200 systems. Doses for peripheral DXA scans are low because: (1) with the thin tissue sections, X-ray beam intensity is smaller; (2) scan fields are smaller than with axial DXA; and (3) there are fewer radiosensitive tissues (Table 8.9)

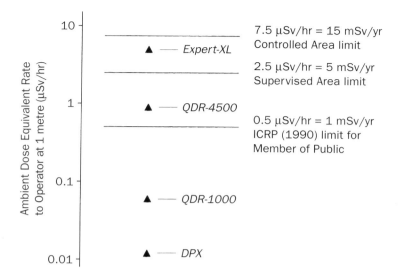

Figure 8.10 Comparison of the time-averaged scatter dose to an operator positioned 1 metre from the centre of the scanning table for four DXA systems. Results show the mean dose equivalent per hour assuming that two patients per hour are scanned on the pencil-beam systems (Lunar DPX and Hologic QDR-1000) and four patients per hour on the fan-beam systems (Lunar Expert-XL and Hologic QDR-4500). Regulatory limits were taken from the United Kingdom Ionising Radiation Regulations[48] and the 1990 recommendations of the ICRP[46] (environmental dose data from Patel et al.[44,45]).

involved, and the fraction of, say, the total bone marrow or bone surfaces irradiated in a forearm or calcaneus scan is much smaller than for a spine scan.

Occupational doses from DXA

Several studies[39,44,45] have evaluated the occupational dose to technologists performing DXA investigations. In the United Kingdom, the maximum permitted annual dose for a non-classified radiation worker is 15 mSv, corresponding to a time-averaged dose rate of 7.5 µSv/hour in the working environment.[48] If dose rates approach this limit, then the working area is defined as a *controlled area*. Radiation monitoring of staff is required, and safe working practice must be detailed in a written *system of work*. At lower dose rates of up to 5 mSv/year (2.5 µSv/hour) the lesser limit of a

supervised area applies. In 1990, the International Commission on Radiological Protection recommended an annual limit of 1 mSv/year for all members of the public.[46] Translated into the workplace, this figure corresponds to 0.5 µSv/hour in the working area. In the author's experience, occupational dose levels below this latter limit are readily achievable for the large majority of hospital staff working with ionizing radiation in radiology or nuclear medicine departments.

Results of the environmental monitoring study at 1 metre from the centre of the scanning table for Hologic QDR-1000, QDR-4500, Lunar DPX and Expert-XL systems reported by Patel et al.[44,45] are shown in Figure 8.10 where they are compared with the controlled area, supervised area and ICRP (1990) limits. These figures assumed scanning loads of two patients/hour for the pencil-beam devices and four patients/hour for the fan-beam systems. For the

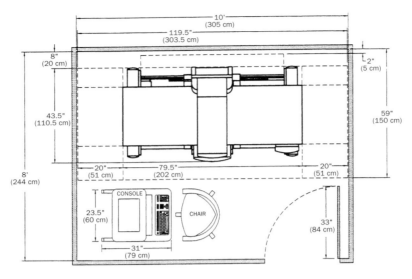

Figure 8.11 Room layout from the manufacturer's data sheet for the Hologic QDR-4500.

two pencil-beam systems, the time-averaged dose to staff from scatter is very low even with the operator sat as close as 1 metre from the patient during scanning. For fan-beam devices, however, scatter dose is considerably higher and, if patient workload approaches the full capacity of the system, occupational exposures may approach the limits set by the regulatory authorities.

With fan-beam systems, therefore, care is needed at installation to ensure the safety of staff. Although very compact room layouts are possible (Figure 8.11), these are not desirable unless the patient workload is very light. Technologists should be protected either by the use of a lead–plastic radiation barrier, or by placing the operator at least 3 metres from the patient.

REFERENCES

1. Wahner HW, Dunn WL, Mazess RB et al. Dual-photon Gd-153 absorptiometry of bone. *Radiology* (1985) **156**: 203–6.

2. Erikson S, Isberg B, Lindgren U. Vertebral bone mineral measurement using dual photon absorptiometry and computed tomography. *Acta Radiologica* (1988) **29**: 89–94.

3. Gotfredsen A, Podenphant J, Norgaard H et al. Accuracy of lumbar spine bone mineral content by dual photon absorptiometry. *J Nucl Med* (1988) **29**: 248–54.

4. Ho CP, Kim RW, Schaffler MB, Sartoris DJ. Accuracy of dual-energy radiographic absorptiometry of the lumbar spine: a cadaver study. *Radiology* (1990) **176**: 171–3.

5. Edmonston SJ, Singer KP, Price RI, Breidahl PD. Accuracy of lateral dual energy x-ray absorptiometry for the determination of bone mineral content in the thoracic and lumbar spine: an in-vitro study. *Br J Radiol* (1993) **66**: 309–13.

6. Sabin MA, Blake GM, MacLaughlin-Black SM, Fogelman I. The accuracy of volumetric bone density measurements in dual X-ray absorptiometry. *Calcif Tissue Int* (1995) **56**: 210–14.

7. Svendsen OL, Hassager C, Skodt V et al. Impact of soft tissue on in-vivo accuracy of bone mineral measurements in the spine, hip and forearm: a human cadaver study. *J Bone Miner Res* (1995) **10**: 868–73.

8. Kuiper JW, van Kuijk C, Grashuis JL et al. Accuracy and influence of marrow fat on quantitative CT and dual-energy X-ray absorptiometry measurements of the femoral neck in vitro. *Osteoporos Int* (1996) **6:** 25–30.

9. Glüer C-C, Blake GM, Lu Y et al. Accurate assessment of precision errors: how to measure the reproducibility of bone densitometry techniques. *Osteoporos Int* (1995) **5:** 262–70.

10. Liberman UA, Weiss SR, Bröll J et al. Effect of oral alendronate on bone mineral density and the incidence of fractures in postmenopausal osteoporosis. *N Engl J Med* (1995) **333:** 1437–43.

11. Patel R, Blake GM, Rymer J, Fogelman I. Long-term precision of DXA scanning assessed in forty postmenopausal women followed over seven years. *Osteoporos Int* (1997) **7:** 288.

12. Faulkner KG, McClung MR, Ravn P et al. Monitoring skeletal response to therapy in early postmenopausal women: which bone to measure? *J Bone Miner Res* (1996) **11**(suppl 1): S96.

13. Christensen C, Ravn P, Alexandersen P, Mollgaard A. A new region of interest (nROI) in the forearm for monitoring the effect of therapy. *J Bone Miner Res* (1997) **12**(suppl 1): S480.

14. Herd RJM, Balena R, Blake GM et al. The prevention of early postmenopausal bone loss by cyclical etidronate therapy: a 2-year double-blind placebo-controlled study. *Am J Med* (1997) **103:** 92–9.

15. Blake GM, Herd RJM, Fogelman I. A longitudinal study of supine lateral DXA of the lumbar spine: a comparison with posteroanterior spine, hip and total body DXA. *Osteoporos Int* (1996) **6:** 462–70.

16. Preston NG, Blake GM, Patel R et al. Monitoring skeletal response to therapy using DXA: which site to measure in the femur? In: Ring EFJ, ed. *Current Research in Osteoporosis and Bone Mineral Measurement V: 1998* (British Institute of Radiology: London, 1998), 35–6.

17. Takada M, Grampp S, Ouyang X et al. A new trabecular region of interest for femoral dual X-ray absorptiometry: short-term precision, age related bone loss and fracture discrimination compared with current femoral regions of interest. *J Bone Miner Res* (1997) **12:** 832–8.

18. Miller CG, Herd RJM, Ramalingam T et al. Ultrasonic velocity measurements through the calcaneus: which velocity should be measured? *Osteoporos Int* (1993) **3:** 31–5.

19. Kanis JA, Melton LJ, Christiansen C et al. The diagnosis of osteoporosis. *J Bone Miner Res* (1994) **9:** 1137–41.

20. Glüer C-C, Blunt B, Engelke M et al. Characteristic follow-up time: a new concept for standardized characterization of a technique's ability to monitor longitudinal changes. *Bone Miner* (1994) **25**(suppl 2): S40.

21. Glüer C-C. How to characterize the ability of a diagnostic technique to monitor skeletal changes. *J Bone Miner Res* (1997) **12**(suppl 1): S378.

22. Nord R, Mazess RB, Hanson JA. Inter-unit variation on 2700 DPX densitometers. *Osteoporos Int* (1997) **7:** 284.

23. Tothill P. Letter to the editor. *Bone* (1996) **19:** 415–17.

24. Gaither KW, Faulkner KG, Ostrem EC et al. Variation in calibration amongst like-manufacturer DXA systems. *J Bone Miner Res* (1996) **11**(suppl 1): S119.

25. *The Ionising Radiation (Protection of Persons Undergoing Medical Examination or Treatment) Regulations 1988* (HMSO: London, 1988).

26. Finkelstein JS, Butler JP, Cleary RL, Neer RM. Comparison of four methods for cross-calibrating dual-energy x-ray absorptiometers to eliminate systematic errors when upgrading equipment. *J Bone Miner Res* (1994) **9:** 1945–52.

27. Laskey MA, Flaxman ME, Barber RW et al. Comparative performance in-vitro and in-vivo of Lunar DPX and Hologic QDR-1000 dual energy x-ray absorptiometers. *Br J Radiol* (1991) **64:** 1023–9.

28. Blake GM. Replacing DXA scanners: cross-calibration with phantoms may be misleading. *Calcif Tissue Int* (1996) **59:** 1–5.

29. Faulkner KG, Glüer C-C, Estilo M, Genant HK. Cross-calibration of DXA equipment: upgrading from a Hologic QDR-1000/W to a QDR-2000. *Calcif Tissue Int* (1993) **52:** 79–84.

30. Blake GM, Fogelman I. Replacing dual x-ray absorptiometry scanners: cross-calibration of a new multidetector array system. *J Bone Miner Res* (1995) **10**(suppl 1): S267.

31. Hanson J. Letter to the editor: standardization of femur BMD. *J Bone Miner Res* (1996) **12:** 1316–17.

32. Looker AC, Wahner HW, Dunn WL et al. Proximal femur bone mineral levels of US adults. *Osteoporos Int* (1995) **5:** 389–409.

33. Looker AC, Wahner HW, Dunn WL et al. Updated data on proximal femur bone mineral levels of US adults. *Osteoporos Int* (1998) (in press).

34. Pye DW, Hannan WJ, Hesp R. Effective dose equivalent in dual X-ray absorptiometry. *Br J Radiol* (1990) **63:** 149.

35. Kalender WA. Effective dose values in bone mineral measurements by photon absorptiometry and computed tomography. *Osteoporos Int* (1992) **2**: 82–7.

36. Rawlings DJ, Faulkner K, Chapple CL. The influence of scan time on patient dose and precision in bone mineral densitometry. In: Ring EFJ, ed. *Current Research in Osteoporosis and Bone Mineral Densitometry II* (British Institute of Radiology: London, 1992), 23–4.

37. Lewis MK, Blake GM, Fogelman I. Patient dose in dual x-ray absorptiometry. *Osteoporos Int* (1994) **4**: 11–15.

38. Lewis MK, Blake GM. Patient dose in morphometric X-ray absorptiometry. *Osteoporos Int* (1995) **5**: 281–2.

39. Njeh CF, Apple K, Temperton DH, Boivin CM. Radiological assessment of a new bone densitometer: the Lunar Expert. *Br J Radiol* (1996) **69**: 335–40.

40. Stewart SP, Milner D, Moore AC et al. Preliminary report on the Lunar Expert-XL imaging densitometer: dosimetry, precision and cross-calibration. In: Ring EFJ, Elvins DM, Bhalla AK, eds. *Current Research in Osteoporosis and Bone Mineral Densitometry IV* (British Institute of Radiology: London, 1996), 101–2.

41. Huda W, Morin RL. Patient dose in bone mineral densitometry. *Br J Radiol* (1996) **69**: 422–5.

42. Bezakova E, Collins PJ, Beddoe AH. Absorbed dose measurements in dual energy X-ray absorptiometry. *Br J Radiol* (1997) **70**: 172–9.

43. Njeh CF, Samat SB, Nightingale A et al. Radiation dose and in vitro precision in paediatric bone mineral density measurement using dual X-ray absorptiometry. *Br J Radiol* (1997) **70**: 719–27.

44. Blake GM, Patel R, Lewis MK et al. New generation dual x-ray absorptiometry scanners increase dose to patients and staff. *J Bone Miner Res* (1996) **11**(suppl 1): S157.

45. Patel R, Blake GM, Batchelor S et al. Occupational dose to the radiographer in dual X-ray absorptiometry: a comparison of pencil-beam and fan-beam systems. *Br J Radiol* (1996) **69**: 539–43.

46. ICRP Publication 60. 1990 recommendations of the International Commission on Radiological Protection. *Ann ICRP* (1991) **21**: Nos 1–3.

47. ICRP Publication 26. Recommendations of the International Commission on Radiological Protection. *Ann ICRP* (1977) **1**: No. 3.

48. *The Ionising Radiation Regulations 1985* (HMSO: London, 1985).

49. Pochin EE. Occupational and other fatality rates. *Community Health* (1974) **6**: 2–13.

50. Parker RP, Smith PHS, Taylor DM. *Basic Science of Nuclear Medicine* (Churchill Livingstone: Edinburgh, 1984), 128.

51. Bouyoucef SE, Cullum ID, Ell PJ. Cross-calibration of a fan-beam X-ray densitometer with a pencil-beam system. *Br J Radiol* (1996) **69**: 522–31.

52. Elvins DM, Ring EFJ. Comparability of hip and spine BMD on the Hologic QDR-1000 and QDR-4500A Acclaim. In: Ring EFJ, Elvins DM, Bhalla AK, eds. *Current Research in Osteoporosis and Bone Mineral Densitometry IV* (British Institute of Radiology: London, 1996), 97–8.

9

Instrument Quality Control and Phantoms for DXA Scanners

Guest chapter by Colin G Miller

CHAPTER OVERVIEW

This chapter familiarizes the reader with the requirements of instrumental quality control (IQC) for dual-energy X-ray absorptiometry (DXA) scanners and the phantoms available for such studies. The daily quality control procedures for Lunar, Hologic and Norland instruments are described, together with details of the manufacturers' phantoms. Some alternative phantoms are described, including the European Spine Phantom. A critique is given of the strengths and weaknesses of the different phantoms currently available. Finally, the development of IQC for multicentre clinical trials is discussed, including the application of Shewhart rules and Cusum charts.

INTRODUCTION

Any medical device delivering ionizing radiation requires testing during installation to ensure that the system is functioning properly and the radiation dose to patients and scatter dose to technologists are within specified limits. For bone densitometers, these tests include checks of bone density calibration, precision and dose, and are carried out routinely by the instrument manufacturer prior to or at the time of installation. Following installation, there are daily quality control procedures which should be performed each day before any patients are scanned. Instrument calibration and, if indicated, radiation dose to the patient should also be checked after each major maintenance or repair. A file should be kept to record the results of these investigations, as well as copies of engineer's reports following all maintenance visits. These different aspects of instrument evaluation and quality control are summarized in Table 9.1.

A determination of the accuracy of bone mass measurements is, in its strictest sense, a difficult task that is not routinely performed. When accuracy studies are undertaken, this should ideally be done by scanning the bone of interest in situ in a cadaver, and comparing the measured bone mineral content (BMC) results with the weight of the properly ashed bones. A short-cut procedure, but one that is still cumbersome to perform, is to scan excised vertebrae (or other bones) immersed in a water tank prior to ashing. The disadvantage of this latter

Table 9.1 Control of instrument performance.

1) *At installation of a new instrument:*
Acceptance testing at time of installation
    performed by manufacturer
    review by user recommended

2) *Routine QC procedures:*
(a) Set up a daily QC procedure and a
    routine recording and review procedure
    (QC log). Most instruments have
    software-supported QC routines.
    Additional QC tests may be needed
b) Start a book to enter any repair or
    malfunction of the instrument, as well
    as results of inspections and
    performance reviews

3) *Evaluation of instrument performance:* Special phantoms and, if still needed, patients
4) *Radiation dose measurements*

INSTRUMENT QUALITY CONTROL

Quality control, or instrument quality control (IQC), is usually taken to mean the evaluation of a bone densitometer's calibration. Its purpose is to allow the operator to assess whether an instrument is operating within well defined limits of its calibration. The phrases 'quality control' and 'quality assurance' are terms that are well understood and used extensively throughout industry. In the field of bone densitometry, the term quality assurance (QA) is usually taken to mean one of two things depending upon the context, either: (1) the review of patient scan data by a quality assurance centre, or (2) the internal calibration of the bone densitometer. Both these areas will be discussed in more detail in the following sections, but for now these definitions provide a framework for the rest of the chapter. The majority of this chapter will concentrate on quality control and will discuss why it is performed and the specific methodologies employed by each manufacturer.

All precision instruments require calibration, and bone densitometers are no exception. Due to the methods used for X-ray generation and detection, a method of ongoing calibration is employed, and records of this can be checked with data that go as far back as the initial calibration of the instrument in the factory. This is achieved by the use of calibration or quality control (QC) phantoms, which are scanned on a regular basis.

Quality control procedures are critical for several reasons. First, they provide information on the health of an instrument. Any changes are suggestive of component failure. Secondly, any change in calibration will affect the accuracy of the measurement and will have implications on the correct interpretation of BMD results. Thirdly, and most critically, for longitudinal assessments (i.e. when patients are coming back for repeat scans months or years later after an initial scan), if the calibration of the instrument has changed, this has to be factored into the interpretation of the patient's follow-up BMD measurements and diagnosis. If known changes went uncorrected, then the wrong conclusion

experimental set-up is that it assumes an idealized uniform soft tissue baseline. Neither of these two methods allows for the measurement of the projected area of bone, which is required for an independent assessment of bone mineral density (BMD). The area is not easy to measure independently from DXA. Therefore accuracy is not normally evaluated when a new DXA system is installed. Instead, the information should be requested from the manufacturer as part of the calibration information provided with the instrument. A more detailed discussion of the accuracy of DXA measurements, including references, is given in Chapter 8.

might be drawn about a patient's bone density result. For example, if the densitometer calibration changed by an increase of 3% between the baseline and follow-up scan for a patient whose absolute BMD remained constant, it might be wrongly concluded that the patient was gaining bone if allowance was not made for the calibration change. Alternatively, if this was an early postmenopausal woman losing bone at 3% per year, the conclusion might be drawn that her bone density was stable. However, once proper allowance is made for the calibration shift, then it would be clear that the patient's BMD had fallen 3% in 12 months, which would be a matter of concern to the clinician and might warrant an alternative patient management strategy. Calibration shifts and changes will be covered in more detail in the section on the conduct of clinical trials, where making appropriate corrections is a major issue.

MANUFACTURERS' PHANTOMS AND INSTRUMENT QUALITY CONTROL

Quality control: Lunar DPX instruments

The Lunar calibration phantom (Lunar Corp., Madison, WI, USA) (Figure 9.1) is a block of tissue-equivalent material with three bone-simulating chambers of known bone mineral content. Each Lunar densitometer is assigned its own phantom (identified by its serial number) in the factory. The phantom is scanned

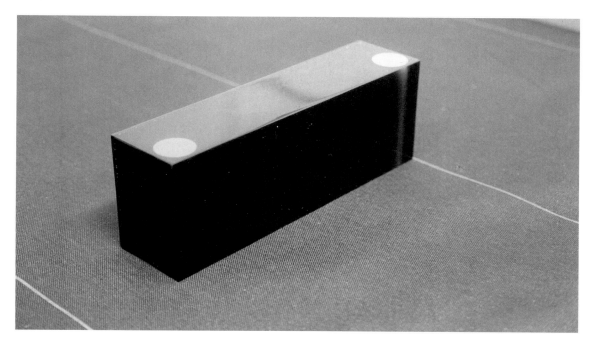

Figure 9.1 Calibration block phantom used for daily quality control studies on Lunar instruments.

daily at a predefined position on the imaging table and the BMC measured for each of the three chambers. At the same time the following additional daily QC tests are conducted as part of the scanning procedure with the calibration phantom: a check of the detector pulse height spectrum; background counts; X-ray shutter operation; cross over of high-energy X-rays into the low-energy window; unattenuated photon count (beam intensity); ratio of photon counts in the low-energy and high-energy channels; scanner mechanics; and a tissue composition measurement of a soft tissue-equivalent cylinder included in the calibration phantom. The QC printout from the Lunar DPX series of instruments is shown in Figure 9.2. A similar

programme is run on the Lunar Expert, but due to the nature of the fan-beam instrument, the details are substantially different. On both instruments, the results of the above QC procedures should be checked daily before patients are scanned.

The Lunar system software provides a pass–fail evaluation for the system tests, flags the mean equivalent BMC of the chambers, and gives figures for the measurement precision if any result is outside a defined range. It also has a fail-safe mechanism that switches the instrument off after 2 weeks if it has not passed a QC procedure. This ensures that patient measurements are only obtained when the instrument is performing within the manufacturer's specified calibration limits.

To pass the daily QC procedure a Lunar DPX system should meet the following conditions: the setting of the pulse height spectrum should be within 50 units of the previous day's value and within a range of 250–750 units; background count should be less than 50 counts/second for each channel; the spillover from the high- to low-energy window should be within the range 6.3–10.0%; the unattenuated counts should be 450 000–900 000 counts/second in the low-energy channel and 270 000–630 000 counts/second in the high-energy channel; the ratio of high-energy to low-energy unattenuated counts should be 0.50–0.70; the transverse mechanics test should be in the range 12 350–12 550 (DPX-L), and the longitudinal mechanics test should be in the range of 19 700–19 800; and the ratio of the low-energy to high-energy attenuation in the soft tissue sector (the R_{st} value, see Chapter 14) should be between 1.302 and 1.320. This value is used to calibrate the system for measurements of percentage fat during body composition studies. The above information is valid at the time of writing, but the user should consult the instrument manual and company literature for recent modifications.

During the scan of the calibration block, five passes or scan lines are performed over the phantom. The measured bone mineral values of the three chambers are used to calculate an index that is used by the system software to

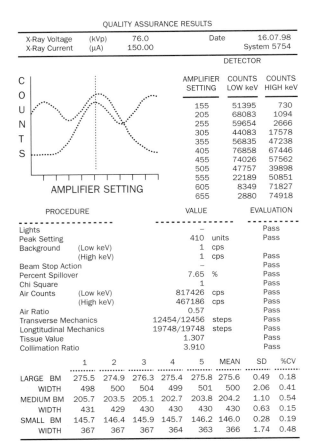

Figure 9.2 Record of daily quality control for a Lunar DPX instrument.

convert patient scan data into calibrated bone mineral values. The mean of the five measurements should be within 2.5% of the expected value entered into the software at installation of the DPX system. The coefficient of variation (CV = (standard deviation/mean) $\times$ 100) calculated from the five measurements should be less than or equal to 2%.

Daily scanning of the Lunar calibration phantom as described above provides only part of the information required for monitoring the system for any possible calibration shifts. To provide a complete assessment, regular scans of a second phantom, the Lunar spine phantom are also required (Figure 9.3). This is important because it provides additional information which is independent of system calibration. Each Lunar instrument is provided with its own spine phantom that should be measured at least once a week. The spine phantom is made of aluminium and has four rectangular 'vertebrae' with a range of BMD values from 0.92 to 1.40 g/cm^2 to test system linearity. To perform a QC scan with the aluminium spine phantom, it must be placed in a water bath with a set depth of water. Since January 1998, however, Lunar has provided purchasers of new DPX systems with an equivalent phantom made of hydroxyapatite and encased in a solid block of tissue-equivalent plastic (Figure 9.4).[1] Like the aluminium phantom, this has four 'vertebrae' with a range of BMD values. This new phantom avoids the inconvenience of having to fill a plastic tank with water. Like the old aluminium spine phantom, the new hydroxyapatite phantom is designed to allow independent tracking of instrument calibration as well as system linearity.

Quality control: Hologic QDR instruments

For Hologic QDR instruments (Hologic Inc., Waltham, MA, USA), daily QC consists of scanning the Hologic spine phantom (Figure 9.5). This consists of four moulded vertebrae (L1–L4) made from hydroxyapatite mixed in epoxy resin, the whole supported and encased in an epoxy-resin block. Each QDR instrument is provided with its own individually numbered phantom in the factory, and the values of BMD, BMC and projected area measured at that time are printed on the side of the phantom.

On Hologic systems, patient scanning is disabled until the instrument passes the daily QC test with the spine phantom. The size of the global region of interest (ROI) utilized for scan analysis of the phantom should remain unchanged from day to day (Figure 9.6). After completing a phantom scan, the results are entered into the QC database provided with the system software. As described in Chapter 3, Hologic QDR densitometers have an internal calibration wheel permanently installed inside the unit which provides the calibration data for the calculation of BMD. The function of this is described in detail in the Appendix to Chapter 3. However, daily scanning of the spine phantom is still required as a precaution against other possible causes of calibration changes or drifts within the instrument. No other daily quality checks are performed on the system.

At the time of installation of a new QDR instrument, 20 scans of the Hologic spine phantom are performed and the data entered into the QC database. The mean BMD, BMC and projected area are calculated and should agree with the values printed on the side of the phantom. If the agreement is outside the limits set by the manufacturer, then the results of the phantom scans are used to recalibrate the system by modifying the area and BMC system calibration factors shown in Figure 9.6. In this event it would be necessary to perform another 20 scans of the spine phantom to check the revised calibration.

Once there is satisfactory agreement with the factory calibration values for the phantom, the measured mean BMD, BMC and area are used to set up the QC plot provided as part of the system QC software (Figure 9.7). The means values are displayed as the central line across each QC plot. The same spine phantom is scanned daily and results added to the QC plot, after which the plot should be inspected for any deviations. The two dashed lines indicate a $\pm$1.5% range of variation about the mean, and

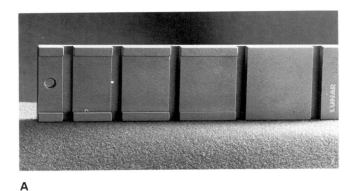

A

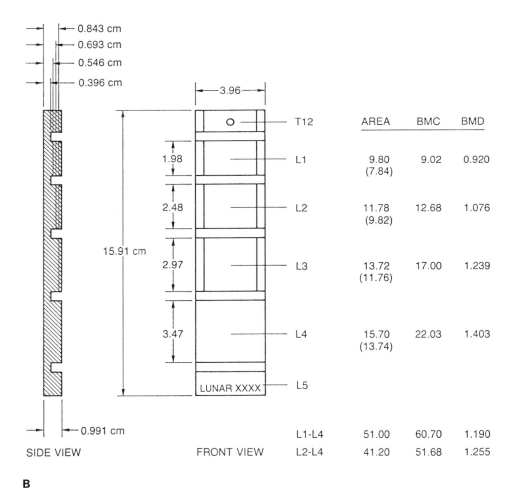

	AREA	BMC	BMD
T12			
L1	9.80 (7.84)	9.02	0.920
L2	11.78 (9.82)	12.68	1.076
L3	13.72 (11.76)	17.00	1.239
L4	15.70 (13.74)	22.03	1.403
L5			
L1-L4	51.00	60.70	1.190
L2-L4	41.20	51.68	1.255

SIDE VIEW   FRONT VIEW

0.843 cm
0.693 cm
0.546 cm
0.396 cm

3.96

15.91 cm

1.98
2.48
2.97
3.47

0.991 cm

LUNAR XXXX

B

Figure 9.3 (A) The aluminium spine phantom used with Lunar DXA instruments. (B) Specifications of the Lunar spine phantom. (Reproduced with permission from Lunar Corp.)

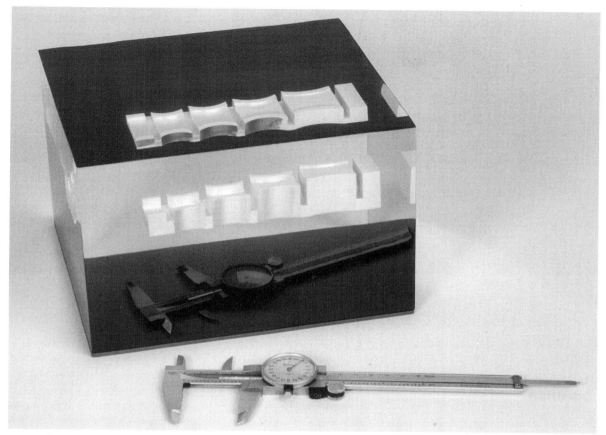

Figure 9.4 The new hydroxyapatite spine phantom developed by Lunar.[1]

values outside these limits require investigation as they indicate a possible QC problem with the system. In the event of such a finding, the phantom should first be scanned again to check the result. If the fault is confirmed, the manufacturer's service department should be contacted before any more patient scans are performed. The size of the day-to-day variations in measured phantom BMD is quantified by the coefficient of variation (CV) which generally lies in the range 0.3–0.7%. Any drifts over a period of time can be examined using a linear regression test provided within the system software (Figure 9.7). In the QDR-2000 and QDR-2000*plus* instruments, it is necessary to

perform daily phantom scans to check both the pencil-beam and fan-beam modes, since calibration drifts may be observed in one, but not the other. Figure 9.8 demonstrates an abrupt change in instrument calibration believed to be due to the scanning arm being struck and the detector knocked out of alignment with the X-ray beam.

The area and BMC calibration factors (CF numbers) given on each scan printout (Figure 9.6) provide a useful check for the status of the system calibration. These numbers should remain constant unless an instrument has been recalibrated after maintenance or repair of a defect. Review of the CF numbers on individual

A

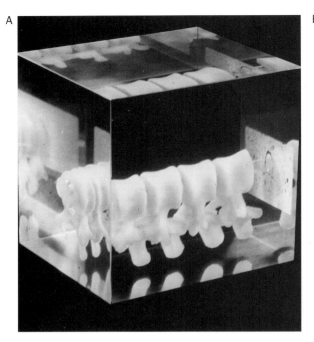

B

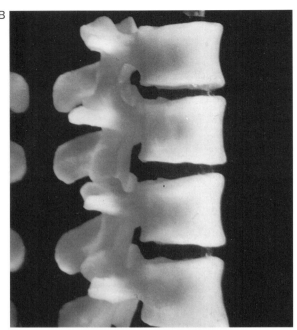

Figure 9.5 (A) Hologic anthropomorphic spine phantom used for calibration and daily quality control scans on QDR-series densitometers. (B) Close-up view of moulded vertebrae in Hologic spine phantom.

scans allows retrospective assessment of whether a scan was performed before or after a calibration change or instrument failure.

Hologic also provide two other phantoms that can be purchased by users interested in other aspects of system QC. The first is a phantom made from a mould of the proximal femur (Figure 9.9). Like the spine phantom, this phantom is embedded in an epoxy-resin block. The femur phantom can be useful for investigating specific aspects of the femur analysis software. Apart from this, femur phantom BMD measurements reflect similar information to that provided by the spine phantom. However, because of the smaller projected area, precision is somewhat poorer. The second additional

phantom is the Hologic block phantom (Figure 9.10). This consists of three rectangular blocks of hydroxyapatite embedded in an epoxy-resin block with uniform BMD values of approximately 0.6, 1.0 and 1.6 g/cm². Although not anthropomorphic as are the Hologic spine and femur phantoms, the block phantom does cover a wide range of bone density values. It may therefore be useful in evaluating any possible variations in the linearity of the BMD scale in a way that is not possible with the spine phantom because each vertebra has the same BMD value of approximately 1.0 g/cm². Therefore for those centres interested in undertaking a more comprehensive QC programme, a weekly scan of the block phantom can provide useful supple-

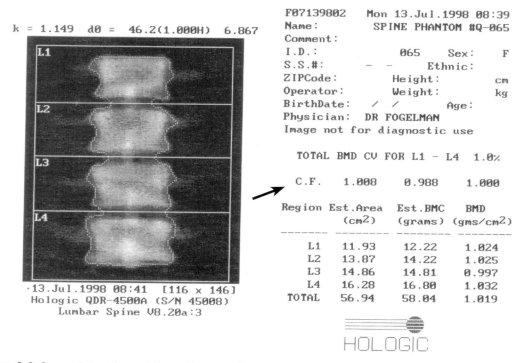

Figure 9.6 Scan printout for a daily quality control scan of the Hologic spine phantom. The height and width of the global ROI box are 146 mm and 116 mm respectively. The arrow points to the two system calibration factors for projected area and BMC respectively.

mentary information in the event of a serious system failure.

Quality control: Norland XR instruments

With Norland XR-series scanners (Norland Medical Systems, Fort Atkinson, WI, USA), a 77-step calibration phantom (Figure 9.11) made of aluminium and acrylic is scanned daily. Scanning this phantom calibrates the coefficients of the equations used to relate the high- and low-energy X-ray attenuation factors to the areal densities of bone mineral and soft tissue. In this way the BMD scale of the system is calibrated over all clinically relevant values of

BMD and soft-tissue thickness. This procedure has the advantage that it eliminates the need for the separate pulse pile-up, cross-over and beam hardening corrections that are generally necessary for X-ray absorptiometry measurements. At the same time that the calibration phantom is scanned, a scan is also performed of a hydroxyapatite spine phantom, and the BMD results are entered into a system QC database. As described above in the discussion of the instrumental QC for Lunar and Hologic densitometers, the important principle here is that regular scans should be performed of a phantom that is independent of the means of system calibration.

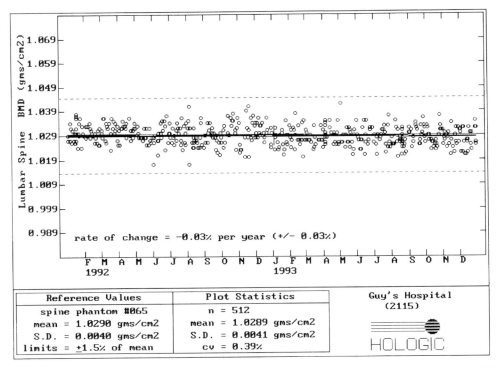

Figure 9.7 Quality control plot for BMD results of daily quality control scans performed on a Hologic QDR-4500 instrument. Any long-term drifts can be detected by the results of linear regression analysis as shown in this plot.

OTHER CROSS-CALIBRATION AND QUALITY CONTROL PHANTOMS

The European Spine Phantom

The European Spine Phantom (ESP) will be familiar to many users of axial DXA scanners because it has been widely used for cross calibration of instruments in multicentre clinical trials.[2] The ESP (Figure 9.12) was developed by Kalender and Felsenberg[3,4] with sponsorship from the European Union under the Committée d'Actions Concerté-Biomedical Engineering (COMAC-BME) programme as part of a wider

agenda for the quantitative assessment of osteoporosis.

The design of the ESP approximates the shape of three human vertebrae of varying thickness and is made of bone-equivalent plastics and hydroxyapatite (Figures 9.13 and 9.14). There are trabecular and cortical structures and cortical walls. The transverse processes are built as ramps to allow a definition of cut-off points for their elimination from spine scans. The aim was to test the bone-edge detection algorithms used by different manufacturers. The three vertebrae have a spongiosa density of 50, 100 and 200 mg/cm^3 and cortical wall thicknesses of 1, 2

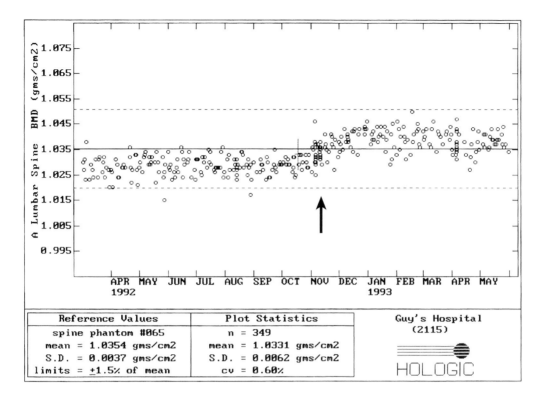

Figure 9.8 Quality control plot for a QDR instrument showing an abrupt change in calibration.

and 3 mm for measurements by QCT. For DXA measurements, the area densities are 0.5, 1.0 and 1.5 g/cm² hydroxyapatite. Exact BMD values vary slightly between phantoms and are listed with the calibration information provided by the manufacturer. End-plates of 1 mm thickness allow good vertebral delineation for lateral scanning with DXA. Detailed specifications of the ESP are given in Table 9.2. A list of physical quantities that can be tested with the ESP including its use for quantitative computed tomography (QCT) studies, is given in Table 9.3.

The introduction of the ESP has raised considerable controversy. Although it was intro-

duced initially to standardize BMD values between different manufacturers' densitometers, the recommendations of the International Committee for Standards in Bone Measurement (ICSBM) for standardization of spine and femur BMD[5-7] have instead been based principally on in vivo cross-calibration studies, with the ESP playing only a minor role. The ICSBM committee recommendations are discussed in detail in Chapters 10 and 12. The decision of the committee to reject the use of any phantom as the basis of BMD standardization was made because no phantom yet built agrees adequately with the differences found in vivo between different manufacturers' equipment.[5,8]

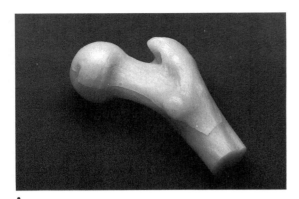

A

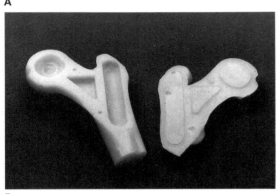

B

Figure 9.9 The hydroxyapatite insert for a Hologic femur phantom shown open (A) and closed (B). The complex bone structure in the proximal femur is imitated by a carved-out triangle at the base of the neck (Ward's triangle) and trochanter.

Other controversial aspects of the ESP include the relatively poor precision of the measurements, which may restrict its usefulness for long-term monitoring of instruments, and debate over the true linearity of the BMD scale established by the phantom.[9]

Perhaps the most important advice about quality control that can be given to users of DXA equipment is that independent phantoms such as the ESP should not be substituted for the daily QC programme recommended by the manufacturer. In the event of a serious failure, the daily phantom measurement programme

recommended by the manufacturer is the only reliable guarantee for the continuity of the system BMD calibration. However, regular scanning of other phantoms such as the ESP in addition to the manufacturers' phantoms may provide further useful data.

The same group of investigators have also developed a forearm phantom, referred to as the European Forearm Phantom (EFP) (Figures 9.15 and 9.16). This phantom has yet to be fully validated and approved.

Bona Fide calcium hydroxyapatite phantom

This phantom (Figure 9.4) was developed to provide a relatively inexpensive alternative to the Lunar aluminium spine phantom (Figure 9.3), but using hydroxyapatite to mimic bone instead of aluminium.[1] By including four different BMD values it also provides a less expensive alternative to the ESP for testing system linearity. However, it is not anthropomorphic and cannot be used in the lateral mode. It consists of a hydroxyapatite 'spine' enclosed in a soft tissue mimic. The overall size of the phantom is 22 cm long × 19 cm wide × 15 cm high. The size of the hydroxyapatite 'spine' is 16 cm long × 4 cm wide × 3 cm high.

A CRITIQUE OF THE AVAILABLE PHANTOMS

There has been considerable debate about the design of a 'useful' phantom. This is in part qualified by which question needs to be answered. For the calibration of an instrument, for example, there are a series of instrument checks being performed and physical items being evaluated. An ideal phantom would exactly mimic a patient. Since such a phantom is not available, then a decision has to be made as to the absolute requirements. Hologic decided that an anthropomorphic phantom of hydroxyapatite would be optimal. The principal limitation of this phantom is that it only measures one point on the BMD calibration scale and therefore cannot be used to check the

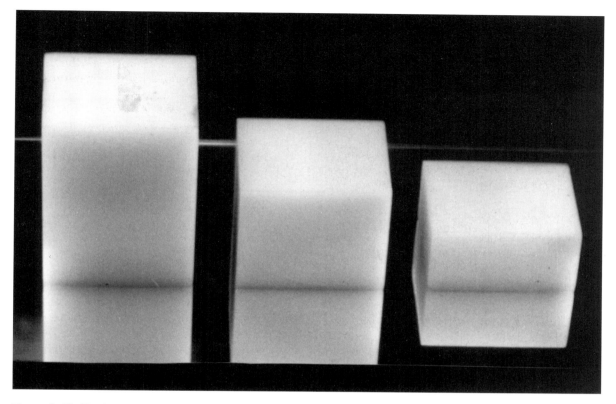

Figure 9.10 The Hologic block phantom used for checking the linearity of BMD measurements on QDR-series instruments. The three hydroxyapatite blocks have BMD values of approximately 0.6, 1.0 and 1.6 g/cm².

system linearity. Also, the soft-tissue equivalent epoxy resin is hyperfatty, and therefore non-physiological.

Lunar concluded that it was important to test linearity, and that a soft tissue medium closer to physiological soft tissue was required. The Lunar spine phantom has four steps (Figure 9.3), is made of aluminium and is scanned in a water bath. From basic physical principles, aluminium is actually quite a close mimic for bone. However, from an aesthetic point of view, the choice was suboptimal, and some regulatory agencies (notably the Food and Drug Administration (FDA)) have suggested that the bone part of phantoms should be made from hydroxyapatite since this is a basic constituent of bone. The Hologic, ESP and Bona Fide phantoms all fulfil this requirement.

The ESP was developed independently of any densitometer manufacturer to overcome the supposed limitations of the other phantoms. A semi-anthropomorphic phantom was developed which measured BMD at three distinct densities. Although the idea was noble, the expectations were not completely fulfilled. The concept was complicated by the phantom being designed to serve as the standard for the newly devised standardized BMD.

The major advantages of the ESP were that it was not manufacturer specific, was made of

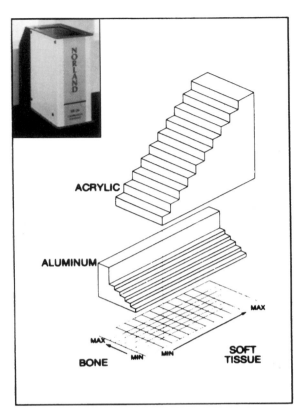

Figure 9.11 The Norland 77-step calibration phantom.

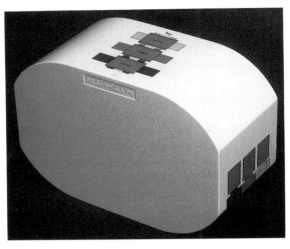

Figure 9.12 The European Spine Phantom. (Courtesy of WA Kalender and D Felsenberg.)

hydroxyapatite, semi-anthropomorphic and gave linearity information. Unfortunately, when scans of the ESP were compared on any two manufacturers' densitometers, the BMD results did not match patient data, and did not lie on the standardized BMD (sBMD) line of identity as determined by in vivo studies.[5] Hence, it could not be used to determine fully the sBMD parameter. The design of the transverse processes made edge detection difficult, giving the phantom rather poor precision. The high cost has also been a major disadvantage for widespread usage.

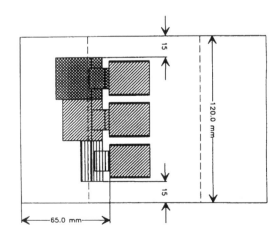

Figure 9.13 Dimensions of the European Spine Phantom from a lateral view. (Courtesy of WA Kalender and D Felsenberg.)

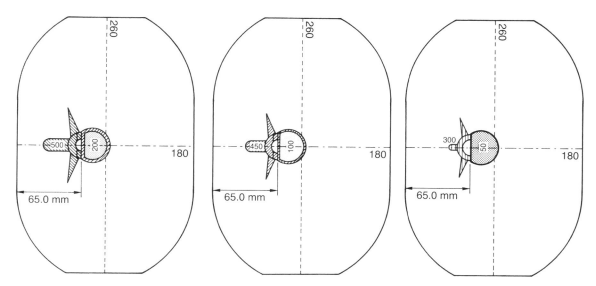

Figure 9.14 Schematic cross-sections through the European Spine Phantom demonstrating the three vertebrae with increasing density of cortical and trabecular bone. Total thickness of the phantom is 180 mm, equal to the average abdominal thickness in patients. The posterior surface of the vertebral body is 65 mm above the table-top, representing the true distance in patients. (Courtesy of WA Kalender and D Felsenberg.)

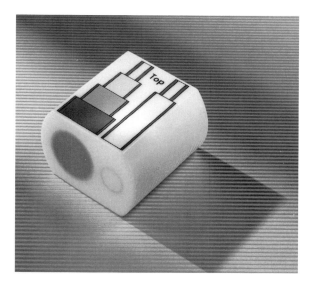

Figure 9.15 The European Forearm Phantom. Both radius and ulna are represented. (Courtesy of WA Kalender and D Felsenberg.)

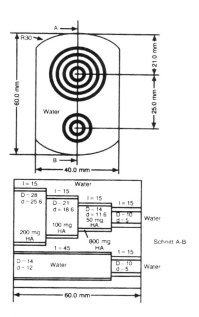

Figure 9.16 Design specifications of the European Forearm Phantom. (Courtesy of WA Kalender and D Felsenberg.)

Table 9.2 Design parameters of the vertebral inserts. (Reproduced with permission from Kalender.[3])

Parameters	Vertebrae		
	Low	Medium	High
Geometry (values in mm)			
Body diameter	36	36	36
Arch diameter	28	28	28
Height	25	25	25
Body wall thickness	1	2	3
End-plate thickness	1	1	1
Arch thickness	5.7	7	8
Spinous process thickness	6	12	12
Spinous process length	8.5	21.6	27.5
Densities (values in mg hydroxyapatite/cm^3)			
Spongiosa	50	100	200
Walls and end-plates	400	400	400
Arch and processes	300	400	500
PA projection of vertebral body			
Area (mm^2)	900	900	900
BMC (g)	4.5	9.0	13.5
BMD (g/cm^2)	0.5	1.0	1.5
Lateral projection of vertebral body			
Area (mm^2)	732.8	732.8	732.8
BMC (g)	2.58	4.17	6.16
BMD (g/cm^2)	0.35	0.57	0.84

The requirements for edge detection in a phantom require further comment. DXA instruments work in part because of well designed software. The ability to distinguish between bone and soft tissue is fully automated, although it can be over-ridden by the operator. The algorithms are very robust and work well except in extreme cases where bone is very osteoporotic. On Hologic instruments, this is compensated by a useful feature allowing the operator to 'paint-in' or 'paint-out' bone if the automatic software algorithms fail. Therefore, testing of an instrument's edge detection algorithms may have some merit, if the phantom can do this with a good physiological mimic.

The Hologic spine phantom is anthropomor-

Table 9.3 Quantities to be tested with the European Spine Phantom (ESP). (Reproduced with permission from Kalender.[3])

1) Projected area of vertebrae (cm²) (DXA)
2) Bone mineral content (g) (DXA)
3) Trabecular and cortical bone mineral density (mg/cm³) (QCT)
4) Cortical thickness (mm) (QCT)
5) Positioning (QCT)

---

phic, but the high BMD value does not effectively test the instrument's edge detection algorithms. However, there has been no documented evidence that any instrument has failed because of this problem. The ESP does challenge the edge-detection algorithms, and is the only phantom that does so, but not physiologically. Unfortunately, this has led to the relatively poor precision of ESP measurements.

Since the spine phantoms described so far test the physics of the instrument from a pseudo-patient standpoint, there have been other phantoms developed to assess other anatomical sites. These are at best poor, and do not really add anything to what is known about an instrument's calibration with the exception of edge-detection algorithms for that particular anatomical site. Since edge-detection algorithms have not been documented to fail, this becomes a moot point. None of the non-spine phantoms available have become widely used.

STANDARDIZED BMD

The ICSBM has attempted to provide a single unified BMD scale that could be reproduced on all densitometers. Due to differences in instrument design, edge-detection algorithms and

system calibration, different manufacturers' densitometers provide different BMD values when used to measure the same site in the body. Therefore, an attempt has been made to bring all the instruments down to a single 'interchangeable' BMD (or standardized BMD (sBMD)) value. For proprietary reasons, sBMD could not be based on one of the calibration indices already in use, and therefore a new independent calibration point was required. Unfortunately, different conversion algorithms for sBMD are required for different sites in the body. The scale for spine BMD is loosely based on the ESP in so far as it is set to ensure that the sBMD values for the middle vertebrae of the ESP on Hologic, Lunar and Norland densitometers average 1.0 g/cm², the nominal BMD for this vertebra. The sBMD algorithms for spine BMD were published in 1995,[6] and for the femur in 1997.[7] Further details are given in Chapters 10 and 12. All the manufacturers represented on the ICSBM committee now offer optional software to provide scan reports in sBMD units, although this has not so far been widely adopted.

Since sBMD is not 'owned' by any individual manufacturer, there has been a reluctance to gravitate towards its use. Although sBMD results can be provided on scan printouts, in the author's experience these have not been used extensively for reporting. With many new sites acquiring DXA instruments without any prior knowledge of this field, this has not become an issue at the point of sale, and many physicians and technologists are unaware of its existence or potential use.

CLINICAL TRIAL IQC

Instrument quality control (IQC) programmes for BMD data required in pharmaceutical clinical trials have had an important influence in raising knowledge and awareness of this issue and its relevance to routine clinical bone densitometry as well as to research studies. The pharmaceutical industry not only demands the optimum, but good clinical practice requires good clear documentation of all events. The thorough types of review that are described below are generally carried out at quality assessment centres, organizations that are specifically set up to undertake the role of 'core laboratories' for DXA equipment. The expectation is that all DXA instruments (regardless of the manufacturer) perform a daily QC BMD measurement. This information is then sent periodically (usually monthly) to the quality assessment centre for review.

Essentially there are two types of calibration changes that have to be guarded against: the rapid shift to a new baseline point, and the more insidious gradual drift. Several statistical solutions have been presented to identify the problem, all of which provide quantification to an 'eye-balled' problem. The most commonly used statistical evaluation of QC data are the adapted Shewhart rules. These were originally introduced for car manufacturing lines to ensure that parts were machined to correct quality. The rules were adapted for use in biochemical assays,[10] and Orwoll and Oviatt[11] applied the idea to DXA IQC. The Shewhart

Table 9.4 Shewhart criteria for the evaluation of quality control charts. These recommendations assume that a measurement on a QC phantom is performed on each day that the instrument is operated. This single measurement is then evaluated against the plot statistics of the instrument. Random error generally is detected with rules 2 and 4, and systematic error by rules 3, 5 and 6. (Modified from Orwoll and Oviatt.[11])

1) *Warning rule:* A phantom measurement may exceed acceptable limits if it is outside + or −1% of the plot mean value. This occurrence should prompt additional inspection of control data with the following rules.

2) *1.5% rule:* A phantom measurement exceeding the plot mean value by ±1.5% indicates the need for instrument evaluation. See rule 7.

3) *1% twice rule:* Two consecutive phantom measurements that exceed the mean by 1% dictate instrument evaluation. See rule 7.

4) *Range of 2% rule:* When the difference between two consecutive measurements exceeds 2% (specifically when one measurement exceeds +1% and another exceeds −1%) the instrument requires evaluation. See rule 7.

5) *Four + or −0.5% rule:* When four consecutive measurements exceed the same limit (+0.5% or −0.5%) instrument evaluation is required. See rule 7.

6) *Mean × 10 rule:* When 10 consecutive control measures fall on the same side of the plot mean value, instrument evaluation is necessary. See rule 7.

7) *Instrument evaluation:* This involves at least five repeated measurements (with repositioning of phantom). If the mean value of these measurements is outside 1% of the plot mean value, inspection or service of the instrument is advised. Smaller differences are acceptable.

rules are summarized in Table 9.4. Several other authors have since described their use in bone densitometry.[12–16]

An alternative to the Shewhart rules which has been adapted by some QC centres is the use of Cusum charts.[15,16] Again, these appear to be reliable and useful. However, like the Shewhart rules, several assumptions are made about the data, including that they are normally distributed. Unless normality is checked as part of the IQC procedure, then a false positive or negative result may be obtained with these algorithms. To overcome this, a third approach has been presented using a multiple graphing analysis.[17] This approach checks QC in several manners, including a review of underlying assumptions, and provides a final number (the control process capability, or CpK) to give an overall evaluation.

Whatever the methodology, the principle behind IQC in clinical trials is to define when an instrument is out of control (OOC), or about to become out of control. Optimally the diagnosis of an instrument that is about to fail is preferable to identifying one that is already OOC. Service engineers will need to be called out for both situations, but the former allows preventative maintenance rather than repair of a system that has already failed. Furthermore, when an instrument is OOC the patient data collected during that time may be unreliable. With a planned preventative maintenance programme in mind, it is possible with Lunar instruments to use the QA data to predict with a high degree of certainty which instruments are likely to fail up to 3 months in advance, knowing how the given variables relate to the instrument's internal working.

One important facet of evaluating instrument drift or change is to check linearity changes. Some phantoms (notably the Hologic spine phantom) provide only a single BMD value. It is often assumed that any changes seen at one BMD will reflect the changes seen at lower or higher BMD values, i.e. that the same percentage changes occur over the entire bone density range. This is not always the case, and any changes seen should be evaluated across a range of densities, particularly if the patient population under investigation is based around a different BMD value from that of the phantom. Otherwise corrections could be applied to the patient data that are incorrect for the population under study. On Hologic densitometers, this can be overcome using the Hologic block phantom which provides BMD results at three different densities. Alternatively, the ESP or Bona Fide phantoms could be used. However, whichever choice is made, the operator is required to scan a second phantom regularly.

SUMMARY AND CONCLUSIONS

Performing IQC is a critically important part of evaluating a DXA instrument's function. It provides the operator with valuable information about the instrument's current calibration and potential future calibration. It should therefore be regarded as an integral part of the instrument's use with sufficient time being allocated daily to ensure this is performed properly before patients are measured. DXA instruments rarely fail or go out of control, but when they do it is vital that this is detected to prevent patient measurement which would compromise ethical and clinical standards.

REFERENCES

1. Nord RH, Bisek JP. A new hydroxyapatite spine phantom. *Osteoporos Int* (1997) **7**: 287.
2. Lees B, Garland SW, Walton C, Stevenson JC. Evaluation of the European spine phantom in a multi-centre clinical trial. *Osteoporos Int* (1997) **7**: 570–4.
3. Kalender WA. A phantom for standardization and quality control in spinal bone mineral measurements by QCT and DXA: design considerations and specifications. *Med Phys* (1992) **19**: 583–6.
4. Kalender WA, Felsenberg D, Genant HK et al. The European spine phantom: a tool for standardization and quality control in spinal bone mineral measurements by DXA and QCT. *Eur J Radiol* (1995) **20**: 83–92.
5. Genant HK, Grampp S, Glüer C-C et al. Universal standardization for dual x-ray absorptiometry: patient and cross-calibration results. *J Bone Miner Res* (1994) **9**: 1503–14.

6. Steiger P. Standardization of measurements for assessing BMD by DXA [letter]. *Calcif Tissue Int* (1995) **57:** 469.

7. Hanson J. Standardization of femur BMD [letter]. *J Bone Miner Res* (1997) **12:** 1316–17.

8. Nord RH. Appropriate use of phantoms in DXA studies. *Osteoporos Int* (1996) **6:** 87.

9. Nord RH. Performance of the European spine phantom – an evaluation from published data. *Osteoporos Int* (1996) **6:** 99.

10. Westgard JO, Barry PL, Hunt MR, Groth T. A multirule Shewhart chart for quality control in clinical chemistry. *Clin Chem* (1981) **27:** 493–501.

11. Orwoll ES, Oviatt SK. Longitudinal precision of dual-energy x-ray absorptiometry in a multicenter study. *J Bone Miner Res* (1991) **6:** 191–7.

12. Orwoll ES, Oviatt SK, Biddle JA. Precision of dual-energy x-ray absorptiometry: development of quality control rules and their application in longitudinal studies. *J Bone Miner Res* (1993) **8:** 693–9.

13. Wahner HW, Looker A, Dunn WI et al. Quality control of bone densitometry in a national health survey (NHANES III) using three mobile examination centers. *J Bone Miner Res* (1994) **9:** 951–60.

14. Faulkner KG, McClung MR. Quality control of DXA instruments in multicenter trials. *Osteoporos Int* (1995) **5:** 218–27.

15. Garland SW, Lees B, Stevenson JC. DXA longitudinal quality control: a comparison of inbuilt quality assurance, visual inspection, multi-rule Shewhart charts and Cusum analysis. *Osteoporos Int* (1997) **7:** 231–7.

16. Pearson D, Cawte SA. Long-term quality control of DXA: a comparison of Shewhart rules and Cusum charts. *Osteoporos Int* (1997) **7:** 338–43.

17. Miller CG. Instrument quality control of DXA in clinical trials. *Osteoporos Int* (1996) **6:** 88.

10

Measurement of Bone Density in the Lumbar Spine: the PA Spine Scan

CONTENTS • Chapter overview • Introduction • Acquisition and analysis of a DXA spine scan • Review of a lumbar spine BMD report • Standardized BMD for lumbar spine DXA scans • Illustrative cases • Appendix

CHAPTER OVERVIEW

This chapter reviews in general terms how postero-anterior (PA) projection dual-energy X-ray absorptiometry (DXA) scans of the lumbar spine are performed. A step-by-step guideline is given for reviewing the computer-generated data provided by the manufacturers' scan report software. These guidelines were designed to achieve optimal precision in longitudinal studies, but also have wider applications for aiding the interpretation of bone mineral density (BMD) results in routine clinical practice. Frequently encountered errors are discussed and relevant points illustrated by case presentations. Normal BMD values are given and the recommendations of the International Committee for Standards in Bone Measurement for the standardization of spinal BMD measurements are discussed.

INTRODUCTION

The lumbar spine is probably the most frequently studied skeletal site for DXA measurements because of its sensitivity to the effects of ageing, the menopause and secondary causes of bone loss. The region of interest (ROI) studied is usually either L1–L4 or L2–L4, and serves as a sampling site for bone mineral estimation in the vertebral column. The total mass of bone mineral in the spine (BMC) is typically about 130 g, of which about 45 g is in the lumbar spine ROI. Thus, about one-third of the total bone mass in the spine is sampled.

In children and young adults, bone mineral, when expressed as BMD, shows a relatively uniform distribution throughout the lumbar spine, gradually increasing from L1 to L4 (Figures 10.1 and 10.2A). BMD values for vertebrae in the thoracic spine are not available from absorptiometry measurements, since the presence of the ribs, sternum and lung fields precludes an accurate estimation of bone density. With advancing age, however, the distribution pattern of bone mineral in the spine becomes less uniform. Spencer et al.[1] studied 236 white women aged 36–85 years, who were examined to rule out osteoporosis, and found that the distribution of BMD along the lumbar spine (L2–L4) showed values within 25% (difference between highest and lowest BMD expressed as a percentage of the mean) in all

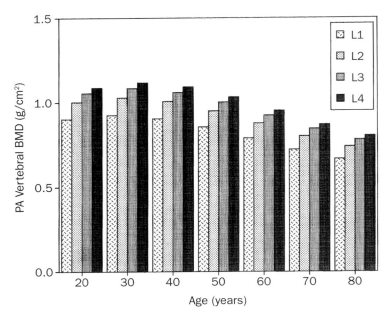

Figure 10.1 Variation of bone mineral density (BMD) in the lumbar spine. BMD data are plotted for the individual vertebrae as a function of age. The figure was prepared using the normal population mean values from the Hologic normal range. Note the gradual decrease in BMD up the spine from L4 to L1.

women under 46 years of age. However, in women over 75 years of age, 40% exceeded the 25% difference level. For the age group 46–75 years, the fraction of the population exceeding the 25% BMD difference increased linearly with age. This inhomogeneity is recognizable on radiographs as well as DXA scan images, and also by reviewing BMD results from individual vertebrae (Figure 10.2B). Vertebrae with varying degrees of compression or with hypertrophic degenerative changes are interspersed with portions of spine with normal appearance. When significant non-uniformity of bone mineral distribution is present, there is less confidence that the BMD measurements are representative of true skeletal status. In elderly patients, spinal abnormalities may be so pronounced that the femur or a peripheral site should be preferred for diagnostic work-up of

patients with suspected osteoporosis or other bone disease.

With DXA, it is usual to measure integral bone mineral and express the results as areal density in units of g/cm^2. However, results can also be expressed as the bone mineral content (BMC) of a given ROI in grams, or as bone mineral (g) per unit of bone volume (cm^3). To obtain this latter result, volume must be estimated for each vertebra from the projected area of the PA spine scan and a vertebral thickness calculated. An example is the bone mineral apparent density (BMAD, units: $g/cm^3)^2$ which appears to be a more robust predictor of CT-measured bone density than BMD.[3] Bone volume can also be estimated by combining PA and lateral projection scans.[4,5] Although volumetric density estimates have been available for many years, recent interest in this measurement

A

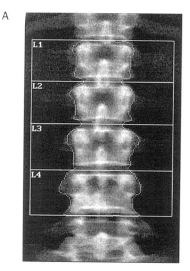

Region	Est Area (cm2)	Est BMC (grams)	BMD (gms/cm2)
L1	14.33	13.77	1.961
L2	15.01	15.74	1.049
L3	17.68	19.34	.094
L4	20.73	23.93	1.154
TOTAL	67.75	72.78	1.074

BMD(L1-L4)   1.074 g/cm2

Region	BMD	T(30.0)		Z	
L1	0.961	+0.33	104%	+0.34	104%
L2	1.049	+0.19	102%	+0.20	102%
L3	1.094	+0.09	101%	+0.10	101%
L4	1.154	+0.35	103%	+0.36	104%
L1-L4	1.074	+0.25	103%	+0.26	103%

B

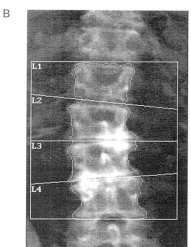

Region	Est.Area (cm2)	Est.BMC (grams)	BMD (gms/cm2)
L1	13.99	8.94	0.639
L2	14.82	12.55	0.847
L3	15.00	16.67	1.112
L4	17.25	17.81	1.033
TOTAL	61.06	55.98	0.917

BMD(L1-L4) = 0.917 g/cm2

Region	BMD	T(30.0)		Z	
L1	0.639	-2.60	69%	-0.50	92%
L2	0.847	-1.65	82%	+0.69	110%
L3	1.112	+0.25	103%	+2.71	137%
L4	1.033	-0.75	93%	+1.78	123%
L1-L4	0.917	-1.18	88%	+1.18	116%

Figure 10.2 (A) Lumbar spine DXA scan image and BMD results in a 31-year-old woman. Note the normal decrease in BMD from L4 to L1 reflected in the uniform T- and Z-score figures. (B) Lumbar spine DXA scan image and BMD results in a 74-year-old woman with extensive degenerative changes in the spine. Note that the obvious changes in the scan image are accompanied by highly discrepant T- and Z-score figures in the individual vertebrae.

unit is based on improved methods of calculation.

The posterior portion of the vertebrae contains primarily compact bone and comprises $45 \pm 6\%$ of total BMC.[3] In the vertebral body, about 40% is compact bone and 60% is trabecular. With advancing age, bone marrow fat increases. The physiological increases in bone marrow fat do not significantly interfere with DXA measurements.[6] It has been shown, however, with phantoms, that the presence of bone marrow decreases BMD in the vertebra by a few per cent.

Recommendations in the manufacturers' manuals on how to perform a bone mineral measurement in the spine, though they are detailed, do not deal with all the problems that may arise. Additional 'rule of thumb' procedures are required to ensure continuity of method at any one centre, and to achieve consistency between centres. The importance of a well trained, dedicated technologist to perform the scans cannot be overemphasized. Centres with a high turnover of staff invariably have problems in the quality of both scan acquisition and analysis. Users' meetings to establish common approaches help to achieve uniformity of technique, as do the technologist training sessions often arranged at the start of multicentre clinical trials. The clinician who is seriously concerned about scan quality will send his or her staff to such meetings. At the Mayo Clinic, all DXA studies are performed by dedicated technologists and less than 1% of studies have to be reanalysed or patients recalled when scans are seen by the reviewing physician. In contrast, in a multicentre study with technologists performing the measurements part time and with a frequent turnover of staff, it was found that 2% of patients needed to be rescanned and that 8–15% of scan images needed to be reanalysed. Adherence to strict guidelines is mandatory if data interpretation is to be based on assumptions of optimal measurement accuracy and precision.

ACQUISITION AND ANALYSIS OF A DXA SPINE SCAN

Patient interview and questionnaire

Prior to performing a DXA study, a short interview establishes that there are no contraindications to the scan. A list of contraindications and interfering conditions can be found in Table 10.1. Pertinent demographic and clinical data should also be obtained at this time as these may be needed for scan interpretation. A sample patient questionnaire is shown in the Appendix to this chapter.

Patient positioning

Before positioning the patient, all metal items should be removed from the clothing. Metal in belts, coins in pockets, wires and hooks in bras, corsets or trusses can all interfere. The recent popularity of naval jewellery has created another type of metal artefact (Figure 10.3).

Acquisition and scan analysis should be performed according to the manufacturers' protocols. These differ in detail on how to operate the instrument and the sequence of steps required. In general, however, all PA spine scans are performed with the patient lying supine on the imaging table. The patient should be aligned in the middle of the table with the spine straight and parallel to the longitudinal table axis. On some systems only a restricted area of the table can be used for scanning the hip or spine. Thus, if both sites are to be scanned, the patient will need to be repositioned between the scans. It is standard practice to use a soft block supplied with the instrument to raise the patient's legs by supporting them under the knees. Raising the legs in this way reduces the physiological spinal lordosis and aligns the disc spaces with the X-ray beam to improve the separation of individual vertebrae on the scan image.

Although the elevated knee position is still the recommended procedure (and was very important with dual photon absorptiometry (DPA) instruments because of the poor image

---

Table 10.1 Contraindications and interfering conditions.

1) *Contraindications to bone mineral measurement at the lumbar spine*
   - Pregnancy (abdominal thickness, radiation)
   - Recent oral contrast media (2–6 days). Intravenous contrast media are rapidly excreted and rarely interfere after a few hours
   - Recent nuclear medicine test (depends on isotope used):

     ^{99m}Tc-MDP bone scan 48 h (6 h half-life)
     ^{99m}Tc-MAA lung scan 24 h
     ^{99m}Tc-SC liver scan 48 h
     ^{131}I more than 4 MBq 72 h or longer if there are bone metastases in the lumbar spine
     ^{99m}Tc-DTPA or Mag3 renal scan 24 h

   - Inability to remain supine on the imaging table for 5 minutes without movement. Fast scan modes may be used for a difficult problem, reducing scan time to less than 1 minute
   - Spinal deformity or disease, orthopaedic hardware in the lumbar spine as diagnosed by radiograph, since results will not be useful for a standard osteoporosis work-up

2) *Interfering conditions or objects*
   - Metal objects such as belt buckles, coins, truss, corset, underwired bra, buttons or zipper should be removed prior to scan
   - Recent ingestion of calcium-containing tablets, which may still be found undissolved in the GI tract
   - Recent ingestion of food is generally not considered to influence the measurement, and a fasting state is not required. If possible, measurements should be performed 2–4 h after the last large meal

---

resolution), the higher image quality of the X-ray systems has meant that in practice there is no significant difference in lumbar spine BMD if the legs are positioned straight on the table. Although it is good practice to adhere to strict guidelines on positioning the patient and setting the start and finishing points of the scan, the relatively large scan field used for lumbar spine DXA studies means that minor deviations from the guidelines are often of little significance, particularly if the patient is studied just once for comparison with the reference range (Figures 10.4 and 10.5). However, strict adherence is necessary for longitudinal studies.

A measurement of abdominal thickness may be helpful if subjects appear unusually obese or thin. Thickness should be measured routinely when the population under study shows significant variation in body weight between scans. For example, patients with liver disease may present with and without ascites on separate occasions, and patients on weight-reducing diets may undergo a significant change in weight. Abdominal thickness should be measured with calipers at the level of the umbilicus. Alternatively, some DXA systems estimate this figure from the attenuation of the radiation beam and print it out routinely on the scan

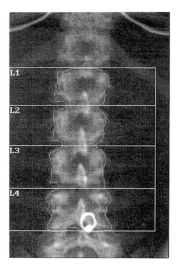

Region	Est.Area (cm^2)	Est.BMC (grams)	BMD (gms/cm^2)
L1	11.58	9.29	0.802
L2	12.28	10.85	0.884
L3	13.97	13.11	0.939
L4	16.55	17.92	1.082
TOTAL	54.39	51.16	0.941

BMD(L1-L4) = 0.941 g/cm^2

Region	BMD	T(30.0)		Z	
L1	0.802	-1.12	87%	-0.75	91%
L2	0.884	-1.31	86%	-0.90	90%
L3	0.939	-1.32	87%	-0.90	91%
L4	1.082	-0.31	97%	+0.14	101%
L1-L4	0.941	-0.97	90%	-0.55	94%

Figure 10.3 PA spine DXA scan for a 44-year-old woman with a metal artefact (a gold navel ring) over L4. The T- and Z-score figures for L4 are increased by approximately 1 SD compared with L1–L3.

report. In patients scanned for suspected osteoporosis abdominal thickness is typically in the range 15–25 cm. These values are within the manfuacturers' range for system calibration for the standard lumbar spine mode. However, scanning thinner (<10 cm) or thicker (>30 cm) body sections may lead to measurement errors depending on the instrument.

It is routine practice to measure patients' weight and height and these may be used to calculate the body mass index (BMI = kg/m^2). In patients with significant obesity (BMI > 30) the precision of the BMD measurements will be significantly poorer than the usually quoted figure of 1% due to the high attenuation of the radiation and the variable soft tissue composition. Most imaging tables for bone mineral measurements support patients up to 160 kg (350 lb). The manufacturer's weight limits should be reviewed before a severely obese subject is scanned. Occasionally the table to detector distance may be too small to fit a patient. Measurements made under such

extreme conditions are of dubious value because of the poor precision and the fact that the instrument is operating well outside the limits of its calibration.

Patient scanning

In the lumbar spine, the region selected for BMD analysis is usually either L1–L4 or L2–L4. However, the start and finish points of the scan should be chosen so that the anatomical landmarks required for reliable identification of the lumbar vertebrae are clearly visible (Figure 10.5).

Scan acquisition should start from a point 2.5–5 cm (1–2 inches) below the anterior margins of the iliac crest and should finish just above the tip of the xiphoid. If L1 is to be included in the BMD analysis, the scan should be lengthened to finish about 4 cm (1.5 inches) above the tip of the sternum to ensure that the scan field includes the entire lumbar spine.

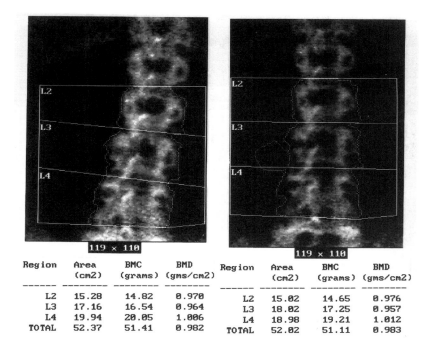

Region	Area (cm2)	BMC (grams)	BMD (gms/cm2)	Region	Area (cm2)	BMC (grams)	BMD (gms/cm2)
L2	15.28	14.82	0.970	L2	15.02	14.65	0.976
L3	17.16	16.54	0.964	L3	18.02	17.25	0.957
L4	19.94	20.05	1.006	L4	18.98	19.21	1.012
TOTAL	52.37	51.41	0.982	TOTAL	52.02	51.11	0.983

Figure 10.4 Poor patient alignment on the imaging table (left). The scan was repeated with better positioning (right). This small position error is tolerable and no difference was noted between scans. However, it should be noted that with fan-beam DXA systems it is more important to ensure that the spine is correctly centred to avoid errors due to image projection.

Normal reference values for both L1–L4 and L2–L4 are available, as well as for each lumbar vertebra individually. Because lumbar BMD is lowest in L1 (Figure 10.1), total BMD is slightly lower when L1–L4 is used. L1 is also a frequent site of compression fracture in older women, and in this circumstance must be excluded from the BMD analysis. In patients with kyphosis or spinal deformity, the sternum is closer to the pelvis, and should be scanned 2.5–5 cm (1–2 inches) higher over the sternum. If the scan direction is towards the head (i.e. from ilium to xiphoid), the scan can be manually terminated when T12 is reached. Important anatomical markers, which should be clearly visible on the scan image, are the upper border of the pelvis and the 12th rib (Figure 10.5). L5 can often be identified by its characteristic 'M' or butterfly shape.

As scanning proceeds and the bone mineral image is displayed on the monitor, the operator should check the emerging image on the monitor and interrupt the scan if the desired anatomical landmarks are not displayed or the spine is markedly off centre in the scan field. The scan can then be restarted after selecting the optimum starting point.

When an earlier scan is available, it is important that the operator reviews the previous scan (either the paper hard copy or a computer dis-

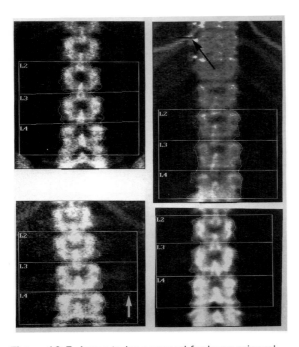

Figure 10.5 Areas to be scanned for bone mineral measurements at the lumbar spine. ***Upper left:*** Optimal scan with rib and pelvic markers visible and sufficient space outside the ROI of L2–L4. This scan would also be acceptable for an ROI of L1–L4. ***Upper right:*** Scan was started too high, and L5 and pelvic markers are not included. It was terminated too late and part of the T-spine is included. At the level of T11 there is a motion artefact, and hooks and eyes on an undergarment are noted. Above are the wire supports of a bra. ***Lower left:*** Scan was started too high and L5 is excluded. The arrow in the lower right side indicates the scan direction. ***Lower right:*** Landmarks are not included and identification of individual vertebrae for correct positioning of ROI is difficult. In all these cases the scans were repeated. Comparison showed that the ROI in the three inadequate cases gave similar results when compared with the adequate scan. Thus, as long as L2–L4 can be clearly identified and there is enough soft tissue space, minor deviations from the optimal scan do not result in significant errors.

play) to ensure that identical ROIs are evaluated. On some instruments a scan comparison option in the analysis software enables the ROI from the original analysis to be quickly and conveniently superimposed on the new scan.

REVIEW OF A LUMBAR SPINE BMD REPORT

The computer-generated scan report obtained with a commercial DXA instrument includes a scan image, the BMD result, biographical data, information on quality control and a normal range plot in which the patient's BMD and age are plotted with respect to reference data matched for age, sex and race. To aid scan interpretation, the report includes T-score and Z-score values generated from the measured BMD and the reference data. Examples of such reports are given in Figures 10.6–10.8. The details included permit an evaluation of instrument performance, a check on whether the acquisition and analysis of the scan were within the guidelines and assistance in the clinical interpretation of the BMD findings. The following guidelines have been developed for review of mailed-in bone mineral scans from a multi-centre research study. These guidelines should be helpful also for a physician generating a clinical report, or occasionally for a physician confronted with a BMD scan result that does not fit the clinical picture of the patient.

Review of quality control features

Comparison of a given measurement with a normal range or with a previously acquired measurement is only meaningful if the interpreter is assured that the instrument performed as expected. If the same Hologic instrument (Hologic Inc., Waltham, MA, USA) was used for two sequential studies, the scan parameters k and $d0$ given just above the scan image (see Figure 10.6) should hardly change. The derivation of these parameters from the Hologic internal reference wheel is explained in the Appendix to Chapter 3. Because of beam-

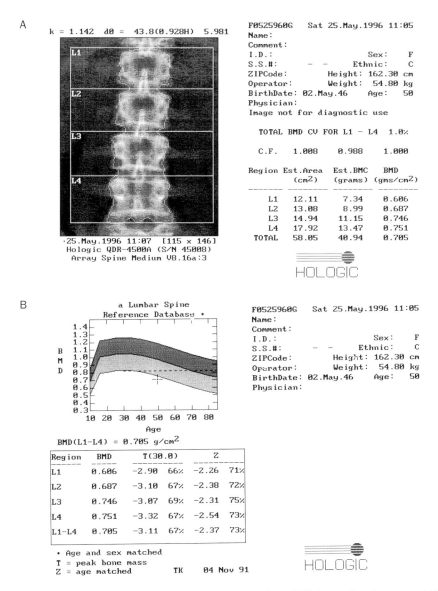

Figure 10.6 Computer printout for a PA spine scan from a Hologic DXA bone densitometer. (A) Scan image, biographical data and information on projected area, BMC and BMD. (B) Scan interpretation with normal range plot, T- and Z-score values and BMD expressed as a percentage of the young adult and age-matched population means.

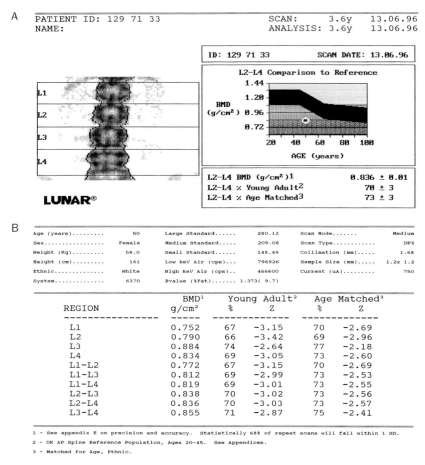

A

| PATIENT ID: 129 71 33 | SCAN: 3.6y 13.06.96 |
| NAME: | ANALYSIS: 3.6y 13.06.96 |

ID: 129 71 33   SCAN DATE: 13.06.96

L2–L4 Comparison to Reference

BMD (g/cm²)

L2–L4 BMD (g/cm²)1	0.836 ± 0.01
L2–L4 % Young Adult2	70 ± 3
L2–L4 % Age Matched3	73 ± 3

LUNAR®

B

Age (years).........	50	Large Standard......	280.12	Scan Mode.......	Medium
Sex.................	Female	Medium Standard.....	209.08	Scan Type...........	DPX
Weight (Kg).........	58.0	Small Standard......	148.49	Collimation (mm).....	1.68
Height (cm).........	161	Low keV Air (cps)...	796926	Sample Size (mm).....	1.2x 1.2
Ethnic.............	White	High keV Air (cps)..	466600	Current (uA)........	750
System.............	6370	Rvalue (%Fat)....... 1.373(9.7)		

REGION	BMD1 g/cm²	Young Adult2 %	Z	Age Matched3 %	Z
L1	0.752	67	-3.15	70	-2.69
L2	0.790	66	-3.42	69	-2.96
L3	0.884	74	-2.64	77	-2.18
L4	0.834	69	-3.05	73	-2.60
L1–L2	0.772	67	-3.15	70	-2.69
L1–L3	0.812	69	-2.99	73	-2.53
L1–L4	0.819	69	-3.01	73	-2.55
L2–L3	0.838	70	-3.02	73	-2.56
L2–L4	0.836	70	-3.03	73	-2.57
L3–L4	0.855	71	-2.87	75	-2.41

1 - See appendix E on precision and accuracy. Statistically 68% of repeat scans will fall within 1 SD.
2 - UK AP Spine Reference Population, Ages 20-45. See Appendices.
3 - Matched for Age, Ethnic.

Figure 10.7 Computer printout for a PA spine scan on a Lunar DPX system for the same subject shown in Figure 10.6. (A) Scan image, biographical data and normal range plot. (B) BMD results, T-score (young adult Z-score), Z-score (age-matched Z-score) values and BMD expressed as a percentage of the young adult and age-matched means. The time difference between the scans in Figures 10.6 and 10.7 was 3 weeks.

hardening effects they are, however, responsive to tissue thickness, and will both decrease slightly if the patient has put on weight. A drastic change, however, is indicative of a serious technical problem. Possible causes might include a patient hitting the C-arm and causing a misalignment of the X-ray beam, or an oil leak from the X-ray tank coolant causing attenuation in the beam. Useful information is also given by the system calibration factors (the numbers labelled CF in Figure 10.6). These should be identical unless the instrument has been recalibrated. Any change in these parameters should prompt a thorough review of the instrument's quality control records (see Chapter 9) and maintenance history to establish the reasons for recalibration.

Equivalent numbers are given on the report sheets of instruments from other manufacturers (Figure 10.7).

Influence of global ROI width on BMD values

Increasing the width of the soft tissue reference area causes a small systematic increase in BMD. This arises mainly because of the gradual increase in percentage body fat when including more soft tissue on either side of the spine. Thus, on Hologic instruments, the BMD value increases slightly as the width of the global ROI is increased, although the exact changes are variable from patient to patient. To avoid this potential small error, an important 'rule of thumb' is always to analyse using the same ROI width. Generally, 115–120 pixels are accepted as the default ROI width, since this gives a sufficient latitude for future scan comparisons and allows for a wide background area for optimal precision in the computer calculation of the tissue baseline.

The same ROI width used for analysing clinical scans should also be used for processing the daily scan of the manufacturer's spine phantom. BMD results from phantom scans also vary very slightly with the width of the global ROI, but in this case due to a small variation of the bone edges with ROI width.

Using non-standard ROI

When spinal *scoliosis* is present, the manufacturer's scoliosis software should be used, since this allows for non-rectangular ROIs with non-horizontal lines defining the intervertebral disc spaces. However, comparison of such results with the reference range may be less reliable, especially as these patients often have additional evidence of degenerative changes. Such BMD data are of more value if a given patient is measured repeatedly to monitor disease process or treatment effect.

If a *compression fracture* or other spinal abnormality exists on the lumbar spine radiograph, this vertebra should be excluded regardless of the appearance of the DXA image or the BMD results of the individual vertebra. BMD in a crushed vertebra may be high, equal or low when compared with the rest of the spine,[7] and the BMD value is often not predictable from the appearance on the image. Crush fractures cannot always be identified on a DXA scan, and radiographic comparison may be helpful if lumbar spine compression fractures are suspected. DXA images do not replace a lumbar spine radiograph, and should not be used to rule out or confirm a compression fracture or other abnormality of the spine for medical decision making. This includes images from a lateral spine DXA scan, on which compressions may be more readily identified. Occasionally, crush fractures or degenerative changes can be identified by inspection of a DXA scan, either by non-uniform BMD results among the individual vertebrae, or by inspection of the image. For research studies (longitudinal or cross-sectional), a standard ROI (L2–L4 or L1–L4) should be used in all patients, but vertebral abnormality should be marked. The decision to include or exclude these areas from the ROI is then made at the time of the final data analysis. This reduces bias when several operators are deciding which vertebrae to exclude. The selected ROI should include at least two vertebrae. However, these should not include L5, since BMD reference range data are not generally available for this vertebra.

Hypertrophic degenerative disease in the lumbar spine can be graded using an image comparison approach similar to that outlined later in Figure 10.17. Again, at the time of data analysis, certain patterns can be excluded. Non-uniformity is the rule rather than the exception in older subjects.[1]

If there are *artefacts overlying bone*, this part of the bone must be excluded from the ROI. Adjusting the brightness and contrast on the monitor can often help to clarify the presence or absence of such artefacts.

Bone sites of previous *surgical intervention*, sites with overlying aortic calcification, primary or secondary bone lesions such as metastasis, Paget's disease and crush fractures should be excluded from the ROI.

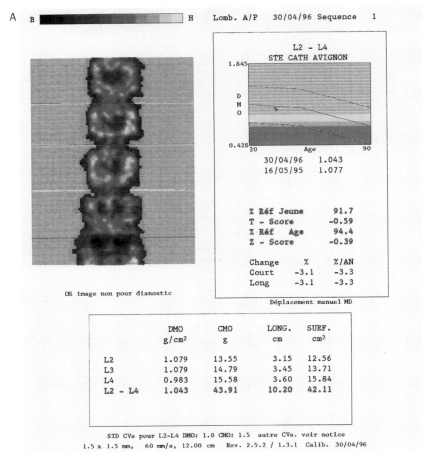

A B ▣ H   Lomb. A/P   30/04/96 Sequence   1

L2 - L4
STE CATH AVIGNON

30/04/96   1.043
16/05/95   1.077

% Réf Jeune	91.7
T - Score	-0.59
% Réf Age	94.4
Z - Score	-0.39

Change	%	%/AN
Court	-3.1	-3.3
Long	-3.1	-3.3

OS image non pour dianostic

Déplacement manuel MD

	DMO g/cm²	CMO g	LONG. cm	SURF. cm²
L2	1.079	13.55	3.15	12.56
L3	1.079	14.79	3.45	13.71
L4	0.983	15.58	3.60	15.84
L2 - L4	1.043	43.91	10.20	42.11

STD CVs pour L2-L4 DMO: 1.0 CMO: 1.5   autre CVs. voir notice
1.5 x 1.5 mm,   60 mm/s, 12.00 cm   Rev. 2.5.2 / 1.3.1 Calib. 30/04/96

Figure 10.8 (A) Computer printout for a PA spine scan on a Norland DXA scanner. (B) Same, but on a DMS Challenger DXA system.

For fracture risk prediction in a given patient, it is better to choose the hip or a site in the peripheral skeleton (forearm or calcaneus) if there is any doubt as to whether an acceptable ROI can be found in the spine.

Comparison of measurements with a reference population

The measured result is then compared with a reference population matched for age, sex and ethnic origin. In many centres, the reference data used will be that provided by the manufacturer. The computer-generated scan report includes a normal range plot in which the

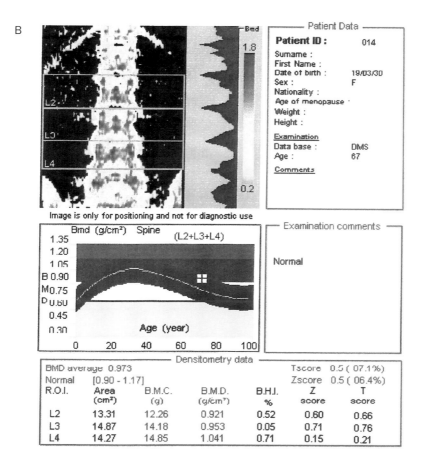

B

Image is only for positioning and not for diagnostic use

Patient Data	
Patient ID :	014
Surname :	
First Name :	
Date of birth :	19/03/30
Sex :	F
Nationality :	
Age of menopause ·	
Weight :	
Height :	
Examination	
Data base :	DMS
Age :	67
Comments	

Examination comments

Normal

Densitometry data

BMD average 0.973					Tscore 0.5 (07.1%)	
Normal [0.90 - 1.17]					Zscore 0.5 (06.4%)	
R.O.I.	Area (cm²)	B.M.C. (g)	B.M.D. (g/cm²)	B.H.I. %	Z score	T score
L2	13.31	12.26	0.921	0.52	0.60	0.66
L3	14.87	14.18	0.953	0.05	0.71	0.76
L4	14.27	14.85	1.041	0.71	0.15	0.21

patient's BMD and age are plotted with respect to the reference population (Figures 10.6–10.8). To interpret the scan result the patient's measured BMD is compared with both age- and sex-matched normal subjects and with normal young adults. The latter group is intended to represent the mean and population standard deviation (SD) of *peak bone mass*, that is the maximum BMD achieved in adult life. The comparison with the young adult and age-matched

reference data is usually expressed by normalizing the differences to the population SD to give the T- and Z-score figures. However, the results may also be expressed as a percentage of the mean value of the reference population. For Hologic (Figure 10.6) and Norland (Figure 10.8) instruments (Norland Medical Systems, Fort Atkinson, WI, USA) the middle line in the normal range plot shows the mean BMD value as a function of age while the upper and lower lines are ±2 SD above and below the mean BMD. For Lunar instruments (Figure 10.7) (Lunar Corp., Madison, WI, USA) the upper and lower lines are the ±1 SD limits.

The computer-generated scan report always includes the results expressed in T- and Z-score units. However, in Lunar instruments, the former is called the young adult Z-score and the latter the age-matched Z-score (Figure 10.7). The T-score is calculated as:

$$\text{T-score} = \frac{\text{Measured BMD} - \text{Young adult mean BMD}}{\text{Young adult standard deviation}}$$

The young adult mean and SD are usually derived from a large group of healthy subjects aged 20–39 years matched for sex and race, since peak bone mass is attained within this age band.

T-scores have assumed considerable importance in the interpretation of bone densitometry studies since the publication of a World Health Organization (WHO) Technical Report that proposed an interpretation of BMD measurements based on dividing patients into four categories on the basis of their T-score results:[8,9]

Normal: A BMD result not more than 1 SD below the young adult mean (T > −1.0) is considered normal.

Osteopenia: A BMD result that lies between 1 and 2.5 SD below the young adult mean (−1.0 > T > −2.5) indicates osteopenia. Such individuals include those in whom the prevention of further bone loss would be most useful.

Osteoporosis: A BMD result more than 2.5 SD below the young adult mean (T < −2.5) is classified as osteoporosis. Such patients are at high risk of fracture.

Established osteoporosis: A BMD result more than 2.5 SD below the young adult mean (T < −2.5) in the presence of one or more fragility fractures is classified as established osteoporosis. With the additional risk factor of previous fracture, such patients are at an especially high risk of further fracture.

The Z-score is similar in concept to the T-score

except that the mean BMD and SD for a healthy age-matched population is used instead of the young normal group as the reference population. The Z-score is calculated from the equation:

$$\text{Z-score} = \frac{\text{Measured BMD} - \text{Age-matched mean BMD}}{\text{Age-matched standard deviation}}$$

and expresses by how many SD the patient differs from the mean value for an age-, sex- and race-matched reference population. Further discussion of the use of T- and Z-scores to interpret BMD results is included in Chapter 16.

Two alternative methods of expressing BMD results are also sometimes useful. Patients in particular may find it easier to understand their BMD results if these are expressed as a *percentage* of the mean values for either the young adult or age-matched populations. Results in this format are routinely given on scan printouts for Hologic, Lunar and Norland instruments (Figures 10.6–10.8). A further method of interpreting BMD results sometimes advocated is to express the Z-score figure as a *percentile* of the healthy age-matched population. This figure indicates the percentage of individuals in the normal population who have BMD results lower than the result being reported. This is a concept familiar to many women because of its use in growth and weight charts in paediatrics. In calculating percentiles, it is usually assumed that the distribution function is a Gaussian curve. The percentile figure can then be calculated from the Z-score figure. Thus, Z = −2 corresponds to the 2.5th percentile, Z = 0 to the 50th percentile and Z = +2 to the 97.5th percentile. The assumption of a Gaussian distribution appears to be a reasonable approximation, although few studies include sufficient data to allow this assumption to be tested in the outer wings in any rigorous way.

Guidelines for reviewing bone mineral scans

Table 10.2 summarizes the guidelines for a systematic review of PA spine DXA scans.

STANDARDIZED BMD FOR LUMBAR SPINE DXA SCANS

It is important that physicians requesting and interpreting DXA studies are aware that results for the same patient measured on different manufacturers' equipment give different BMD figures. These differences arise from differences in scanner design, edge-detection algorithms and calibration. For clinicians presented with results from different systems, this can cause confusion.

The disagreement between different manufacturers' BMD results has caused considerable controversy. To resolve this problem, the International Committee for Standards in Bone Measurement (ICSBM) was established to recommend appropriate methods of cross calibration. A study was undertaken in the UCSF Osteoporosis Research Group of 100 healthy women evenly distributed over the age range 20–80 years on whom DXA studies were

acquired on a Norland XR-26 Mark II, a Lunar DPX-L and a Hologic QDR-2000 system.[10,11] In addition to these in vivo measurements, the European Spine Phantom (ESP)[12] and the Hologic, Lunar and Norland manufacturers' phantoms were scanned on all three systems. The in vivo BMD data were plotted pairwise for the three systems and analysed using linear regression. An important conclusion of this study was that none of the phantom data lay close enough to the regression lines derived from the in vivo measurements for any of the phantoms to be recommended as the basis of the cross-calibration standard.

Of the phantom results, the middle vertebra of the ESP (nominal BMD: $1.0\,g/cm^2$) came closest to the in vivo regression lines. The ICSBM committee therefore derived the relative calibration between the different manufacturers' systems by fitting the in vivo data with regression lines forced through the origin. However, the absolute BMD scale was estab-

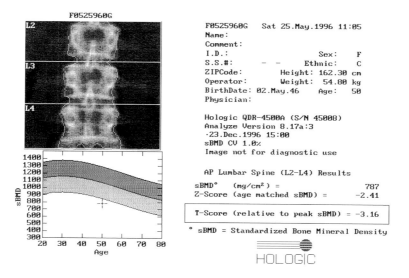

Figure 10.9 Scan results from Figure 10.6 expressed as standardized bone density (sBMD) values. The sBMD figures are given for L2–L4 in units of mg/cm². Note the simplified presentation compared with Figure 10.6.

Table 10.2 Guidelines for a systematic review of PA spine DXA scans.

1) INSPECT BIOGRAPHIC DATA	Action	Remarks
Are obesity or ascites present? Weight, height, sex	Measure abdominal thickness in cm at mid-abdomen if patient is obese (over 90 kg/200 lbs) or small (under 36 kg/80 lbs)	If significant changes between scans occurred, such as with ascites, comparison may not be possible
2) INSPECT PRINTOUT		
Bone mineral image	*Action in processing*	*Remarks*
Is the brightness of the scans properly adjusted?	Adjust contrast and brightness settings	May obscure compression fractures or hypertrophy (Figure 10.10)
Check if patient is aligned straight on the image	Patient should be aligned with the mid-line of the table. Repeat scan if gross misalignment	Interspaces should be perpendicular to axis of scan table for optimal ROI position. Non-standard separation of vertebrae is possible with scoliosis software (Figure 10.4)
Are landmarks included for ROI selection?	Repeat scan if L2–L4 (or L1–L4) cannot be clearly identified	Figure 10.5
Are the bone borders clearly defined?	Attention when processing. Enlarging global ROI or manual border delineation are options	Special processing considerations are needed (Figure 10.11)
Artefacts in ROI overlying bone	Repeat scan after removal of artefact	If repeating scan is not possible, exclude artefact by using smaller ROI (Figure 10.12)
Artefact within ROI but outside bone	Algorithm allows elimination of artefact Repeat scan if it is metal object in pocket or other external object	If artefact is small, it may not affect scan result (Figure 10.13)
Artefact outside the ROI over bone or soft tissue	Does not affect scan	Figure 10.14
Check for transverse processes included as bone	If only a small portion of a process is included, no action is required. Occasionally, there is one very prominent process	The rule of thumb is not to change arbitrarily transverse process delineation if they are attached to the vertebral body. If a portion of a transverse process is detached, this should be eliminated. Check this when comparing successive scans (Figures 10.15A–C)

Table 10.2 continued

Look for spinal rotation. Spinal processes should be centred along the vertebrae	If spinal processes are not centred, check for poor positioning and repeat scan if possible	If not due to scoliosis or spine deformity, scan should not be accepted. Rotation increases the projected area while bone mineral remains constant resulting in lower BMD (Figure 10.16). Extreme rotation may project the transverse processes into the vertebral body, which increases BMC
Inspect for uniformity of bone distribution in ROI	Laminectomy, compression fractures, aortic calcification, degenerative disease, orthopaedic devices, scoliosis and lordosis in the ROI should be identified. Uniformity of bone mineral distribution should be established	Establish criteria for acceptable uniformity of bone mineral distribution (Figure 10.17)
Selection of ROI	Should be L2–L4 (or L1–L4) if bone mineral is uniform. Omit from ROI clearly abnormal high or low foci of bone mineral	Selection of different ROI in a study enters a subjective bias into the measurement and should not be done in research studies without clear guidelines. Establish criteria for ROI selection
Check if ROI has sufficient width and contains tissue space equal on both sides	Some asymmetry in position of spine in ROI is acceptable. ROI limits should not coincide with upper and lower limits of scan image	Upper and lower margins should go through middle of disc space (Figure 10.18)
Check k and $d0$ factors (Hologic instruments) or equivalent numbers	If a sudden change is noted, a service call may be necessary. Check for misalignment of C-arm	$d0$ values below 85 on Hologic QDR 1000 or below 40 on QDR 4500 suggest massive obesity
Check calibration factor		Calibration factor should be identical in scans obtained with the same instrument if no recalibration occurred
Check BMD results for reasonable numbers	BMD should vary between 0.4 and 1.6 g/cm^2. Higher or lower numbers are rarely seen as true measurement results	If outside this range, a review is needed

lished relative to the middle vertebra of the ESP by making the mean of the corrected BMD values for all three systems equal to the nominal BMD of 1.0 g/cm².[10,11]

Standardized PA spine (L2–L4) BMD results (denoted sBMD and expressed in units of mg/cm² to differentiate them clearly from conventional BMD measurements) are derived from the manufacturers' existing BMD figures (expressed in units of g/cm²) using the following conversion equations:[10,11,13]

For Hologic instruments:

$$sBMD = 1000(BMD_{Hologic} \times 1.0755)$$

For Lunar instruments:

$$sBMD = 1000(BMD_{Lunar} \times 0.9522)$$

For Norland instruments:

$$sBMD = 1000(BMD_{Norland} \times 1.0761)$$

The manufacturers have recently issued software giving users the option of giving reports in sBMD units (Figure 10.9). Clearly the conversion equations given above represent results derived for three particular DXA instruments in use in San Francisco, USA, and had the study been conducted on three similar instruments anywhere else in the world the values of the coefficients might have been slightly different. In general, sBMD values obtained by scanning a patient on one of these three manufacturers' systems anywhere else are expected to agree to within 2–5%.[13]

The equations for generating sBMD values issued by the ICSBM committee were derived from linear regression lines forced through the origin. It is clear that this masks the effect of small non-linearities in the BMD scales. This issue has been discussed by Hui and colleagues[14] who have derived an optimal procedure for cross calibrating two or more bone densitometers using in vivo data.

ILLUSTRATIVE CASES

A few points discussed only briefly in the above outline are illustrated and discussed in more detail in the following examples (Figures 10.10–10.39). It should be emphasized again that DXA scan images cannot replace radiographs. There is, however, much information in these images which can assist in the meaningful interpretation of BMD results.

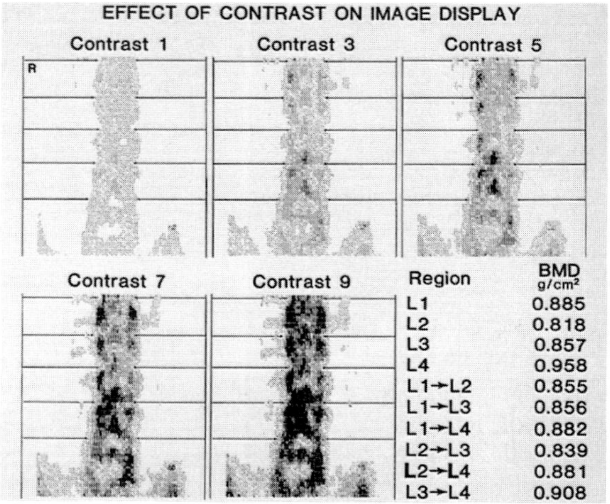

EFFECT OF CONTRAST ON IMAGE DISPLAY

Region	BMD g/cm²
L1	0.885
L2	0.818
L3	0.857
L4	0.958
L1→L2	0.855
L1→L3	0.856
L1→L4	0.882
L2→L3	0.839
L2→L4	0.881
L3→L4	0.908

Figure 10.10 Effect of contrast setting on the image display. Nine steps of contrast are tested. Generally an intermediate step is selected – contrast 7 is about optimal for this image. Degenerative disease or crush fractures can be overlooked or overdiagnosed with poor contrast settings, and interspaces can be missed. The BMD values themselves are not affected by poor contrast settings.

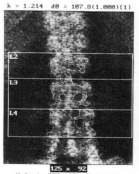

k = 1.214 d0 = 107.8(1.000)[1]

```
L2
L3
L4
```

125 x 92

Hologic QDR 1000 (S/N 190)
Lumbar Spine Version 4.01

TOTAL BMD CV FOR L1 - L4 1.0%

C.F.   1.004   1.037   1.000

Region	Area (cm2)	BMC (grams)	BMD (gms/cm2)
L2	6.14	2.45	0.399
L3	9.00	3.58	0.397
L4	10.85	5.05	0.466
TOTAL	25.99	11.08	0.426

A

k = 1.214 d0 = 107.6(1.000)[1]

```
L2
L3
L4
```

125 x 92

Hologic QDR 1000 (S/N 190)
Lumbar Spine Version 4.01

TOTAL BMD CV FOR L1 - L4 1.0%

C.F.   1.004   1.037   1.000

Region	Area (cm2)	BMC (grams)	BMD (gms/cm2)
L2	8.11	2.82	0.347
L3	11.06	3.95	0.357
L4	12.21	5.31	0.435
TOTAL	31.39	12.08	0.385

Figure 10.11 Very low bone mineral. When BMD approaches 0.4–0.5 g/cm^2, density differences between background and bone become too small for determination of bone edges. Three approaches can be used: (1) report a value of lower than 0.5 g/cm^2; (2) reanalyse the scan by manually determining the bone outline and filling in bone inside this outline. This will further decrease BMD, since area is added with little bone (this approach requires a subjective interaction and loss of precision); and (3) change the threshold value in the software until an anatomical bone outline is achieved. Again, this approach is not objective and may result in using inadvertently different threshold levels in subsequent scans if this level is changed at will. This approach is not recommended. (A) Apparent bone defects in the centre of the vertebra must be filled in during data processing. (B) A greater problem is incompleteness of bone contour borders. In this case, the missing bone edges can be drawn in manually.

k = 1.223 d0 = 94.2(1.000)[1]

```
L2
L3
L4
```

116 x 93

Hologic QDR 1000 (S/N 002)
Lumbar Spine Version 4.20

```
B
M  1.4
D  1.3
   1.2
   1.1
   1.0
   0.9
   0.8
   0.7
   0.6
   0.5
   0.4
      20  30  40  50  60  70  80
              Age
```

BMD(L2-L4) = 0.442 g/cm^2

Region	BMD	T(30.0)		Z	
N/A					
L2	0.358	-6.69	33%	-6.39	34%
L3	0.468	-5.77	42%	-5.46	44%
L4	0.457	-6.25	40%	-5.94	41%
L2-L4	0.442	-6.12	40%	-5.81	41%

* Age and sex matched
Reference Curve for Males
TK   10/13/89

B

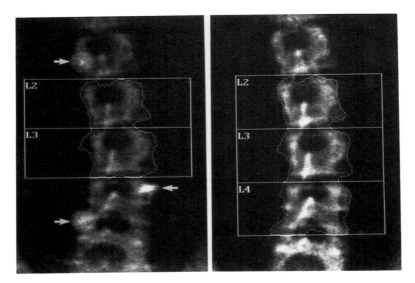

Figure 10.12 The left panel shows a scan of the lumbar spine (L1–L4). Two buttons and a metal hook were attached to an undergarment. These were then removed and the repeat scan is in the right panel. In addition, this scan shows rotation with eccentric position of the spinous processes and mild scoliosis. The image intensity was increased in the display on the right.

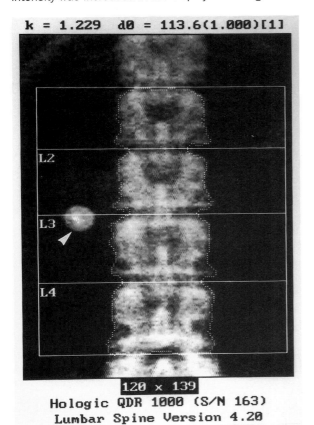

Figure 10.13 An artefact (a calcium-containing tablet) in the GI tract. Since this feature lies over the soft tissue area in the global ROI, the scan analysis software should automatically exclude it from both the soft tissue baseline and the BMD analysis.

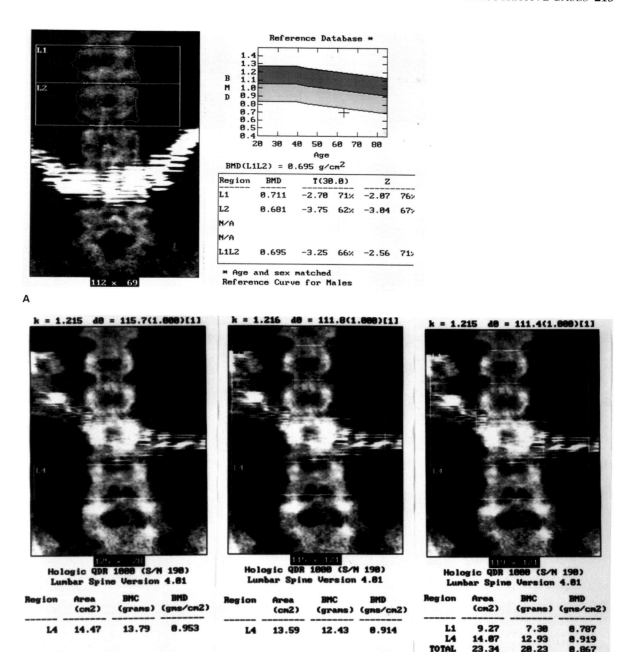

Figure 10.14 (A) Contrast media from a recent barium swallow is seen in the transverse colon. The global ROI does not include the barium and BMD measurements of L1–L2 are unaffected. (B) Alternative approaches to selection of the global ROI in case of contrast medium in the abdomen illustrate how results can be affected. *Left:* Global ROI is selected to include only L4. This is an acceptable compromise. *Middle:* Standard global ROI. The contrast medium is counted as bone and does not affect the soft tissue baseline. BMD in L4 is close to that in the left panel. *Right:* Standard global ROI. Contrast medium is counted as soft tissue and the soft tissue baseline is affected. As a result BMD in L4 is falsely low. The first analysis is preferred.

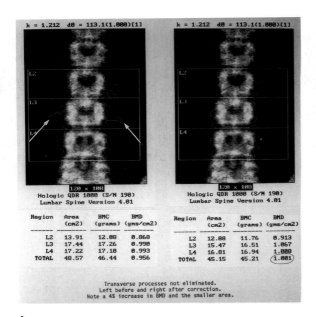

Region	Area (cm2)	BMC (grams)	BMD (gms/cm2)
L2	13.91	12.08	0.868
L3	17.44	17.26	0.990
L4	17.22	17.10	0.993
TOTAL	48.57	46.44	0.956

Region	Area (cm2)	BMC (grams)	BMD (gms/cm2)
L2	12.88	11.76	0.913
L3	15.47	16.51	1.067
L4	16.81	16.94	1.008
TOTAL	45.15	45.21	(1.001)

Transverse processes not eliminated.
Left before and right after correction.
Note a 4% increase in BMD and the smaller area.

A

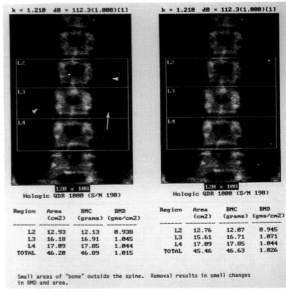

Region	Area (cm2)	BMC (grams)	BMD (gms/cm2)
L2	12.93	12.13	0.938
L3	16.18	16.91	1.045
L4	17.09	17.85	1.044
TOTAL	46.20	46.89	1.015

Region	Area (cm2)	BMC (grams)	BMD (gms/cm2)
L2	12.76	12.07	0.945
L3	15.61	16.71	1.071
L4	17.09	17.85	1.044
TOTAL	45.46	46.63	1.026

Small areas of "bone" outside the spine. Removal results in small changes
in BMD and area.

B

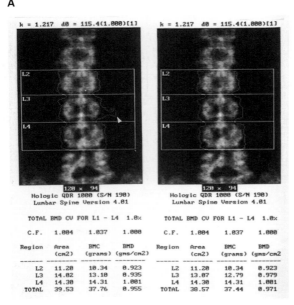

TOTAL BMD CV FOR L1 - L4 1.0%   TOTAL BMD CV FOR L1 - L4 1.0%

C.F.   1.004   1.037   1.000   C.F.   1.004   1.037   1.000

Region	Area (cm2)	BMC (grams)	BMD (gms/cm2)
L2	11.20	10.34	0.923
L3	14.02	13.10	0.935
L4	14.30	14.31	1.001
TOTAL	39.53	37.76	0.955

Region	Area (cm2)	BMC (grams)	BMD (gms/cm2
L2	11.20	10.34	0.923
L3	13.07	12.79	0.979
L4	14.30	14.31	1.001
TOTAL	38.57	37.44	0.971

C

Figure 10.15 (A) Several transverse processes are not completely eliminated. In this case, this should be corrected. Because of the low BMD in the visualized transverse processes, when they are erased BMD shows a slight increase. As expected from the images, BMD of L3 is most affected. (B) Remnants of bone in the transverse processes which were deleted. No significant difference in BMD resulted from this small change, but improved precision in longitudinal studies may occur. (C) Single prominent transverse process. Correction is not recommended by the manufacturer. However, some centres would correct as indicated.

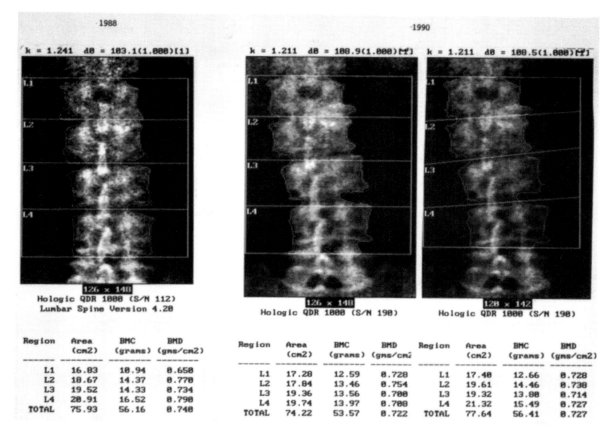

Region	Area (cm2)	BMC (grams)	BMD (gms/cm2)
L1	16.83	10.94	0.650
L2	18.67	14.37	0.770
L3	19.52	14.33	0.734
L4	20.91	16.52	0.790
TOTAL	75.93	56.16	0.740

Region	Area (cm2)	BMC (grams)	BMD (gms/cm2)	Region	Area (cm2)	BMC (grams)	BMD (gms/cm2)
L1	17.28	12.59	0.728	L1	17.40	12.66	0.728
L2	17.84	13.46	0.754	L2	19.61	14.46	0.738
L3	19.36	13.56	0.700	L3	19.32	13.80	0.714
L4	19.74	13.97	0.708	L4	21.32	15.49	0.727
TOTAL	74.22	53.57	0.722	TOTAL	77.64	56.41	0.727

Figure 10.16 *Left:* Off-centre position of spinous processes due to spinal deformity. This could not be corrected by repositioning. *Middle:* Incorrect position of the global ROI, poor positioning on the table and poor outline of individual vertebrae. The latter is of no consequence when only the entire ROI is evaluated. *Right:* Poor position on the table but correct setting of the ROI limits. Note that the height of the ROI is smaller by 6 pixels. The patient had lost 1 cm in height in the interval of 2 years.

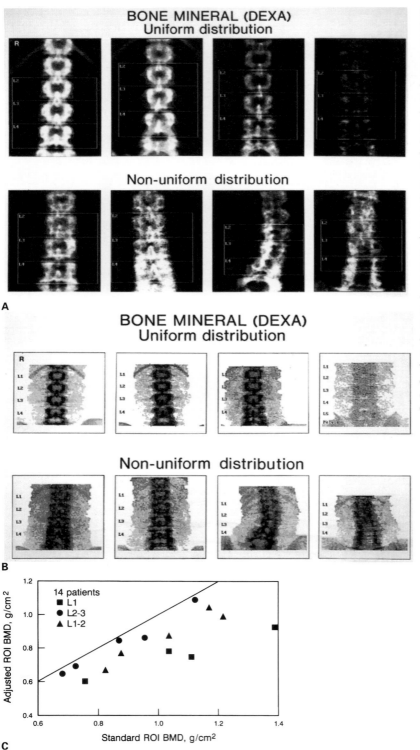

Figure 10.17 Patterns of spinal bone mineral distribution in the lumbar spine, showing uniform and non-uniform distribution. Hard copies from different companies. (A) Scan images obtained with a Hologic QDR-1000. (B) The same patients measured on the same day with a Lunar DPX. (Images from the Lunar instrument were in colour and have lost detail in reproduction.) (C) Effect on BMD of changing the vertebrae included in the analysis in patients with non-uniform BMD in the lumbar spine. BMD in the standard ROI (L2–L4) on the horizontal axis is compared with BMD for an adjusted ROI that excludes the vertebrae with abnormal BMD. The diagonal line is the line of identity. In every case the adjusted ROI resulted in a lower BMD. The BMD values were generally lowest if L1 was chosen as the adjusted ROI (unpublished data from Mayo Clinic).

SPINE BMD
Changing width of ROI

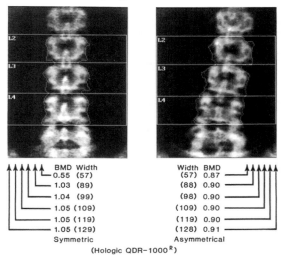

BMD	Width		Width	BMD
0.55	(57)		(57)	0.87
1.03	(89)		(88)	0.90
1.04	(99)		(98)	0.90
1.05	(109)		(109)	0.90
1.05	(119)		(119)	0.90
1.05	(129)		(128)	0.91
	Symmetric		Asymmetrical	

(Hologic QDR-1000 R)

Figure 10.18 Effect of varying the width of the soft tissue reference area on the BMD result. ***Left:*** The arrows show the position of the lateral border of the global ROI and its width is given in parentheses together with the BMD obtained. A width of the global ROI of 120 mm appears optimal. ***Right:*** This study began with an optimal global ROI setting of 119 mm and the left side only was progressively reduced, as shown by the arrows. This shows the effect of an unequal soft tissue amount about the spine.

Bone mineral measurements in degenerative, osteoporotic and primary bone disease

A

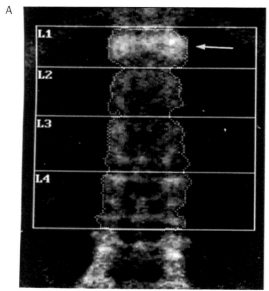

Comment:		SCREENING
I.D.:		Sex: F
S.S.#:	– –	Ethnic: C
ZIPCode:	Height:	135.00 cm
Scan Code:	Weight:	48.00 kg
BirthDate:		Age: 61
Physician:		

TOTAL BMD CV FOR L1 - L4   1.0%

C.F.   0.996   1.031   1.000

Region	Area (cm2)	BMC (grams)	BMD (gms/cm2)
L1	8.81	5.85	0.665 ◀
L2	9.43	3.74	0.396
L3	12.43	5.41	0.435
L4	14.50	7.63	0.526
TOTAL	45.17	22.63	0.501

Figure 10.19 Recent compression fracture and low spinal bone mineral in a 61-year-old woman with Type I osteoporosis. (A) Bone mineral image shows a compression in L1 with high BMD and small bone area when compared with the rest of the vertebrae. L1 should be excluded from the BMD analysis. (B) A ^{99m}Tc-MDP bone scan shows increased uptake in L1, consistent with a recent vertebral crush fracture.

B

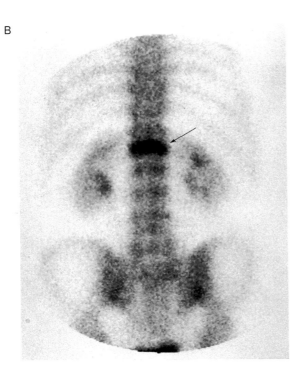

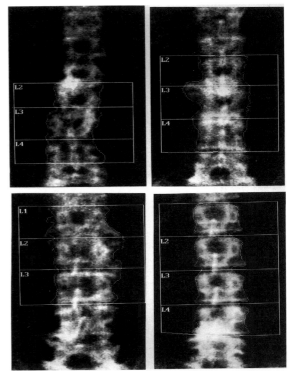

Figure 10.20 Patterns of non-uniform distribution of bone mineral in the lumbar spine due to osteoporotic compression fractures and hypertrophic osteoarthritic changes. In such cases, the lumbar spine is of limited value for diagnosis of osteoporosis or fracture risk. BMD values are generally high or normal despite low BMD at other skeletal sites. BMD in the hip or forearm should be measured instead.

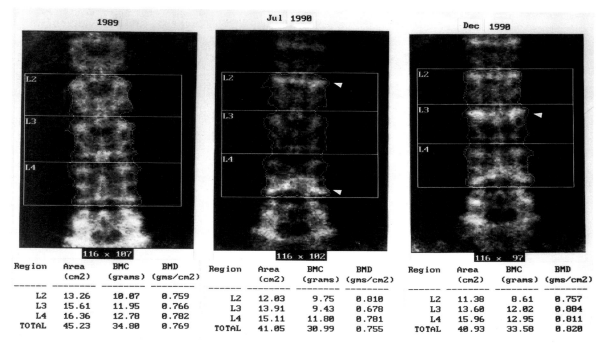

Region	Area (cm2)	BMC (grams)	BMD (gms/cm2)
L2	13.26	10.07	0.759
L3	15.61	11.95	0.766
L4	16.36	12.78	0.782
TOTAL	45.23	34.80	0.769

Region	Area (cm2)	BMC (grams)	BMD (gms/cm2)
L2	12.03	9.75	0.810
L3	13.91	9.43	0.678
L4	15.11	11.80	0.781
TOTAL	41.05	30.99	0.755

Region	Area (cm2)	BMC (grams)	BMD (gms/cm2)
L2	11.38	8.61	0.757
L3	13.60	12.02	0.884
L4	15.96	12.95	0.811
TOTAL	40.93	33.58	0.820

A

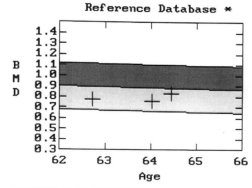

Reference Database *

Region	Rate of Change	±SD	% Change	±% Dev
L2–L4	+0.0199	0.0139	+2.58	1.80

Date of Scan	Age	BMD(L2–L4)
03/23/89	62.7	0.769
07/11/90	64.0	0.755
12/13/90	64.4	0.820

* Age and sex matched
Reference Curve for Females

B

Figure 10.21 (A) A series of three bone mineral images showing bone loss and new compression fractures in a 62-year-old Caucasian female with primary biliary cirrhosis. **Left:** Scan in August 1989 shows uniform mineral distribution in L2–L4 and a dense body at L5, a radiographically proven compression fracture. **Middle:** Scan in July 1990 shows increased bone mineral at the upper end-plate of L2 and the lower portion of L4, consistent with new crush fractures. The global ROI is smaller, consistent with compression. **Right:** Scan in December 1990 shows a new compression fracture in L3. From left to right, there is a decrease in height of the L2–L4 ROI corresponding with the measured loss of the patient's height. The general bone loss (seen in L3 in left and middle pictures) is obscured by the crush fractures when the full ROI (L2–L4) is used for all scans. (B) Graphical display of BMD data from (A). The bone loss is obscured by the occurrence of new compression fractures. There is an apparent increase in BMD with time. This demonstrates the need for inspection of the scan images when data are interpreted. Images and ROI size should be compared.

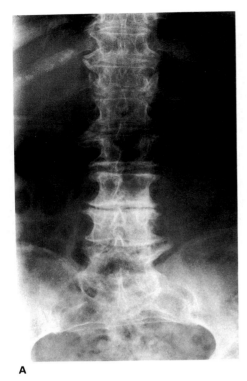

A

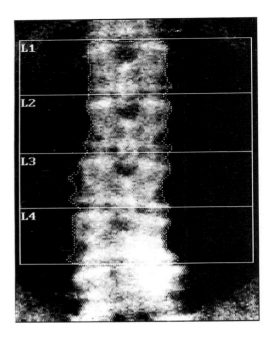

B

Figure 10.22 A 57-year-old Caucasian female with known osteoporosis (Type I). (A) Radiograph of the L-spine shows severe hypertrophic osteoarthritic changes, demineralization and compression. (B) A bone mineral image performed on the same day shows similar changes. The hypertrophic changes are not appreciated since these outgrowths are removed by the algorithm as are transverse processes. The demineralization is obscured by the osteoarthritic changes. The limitations of the bone mineral image in comparison with the radiograph are apparent.

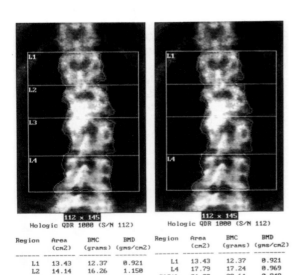

Hologic QDR 1000 (S/N 112)   Hologic QDR 1000 (S/N 112)

Region	Area (cm2)	BMC (grams)	BMD (gms/cm2)
L1	13.43	12.37	0.921
L2	14.14	16.26	1.150
L3	17.35	17.87	1.030
L4	17.79	17.24	0.969
TOTAL	62.71	63.74	1.016

Region	Area (cm2)	BMC (grams)	BMD (gms/cm2)
L1	13.43	12.37	0.921
L4	17.79	17.24	0.969
TOTAL	31.22	29.61	0.948

Figure 10.23 Local degenerative changes increase the BMD in L2–L3. This can be appreciated on the images as well as by a review of the BMD values. An alternative ROI, including L1 and L4, was used in this case.

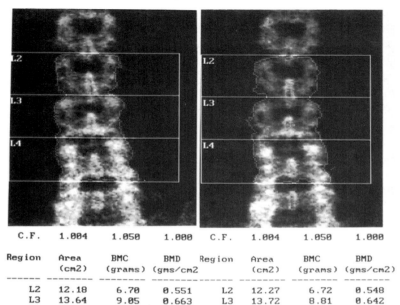

Figure 10.24 Bone mineral changes with age and osteoarthritis are seen in these scans made 1 year apart. There is degenerative disease in L4, L5 and the inferior end-plate of L3. Bone mineral in L1–L3 is essentially uniform. The right scan performed 1 year later shows no significant change in BMD in L2 and L3. Progression of the degenerative process in L4 resulted in an increase in L4. If a standard ROI of L4 is used there is increased BMD. L4 should be excluded.

C.F.	1.004	1.050	1.000	C.F.	1.004	1.050	1.000
Region	Area (cm2)	BMC (grams)	BMD (gms/cm2	Region	Area (cm2)	BMC (grams)	BMD (gms/cm2)
L2	12.18	6.70	0.551	L2	12.27	6.72	0.548
L3	13.64	9.05	0.663	L3	13.72	8.81	0.642
L4	15.48	11.46	0.740	L4	16.39	13.27	0.810
TOTAL	41.29	27.21	0.659	TOTAL	42.38	28.81	0.680

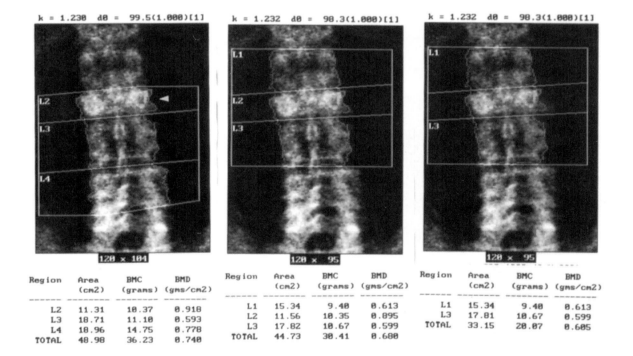

| k = 1.230 | dθ = | 99.5(1.000)[1] | | k = 1.232 | dθ = | 98.3(1.000)[1] | | k = 1.232 | dθ = | 98.3(1.000)[1] |

Region	Area (cm2)	BMC (grams)	BMD (gms/cm2)	Region	Area (cm2)	BMC (grams)	BMD (gms/cm2)	Region	Area (cm2)	BMC (grams)	BMD (gms/cm2)
L2	11.31	10.37	0.918	L1	15.34	9.40	0.613	L1	15.34	9.40	0.613
L3	18.71	11.10	0.593	L2	11.56	10.35	0.895	L3	17.81	10.67	0.599
L4	18.96	14.75	0.778	L3	17.82	10.67	0.599	TOTAL	33.15	20.07	0.605
TOTAL	48.98	36.23	0.740	TOTAL	44.73	30.41	0.680				

Figure 10.25 Lumbar spine bone mineral scan with multiple compression fractures. Several ROIs are displayed. The image on the right could be acceptable for patient management but radius or hip would be better choice.

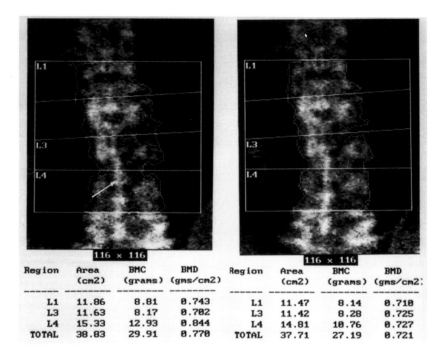

Region	Area (cm2)	BMC (grams)	BMD (gms/cm2)	Region	Area (cm2)	BMC (grams)	BMD (gms/cm2)
L1	11.86	8.81	0.743	L1	11.47	8.14	0.710
L3	11.63	8.17	0.702	L3	11.42	8.28	0.725
L4	15.33	12.93	0.844	L4	14.81	10.76	0.727
TOTAL	38.83	29.91	0.770	TOTAL	37.71	27.19	0.721

Figure 10.26 Abnormal bone mineral distribution pattern with rotation around the longitudinal axis (asymmetric position of spinous processes) and compressions. Scans were performed on subsequent days. Precision is poor because of the difficulty in obtaining identical ROIs. Slight variations in bone edge outline are noted (right border of L2–L3).

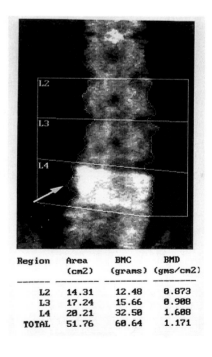

Region	Area (cm2)	BMC (grams)	BMD (gms/cm2)
L2	14.31	12.48	0.873
L3	17.24	15.66	0.908
L4	20.21	32.50	1.608
TOTAL	51.76	60.64	1.171

Figure 10.27 Paget's disease of L4. Bone area, BMC and BMD are high. There is degenerative disease in the right facet joint of L5. An ROI of L1–L3 or L2–L3 should be selected.

Bone mineral measurements in the presence of postoperative changes and orthopaedic appliances

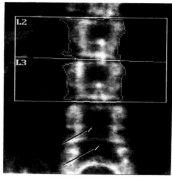

Region	Area (cm2)	BMC (grams)	BMD (gms/cm2)
L2	13.37	9.32	0.697
L3	13.90	10.37	0.746
TOTAL	27.26	19.70	0.722

Figure 10.28 Laminectomy L4–L5. Note the absence of the posterior arch and spinal processes. Ribs are very low because of thoracic kyphosis. Calcification of costochondral junctions is seen. Absence of the posterior arch decreases BMC and BMD when compared with normal data.

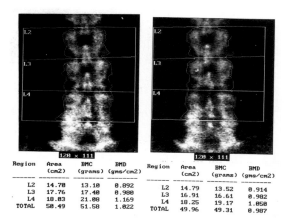

Region	Area (cm2)	BMC (grams)	BMD (gms/cm2)	Region	Area (cm2)	BMC (grams)	BMD (gms/cm2)
L2	14.70	13.10	0.892	L2	14.79	13.52	0.914
L3	17.76	17.40	0.980	L3	16.91	16.61	0.982
L4	18.03	21.08	1.169	L4	18.25	19.17	1.050
TOTAL	50.49	51.58	1.022	TOTAL	49.96	49.31	0.987

Figure 10.29 *Left:* Degenerative changes in L4 and some in L3. BMD in L4 is high when compared with the other vertebrae. *Right:* Repeat scan 1 year later and 3 months after a laminectomy L4–L5. Slight decrease in BMD in L4 is noted, but the laminectomy is not readily recognizable on the image. This emphasizes the need for a short history taken at the time of the scan or a review of a spinal radiograph when the results are interpreted. Even with the best printout the bone mineral images do not replace a spinal radiograph.

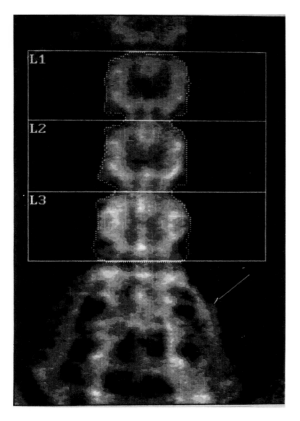

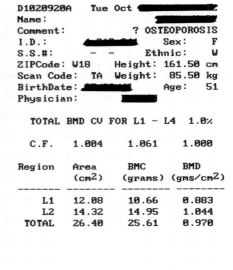

k = 1.221 d0 = 95.9(1.000)[1]   k = 1.211 d0 = 86.4(1.000)[1]

Region	Area (cm2)	BMC (grams)	BMD (gms/cm2)
L1	13.50	22.87	1.694
L2	14.17	26.46	1.867
L3	13.68	25.41	1.857
L4	15.97	28.38	1.777
TOTAL	57.32	103.12	1.799

Region	Area (cm2)	BMC (grams)	BMD (gms/cm2)
L5	13.90	10.02	0.721

Figure 10.31 Harrington rods in the lumbar spine. Interference by metal excludes valid measurements. Another skeletal site should be selected.

Figure 10.30 Spinal fusion L4–S1.

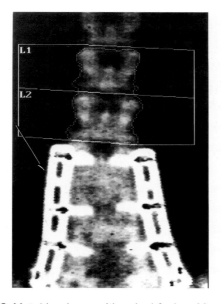

D1020920A   Tue Oct
Name:
Comment: ? OSTEOPOROSIS
I.D.:   Sex: F
S.S.#:   -   -   Ethnic: W
ZIPCode: W18   Height: 161.50 cm
Scan Code: TA Weight: 85.50 kg
BirthDate: Age: 51
Physician:

TOTAL BMD CV FOR L1 - L4   1.0%

C.F.   1.004   1.061   1.000

Region	Area (cm²)	BMC (grams)	BMD (gms/cm²)
L1	12.08	10.66	0.883
L2	14.32	14.95	1.044
TOTAL	26.40	25.61	0.970

Figure 10.32 Metal hardware with spinal fusion. Measurement of BMD in adjacent vertebrae may at times give useful clinical information.

Bone mineral measurements in scoliosis

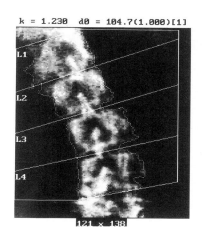

```
k = 1.230   d0 = 104.7(1.000)[1]
```

```
A08198802   Fri Aug 19 12:15 1988
Name:                  Scoliosis #1
Comment:
I.D.:              1    Sex:  / F
S.S.#:        -   -    Ethnic:   C
ZIPCode: ALH   Height: 162.56 cm
Scan Code:     Weight:  59.47 kg
BirthDate:             Age:   68
Physician:

   TOTAL BMD CV FOR L1 - L4   1.0%

   C.F.   1.004     1.036     1.000
```

Region	Area (cm2)	BMC (grams)	BMD (gms/cm2)
L1	13.97	11.22	0.803
L2	13.25	10.55	0.796
L3	14.05	10.32	0.734
L4	14.75	11.84	0.803
TOTAL	56.02	43.92	0.784

Figure 10.33 Severe lumbar scoliosis. Spinous processes are not centred, bone mineral is dense at the concave side and the vertebral end-plates are not clearly visible and not horizontal. The scan was analysed using the scoliosis software, which allows the vertebral spaces to be marked with lines that are not horizontal.

Artefacts in soft tissue or overlying bone

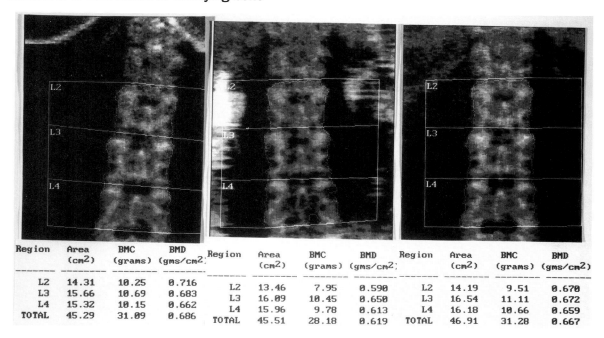

Region	Area (cm2)	BMC (grams)	BMD (gms/cm2)	Region	Area (cm2)	BMC (grams)	BMD (gms/cm2)	Region	Area (cm2)	BMC (grams)	BMD (gms/cm2)
L2	14.31	10.25	0.716	L2	13.46	7.95	0.590	L2	14.19	9.51	0.670
L3	15.66	10.69	0.683	L3	16.09	10.45	0.650	L3	16.54	11.11	0.672
L4	15.32	10.15	0.662	L4	15.96	9.78	0.613	L4	16.18	10.66	0.659
TOTAL	45.29	31.09	0.686	TOTAL	45.51	28.18	0.619	TOTAL	46.91	31.28	0.667

Figure 10.34 Effect of grossly non-uniform attenuation within the soft tissue reference region. **Left:** Baseline study. Note artefact due to bra support wires. **Middle:** A scan 15 months later shows residual barium in the GI tract which is included in the global ROI. This results in a false BMD. **Right:** A repeat scan performed 2 days later.

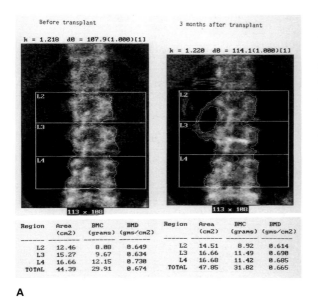

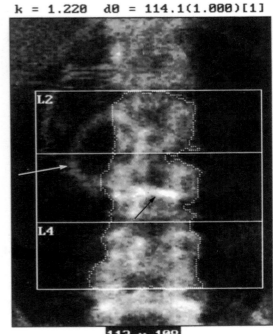

Region	Area (cm2)	BMC (grams)	BMD (gms/cm2
L2	12.18	8.01	0.657
L4	16.94	11.45	0.676
TOTAL	29.12	19.46	0.668

B

Figure 10.35 (A) Bone mineral scan of the lumbar spine. **Left:** Acceptable scan prior to a liver transplant. **Right:** Scan 3 months after transplant shows T-tube drain on the right side of L2–L3 and overlying it. Multiple small areas within the confines of the anatomical bone are not recognized as bone. (B) The scan was processed by excluding the T-tube from the bone area and filling in the bone along the spine. Only L2 and L4 were selected for the ROI. In this case, the T-tube did not significantly effect the BMD measurements.

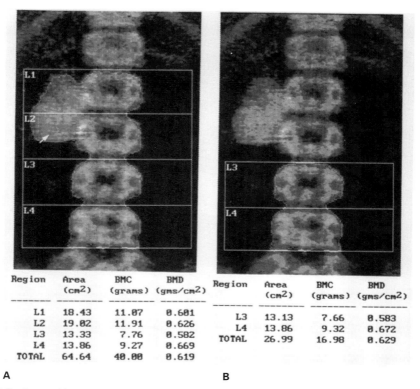

Region	Area (cm^2)	BMC (grams)	BMD (gms/cm^2)
L1	18.43	11.07	0.601
L2	19.02	11.91	0.626
L3	13.33	7.76	0.582
L4	13.86	9.27	0.669
TOTAL	64.64	40.00	0.619

Region	Area (cm^2)	BMC (grams)	BMD (gms/cm^2)
L3	13.13	7.66	0.583
L4	13.86	9.32	0.672
TOTAL	26.99	16.98	0.629

A B

Figure 10.36 (A) Radiographic contrast medium in the gall bladder. The contrast material is not distinguished from bone. (B) A useful ROI here would be L3–L4.

Bone mineral measurements in obesity

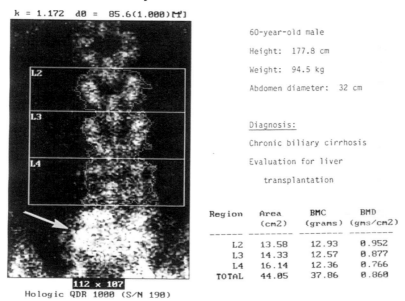

k = 1.172 d0 = 85.6(1.000)[Y]

60-year-old male

Height: 177.8 cm

Weight: 94.5 kg

Abdomen diameter: 32 cm

Diagnosis:

Chronic biliary cirrhosis

Evaluation for liver

    transplantation

Region	Area (cm2)	BMC (grams)	BMD (gms/cm2)
L2	13.58	12.93	0.952
L3	14.33	12.57	0.877
L4	16.14	12.36	0.766
TOTAL	44.05	37.86	0.860

112 × 107

Hologic QDR 1000 (S/N 190)

Figure 10.37 Traumatic compression fracture of L5. The remainder of the lumbar spine shows uniform bone mineral distribution. The abdominal diameter was 32 cm owing to ascites. The image appears grainy due to the high soft tissue attenuation.

Figure 10.38 Bone mineral scan in a patient with primary biliary cirrhosis and severe ascites. Abdominal diameter was 38 cm and the high attenuation gives a very grainy image and an unusually low value of *d*0 (59.0). This is not a valid measurement.

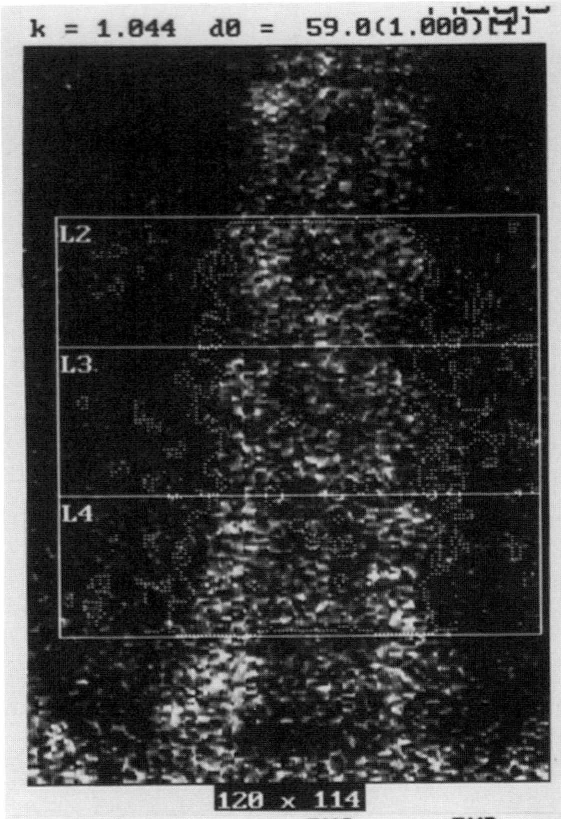

k = 1.044 d0 = 59.0(1.000)
L2
L3
L4
120 x 114

Region	Area (cm2)	BMC (grams)	BMD (gms/cm2)
L2	18.92	27.22	1.439
L3	24.88	33.75	1.357
L4	23.82	36.00	1.511
TOTAL	67.62	96.97	1.434

Variations in spinal anatomy

L1
L2
L3
L4

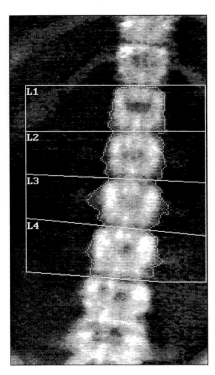

Figure 10.39 PA spine scan showing six lumbar vertebrae.

APPENDIX

Table A1 Example of a questionnaire used by the technologist to obtain information useful in setting up the scanning procedure as well as in scan interpretation. The questions also serve to alert the technologist if there are contraindications to the performance of the scan.

CLINIC NUMBER: _____

NAME: _____

DATE: _____

Mayo Clinic
Department of Radiology
Nuclear Medicine
Charlton 2N

<u>BONE MINERAL ANALYSIS</u>
<u>CHECKLIST</u>

Routine	Study

<u>INTERFERING DIAGNOSTIC STUDIES:</u>

Yes   No   1. Any X-ray studies performed in the last 5 days with oral contrast media?
                   [   ] CT   [   ] Stomach or colon X-ray
                   [   ] EXU   [   ] Other (myelogram) (specify):
                   _____

Yes   No   2. Any radioactive study in the last 3 days?
                   Specify: _____

<u>INTERFERING MEDICAL CONDITIONS:</u>

Yes   No   3. Any lower back surgery?
                   Type: _____ Date: _____

Yes   No   4. Metal objects in the abdominal area or in the back?
                   Specify: _____

               5. Pregnant   Yes   No
               6. FEMALES: Menopause (age:)   Yes   No
                              Hysterectomy (age:)   Yes   No

If any answer (1–5) is yes, check with physician.

<u>INTERFERING DRUGS</u>

               7. DRUG HISTORY _____

Yes   No   Estrogen _____
Yes   No   Steroids _____
Yes   No   Calcium _____
Yes   No   Vitamin D _____
Yes   No   Calcitonin _____
Yes   No   Sodium Fluoride _____
Yes   No   Diphosphonate _____

<u>CLINICAL INFORMATION</u>

<u>Reason for referral:</u>   Known osteoporosis
                          Suspected osteoporosis
                          Risk factors
                          Other _____

Previous bone mineral   Yes (date: _____)   No

_____
Signature of Technologist

Table A2 Normal values (females): Hologic instruments. (Reproduced with permission from Peter Steiger, Senior Scientist, Hologic Inc., Waltham, MA, USA)

Spine (L1–L4)			Spine (L2–L4)		
Age (years)	BMD (g/cm^2)	SD (g/cm^2)	Age (years)	BMD (g/cm^2)	SD (g/cm^2)
00	0.336	0.035	–	–	–
01	0.399	0.040	–	–	–
04	0.512	0.053	–	–	–
07	0.607	0.070	–	–	–
10	0.677	0.085	–	–	–
13	0.838	0.099	–	–	–
16	1.010	0.110	–	–	–
18	1.015	0.110	–	–	–
20	1.019	0.110	20	1.051	0.110
25	1.040	0.110	25	1.072	0.110
30	1.047	0.110	30	1.079	0.110
35	1.041	0.110	35	1.073	0.110
40	1.024	0.110	40	1.056	0.110
45	0.999	0.110	45	1.030	0.110
50	0.967	0.110	50	0.997	0.110
60	0.892	0.110	55	0.960	0.110
70	0.815	0.110	60	0.920	0.110
80	0.752	0.110	65	0.878	0.110
85	0.731	0.110	70	0.840	0.110
			75	0.805	0.110
			80	0.775	0.110
			85	0.754	0.110

Table A3 Normal values (males): Hologic instruments. (Reproduced with permission from Peter Steiger, Senior Scientist, Hologic Inc., Waltham, MA, USA)

Spine (L1–L4)			Spine (L2–L4)		
Age (years)	BMD (g/cm^2)	SD (g/cm^2)	Age (years)	BMD (g/cm^2)	SD (g/cm^2)
00	0.336	0.035	–	–	–
01	0.399	0.040	–	–	–
04	0.512	0.053	–	–	–
07	0.607	0.070	–	–	–
10	0.677	0.085	–	–	–
13	0.838	0.099	–	–	–
16	1.010	0.110	–	–	–
18	1.050	0.110	–	–	–
20	1.091	0.110	20	1.115	0.110
25	1.091	0.110	25	1.115	0.110
35	1.091	0.110	30	1.115	0.110
45	1.068	0.110	35	1.115	0.110
50	1.053	0.110	40	1.115	0.110
55	1.038	0.110	45	1.091	0.110
60	1.023	0.110	50	1.076	0.110
65	1.008	0.110	55	1.061	0.110
70	0.993	0.110	60	1.045	0.110
75	0.978	0.110	65	1.030	0.110
80	0.963	0.110	70	1.015	0.110
85	0.947	0.110	75	0.999	0.110
			80	0.984	0.110
			85	0.968	0.110

Table A4 Normal values (spine L1–L4): Lunar instruments. (Reproduced with permission from Howard S Barden, Senior Scientist, Lunar Corp., Madison, WI, USA.)

Caucasian females			Caucasian males		
Age (years)	n	BMD mean (g/cm²)	Age (years)	n	BMD mean (g/cm²)
20–29	672	1.200	20–29	85	1.255
30–39	916	1.214	30–39	106	1.215
40–49	1630	1.180	40–49	73	1.174
50–59	2472	1.096	50–59	67	1.161
60–69	1942	1.016	60–69	63	1.183
70–79	1273	0.988	70–79	51	1.178

Table A5 Normal values (BMD): Norland XR-36. (Reproduced with permission from Keith Nelson, Norland Medical Systems, Fort Atkinson, WI, USA.)

Caucasian females[a]			Caucasian males[a]		
Age group (years)	Spine (L1–L4) BMD (g/cm²)		Age group (years)	Spine (L2–L4) BMD (g/cm²)	
	Mean	SD		Mean	SD
20	1.183	0.162	20	1.109	0.167
50	1.015	0.162	80	0.947	0.167
90	0.815	0.162			

[a]Population is from north-west and central states of the USA.

REFERENCES

1. Spencer RP, Hosain F, Yoosujani KA. Bone density variation within lumbar vertebrae in apparently normal women. *Int J Rad Appl Instrum* (1992) **19:** 83–5.
2. Carter DR, Bouxsein ML, Marcus R. New approaches for interpreting projected bone densitometry data. *J Bone Miner Res* (1992) **7:** 137–45.
3. Bouxsein ML, Bassman LC, Marcus R et al. Comparisons of bone mineral measures from dual energy X-ray absorptiometry, computed tomography and ash content. *J Bone Miner Res* (1992) **7**(suppl 1): S138.
4. Sabin MA, Blake GM, MacLaughlin-Black SM, Fogelman I. The accuracy of volumetric bone density measurements in dual x-ray absorptometry. *Calcif Tissue Int* (1995) **56:** 210–14.
5. Jergas M, Breitenseher M, Glüer C-C et al. Estimates of volumetric bone density from projectional measurements improve the discriminatory capability of dual x-ray absorptiometry. *J Bone Miner Res* (1995) **10:** 1101–10.
6. Wahner HW, Dunn WL, Mazess RB et al. Dual photon Gd-153 absorptiometry of bone. *Radiology* (1985) **156:** 203–6.
7. Ryan PJ, Evans P, Blake GM, Fogelman I. The effect of vertebral collapse on spinal bone mineral density measurements in osteoporosis. *Bone Miner* (1992) **18:** 267–72.
8. WHO Technical Report Series 843. Assessment of fracture risk and its application to screening for postmenopausal osteoporosis (World Health Organization: Geneva, 1994).
9. Kanis JA, Melton LJ, Christiansen C et al. The diagnosis of osteoporosis. *J Bone Miner Res* (1994) **9:** 1137–41.
10. Genant HK, Grampp S, Glüer C-C et al. Universal standardization of dual x-ray absorptiometry: patient and phantom cross-calibration results. *J Bone Miner Res* (1994) **9:** 1503–14.
11. Genant HK. Universal standardization of dual x-ray absorptiometry: patient and phantom cross-calibration results [letter]. *J Bone Miner Res* (1995) **10:** 997–8.
12. Kalender WA, Felsenberg D, Genant HK et al. The European spine phantom: a tool for standardization and quality control in spinal bone density measurements by DXA and QCT. *Eur J Radiol* (1995) **20:** 83–92.
13. Steiger P. Standardization of measurements for assessing BMD by DXA [letter]. *Calcif Tissue Int* (1995) **57:** 469.
14. Hui SL, Gao S, Zhou X-H et al. Universal standardization of bone density measurements: a method with optimal properties for calibration among several instruments. *J Bone Miner Res* (1997) **12:** 1463–70.

11

Measurement of Bone Density in the Lumbar Spine: the Lateral Spine Scan

CHAPTER OVERVIEW

This chapter reviews the reasons for performing lateral projection dual energy X-ray absorptiometry (DXA) studies of the lumbar spine. Lateral scans isolate the cancellous bone in the vertebral body from the cortical bone in the posterior elements. They therefore better approximate one of the principal objectives of bone densitometry, that of measuring a site of trabecular bone free of any artefacts. However, the advantage of access to one of the most metabolically active sites in the skeleton must be balanced against the significantly larger errors caused by the greater thickness and inhomogeneity of the overlying soft tissue. This chapter discusses the relative advantages and disadvantages of conventional postero-anterior (PA) and lateral DXA spine scans and makes recommendations for the use of lateral projection scans.

INTRODUCTION

As described in Chapter 10, the spine is generally the preferred site for measurements of bone mineral density (BMD), and the PA projection scan of the lumbar spine is probably still the most widely used clinical study performed with DXA instruments. However, DXA is a projectional technique that measures the mass of bone mineral in unit cross-sectional area (units: g/cm^2), and the conventional PA spine scan includes not only the metabolically active trabecular bone of the vertebral body, but also substantial amounts of cortical bone, especially in the posterior elements. Degenerative and hypertrophic changes in the spine, such as osteoarthritis of the articular facets, hypertrophy of the spinous processes and degenerative sclerosis of the end-plates, all lead to increases in BMD as measured by PA projection DXA scans such that the BMD measurements may no longer be representative of a patient's true skeletal status.[1–5]

For this reason there has always been interest in spinal DXA studies using the lateral instead of the PA projection.[6–10] Lateral scans isolate the vertebral body from the posterior elements (Figure 11.1) and better approximate the ideal objective of a measurement site with a higher percentage of trabecular bone that is less

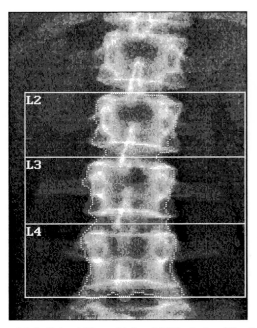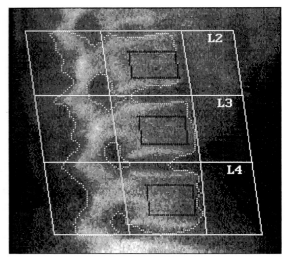

Figure 11.1 Paired PA and lateral DXA study of the lumbar spine showing the scan analysis for L2–L4. Because of the use of the supine lateral technique with a rotating C-arm, there is an exact line-by-line match between the two scans. Vertebral body BMD is measured on the lateral projection scan anterior to the vertical line intersecting the neural arches. Mid-vertebral BMD is measured inside the black ROIs within each vertebral body. Width-adjusted (WA) vertebral body and mid-vertebral body BMD are obtained by dividing each of the two lateral areal BMD measurements by the mean vertebral width measured on the PA scan.

affected by artefacts than the conventional PA spine scan. The first studies of lateral spine BMD used the technique of dual photon absorptiometry (DPA) based on a [153]Gd radionuclide source.[11] Patients were scanned in the lateral decubitus position on the imaging table. However, the intensity of the photon beam from DPA instruments proved too low for the task, resulting in long scanning times,

relatively large precision errors and poor images.

With the widespread introduction of DXA-based instruments in the late 1980s, several studies re-examined the practicality and clinical utility of lateral projection BMD scans using the decubitus position.[6–10,12] For example, Wilson[12] modified the collimator of a standard Hologic QDR-1000 instrument (Hologic Inc.,

Waltham, MA, USA) to achieve a fourfold increase in beam intensity and obtained reasonable quality images with scan times of less than 10 minutes. However, such modifications were not possible in commercial instruments in the field, and early software for the lateral BMD application required scan times of 20–30 minutes. Over such times the lateral decubitus position can be very uncomfortable for patients. Combined with the poor precision, the difficulty of accurately repositioning subjects and the lack of anatomical landmarks for identifying vertebrae, these disadvantages meant that the decubitus lateral DXA scan never found widespread acceptance in clinical practice.

The major technical development that has sustained interest in lateral spine BMD measurements in recent years was the introduction of a new generation of fan-beam DXA bone densitometers with a rotating C-arm design that allows for a 90° rotation of the X-ray tube and detector assembly around the patient during scanning.[13] In this technique, PA and lateral projection scans of the lumbar spine can be acquired in matched pairs (Figure 11.1). After completion of the PA scan, the C-arm is rotated through 90° and a lateral study performed without the subject moving from the supine position. As well as the comfort and ease of repositioning the patient, scan times are greatly shortened because of the fan-beam and multidetector array, and appropriate collimation ensures adequate beam intensity to match the increased tissue thickness of the lateral projection.

The chief technical limitation that may prevent lateral spine BMD measurements from achieving their theoretical advantage over PA DXA scanning is the effect of the variable composition of the soft tissue reference baseline on the accuracy of the BMD measurements.[14–18] Many of the issues centred on the relative advantages and disadvantages of PA and lateral scanning remain unresolved. While some reports of the comparative accuracy of lateral DXA suggest that it may be superior to PA spine DXA for identifying patients with osteoporosis,[19–22] other studies have reached the opposite conclusion.[23–25] Table 11.1 summarizes

Table 11.1 Some methods for comparing postero-anterior (PA) and lateral BMD scans.
Age-related losses in healthy subjects
Longitudinal studies of glucocorticoid treatment
Longitudinal studies of anti-resorptive treatment
Precision and longitudinal sensitivity
Percentage differences in BMD between healthy subjects and patients with established osteoporosis
Differences in Z-score between healthy subjects and patients with established osteoporosis
ROC analysis of BMD values for healthy subjects and patients with established osteoporosis
Correlations with biomechanical studies of vertebral body strength
Prospective studies of incident fractures

some methods for making a comparative evaluation of the clinical utility of PA and lateral spine DXA that have appeared in the literature, and these will form the basis of discussion on this issue throughout the chapter. For a comprehensive review, the reader is also referred to the article by Jergas and Genant.[26]

THE ADVANTAGES OF LATERAL SPINE DXA

There are several reasons for wishing to measure BMD from a lateral projection scan of the vertebral body. First, calcium deposits in the abdominal aorta and degenerative changes around the facet joints, which are both included in the PA spine scan, are projected outside the region of interest (ROI) used for measuring vertebral body BMD on lateral DXA studies. Degenerative changes along the end-plates, such as Schmorl's and Junghann's nodes and osteophytes, can also often be excluded.[7]

Secondly, bone composition is not uniform throughout a vertebra. The vertebral body is the site of osteoporotic crush fractures and is predominantly composed of trabecular bone. In contrast, the posterior elements of the vertebrae are mainly composed of cortical bone. While the posterior portion is occasionally the site of stress fractures, congenital defects or traumatic fractures, the posterior portion of a vertebra does not play an important role in osteoporotic vertebral crush fractures. The fraction of trabecular bone expressed as a percentage of ash weight has been estimated as 42% in the vertebral body, 10% in the vertebral arch and 24% in the whole vertebra.[27] Higher estimates (about 60%) of trabecular bone in the vertebral body have also been reported.

Lastly, bone loss with age and disease differs in trabecular and cortical bone. In oophorectomized women, the rate of bone loss in trabecular bone of the anterior vertebral body measured with quantitative computed tomography (QCT) was twice that in the total vertebra.[28] In the vertebral body (also measured with QCT), the average decrease of BMD in a lifetime is about 50%, but only 25% in the posterior elements.[29] Normal men show almost as much trabecular bone loss as women during a lifetime, but, unlike women, a man's cortical bone mass remains almost unchanged.[30] This loss of bone mass from the vertebral body is associated with a reduction in bone strength and with increased risk of non-traumatic fractures.[31-34]

PATIENT POSITIONING FOR LATERAL DXA SCANS

The optimum technique for performing lateral spine DXA studies is to use an instrument with a rotating C-arm so the patient can be scanned in the supine position. Patient positioning is similar to that required for a PA projection scan (Chapter 10). The patient should be aligned in the middle of the scanning table with the spine straight and parallel to the longitudinal axis. A soft block is placed under the calves to raise the legs and reduce lumbar lordosis. The patient's arms should be raised above the shoulders so they do not obstruct the view of the spine on the lateral image. If a conventional PA projection scan is performed first, the arms should be raised before starting the PA study to avoid any movement between the PA and lateral studies. On completing the PA scan, the patient should be instructed to keep as still as possible while the C-arm is rotated for the lateral scan.

The supine lateral position is preferable because it is more comfortable for the patient, results in more reproducible positioning, and usually allows more vertebrae to be included in the scan analysis ROI without obscuration by overlying rib or pelvic bone.[35] Finally, combined PA and lateral scans permit unambiguous identification of the lumbar vertebrae.

The alternative lateral position, the decubitus scan, is now seldom used. In this position, the patient is placed in the left lateral decubitus position with hips and knees flexed. Positioning is helped by aligning the pelvis perpendicular to the margin of the scanning table and by using a support for head, knees and pelvis. Custom-made supports to assist in maintaining a lateral position are supplied with instruments from the various manufacturers. As a minimum, a back and shoulder support is needed to prevent the patient from moving out of the desired lateral position. Images of the lumbar spine in an oblique position cannot be interpreted, since the projected area in the oblique view is of a different bone region when compared with the proper lateral position (Figure 11.2). Compared with a supine lateral scan, reproducible positioning of the patient for a decubitus scan is quite difficult, even using the special positioning aids. Since the starting points of the PA and lateral scans are not linked, reliable identification of vertebral levels is more difficult since the anatomical landmarks are less obvious on lateral than on conventional PA scans. Aside from the implications for reproducibility, from a practical point of view

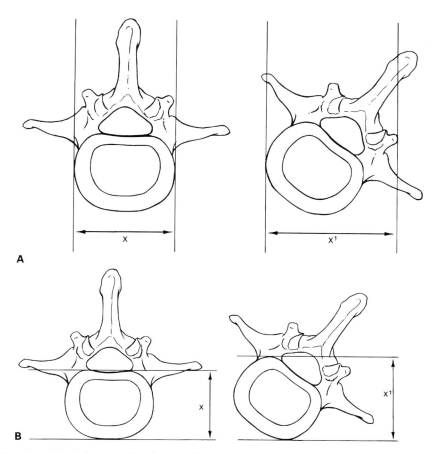

Figure 11.2 This shows the influence of spine position during scanning on BMD results. X is the width of the projected area scanned and used in the calculations of BMD (g/cm^2). (A) In the standard PA scan, the oblique position increases the projected area, portions of the transverse processes are included and the tip of the spinous process may be excluded. (B) In the lateral scan, the oblique position includes progressively more of the posterior elements and the projected area increases.

and compared with other DXA procedures, lateral decubitus scans are time consuming and difficult to perform.[26]

INSTRUMENTS AND DATA PRESENTATION

Lateral lumbar spine scans obtained with three different commercial DXA instruments are shown in Figure 11.3. The data printout for all

instruments shows the total area scanned, the ROI selected by the computer algorithm or the operator, and results for BMD, BMC and the projected area. This is given for each vertebra separately, as well as for the total ROI. As mentioned above, the overlap of the vertebral bodies by rib and pelvic bone is one of the principal issues in the interpretation of lateral spine DXA scans.[35] Blake et al. reported on a group of 131 patients enrolled in a clinical trial and followed up with supine lateral DXA scan-

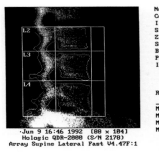

A

REGION	BMD g/cm²	% Young Whites	% Age Matched
B2	0.409 ± 0.03	55	63
B3	0.536 ± 0.03	72	83
M2	0.364 ± 0.03	53	61
M3	0.470 ± 0.03	68	79
B2–B3	0.472 ± 0.02	64	67
M2–M3	0.417 ± 0.01	61	64

B

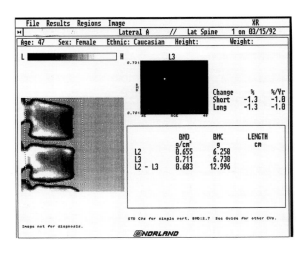

C

Figure 11.3 Data output for lateral spine scans from different commercial manufacturers' instruments showing scan image, regions of interest and measurement results. (A) Hologic Inc.; (B) Lunar Corp.; and (C) Norland Medical Systems.

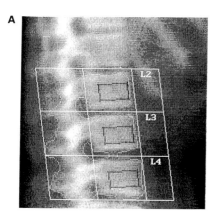
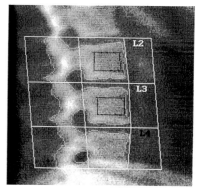
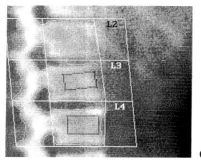

Figure 11.4 Examples of rib and pelvic overlay of a vertebral body on a supine lateral BMD scan. (A) No rib or pelvic overlay, and the maximum ROI (L2–L4) can be used; (B) example of pelvic overlay of L4. Only L2–L3 can be used; (C) example of rib overlay of L2. Only L3–L4 can be used.

ning.[36] Eighty-one subjects (62%) had lateral BMD measurements for L2–L4 (Figure 11.4A), 49 (37%) for L2–L3 because of the pelvis overlying L4 (Figure 11.4B) and one (1%) for L3–L4 because of prominent rib overlay of L2 (Figure 11.4C).

Some guidelines for using and interpreting lateral spine DXA scans are listed in Tables 11.2 and 11.3.

REGIONS OF INTEREST FOR LATERAL DXA SCANS

Because of the overlap of ribs and pelvis, lateral BMD measurements of the lumbar vertebrae L2 and L4 are regarded as unreliable by some authors.[35] Hence, BMD measurements of L3 alone, or a combination of L2 and L3, have been used in several studies.[8,23,24,37,38] It is likely that the effect of any overlap of L2 or L3 by ribs on the diagnostic accuracy of the BMD scan is negligible.[26,39] In contrast, the inclusion of L4, which is overlapped by pelvis in 30–50% of patients,[26,36] is more difficult because it may falsely increase the BMD measurement and affect the interpretation of the scan. Jergas and colleagues concluded that, when L4 was not overlapped by the pelvis, the use of the L2–L4 ROI improved both the diagnostic sensitivity and the precision of lateral DXA.[26,39]

Table 11.2 Exclusion criteria for lateral spine scan.

1) *From pretest spinal radiograph*
   Severe scoliosis
   Severe thoracic spinal deformity
   Compression fracture L2, L3
   Congenital or postoperative changes in L-spine
   Marked obesity (tolerable thickness 15–30 cm)

2) *From inspection of scan image*
   Same as above +
   Ribs projected on L2
   Ilium projected on L3

Within the vertebral body, a number of measurement sites have been used by different investigators, or are available on different commercial instruments. Selection is partly based on experience gained from QCT studies. At this time, no single ROI has been found to be clearly superior for clinical or research use. Figure 11.5 illustrates schematically the position of some different lateral ROIs that have been used. The largest ROI includes the entire vertebral body anterior to the neural arch (ROI 1 in Figure 11.5). The line of separation here is critical and should run closely adjacent to the posterior wall of the vertebral body, where it is seen in the area of the intervertebral foramina (Figure 11.1). This ROI includes the entire cortical shell of the vertebral body and all of the trabecular bone. Degenerative changes at the vertebral end-plates will mostly be included. BMD mea-

---

Table 11.3 Review of lateral spine bone mineral scans.

1) *Satisfactory positioning of scan*
   Is accurate lateral projection of spine achieved?
   Can L2 and L3 be identified?

2) *Satisfactory position of ROI*
   Is relationship of spinal anatomy to borders of ROI accurate?

3) *Is bone (rib) or other dense material present in the region outside the bone that is used for estimating the background?*
   Consult manufacturer's manual for details on how to handle this. This area has to be excluded from the background on some machines.

4) *Rib projected on L2*
   (a) Rescan with arms higher up.
   (b) Omit L2 from ROI and use L3 only. (Mean BMD in L2 is about 8% lower than L3.)

5) *Iliac crest projected on L3*
   (a) Repositioning is generally not helpful if the patient was well positioned.
   (b) Omit L3 from ROI and use L2.

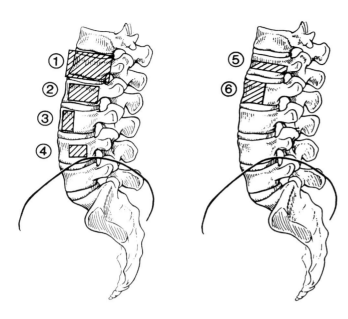

Figure 11.5 Schematic illustrations of ROI locations that have been used in lateral spine scanning. BMD results depend on ROI location because of the different amount of cortical and trabecular bone included in the ROI, and because trabecular bone is not lost uniformly from the vertebral body.

surements in this ROI will be referred to as *vertebral body BMD*.

Another measurement site represents the largest rectangular area that can be fitted into the vertebral body, omitting the cortical rim (ROI 2 in Figure 11.5). This ROI excludes the anterior and posterior cortical surfaces of the vertebral body, as well as the end-plates (Figure 11.1), but does include the lateral cortical surfaces (Figure 11.6). In most cases, degenerative changes at the site of the vertebral end-plates are excluded. BMD measurements in this ROI will be referred to as *mid-vertebral body BMD*.

An interesting development made possible by supine lateral DXA is the combination of PA and lateral data to infer a *volumetric bone density* (VBMD) figure which, in analogy to a QCT measurement, is an estimate of the true physical density. As data from only two projections are available, it is not possible to perform a tomographic reconstruction. Instead, it is necessary to assume that the lumbar vertebral body has a fixed geometric shape, for example an elliptical cylinder. With this assumption, the

projected areas on the PA and lateral images may be combined to estimate vertebral body volume, and the vertebral body bone mineral content (BMC) measured on the lateral scan is divided by volume to give VBMD. A descrip-

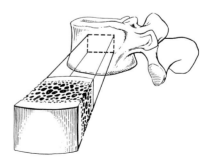

Figure 11.6 Schematic illustration of a bone sample measured with a lateral scan of a vertebral body. Note the cortical rim on both sides of the trabecular bone sample.

tion of the algorithm used to infer volume is given in the Appendix to this chapter. Further mathematical details can be found in other reports.[22,23,40]

If the issue of the exact geometric shape is ignored, the VBMD calculation can also be described as the division of the vertebral body and mid-vertebral body BMD figures by the mean width of the spine measured on the PA projection scan to derive two width-adjusted (WA) volumetric BMD parameters. For this reason, the VBMD figures will be referred to as the *WA vertebral body BMD* and *WA mid-vertebral body BMD* respectively.

Other smaller areal BMD sites have been proposed, one in the anterior aspect of the vertebral body, either including or excluding the cortical shell (ROI 3 in Figure 11.5), and the other in the centre (ROI 4 in Figure 11.5). A region of interest consisting of a slice of the entire vertebral body (cortex and trabecular bone) representing the middle one-third has also been used (ROI 5 in Figure 11.5, see also Figure 11.3). Because the posterior aspect of the vertebral body contains vascular spaces and supporting bone for the neural arch, areas in the anterior aspect of the vertebral body may show greater sensitivity to trabecular bone loss (ROI 6 in Figure 11.5).

It is also possible to measure the average BMD over the entire vertebra (i.e. the vertebral body and the posterior elements) on the lateral scan, a measurement that will be referred to as the *total lateral BMD*. This latter ROI will, of course, not contain any diagnostic information different from the PA projection scan. However, total lateral BMD has been found helpful in the baseline compensation algorithm, a technique used to improve the precision of vertebral body BMD measurements in longitudinal studies.[41] Mathematical details of this technique are given in the Appendix to this chapter.

PRECISION AND ACCURACY OF LATERAL DXA SCANS

As described above, the initial studies of lateral spine DXA used the decubitus scan, in which a patient lies on their side. Table 11.4 lists published studies of the decubitus technique that

Table 11.4 Precision of vertebral body BMD using the decubitus lateral scan.

Precision study	Year of publication	CV for vertebral body BMD (with degrees of freedom)[a]
Mazess et al.[42]	1990	2.0% (35)
Slosman et al.[7]	1990	2.8% (10)
Lilley et al.[43]	1992	3.6% (36)
Banks et al.[44]	1992	3.8% (20)
Larnach et al.[9]	1992	3.8% (100)
Pye et al.[45]	1992	5.2% (10)
Economou et al.[46]	1993	5.9% (10)
Devogelaer et al.[47]	1993	6.9% (15)

[a]The degrees of freedom is the number of independent items of information used in the calculation of the coefficient of variation (CV) and indicates the statistical weighting of the study (see Chapter 8).

Table 11.5 Precision of vertebral body BMD using the supine lateral scan with baseline compensation.

Precision study	Year of publication	CV for vertebral body BMD (with degrees of freedom)[a]
Steiger et al.[13]	1990	0.9% (24)
Slosman et al.[48]	1992	1.0% (51)
Devogelaer et al.[49]	1993	1.2% (13)
Blake et al.[41]	1994	1.2% (48)

[a]The degrees of freedom is the number of independent items of information used in the calculation of the coefficient of variation (CV) and indicates the statistical weighting of the study (see Chapter 8).

have included a figure for the precision of the BMD results expressed as the coefficient of variation (CV).[7,9,42–47] While early reports gave CV values of 2–3%, later studies suggest much poorer precision, with CV figures in the range of 5–6%. As emphasized above, the poor precision of the decubitus scan is partly the result of the difficulty in reproducing patients' positions on follow-up scans, which leads to variations in the thickness and composition of the soft tissue baseline,[14–18] as well as projection errors (Figure 11.2). A further limitation is that in some studies only the L3 vertebral body may have been measured due to concerns over the effects of overlay of L2 and L4 by rib and pelvic bone.[35] As a general rule, use of a smaller ROI is always associated with greater relative errors.[26]

For supine lateral BMD studies, the use of paired PA/lateral DXA scans has led to a major improvement in measurement precision. This is achieved by using information from both the PA and lateral scans to compute the changes in vertebral body BMD. This technique, referred to as *baseline compensation*, corrects for the effects of variable thickness and composition of soft tissue in the lateral scanning field. A description of two alternative algorithms for performing baseline compensation is given in the Appendix to this chapter. In multiplicative

baseline compensation, a correction factor is derived that is applied to each lateral BMD parameter, while in additive baseline compensation the correction is added to each BMD figure.[41] Initial studies of paired PA and supine lateral measurements of vertebral body BMD report CV figures of about 1% for L2–L4 (Table 11.5).[13,41,48,49] Rather larger precision errors are found if: (1) fewer than three vertebrae are included in the measurement ROI; (2) smaller measurement sites are used (for example, mid-vertebral body BMD instead of vertebral body BMD); and (3) the baseline compensation correction is omitted. Details of these differences are given in Tables 11.6 and 11.7.

Another advantage of paired PA and supine lateral BMD measurements is the exact line-by-line registration achieved between the PA and lateral images (Figure 11.1). This removes the possibility of erroneous identification of vertebrae and the consequent accuracy errors.

Sabin et al. reported a cadaver study that examined the accuracy of paired PA and supine lateral DXA measurements of vertebral body and whole vertebrae BMC, vertebral body volume, and volumetric BMD.[40] A summary of the findings is given in Table 11.8. Accuracy errors, as expressed by the RMSE errors about the regression lines, had a CV of between 3.1% and

Table 11.6 Short-term precision for the postero-anterior (PA) and the different lateral BMD measurement ROIs for the paired PA and lateral scan mode on a Hologic QDR-2000. All measurements are for L2–L4. Results are shown with and without baseline compensation.[41]

Measurement ROI (L2–L4)	Coefficient of variation (CV) (95% confidence interval)	
	With baseline compensation (%)	Without baseline compensation (%)
PA spine	0.80 (0.66–1.00)	–
Vertebral body	1.20 (0.72–1.54)	2.11 (1.75–2.64)
Mid-vertebral body	2.44 (2.03–3.05)	3.00 (2.49–3.75)
WA vertebral body	1.54 (1.26–1.90)	2.45 (1.57–3.08)
WA mid-vertebral	2.48 (2.06–3.10)	3.28 (2.72–4.10)
Total lateral	0.80 (0.66–1.00)	1.95 (1.62–2.44)

WA, width adjusted.

Table 11.7 Short-term precision for different combinations of vertebrae for postero-anterior (PA) and lateral (vertebral body ROI) BMD measurements on a Hologic QDR-2000.[41]

Vertebrae included	CV for PA BMD (%) (95% confidence interval)	CV for vertebral body BMD (%) (95% confidence interval)
L2–L4	0.80 (0.66–1.00)	1.20 (0.72–1.54)
L3–L4	–	1.53 (1.27–1.91)
L2	1.35 (0.74–1.75)	2.58 (1.03–3.50)
L3	1.13 (0.94–1.41)	1.81 (1.21–2.25)
L4	1.48 (1.23–1.85)	2.37 (1.10–3.17)

4.9%. Although vertebral body volumes estimated from the DXA study underestimated the true volumes, this simply reflects an error in the geometric shape factor derived from the elliptical cylinder model (see Appendix). Absolute accuracy errors were larger for vertebral body BMC than for the whole vertebra BMC derived from the PA scan, a finding that appeared to reflect the relatively greater organic fraction in the vertebral body composition.[40]

LONGITUDINAL BMD CHANGES WITH AGEING AND TREATMENT

Figures for lifetime bone loss in normal white women (Table 11.9) show losses that relate to the trabecular bone content.[50] As would be expected from Table 11.9, DXA studies comparing age-related changes in PA and lateral BMD confirm that the decrease in lateral BMD is around 50% greater than for PA BMD.[6,7,19–21,23,51]

Table 11.8 Comparison of lateral DXA scanning and ashing measurements in 12 cadaver spines.[40]

Variable	Mean ashed data (L2–L4)[a]	DXA/ashed ratio[b]	RMSE[c]	CV (%)[d]
PA BMC	45 g	0.86	2.2 g	4.9
Vertebral body BMC	23 g	0.67	1.0 g	4.3
Vertebral body volume	137 cm^3	0.77	5.1 cm^3	3.7
Volumetric BMD	0.16 g/cm^3	0.88	0.005 g/cm^3	3.1

[a]The mean results of the ashing data for the 12 cadaver spines (L2–L4).
[b]The mean ratio of DXA to ashing measurements.
[c]The RMSE for predicting ashing measurements from DXA data using linear regression.
[d]The coefficient of variation (CV) obtained by dividing the RMSE by the mean ashed data.

Table 11.9 Lifetime bone loss in normal white women.

Bone site	Bone composition	Method	Lifetime loss (%)
Iliac crest	40–60% trabecular bone	Biopsy	41
Lateral spine (vertebral body)	About 50% trabecular bone	DXA	44
PA spine	About 30%	DXA	30
Centre of vertebra	Pure trabecular bone	QCT	80

There is also considerable evidence that the effects of treatment are greater for lateral than for PA BMD. Reid et al.[37] and Finkelstein et al.[21] both reported an apparently greater percentage loss in bone mass for lateral compared with PA projection BMD scans for patients on glucocorticoid therapy when interpreted using the manufacturer's reference data. Blake et al. reported on the effect of 2 years of treatment with cyclical etidronate therapy in recently post-menopausal women.[36] The total treatment effect, defined as the difference in the percentage change from baseline in the etidronate-treated and placebo groups, was 4.00 ± 0.63% for PA spine BMD, 5.50 ± 0.84% for vertebral body BMD, and 7.71 ± 1.49% for mid-vertebral

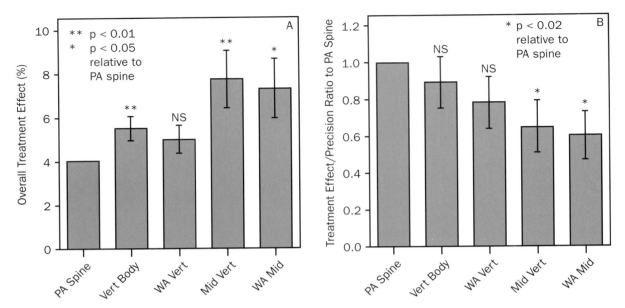

Figure 11.7 (A) Comparison of the total treatment effect (defined as the difference in the percentage change in BMD in the treated and control groups at 2 years) for PA and lateral BMD measurements in postmenopausal women in a clinical trial of cyclical etidronate therapy.[36] The error bars (± 1 SE) show the error in the difference in treatment effect between each site and the PA spine measurement. NS, not statistically significantly different from the PA spine result. (B) Comparison of the longitudinal sensitivity of the different spine BMD sites obtained by dividing the total treatment effect by the long-term precision of the BMD measurements. The results show this ratio normalized to PA spine BMD. The error bars are ± 1 SE. NS, ratio not statistically significantly different from unity.

body BMD (Figure 11.7A). However, when the longitudinal sensitivity was calculated by dividing the treatment effect by precision, the larger precision errors for lateral BMD cancelled any significant advantage of the greater treatment effect (Figure 11.7B). At present, there is no evidence that lateral BMD measurements have an advantage for longitudinal studies.

LATERAL BMD AND VERTEBRAL BODY STRENGTH

The major purpose of bone densitometry is to predict fracture risk, and therefore biomechanical studies of the relationship between compressive strength and BMD in cadaver specimens may give useful information. Myers et al. reported significant correlations between both PA ($r^2 = 0.444$; $p < 0.001$) and lateral ($r^2 = 0.615$; $p < 0.001$) BMD over a wide range of vertebral body strength.[52] Vertebral body BMD from the lateral scan predicted the compressive strength of the vertebral body better than BMD from the conventional PA spine scan, predicting respectively 62% and 44% of the variation in vertebral strength. In contrast, Wilson et al.[53] found similar correlation coefficients for both PA and lateral BMD with compressive strength ($r^2 = 0.69$ versus $r^2 = 0.61$ respectively), a finding they attributed to the high correlation between bone mass in vertebral body and posterior elements. Similar agreement between PA and lateral BMD and vertebral body strength was reported by Moro et al.[54] In an interesting study, Bjarnason et al. performed BMD measurements in situ before excising the vertebral bodies and measuring bone density again.[55] They found that lateral BMD measured in situ correlated less well with compressive strength than did PA BMD, while after excision this finding was reversed, a result they attributed to the effect of overlying soft tissue on the accuracy errors of the lateral measurements. Overall, it would seem that any differences between PA and lateral spine BMD for the prediction of vertebral body strength are marginal, perhaps for the reasons suggested by Wilson et al.[53] This explanation is supported by an interesting study by Seeman et al.,[56] who also reported evidence for comparable losses in the vertebral body and posterior processes associated with ageing and osteoporosis. The implications of these findings are potentially very important for the clinical application of PA and lateral DXA. If the posterior process and vertebral body do indeed lose bone to an equal extent with ageing, then measurements of PA and lateral BMD provide equivalent diagnostic information. The controversial nature of such results emphasizes the need for further studies in this field.

LATERAL BMD AND THE DIAGNOSIS OF OSTEOPOROSIS

Another method of investigating the clinical utility of lateral DXA scanning is to compare the relative differences in bone loss and Z-score between fractured and non-fractured subjects for PA and lateral BMD (Table 11.10).[26] As can be seen from Table 11.10, percentage BMD losses in established osteoporosis are significantly larger for lateral than for PA BMD, a finding that is consistent with the discussion given above of the greater age- and treatment-related changes for lateral BMD reported in cross-sectional and longitudinal studies. The same finding is shown graphically in Figure 11.8. However, because the population standard deviation is larger for lateral than for PA BMD, when the differences between PA and lateral BMD are expressed in terms of Z-scores they become relatively small and may be negligible in clinical practice (Table 11.10). To date, there are no prospective studies relating lateral DXA to fracture occurrence.

THE CLINICAL USEFULNESS OF LATERAL DXA SCANS

Measurements of BMD on the lateral spine with state-of-the-art equipment can now be performed with a small precision error, allowing repeated measurements for longitudinal studies and estimation of the rate of bone loss. However, it is not clear at present whether lateral spine scans will be of greater diagnostic sensitivity for fracture prediction than more commonly used measurement sites such as the PA spine, femur, forearm or calcaneus.

Possible advantages of lateral DXA for clinical and research applications are derived from the following observations:

1) The age-related bone loss for lateral spine BMD is about 50% larger than that for the PA projection. The difference is due to the greater trabecular bone content of the vertebral body.
2) Differences between fractured and non-fractured subjects are greater for lateral BMD when expressed in percentage terms. However, the differences are more marginal when expressed in terms of Z-scores.
3) Changes in older patients due to degenerative disease may have less effect on lateral than PA BMD.

Table 11.10 Discrimination between fractured and non-fractured women using postero-anterior (PA) and lateral DXA of the lumbar spine as found in various studies.[a] (Reproduced with permission from Jergas and Genant.[26])

Authors	PA BMD		Lateral BMD	
	% difference	Z-score	% difference	Z-score
Uebelhart et al.[11]	−22.8	−1.6	−27.8	−0.88
Slosman et al.[7]	−15.9	−0.83	−23.0	−0.61
Peel et al.[23]	−23.0	−1.47	−34.3	−1.33
Duboeuf et al.[51]	− 9.0	−0.66	−21.0	−1.08
Guglielmi et al.[19]	−16.8	−0.99	−24.7	−1.01
Bjarnason et al.[24]	−16.0	−0.80	−17.4	−0.65
Yu et al.[57]	− 8.0	−0.5	−10.9	−0.79

[a]Data are given as the per cent difference between the means, as well as the respective Z-scores.

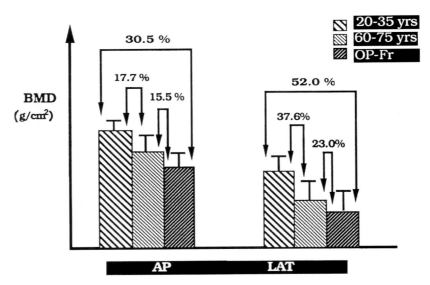

Figure 11.8 Bone mineral density (BMD) determined in AP (entire vertebra less transverse processes) and lateral view (entire vertebral body) is compared in two groups of normal women of different age and a group of older women with established osteoporosis (presence of crush fractures). Differences between mean values are listed. Statistically significant differences are seen in mean BMD. (From: Slosman DO. Non-invasive measurement of focal or whole body mass and body composition by dual X-ray absorptiometry. Thèse de Privat-Docent, Division de Médecine Nucléaire, Department de Radiologie, Hôpital Cantonal Universitaire, Genève-Suisse, 1991. Reproduced with permission.)

In contrast, factors that may reduce the value of lateral scans are as follows:

1) Although precision for vertebral body BMD may approach the precision of PA scans in young normal subjects, it is inferior in older patients.
2) The sampling volume for the vertebral body ROI is smaller than for the PA scan. Therefore, local changes not representative of the entire spine are more likely to influence the outcome.
3) The population standard deviation appears larger for lateral BMD than for PA BMD.
4) Spinal deformity and obesity may significantly interfere with the interpretation of lateral BMD scans, while such patients may still be assessed using the PA scan mode.
5) Lateral spine DXA scans are more seriously affected by inhomogeneity of fat distribution than PA scans. This may compromise the accuracy of lateral BMD results and lead to misinterpretation of the scan.

In summary, after some 10 years of study, lateral DXA has yet to establish itself as a routine measurement site for bone densitometry studies. However, there may be specific indications for the application of lateral DXA. These include its use as a research tool in epidemiological studies, clinical drug trials and for monitoring patients receiving drugs known to affect bone mineral metabolism. In the latter case, however, the greater precision error may offset the benefits of direct measurements of the vertebral body. At the present time, a lack of relevant prospective studies prevents a final judgement being reached on the status of lateral spine DXA as a technique for determining a patient's risk of osteoporotic fracture compared with conventional PA and femur scans.

ILLUSTRATIVE CASES

The cases shown in Figures 11.9–11.15 are presented to illustrate some of the points discussed on data analysis and interpretation. Positions of the ROI are shown. Scans obtained in pencil-beam mode and in lateral decubitus position are contrasted with scans obtained in fan-beam mode and supine position. Technical limitations are demonstrated.

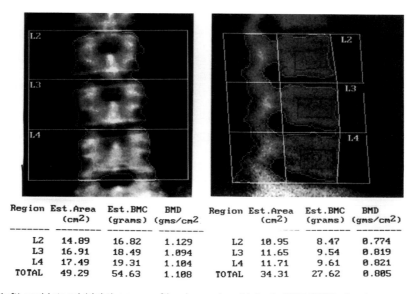

Region	Est.Area (cm2)	Est.BMC (grams)	BMD (gms/cm2)	Region	Est.Area (cm2)	Est.BMC (grams)	BMD (gms/cm2)
L2	14.89	16.82	1.129	L2	10.95	8.47	0.774
L3	16.91	18.49	1.094	L3	11.65	9.54	0.819
L4	17.49	19.31	1.104	L4	11.71	9.61	0.821
TOTAL	49.29	54.63	1.108	TOTAL	34.31	27.62	0.805

Figure 11.9 PA (left) and lateral (right) scans of lumbar spine (Hologic QDR-2000, fan-beam mode). On the lateral scan, the data given refer to the large ROI. A separate printout is available for different ROIs.

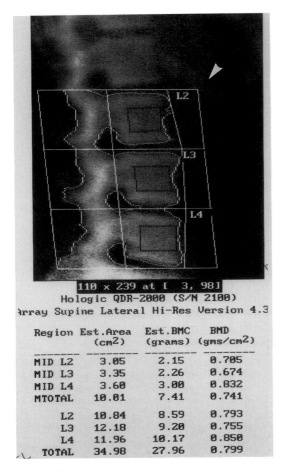

```
           110 x 239 at [  3, 98]
        Hologic QDR-2000 (S/N 2100)
   Array Supine Lateral Hi-Res Version 4.3

   Region  Est.Area   Est.BMC    BMD
             (cm2)    (grams)  (gms/cm2)

   MID L2     3.05      2.15     0.705
   MID L3     3.35      2.26     0.674
   MID L4     3.60      3.00     0.832
   MTOTAL    10.01      7.41     0.741

       L2   10.84      8.59     0.793
       L3   12.18      9.20     0.755
       L4   11.96     10.17     0.850
    TOTAL   34.98     27.96     0.799
```

Figure 11.10 Lateral spine scan (fan-beam mode) shows L1–L4. The 12th rib is seen crossing L1. Results on BMD for the entire vertebral body and the central (mid) ROI are shown. The position of the posterior border of the large ROI is critical. BMD values will be higher if portions of the neural arch are included. On repeated scans, the compare feature should be used to assure similar ROIs. The central ROI should always show a lower BMD.

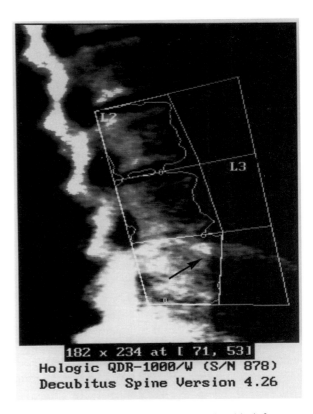

```
     182 x 234 at [ 71, 53]
  Hologic QDR-1000/W (S/N 878)
  Decubitus Spine Version 4.26
```

Figure 11.11 Lateral spine scan obtained in left lateral decubitus position. L4 is obscured by the ilium.

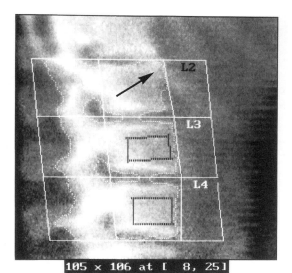

```
105 x 106 at [   8, 25]
Hologic QDR-2000 (S/N 2100)
Array Supine Lateral Fast Version 4.37I
```

Figure 11.12 Lateral spine scan obtained with fan-beam mode. The patient is in the supine position. This scan illustrates the proper positioning of the global ROI. L3 and L4 are used. The anterior tip of L2 is superimposed by the 12th rib, making it difficult to delineate its anterior border.

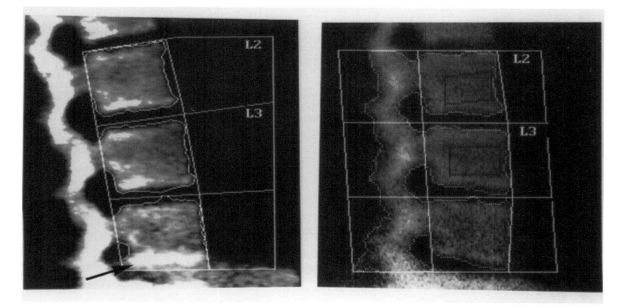

Figure 11.13 Comparison of lateral scans of the lumbar spine obtained in the left lateral decubitus position in pencil-beam mode (left panel) and supine lateral position in fan-beam mode (right panel) (Hologic QDR-2000). On the decubitus scan, the inferior portion of L4 is superimposed on the iliac crest. The supine lateral scan more frequently shows useful images of L2 and L4.

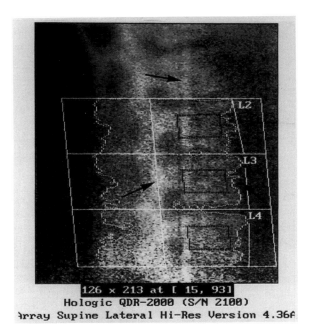

Hologic QDR-2000 (S/N 2100)
Array Supine Lateral Hi-Res Version 4.36f

Figure 11.14 Lateral spine scan of an obese subject (115 kg) showing the limitation of the technique. Note the false position of the posterior limit of the large ROI. This can be manually corrected. There are problems in delineation of the anterior vertebral border. Note the vertical artefact across the centre of the scan. The measurement results are not reliable.

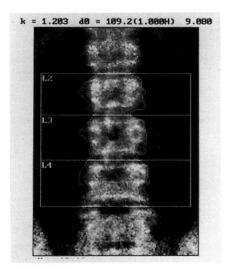

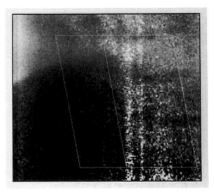

Figure 11.15 PA and lateral spine images in an obese subject (148 kg, abdominal thickness 33 cm). While the PA scan (left panel) is still technically acceptable, a lateral scan (right panel) cannot be performed because of the abnormal distance from the scanning table and the high attenuation.

APPENDIX

Estimate of vertebral body volume from paired PA and lateral DXA scans

Vertebral body volume is estimated from the paired PA and lateral DXA scans by assuming that the vertebral body is an elliptical cylinder (Figure 11.A1). Let a be the length of the major axis of the ellipse, b the minor axis and h the height of the cylinder. The projected area on the PA scan is given by:

$$A_{PA} = ah \qquad (A1)$$

and the projected area of the vertebral body measured on the lateral scan by:

$$A_{LAT} = bh \qquad (A2)$$

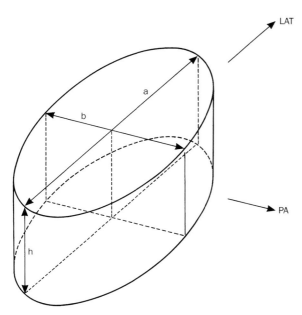

Figure 11.A1 Elliptical cylinder model of the vertebral body used in the calculation of volumetric BMD from paired PA and lateral DXA data.

The volume of the elliptical cylinder is given by:

$$\text{Volume} = \frac{\pi}{4} abh \qquad (A3)$$

After substituting the projected areas for the major and minor axes, the equation for volume becomes:

$$\text{Volume} = \frac{\pi}{4} \frac{A_{PA} A_{LAT}}{h} \qquad (A4)$$

The baseline compensation algorithm

For repeated paired PA and lateral DXA scans, information from the PA projection scan may be used to correct lateral BMD measurements for the errors resulting from variability in thickness and composition of the soft tissue reference baseline. The correction is made to improve the precision of BMD results derived from the lateral scan. Let TLAT BMD be the BMD figure for the lateral scan over the total projected area of bone (i.e. to include both the vertebral bodies and the posterior elements) of the vertebrae being analysed, and PA BMD the BMD figure for the same vertebrae on the PA scan. Let subscripts '0' and 'f' represent the baseline and follow-up scans, and a superscript '*' distinguish corrected from uncorrected lateral BMD figures.

Because any change in the total vertebral bone mineral content (BMC) will affect the measurements on both the PA and lateral projection scans, the change measured in PA BMD must be reflected in a proportionally equal change in TLAT BMD. Hence, the corrected value of TLAT BMD on the follow-up scan is given by:

$$\text{TLAT BMD}_f^* = \text{TLAT BMD}_0 \times \frac{\text{PA BMD}_f}{\text{PA BMD}_0} \qquad (A5)$$

The uncorrected value of TLAT BMD will therefore be in error by a factor F given by:

$$F = \frac{\text{TLAT BMD}_f^*}{\text{TLAT BMD}_f}$$

$$= \frac{\text{TLAT BMD}_0}{\text{TLAT BMD}_f} \times \frac{\text{PA BMD}_f}{\text{PA BMD}_0} \qquad (A6)$$

The correction factor F can be derived directly from the PA and total lateral BMDs on the baseline and follow-up scans. Two different ways of applying this correction can now be considered:

1) Multiplicative baseline compensation is the correction used in Hologic (Hologic Inc., Waltham, MA, USA) software for supine lateral BMD. In this algorithm it is assumed that the correction factor F derived from the total lateral BMD in equation A6 may be applied to correct the BMD of any regional part of the lateral scan. Therefore, all uncorrected vertebral body BMD results are adjusted by multiplying by F. For example, if VB BMD is the vertebral body BMD, the corrected and uncorrected values on the follow-up scan are related by:

$$\text{VB BMD}_f^* = \text{VB BMD}_f \times F \qquad (A7)$$

$$= \text{VB BMD}_f \times \frac{TLAT\ BMD_0}{TLAT\ BMD_f} \times \frac{PA\ BMD_f}{PA\ BMD_0}$$
$$(A8)$$

The significance of equation A8 becomes clearer if it is rewritten in the form:

$$\text{VB BMD}_f^* = \frac{\text{VB BMD}_f}{\text{TLAT BMD}_f} \times \text{PA BMD}_f \times$$

$$\frac{\text{TLAT BMD}_0}{\text{PA BMD}_0} \qquad (A9)$$

when it is clear that the essential information being derived from the follow-up lateral scan is the ratio of vertebral body to total lateral BMD.

2) In additive baseline compensation it is assumed that the difference between the corrected and uncorrected total lateral BMD results:

$$\Delta \text{ TLAT BMD} = \text{TLAT BMD}_f^* - \text{TLAT BMD}_f$$
$$= (F - 1) \times \text{TLAT BMD}_f$$
$$(A10)$$

should be added to the BMD of any regional part of the lateral scan. Therefore, all uncorrected vertebral body BMD and mid-vertebral body BMD results are adjusted by adding Δ TLAT BMD.

REFERENCES

1. Reid IR, Evans MC, Ames R, Wattie DJ. The influence of osteophytes and aortic calcification on spinal bone mineral density in post-menopausal women. *J Clin Endocrinol Metab* (1991) **72:** 1372–4.
2. Drinka PJ, DeSmet AA, Bauwens SF, Rogot A. The effect of overlying calcification on lumbar bone densitometry. *Calcif Tissue Int* (1992) **50:** 507–10.
3. Ito M, Hayashi K, Yamada M et al. Relationship of osteophytes to bone mineral density and spinal fracture in men. *Radiology* (1993) **189:** 497–502.
4. Yu W, Glüer C-C, Fuerst T et al. Influence of degenerative joint disease on spinal bone mineral measurements in postmenopausal women. *Calcif Tissue Int* (1995) **57:** 169–74.
5. Rand Th, Seidl G, Kainberger F et al. Impact of spinal degenerative changes on the evaluation of bone mineral density with dual energy x-ray absorptiometry (DXA). *Calcif Tissue Int* (1997) **60:** 430–3.
6. Rupich R, Pacifici R, Griffin M et al. Lateral dual energy radiography: a new method for measuring vertebral bone density: a preliminary study. *J Clin Endocrinol Metab* (1990) **70:** 1768–70.
7. Slosman DO, Rissoli R, Donath A, Bonjour J-P. Vertebral bone mineral density measured laterally by dual-energy X-ray absorptiometry. *Osteoporos Int* (1990) **1:** 23–9.
8. Mazess RB, Gifford CA, Bisek JP et al. DEXA measurement of spine density in the lateral projection. I. Methodology. *Calcif Tissue Int* (1991) **49:** 235–9.
9. Larnach TA, Boyd SJ, Smart RS et al. Reproducibility of lateral spine scans using dual energy x-ray absorptiometry. *Calcif Tissue Int* (1992) **51:** 255–8.
10. Lilley J, Eyre S, Walters B et al. An investigation of spinal bone mineral density measured laterally: a normal range for UK women. *Br J Radiol* (1994) **67:** 157–61.
11. Uebelhart D, Duboeuf F, Meunier PF, Delmas PD. Lateral dual photon absorptiometry: a new technique to measure the bone mineral density at the lumbar spine. *J Bone Miner Res* (1990) **5:** 525–31.
12. Wilson CR, Fogelman I. Lateral lumbar BMD with dual energy absorptiometry. In: Ring EFJ, ed. *Current Research in Osteoporosis and Bone Mineral Measurement I* (British Institute of Radiology: London, 1990), 15–17.

13. Steiger P, von Stetten E, Weiss H, Stein JA. Paired AP and lateral supine dual X-ray absorptiometry of the spine: initial results for a 32 detector system. *Osteoporos Int* (1991) **1:** 190.

14. Hangartner TN, Johnston CC. Influence of fat on bone measurements with dual-energy x-ray absorptiometry. *Bone Miner* (1990) **9:** 71–81.

15. Tothill P, Pye DW. Errors due to fat in lateral spine DPA. In: Ring EFJ, ed. *Current Research in Osteoporosis and Bone Mineral Measurement I* (British Institute of Radiology: London, 1990), 19.

16. Tothill P, Pye DW. Errors due to non-uniform distribution of fat in dual X-ray absorptiometry of the lumbar spine. *Br J Radiol* (1992) **65:** 807–13.

17. Tothill P, Avenell A. Errors in dual-energy X-ray absorptiometry of the lumbar spine owing to fat distribution and soft tissue thickness during weight change. *Br J Radiol* (1994) **67:** 71–5.

18. Formica C, Loro M-L, Gilsanz V, Seeman E. Inhomogeneity in body fat distribution may result in inaccuracy in the measurement of vertebral bone mass. *J Bone Miner Res* (1995) **10:** 1504–11.

19. Guglielmi G, Grimston SK, Fischer KC, Pacifici R. Osteoporosis diagnosis with lateral and posteroanterior dual x-ray absorptiometry compared with quantitative CT. *Radiology* (1994) **192:** 845–50.

20. Mazess RB, Barden HS, Eberle RW, Denton MD. Age changes in spine density in posterior-anterior and lateral projections in normal women. *Calcif Tissue Int* (1995) **56:** 201–5.

21. Finkelstein JS, Cleary RL, Butler JP et al. A comparison of lateral *versus* anterior-posterior spine dual energy x-ray absorptiometry for the diagnosis of osteopenia. *J Clin Endocrinol Metab* (1994) **78:** 724–30.

22. Jergas M, Breitenseher M, Glüer C-C et al. Estimates of volumetric bone density from projectional measurements improve the discriminatory capability of dual x-ray absorptiometry. *J Bone Miner Res* (1995) **10:** 1101–10.

23. Peel NF, Eastell R. Diagnostic value of estimated volumetric bone mineral density of the spine in osteoporosis. *J Bone Miner Res* (1994) **9:** 317–20.

24. Bjarnason K, Nilas L, Hassager C, Christiansen C. Dual energy x-ray absorptiometry of the spine – decubitus lateral versus anteroposterior projection in osteoporotic women: comparison to single energy x-ray absorptiometry of the forearm. *Bone* (1995) **16:** 255–60.

25. Del Rio L, Pons F, Huguet M et al. Anteroposterior versus lateral bone mineral density of spine assessed by dual x-ray absorptiometry. *Eur J Nucl Med* (1995) **22:** 407–12.

26. Jergas M, Genant HK. Lateral dual x-ray absorptiometry of the lumbar spine: current status. *Bone* (1997) **20:** 311–14.

27. Nottestad SY, Baumel JJ, Kimmel DB et al. The proportion of trabecular bone in human vertebrae. *J Bone Miner Res* (1987) **2:** 221–9.

28. Cann C, Genant H, Ettinger B et al. Spinal mineral loss in oophorectomized women. *JAMA* (1980) **244:** 256–9.

29. Jones CD, Laval-Jeanet AM, Laval-Jeanet MH et al. Importance of measurement of spongious vertebral bone mineral density in the assessment of osteoporosis. *Bone* (1987) **8:** 201–6.

30. Kalender W, Felsenberg D, Louis O et al. Reference values for trabecular and cortical vertebral bone density in single and dual-energy quantitative computed tomography. *Eur J Radiol* (1989) **9:** 75–80.

31. Bergot C, Laval-Jeanet AM, Preteux F et al. Measurements of anisotopic vertebrae trabecular bone loss during aging by quantitative image analysis. *Calcif Tissue Int* (1988) **43:** 143–9.

32. Bell GH, Dunbar O, Beck JS et al. Variations in strength of vertebrae with age and their relation to osteoporosis. *Calcif Tissue Res* (1967) **1:** 75–86.

33. Kleerekoper M, Villaneuva AR, Stanciu J et al. The role of three-dimensional trabecular microstructure in the pathogenesis of vertebral compressive fractures. *Calcif Tissue Int* (1985) **37:** 594–7.

34. Podenphant J, Herss Nielsen VA, Riis BJ et al. Bone mass, bone structure and vertebral fractures in osteoporotic patients. *Bone* (1987) **8:** 127–30.

35. Rupich RC, Griffin MG, Pacifici R et al. Lateral dual-energy radiography: artifact error from rib and pelvic bone. *J Bone Miner Res* (1992) **7:** 97–101.

36. Blake GM, Herd RJM, Fogelman I. A longitudinal study of supine lateral DXA of the lumbar spine: a comparison with posteroanterior spine, hip and total-body DXA. *Osteoporos Int* (1996) **6:** 462–70.

37. Reid IR, Evans MC, Stapleton J. Lateral spine densitometry is a more sensitive indicator of glucocorticoid-induced bone loss. *J Bone Miner Res* (1992) **7:** 1221–5.

38. Matkovic V, Jelic T, Wardlaw GM et al. Timing of peak bone mass in caucasian females and its implication for the prevention of osteoporosis. *J Clin Invest* (1994) **93:** 799–808.

39. Jergas M, Breitenseher M, Glüer C-C et al. Which vertebrae should be assessed using lateral dual x-ray absorptiometry of the lumbar spine? *Osteoporos Int* (1995) **5:** 196–204.

40. Sabin MA, Blake GM, MacLaughlin-Black SM, Fogelman I. The accuracy of volumetric bone density measurements in dual x-ray absorptiometry. *Calcif Tissue Int* (1995) **56:** 210–14.

41. Blake GM, Jagathesan T, Herd RJM, Fogelman I. Dual x-ray absorptiometry of the lumbar spine: the precision of paired antero-posterior/lateral studies. *Br J Radiol* (1994) **67:** 624–30.

42. Mazess RB, Hanson J, Gifford C et al. Measurement of spinal density in the lateral projection. In: Ring EFJ, ed. *Current Research in Osteoporosis and Bone Mineral Measurement I* (British Institute of Radiology: London, 1990), 17–18.

43. Lilley J, Eyre S, Heath DA. *In-vivo* and *in-vitro* precision for BMD of the spine measured laterally using DEXA. In: Ring EFJ, ed. *Current Research in Osteoporosis and Bone Mineral Measurement II* (British Institute of Radiology: London, 1992), 27–8.

44. Banks LM, Lees B, Stevenson JC. Comparison of bone density measurements assessed by lateral DXA and QCT. In: Ring EFJ, ed. *Current Research in Osteoporosis and Bone Mineral Measurement II* (British Institute of Radiology: London, 1992), 26–7.

45. Pye DW, Bassey EJ, Armstrong A. Precision in practice: experience with a Lunar DPX-L densitometer. In: Ring EFJ, ed. *Current Research in Osteoporosis and Bone Mineral Measurement II* (British Institute of Radiology: London, 1992), 21–2.

46. Economou G, Rushton S, Adams JE, Whitehouse RW. Precision of lateral DXA and correlation with QCT. *Calcif Tissue Int* (1993) **52:** 159.

47. Devogelaer JP, Baudoux C, Nagent de Deuxchaisnes C. Lack of precision of the lumbar spine BMD measurements with the QDR-1000/W when patients are lying in the lateral position. *Calcif Tissue Int* (1993) **52:** 163.

48. Slosman DO, Rissoli R, Donath A, Bonjour J-P. Bone mineral density of lumbar vertebral body determined in supine and lateral decubitus: study of precision and sensitivity. *J Bone Miner Res* (1992) **7**(suppl 1): S192.

49. Devogelaer JP, Baudoux C, Nagent de Deuxchaisnes C. Reproducibility of BMD measurements on the QDR-2000. *Calcif Tissue Int* (1993) **52:** 164.

50. Delmas PD, Fontanges E, Duboeuf F et al. Comparison of bone mass measured by histomorphometry on iliac biopsy and by dual photon absorptiometry of the lumbar spine. *Bone* (1988) **9:** 209–13.

51. Duboeuf F, Pommet R, Meunier PJ, Delmas PD. Dual-energy X-ray absorptiometry of the spine in anteroposterior and lateral projections. *Osteoporos Int* (1994) **4:** 110–16.

52. Myers BS, Arbogast KB, Lobaugh B et al. Improved assessment of lumbar vertebral body strength using supine lateral dual-energy X-ray absorptiometry. *J Bone Miner Res* (1994) **9:** 687–93.

53. Wilson CR, Yoganandan N, Collier BD. The relationship between frontal and lateral DPA measurement of the lumbar spine and the strength of the vertebral body. In: Ring EFJ, ed. *Current Research in Osteoporosis and Bone Mineral Measurement II* (British Institute of Radiology: London, 1992), 25.

54. Moro M, Hecker AT, Bouxsein ML, Myers ER. Failure load of thoracic vertebrae correlates with lumbar bone mineral density measured by DXA. *Calcif Tissue Int* (1995) **56:** 206–9.

55. Bjarnason K, Hassager C, Svendesen OL et al. Anteroposterior and lateral spinal DXA for the assessment of vertebral body strength: comparison with hip and forearm measurements. *Osteoporos Int* (1996) **6:** 37–42.

56. Seeman E, Formica C, Mosekilde L. Equivalent deficits in bone mass of the vertebral body and posterior processes in women with vertebral fractures: implications regarding the pathogenesis of spinal osteoporosis. *J Bone Miner Res* (1995) **10:** 2005–10.

57. Yu W, Glüer C-C, Grampp S et al. Spinal bone mineral assessment in postmenopausal women: a comparison between dual X-ray absorptiometry and quantitative computed tomography. *Osteoporos Int* (1995) **5:** 433–9.

12

Measurement of Bone Density in the Proximal Femur

CONTENTS • **Chapter overview** • **Introduction** • **Structural anatomy and trabecular architecture in the proximal femur** • **Summary of measurement techniques in the proximal femur** • **Acquisition and analysis of a femur DXA scan** • **Review of a femur DXA report** • **Standardized BMDs for femur DXA scans** • **Illustrative cases**

CHAPTER OVERVIEW

This chapter reviews the techniques for performing and analysing DXA scans of the proximal femur. The Singh index is reviewed first, since it represents a useful approach to understanding trabecular structure in the hip. Guidelines are then given on how to perform, analyse and interpret a femur dual-energy X-ray absorptiometry (DXA) study, and frequently encountered practical problems are discussed. The controversy over reference range data for femur bone mineral density (BMD) is described, and the recommendation by the International Committee for Standards in Bone Measurements that DXA femur studies should be interpreted using the total hip site with reference ranges derived from the NHANES III study is discussed. Case examples illustrate pitfalls and problems in data interpretation.

INTRODUCTION

Hip fracture is widely recognized as the most serious consequence of osteoporosis. In white women aged 65–84 years old, 90% of hip frac-

tures are believed to be due to osteoporosis.[1] It is estimated that in the USA in 1995 the total healthcare costs attributable to osteoporotic fractures exceeded $13 billion, of which two-thirds was due to hip fractures.[2] A quarter of hip fracture patients die within a year following their fractures, and survivors frequently suffer sustained disability and loss of independence leading to institutionalization.[2]

Until the commercial development of dual photon absorptiometry (DPA) scanners in the early 1980s, information about bone loss in the hip was based mainly on changes in trabecular structure and cortical thickness which was assessed by visual evaluation of radiographs. Since the late 1980s, however, technical improvements and the widespread availability of DXA systems have made it possible to quantify BMD in the hip routinely with good accuracy and precision. These developments have stimulated further research into the understanding of osteoporosis in the hip, and the clinical utility of measurements of femur BMD. After the spine, the hip is the most frequently studied skeletal site for research and clinical applications of bone densitometry. Indeed, a strong case can be made that a measurement of femur BMD is actually the single most reliable variable for the prediction of hip fracture,[3,4] the prevention of which must surely be the principal aim of the new therapeutic strategies for prevention of osteoporosis now being developed.

In addition to bone mass, the integrity of trabecular structure in the proximal femur is also an important factor in bone strength. This should be appreciated when using BMD measurements to estimate fracture risk. Present approaches to bone mineral measurement in the hip recognize this. Rather than using a BMD value for the entire proximal femur in a single region of interest (ROI), localized ROIs in the femur that reflect structurally important sites are identified and measured. As an introduction to the complexity of bone structure in the hip, an understanding of the anatomy of the proximal femur and the changes in bone structure and mass that occur during life is required. As previously stressed for the spine, it is perhaps even more true for the hip that the skill and training of the technologist performing the DXA scan are vitally important for high quality studies. Reproducibility of patient positioning, awareness of the special difficulties in scanning and analysing this area, and knowledge of the range of anatomical variations will prevent many frustrations when BMD scans are interpreted.

STRUCTURAL ANATOMY AND TRABECULAR ARCHITECTURE IN THE PROXIMAL FEMUR

Developmental changes during childhood

In a newborn human baby only the shaft of the femur is ossified, whereas the femoral head and neck, the intertrochanteric crest and the trochanters consist of epiphyseal cartilage. At 3 years of age, bony lamellae are present in the region of the base of the lesser trochanter, the earliest signs of the calcar femorale. Bony lamellae become more abundant, and the trochanter and the intertrochanteric crest develop by budding out from the original oval diaphysis. The trabecular structure and the cal-

car femorale reach maximal size and density in early adulthood.

The medial angle between the shaft and the neck decreases during active growth and ranges between 110° and 145° in adulthood. However, after adulthood is reached, the angle remains constant into old age. The medial and backward deviation of the femoral neck produces maximal pressure stresses on the inner posterior surfaces of the upper-fourth of the shaft, and the calcar femorale reinforces the bone in this region (Figure 12.1).

Age-related bone loss in the proximal femur

With old age, there is progressive thinning of the cortex and trabeculae, and the space resulting from the reduction in trabecular bone mass is filled with fat. In addition, there is a change from red bone marrow to yellow marrow. These alterations result in a significant change in intraosseous fat content of the proximal femur during life. In 60% of a group of 110 persons 75 years old or older, Harty[5] found that the Ward's triangle contained no trabecular bone, but was occupied entirely by yellow marrow.

The internal architecture of the proximal femur is composed of two major trabecular systems arranged along the lines of compressive and tensile stresses produced during weight-bearing (Figure 12.2). A central region defines a neutral axis where tensile and compressive forces balance each other. Secondary compressive and tensile groups of trabeculae can be seen. Changes in the appearances of these groups of trabeculae with ageing are the basis of the grading scheme proposed by Singh (the Singh index, Figure 12.3).[6]

Adaptive alterations of these patterns occur by bone remodelling as a result of changes in the direction of the stress forces. Variations in the external configuration of the proximal femur, as well as variations in the trabecular pattern between individuals, are explained by genetic factors as well as these forces.

Bone loss with age in the proximal femur is different from that in the spinal column.[7] In the latter, bone loss starts with loss of horizontal

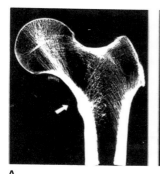 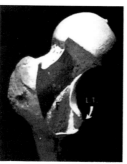

A

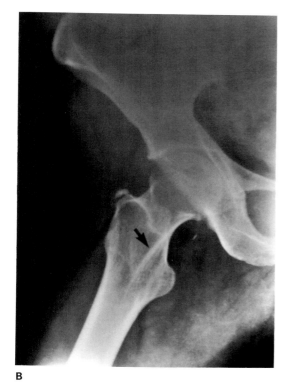

B

Figure 12.1 Strength is given to the femoral neck by the calcar femorale, which reinforces bone at a site of major stress. (A) Ashed bone specimen of proximal femur showing Ward's triangle in the centre of the neck, the medial compressive buttress (arrow) (left), the calcar femorale (F) (right) and the lesser trochanter (LT). (Reproduced with permission from ref. 5.) (B) Radiograph of the proximal femur shows the calcar femorale (arrow).

trabeculae, which results in increased pressure and hypertrophy of the remaining vertical trabeculae. In time, this leads to a decrease in the specific surface of trabecular bone (i.e. the trabecular bone surface area per unit volume of trabeculae).[8] Microfractures, repair and hypertrophy constitute a chronic process that ultimately results in end-plate deformities and compression fractures.

In the proximal femur, however, bone loss follows a different pattern that reflects a hierarchy of trabecular groups in order to meet the mechanical demands of weight-bearing. Secondary trabeculae are resorbed first, and in time Ward's triangle becomes well defined and enlarges (Figure 12.2). Next, there is a loss of tensile trabeculae which starts centrally, with the primary tensile group being the last to be absorbed (Figure 12.3).[6] Trabecular hypertrophy is not observed. Also in the hip, the decreasing mean trabecular diameter leads to an increase in the specific surface area of trabecular bone with age.[8] This sequence of events is shown in the schematic illustrations of the femoral grading patterns referred to as the Singh index (Figure 12.3).

A question often asked is whether cancellous or cortical bone is more important for bone strength of the proximal femur. In cancellous bone from excised specimens of the proximal femur, there is a significant correlation between mechanical properties and bone mineral.[9] Removal of the central trabecular bone portion from a proximal femur specimen reduces the strength for impact loading by about 50%. This reduction suggests trabecular bone has a major role in bone strength, but that cortical bone also has structural importance. Variations in compressive strength and elastic modulus within and between femoral bone samples are larger than those seen in the spinal column. This suggests that age-related bone loss in the hip is modulated more effectively by certain factors (exercise, lifestyle, nutrition, squatting) than is bone loss in the spinal column. Bone density alone does not fully account for the wide variation in mechanical properties, and macro- and microstructure have prominent roles in mechanical behaviour. This is the reason for the

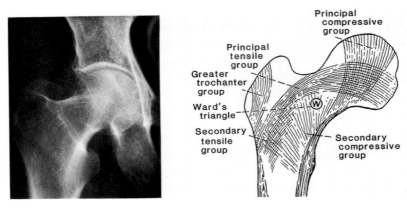

Figure 12.2 Schematic illustration of the trabecular structure in the proximal femur as observed in the trabecular grading pattern proposed by Singh. (Reproduced with permission from ref. 6.)

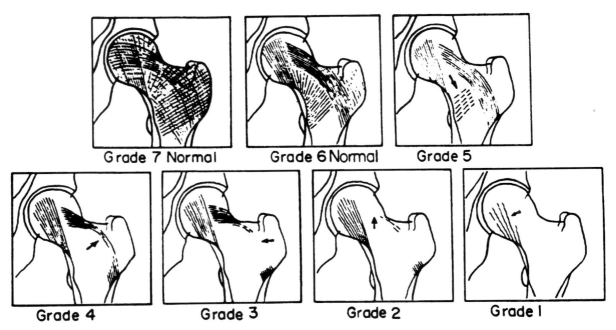

Figure 12.3 Schematic illustration of trabecular grading patterns proposed by Singh. (Reproduced with permission from ref. 6.)

relatively low correlation between the trabecular pattern (Singh index) in the femur and either cortical bone mass in the forearm or trabecular bone mass in the spine.[10,11] Optimal estimation of bone strength could probably be achieved if both trabecular structure and bone mass could be measured.

In addition to these age-related changes in bone and bone marrow, the fat content of the body increases with age, with particular accumulation in the hip region. These changes may occasionally affect the measurements when marked obesity is present (Figure 12.4).

The Singh index and the assessment of structural changes in the proximal femur

The most readily available approach to study the structural changes with age in the proximal femur is by means of the Singh index, which has been described above. This requires radiographs of the hip with careful attention given to correct positioning. A set of reference radiographs should be available to ensure reproducible readings of the grading patterns. Prior to the introduction of DPA, the Singh index was proposed as a test for the diagnosis of osteoporosis.[6,12–16] All healthy men and women aged 40 years and under can be classified as grades 6 or 7, which are considered normal. Lower grades indicate trabecular bone loss (Figure 12.5). However, the test has not found general acceptance because of the subjective aspects of interpretation, the relatively high radiation dose, the inability to quantify results and the need for radiographic standards for comparison.

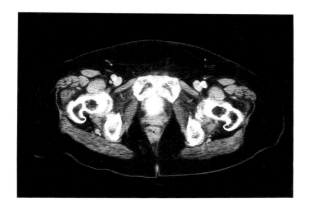

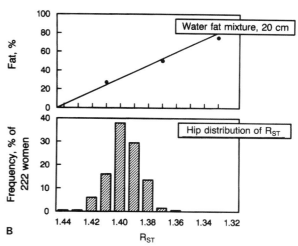

A

B

Figure 12.4 (A) Cross-section of pelvis at hip level. CT image of a 62-year-old woman. Note the fat and muscle distribution in the soft tissue surrounding the proximal femur. (B) Estimation of fat content in the soft tissue surrounding the proximal femur in 222 women aged 30–80 years seen at the Mayo Clinic for osteoporosis-related problems. The R-values given on Lunar instruments ranged from 1.36 to 1.44 with a median value of 1.40. The upper panel shows a standard curve obtained with water–oil mixtures, relating R-values to per cent fat. By using this standard curve and the R-value of a given patient, the fat content of the soft tissue surrounding the proximal femur can be calculated. The two graphs have the same horizontal axis. (For explanation of the R-value, see the Appendix to Chapter 14.)

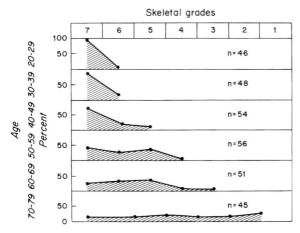

Skeletal grading in 300 normal subjects

Figure 12.5 Distribution of Singh index grades as a function of age. Young adults are all grade 6 or 7. With progressive ageing, lower grades are observed in most but not all subjects. (Reproduced with permission from ref. 6.)

SUMMARY OF MEASUREMENT TECHNIQUES IN THE PROXIMAL FEMUR

Apart from DPA and DXA, several procedures have been used to study bone changes in the hip in vivo (Table 12.1). Earlier tests based on radiographs of the hips concentrated on structural information. As discussed above, early attempts to quantify trabecular bone changes in the hip resulted in the Singh index.[6]

Other radiographic methods have included assessment of the calcar femorale, and the cortical index of the femoral neck and shaft.[16,17] Also of interest are newer experimental imaging and image-processing techniques based on axial tomograms obtained with CT scanners.[18–20] These techniques image the cross-sectional distribution of trabeculae, including the femoral head and acetabulum. More recently, the report by Faulkner et al.[21] that hip-axis length is an independent predictor of hip fracture risk has revived interest in simple geometrical measurements made from radiographs.[22]

ACQUISITION AND ANALYSIS OF A FEMUR DXA SCAN

Bone density measurement sites in the proximal femur

Until very recently there was a widely accepted convention to base the clinical interpretation of DXA scans of the hip on the BMD measurement in the femoral neck ROI (Figure 12.6). Other sites considered of interest were Ward's triangle and the trochanter region. BMD measurements at all three ROIs were routinely available using the scan analysis software provided by the principal commercial manufacturers. However, the decision of the International Committee for Standards in Bone Measurement (ICSBM) to recommend that the various manufacturers should standardize BMD measurements on a common scale using the total hip ROI,[23] and the recent controversy over the accuracy of femur reference ranges,[23–25] has led to a reappraisal of clinical practice. At present there is no clear consensus, but it seems likely that in the near future total hip BMD will become the most widely used measurement for scan interpretation.

The different ROI sites available in the femur (Figure 12.6) were selected to represent critical points in the hip where fractures occur (Figure 12.7). The femoral neck is the site of subcapital, mid-cervical and basicervical fractures, which together constitute 63% of all proximal femur fractures. The trochanter is the site of the remaining 37% of hip fractures. Ward's triangle at the base of the femoral neck is the site of the earliest trabecular bone loss, as was discussed above in relation to the Singh index. However, early bone loss does not necessarily prove that this site is a good marker for fracture prediction, since bone may be lost first from sites with little structural importance. The fracture study of Cummings et al.[3] suggests there is relatively little difference between the different femur ROIs in terms of fracture prediction (Figure 12.8). The inferior precision of BMD measurements at the Ward's triangle ROI (CV: 3.0–3.5%) when compared with femoral neck (CV: 1.5–2.0%) or total hip BMD (CV: 1.0–1.5%)

Table 12.1 Methods used for non-invasive estimation of bone loss at the hip.		
Principal approach	*Information available*	*Technique*
Imaging procedures (descriptive)	Description of trabecular structure and/or cortical bone thickness	Radiography; computed X-ray tomography; magnetic resonance imaging
Semi-quantitative procedures	Grading of trabecular bone pattern in proximal femur (Singh index)	Radiographs of hips; inward rotation
	Thickness of calcar femorale; cortical index	Frog, lateral view
Quantitative	Area density at different sites of the proximal femur; integral[a] bone area density (g/cm^2)	DXA
	Trabecular and/or integral[a] bone density (mg/mm^3)	Quantitative computed tomography Transverse slice technique; histogram analysis technique; three-dimensional reconstruction technique

[a]Integral bone density refers to measurements in which trabecular and cortical bone are not separated.

makes it a less suitable site for longitudinal studies.

The scan analysis software provided by the manufacturers is based on automatic identification of the femur ROIs with a minimum of operator intervention. However, apart from the total hip ROI the approach is not standardized, and significant differences exist between different makes of equipment. The exact location of the ROIs is based on anatomical markers used by the algorithms to ensure that equivalent locations in the femur are evaluated in different subjects. Follow-up scans are analysed using a scan comparison option which matches the ROIs to the baseline scan.

Performing a femur DXA scan

As previously stated for the spine (Chapter 10), details of scan acquisition and scan analysis vary between manufacturers and strict adherence to the manufacturer's recommendations is advised. A few general comments follow:

1) In performing a hip BMD measurement, *patient positioning* and the specific positioning of the legs is of great importance for achieving high measurement precision. Similarly, in scan analysis, careful positioning of the ROIs is of equal importance. As with spine measurements, the patient lies supine on the imaging table. The legs should be flat on the table with the feet

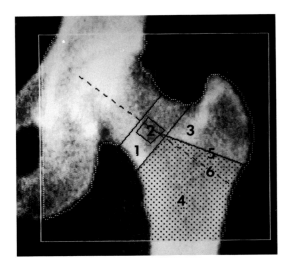

Figure 12.6 Bone mineral image of the left proximal femur. The ROIs as defined on Hologic instruments are shown: 1, femoral neck ROI; 2, Ward's triangle ROI; 3, trochanter ROI; 4, intertrochanteric ROI; 5, inferior border of trochanter ROI; 6, central axis of femoral neck. The entire area covered by femoral neck, trochanter and intertrochanteric ROIs is called the total hip ROI.

(shoes removed) strapped to a footholder to ensure proper inward rotation of the leg and a reproducible position of the proximal femur. It is important to stress that the entire leg should be rotated, and not just the foot or lower leg. Several studies have evaluated the influence of the position of the proximal femur on BMD results.[26] Rotation around the long axis of the femur, abduction or adduction and (rarely) flexion must be controlled. The leg is flat on the table, which generally ensures a reproducible position in the frontal plane (flexion-extension). The patient is aligned with the mid-line of the scanning table (Figure 12.9A), as is the footholder. This ensures a constant angle of abduction. A footholder fixes the foot in a firm position with a small inward rotation (Figure 12.9B). This controls the rotational angle. The angle varies slightly between manufacturers, but is typically in the range 25° to 30°.

2) Given good positioning, there are still significant *anatomical variations* of the proximal

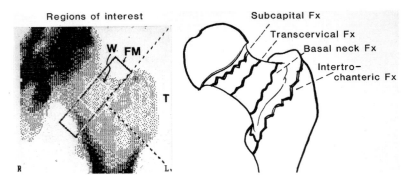

Figure 12.7 Relationship between sites of fracture and ROIs in the proximal femur. W, Ward's triangle ROI; T, trochanter ROI; FM, femoral neck ROI. This figure demonstrates the placement of ROIs in Lunar instruments (scan image from a DP3 DPA system).

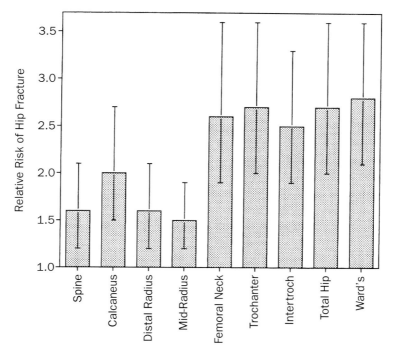

Figure 12.8 Risk ratios for hip fracture for DXA bone density measurements at five sites in the proximal femur and the spine, as well as SPA measurements in the radius and calcaneus. Error bars show the 95% confidence intervals. (Data from Cummings et al.[3])

femur that influence the measurements. These need to be recognized because they cannot be corrected by repeated positioning. Another skeletal site may have to be selected.

3) *Scan acquisition* occurs in a single direction, which is either cranio-caudal or side to side, depending on the instrument. Line spacing and resolution are about 1 mm. The monitor displays the scanned area. In the case of poor positioning or patient movement, the scan should be stopped and restarted as soon as the problem is recognized on the monitor. This requires the technologist to observe the monitor during the entire scanning procedure, which may be up to 5 minutes for pencil-beam systems. With training, repositioning after initiating the

scan is needed in less than 3% of scans. The area scanned should include the entire femoral head, the greater trochanter and the proximal end of the femoral shaft at least 2.5 cm (1 inch) below the lesser trochanter. For the detection of osteoporosis, and for estimation of fracture risk in patients with suspected or known osteoporosis, one hip, usually the left (non-dominant), is scanned. There may be specific reasons to scan either the right hip or both hips, such as when hip disease is evaluated, or in the case of prior fracture, congenital disease or hip replacement on the left side. BMD results from the two hips may not be identical, and both hips should be scanned if a specific hip-related problem is being investigated.

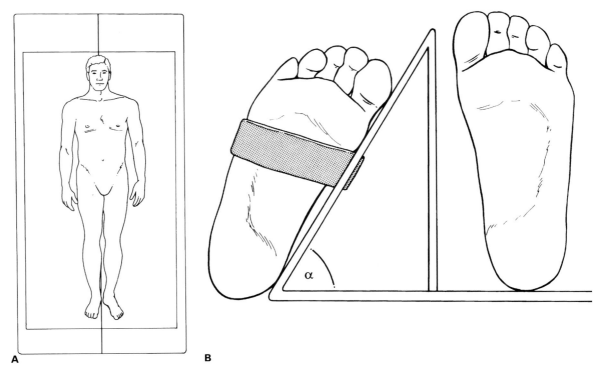

Figure 12.9 (A) Position of the patient on the imaging table. The central axis of the patient should be aligned with the mid-line of the table. (B) A footholder for reproducible foot positioning is provided by the manufacturer of the instrument. The angle (α) varies slightly between instruments, and results in an inward rotation of the foot between 25° and 30°.

Analysing a femur DXA scan

All instruments use semi-automated scan analysis software to reduce operator subjectivity in ROI placement. However, because of anatomical variations, and other factors, manual adjustments occasionally have to be made. These manual corrections are made according to predetermined guidelines which define where the ROIs should be located. The automated positioning of ROIs is a robust technique on most instruments, and suffices for the majority of studies where a single test is performed for an osteoporosis work-up or fracture risk prediction. However, in longitudinal studies exact and reproducible positioning of ROIs is mandatory to achieve optimum results. Each

manufacturer has its own recommendations on how to proceed, and these must be followed. There are, however, general rules to assist in quality control efforts, and in reviewing and interpreting scan results. These will now be reviewed.

(a) The global ROI

The placement of the global ROI is an important aspect of scan analysis on Hologic instruments (Hologic Inc., Waltham, MA, USA). The global ROI is a rectangular area placed around the proximal femur and adjacent pelvic bone structures. It is smaller than the area scanned and ensures that with repeated scans exactly the same volume of tissue is used to calculate the soft tissue reference area. Positioning of the

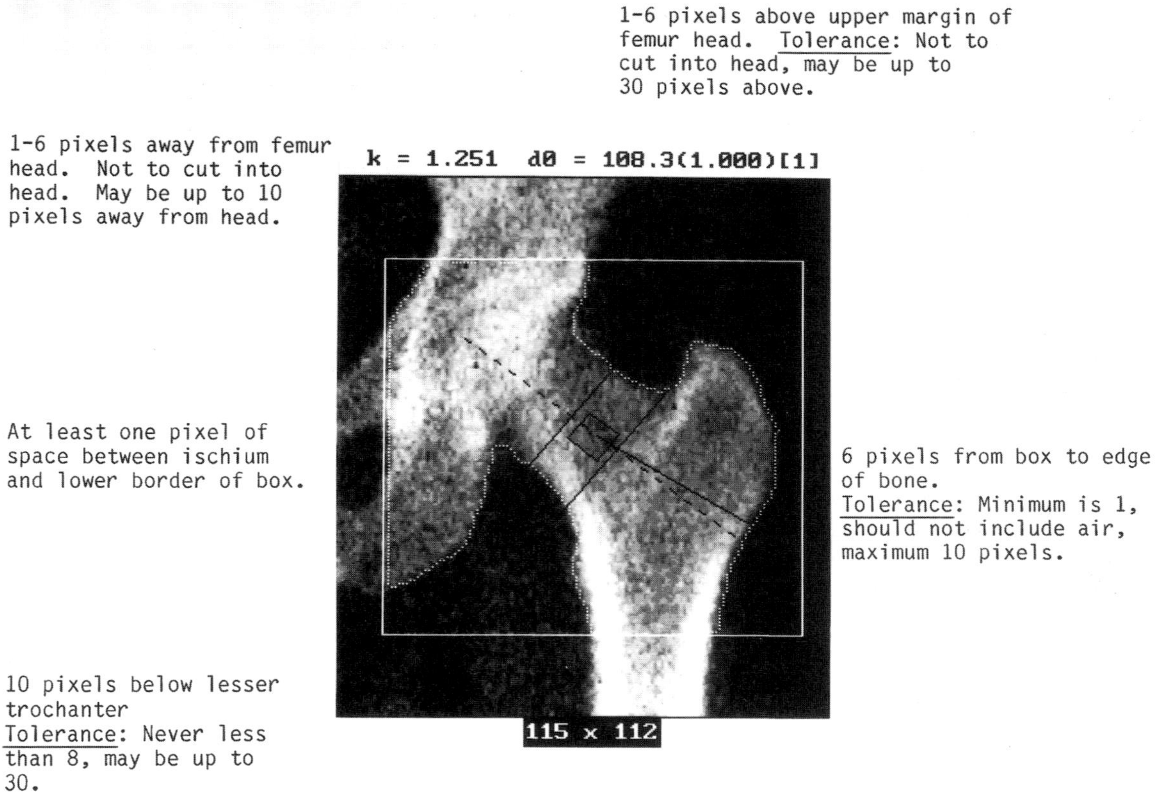

1-6 pixels above upper margin of femur head. <u>Tolerance</u>: Not to cut into head, may be up to 30 pixels above.

1-6 pixels away from femur head. Not to cut into head. May be up to 10 pixels away from head.

`k = 1.251  d0 = 108.3(1.000)[1]`

At least one pixel of space between ischium and lower border of box.

6 pixels from box to edge of bone.
<u>Tolerance</u>: Minimum is 1, should not include air, maximum 10 pixels.

10 pixels below lesser trochanter
<u>Tolerance</u>: Never less than 8, may be up to 30.

`115 x 112`

Figure 12.10 Recommendations and tolerance limits for positioning the global ROI at the proximal femur, as used in Hologic QDR instruments.

global ROI requires care to ensure inclusion of the entire head of femur and both trochanters (Figure 12.10). Borders are 5–10 pixels (5–10 mm) above and medial to the femoral head and 10 pixels (10 mm) below the lesser trochanter. Deviations from the standard size of the global ROI can result in errors in BMD measurements and positioning of the ROIs. Errors are due to an inability to define the soft tissue area accurately for background calculations and to delineate bone edges. The latter is important for the algorithm to identify correctly the locations of the ROIs. Data outside the global ROI are excluded from the calculations. On other

manufacturers' instruments, where there is no global ROI, the entire area scanned should be considered as within the global ROI with respect to artefacts as described below.

(b) The femoral neck ROI
With the exception of the total hip region, this is the most reproducible ROI in the femur, and shows the least difference in size and position between different commercial instruments. The proportion of trabecular and cortical bone at this site is about equal. In order to position the ROI in the femoral neck, the algorithm first sets a straight line through the central axis of the

femoral neck. The recognized bone edges of the femoral neck are used for positioning the mid-line. If there are problems with edge detection in the femoral neck, the line may not be properly centred (see Figure 12.31). Problems with the proper positioning of the mid-line arise occasionally in patients with very short femoral necks, or inadequate leg abduction results in a small femoral angle. When this occurs, the technologist should reposition the patient and attempt to widen the angle by further abduction of the leg.

The femoral neck ROI box should be perpendicular to the central axis of the femur neck. It should include the bone of the femoral neck and should extend into soft tissue at either end of the box. It should not include bone from the trochanter or ischium. In Hologic instruments, the neck ROI includes 15 mm of the length of the femoral neck, with its lower lateral border anchored at the base of the neck. Manual positioning is frequently required, which involves moving the femoral neck box distally until it touches the medial border of the greater trochanter (Figure 12.10). This is important, because in some patients there is a pronounced gradient of BMD along the central axis with bone density decreasing distally (Figure 12.11).

A narrower ROI may occasionally be necessary when the femoral neck is unusually short or the ischio-femoral angle is small. By convention, the width of the neck ROI should not be adjusted from the default value of 15 mm unless unavoidable. When different scans from the same patient are compared, only ROIs exactly matched for size and position should be compared. In a satisfactory scan, with good positioning, the ROIs can be matched using the ROI co-ordinates available on the scan image. With Lunar instruments (Lunar Corp., Madison, WI, USA), the ROI at the femoral neck is centred around the mid-point of the femoral neck. This positions the box a few millimetres more proximal in the neck than in Hologic instruments.

(c) The Ward's triangle ROI
In the recommended leg position, Ward's triangle is located in the mid-portion of the femoral

neck (Figures 12.2 and 12.6). It is the femur ROI with the highest proportion of trabecular bone.

With Hologic instruments an ROI of 10.5 mm × 10.5 mm is used. The algorithm searches for the area of lowest BMD within a search region that encompasses the femoral neck (Figure 12.12A). In cases where BMD is uniform, early software versions located the Ward's triangle ROI in a default location at position 3 (Figure 12.12B). Newer software (version 6.10 and later) has a default location at position 5. The default is most often seen in young adults or very old patients. The Lunar approach uses a varying size ROI depending on the size of the femoral neck, and positions the box in the centre of the neck using the mid-line and femoral neck outline as reference. There is no operator interaction. Regardless of whether a region of minimum BMD is recognizable, a measurement is taken at a fixed location.

(d) The trochanter ROI
All commercial instruments include a measurement ROI encompassing the greater trochanter. However, differences between instruments exist in the positioning of the inferior border of this ROI. The Hologic software uses the point of inflexion on the lateral bone edge where the trochanter blends into the shaft (Figure 12.6). In contrast, Lunar software uses an extension of the straight line through the central axis of the femoral neck. The trochanter ROI has a high proportion of trabecular bone.

(e) The intertrochanteric ROI
This ROI is only available with Hologic software. Precision is generally good because of the relatively large bone mass measured. However, since the inferior border of the global ROI is determined subjectively by the operator (it should be set 10 pixels below the lesser trochanter), large variations in BMD can be expected if strict recommendations are not followed. Among the ROIs in the proximal femur, the intertrochanter region has the highest proportion of cortical bone.

(f) The total hip ROI
Total hip BMD is the area weighted mean of the femoral neck, trochanter and intertrochanteric

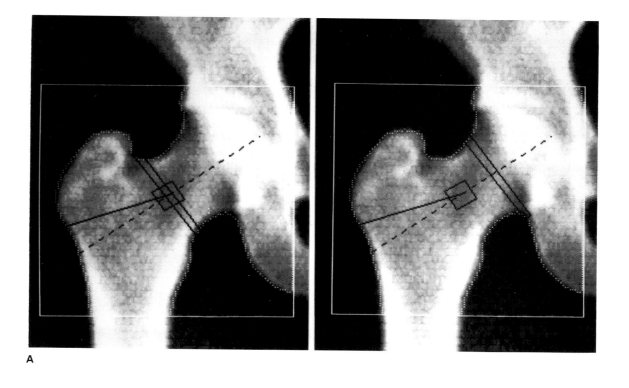

A

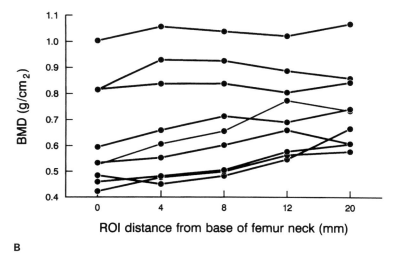

B

Figure 12.11 (A) A small (4-mm-wide) ROI is set at the base of the femoral neck. This position is the origin of the graphic display shown in the plot below. The ROI was moved proximally along the femoral neck axis. (B) Distribution of BMD values along the femoral neck. An increase in BMD is noted towards the femur head for the lower BMD values.

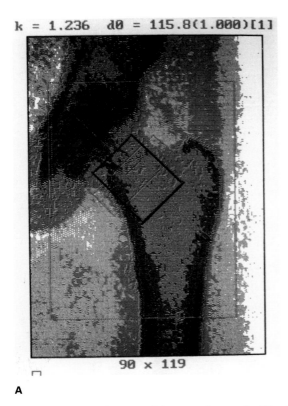

k = 1.236 d0 = 115.8(1.000)[1]

90 × 119

A

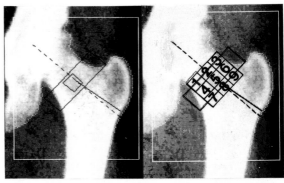

B

Ward's triangle 0.508 g/cm²

Box position	BMD (g/cm²)	BMC (g)	Area (mm²)
1	0.918	0.48	0.52*
2	0.553	0.30	0.54*
3	0.647	0.33	0.51*
4	0.598	0.64	1.07
5	0.508	0.51	1.07
6	0.641	0.68	1.11
7	0.770	0.82	1.07
8	0.677	0.75	1.11
9	0.569	0.61	1.11

* Outside search area

Figure 12.12 (A) Outline of the search area for Ward's triangle. (B) Ward's triangle in a Hologic instrument is positioned at the lowest point of the bone mineral distribution in a search area which includes most of the femoral neck. The search area can be divided into nine sectors as outlined. An inspection of the BMD data below the scan shows that the lowest BMD is in sector 5 where the Singh index grades suggest that Ward's triangle should be.

ROIs (Figure 12.6). Formerly, this site was only available with Hologic software, but is now generally available following the decision of the ICSBM committee to recommend the standardization of femur BMD using this region, and that femur scans should be interpreted using total hip reference data from the NHANES III study.[23,25,27] The principal contribution to total hip BMD is from the intertrochanteric ROI, and thus overall this site is dominated by the contribution from cortical bone. However, the potential disadvantages of this are balanced by the large projected area which helps ensure good measurement precision.

(g) Other femur sites
Several other femur ROIs have been proposed. Takada et al.[28] described a new trabecular ROI (the central hip site) generated by expanding the Ward's triangle analysis box to include a large area of the neck and trochanter centred on the femoral neck axis. Such an ROI might combine the sensitivity to change of Ward's triangle site with improved precision due to the inclusion of

a larger area included in the BMD measurement. Other possible ROIs include a section across the femur shaft representing cortical bone.

REVIEW OF A FEMUR DXA REPORT

The computer-generated report for a femur scan obtained with a commercial DXA instrument includes a scan image overlain with the various software-generated ROI boxes in the hip, BMD results for the different measurement sites, biographical data, information on quality control, and a normal range plot in which BMD data for one of the ROI sites are plotted with

respect to reference data matched for age, sex and race. Scan interpretation is aided by T-score and Z-score values generated from the measured BMD and the reference data. Some examples of femur scan reports from different commercial instruments are shown in Figures 12.13–12.15. The information provided allows a check of whether scan acquisition and analysis are within the guidelines, and assistance with the clinical interpretation of the BMD results.

As emphasized earlier in this chapter, there are sometimes special difficulties in acquiring and analysing femur DXA studies. Careful evaluation is required to spot irregularities in acquisition or scan analysis that may reduce the

A
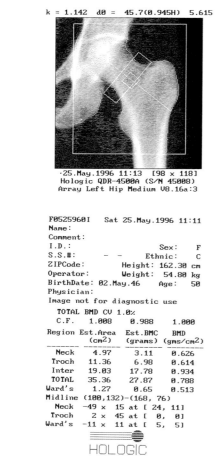

B
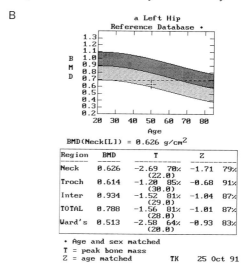

Figure 12.13 Computer printout for a proximal femur scan from a Hologic DXA bone densitometer. (A) Scan image with femur ROIs superimposed, biographical data, and information on projected area, BMC and BMD; (B) scan interpretation with normal range plot, T- and Z-score values, and BMD values expressed as percentages of the young adult and age-matched population means.

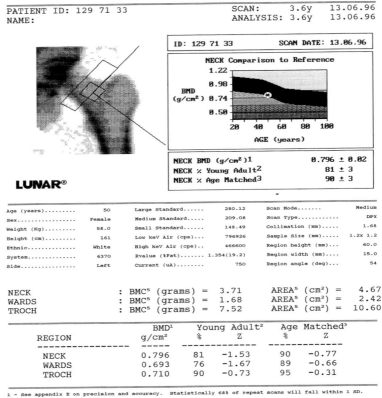

```
PATIENT ID: 129 71 33                        SCAN:        3.6y   13.06.96
NAME:                                        ANALYSIS:    3.6y   13.06.96
```

```
ID: 129 71 33                    SCAN DATE: 13.06.96

          NECK Comparison to Reference
         1.22
         0.98
  BMD
(g/cm²)  0.74
         0.50
              20    40    60    80    100
                    AGE (years)

NECK BMD (g/cm²)1              0.796 ± 0.02
NECK % Young Adult2              81 ± 3
NECK % Age Matched3             90 ± 3
```

LUNAR®

```
Age (years)........   50      Large Standard......   280.12    Scan Mode.......        Medium
Sex................  Female    Medium Standard.....   209.08    Scan Type...........      DPX
Weight (Kg)........   58.0     Small Standard......   148.49    Collimation (mm).....    1.68
Height (cm)........   161      Low keV Air (cps)...   796926    Sample Size (mm).....  1.2x 1.2
Ethnic.............  White     High keV Air (cps)..   466600    Region height (mm)...    60.0
System.............   6370     Rvalue (%Fat)....... 1.354(19.2) Region width (mm)....    15.0
Side...............   Left     Current (uA)........   750       Region angle (deg)...     54
```

```
NECK     : BMC⁵ (grams) =  3.71    AREA⁵ (cm²) =   4.67
WARDS    : BMC⁵ (grams) =  1.68    AREA⁵ (cm²) =   2.42
TROCH    : BMC⁵ (grams) =  7.52    AREA⁵ (cm²) =  10.60
```

REGION	BMD[1] g/cm²	Young Adult[2] %	Z	Age Matched[3] %	Z
NECK	0.796	81	-1.53	90	-0.77
WARDS	0.693	76	-1.67	89	-0.66
TROCH	0.710	90	-0.73	95	-0.31

1 - See appendix E on precision and accuracy. Statistically 68% of repeat scans will fall within 1 SD.
2 - UK Femur Reference Population, Ages 20-45. See Appendices.
3 - Matched for Age, Weight(males 50-100kg; females 35-80kg), Ethnic.
5 - Results for research purposes, not clinical use.

Figure 12.14 Computer printout for a proximal femur scan from a Lunar DPX DXA bone densitometer.

diagnostic quality of studies. Guidelines for such a systematic review are outlined in Table 12.2. Table 12.3 details the reasons for rejecting a particular scan because of failures in technique or abnormal bone structures. These guidelines were originally developed for multicentre research studies with particular emphasis on scan interpretation in longitudinal studies, but they also have a wider applicability in assessing the reliability of femur DXA studies.

The effect of leg positioning on femur BMD measurements

Wilson et al.[26] evaluated the effect of varying the angles of rotation and abduction of the leg on BMD results obtained with a Hologic QDR-1000 instrument. To examine the effect of different angles of rotation, the foot was rotated from the zero position (defined as having the leg relaxed with the toes upwards) by ±27°; 27° inward rotation being the standard position recommended by the manufacturer. Compared with the standard position, the largest error occurred at 27° outward rotation, when BMD generally was increased in the femoral neck and Ward's triangle regions, with lesser errors noted in the trochanter. Careless positioning of patients, defined as variations in position between toes up, 13° and 27° inward rotation in eight patients, resulted in errors from 0.9% to 4.5% (mean ± SD: 2.7 ± 1.5%) at the femoral

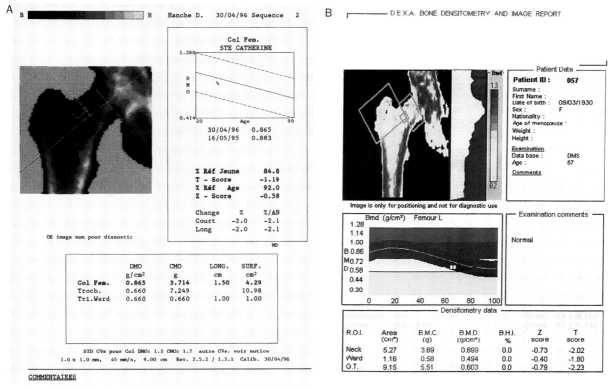

Figure 12.15 (A) Computer printout for a proximal femur scan from a Norland DXA system. (B) Same, but for a DMS Challenger DXA system.

neck, 1.0% to 6.7% (4.9 ± 1.9%) at Ward's triangle and 0.4% to 3.1% (1.7 ± 0.8%) for the trochanter ROI.

At the same time, the authors also evaluated the effect of leg abduction (6° outward) or adduction (6° inward). Compared with the standard 0° position, careless leg positioning introduced an error of 3.5 ± 2.8% for femoral neck BMD, 2.6 ± 1.0% for Ward's triangle and 1.6 ± 1.0% for the trochanter.

It appears that for diagnostic applications extreme care in foot and leg positioning is unnecessary (as long as there is no outward rotation) because the errors are small compared

with the normal intrapopulation variance in BMD. For longitudinal studies, however, careful repositioning of follow-up scans is necessary to achieve an optimum precision.

Reference data for femur BMD

The accuracy of reference data is fundamental to the reliable interpretation of bone densitometry studies. However, this is an issue that continues to generate controversy. A good example of the potential problem is shown by the study by Faulkner et al.[24] comparing T-score results

Table 12.2 Guide to processing bone mineral scans of the hip.

Inspection of scan printout	Description of effect	Decision (accept/reject)
(1) Screen image		
(a) Setting of intensity or brightness adequate for image evaluation?	False setting may impair scan evaluation but does not effect BMD results	Reprocess scan with optimal settings
(b) Entire proximal femur included in scan?	Only the standard global ROI is acceptable	Reject if the ROI is incomplete
(c) Artefacts *outside* the global ROI over bone or soft tissue	No effect on results	Accept scan
Artefacts *within* the global region of interest:		
— over bone within specific ROIs	Artefact will alter BMD value	Repeat scan after removal of artefact or exclude from specific ROI
— over bone outside specific ROIs	No effect on BMD	Accept scan
— over soft tissue	May alter tissue readings and consequently BMD	Programme allows manual deletion of pixels that contain the artefact information
(d) Missing bone (gaps in BMC image) in global region of interest (usually trochanter region and base of neck)	If the automatic analysis fails to fill in all the bone, the first approach is to enlarge the global ROI upwards and reanalyse. Then enlarge the ROI medially. If still not corrected, manually draw bone borders and fill in bone gaps	Reject or exclude from ROI if major problems exist after enlarging global ROI
(e) Motion artefacts within femoral neck, Ward's triangle or trochanter region		Reject scan
(f) Motion artefacts outside global ROI		Accept scan if small artefacts
(g) Check *d0*- and *k*-values	$k = 1.120–1.240$ (Hologic) $d0 = 97.0–120.0$ (QDR 1000) $d0 = 44.0–50.0$ (QDR 4500)	If outside limits, needs explanation: obesity, thin patient, technical problems. Make decision on acceptance based on explanation

Table 12.2 continued

(h) Check BMD result for reasonable numbers

For neck, trochanter, WT, 0.2–1.3 g/cm^2; for total and intertrochanter, 0.7–1.3 g/cm^2

(i) Check position of femur on scan. Shaft should show axis running straight down. If the leg is adducted, the ischial femur angle will be smaller than optimal

If leg is straight or lateral towards the edge of the global ROI, the ischial/femoral angle is more likely to be open. Note that the centre of the foot positioning device has to be centred with the mid-line of the patient

Reject scan if neck box cannot be positioned

(j) Unusual anatomy, such as very short neck or unusual angle of neck. This may be due to faulty position or patient's anatomy

Repeat with better positioning. If no change, this should be dealt with as outlined for neck and Ward's triangle ROI, i.e. the criteria for these ROI should be acceptable

See below

(2) Femoral neck ROI

Desired position: perpendicular to femoral neck mid-line; medial border of neck should touch the greater trochanter; does not cut into trochanter or base of head

Change borders of box to criteria outlined.

Reject if box width is less than 10 pixels (1 cm). Desired box width is 16 pixels (1.6 cm)

(3) Ward's triangle (WT)

Usual position is the anatomical site on the Singh index. Region of interest is 1.0 cm^2. Other positions are occasionally encountered

ROI may be outside the general area of the WT

No action necessary. Manual restriction of search area only if WT is outside the femoral neck, i.e. trochanter of shaft

(4) Trochanter

Includes the greater trochanter only. Upper border is lower border of the neck box. Inferior border goes from mid-line intersect of neck box (inferior border) to a point where the greater trochanter changes into the shaft

This is the least variable ROI. Adjustment needed only if not set appropriately

Intertrochanter and total regions result from above

Requires no special adjustments

Table 12.3 Bone mineral measurements: evaluation of proximal femur (Hologic QDR instruments). Rejection criteria for multicentre study.

1) Incomplete scan, bone structures required for global ROI not included
2) Abnormal configuration of proximal femur, specific ROI cannot be placed
3) Abnormal angle of femur, inward or outward rotation of femur axis not allowing proper placement of ROI
4) Faulty mid-line position through femur head that cannot be changed
5) Motion and artefacts that interfere with ROI settings
6) Technical problem in processing
7) Body thickness exceeds limits (>25 cm)

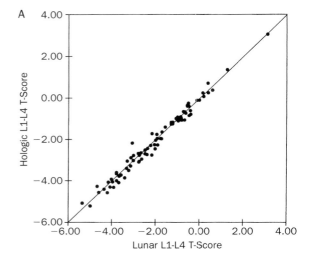

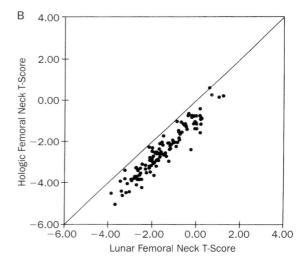

Figure 12.16 Comparison of T-score results measured on a Lunar DPX and a Hologic QDR-1000/W and calculated using the respective manufacturers' reference ranges. (A) Results for PA spine (L1–L4) scans in 83 women; (B) results for the femoral neck in 120 women. (Reproduced with permission from ref. 24.)

based on the Lunar and Hologic manufacturers' reference ranges. Scans were obtained on a Lunar DPX and a Hologic QDR-1000/W system in 83 women for PA spine (L1–L4) BMD and 120 women for femoral neck BMD. T-score figures derived from the respective manufacturers' normative databases were compared in scatter plots (Figure 12.16). Although the slopes were consistent with unity within the 95% confidence intervals, the mean differences in T-score (Hologic − Lunar) were −0.05 ($p = 0.02$) for the spine and −0.93 ($p < 0.001$) for the femoral neck. The difference for the spine is too small to have clinical significance, but that for the hip indicates a major discrepancy in scan interpretation on the two systems.

Few independent studies provide an adequate body of data for comparison with the manufacturers' databases. However, one very influential study has been the recently conducted third National Health and Nutrition

Survey (NHANES III), which includes a DXA examination of the proximal femur conducted using mobile Hologic QDR-1000 densitometers.[25] Scans were acquired across the USA between 1988 and 1994. The combined phase 1 and phase 2 data from this study have allowed the compilation of a nationally representative sample of 14 646 men and women aged 20 years and older.[27] Unlike many surveys limited to white Caucasian patients, NHANES III includes approximately equal numbers of non-Hispanic white, non-Hispanic black and Mexican Americans. The survey of non-Hispanic white women included 3251 subjects. Mean femoral neck BMD (0.858 g/cm²) in the youngest group (aged 20–29 years, $n = 409$) was significantly lower than the Hologic's own young adult figure (0.895 g/cm²), corresponding to a T-score difference (NHANES – Hologic) of 0.37. The population standard deviation from the NHANES III study was larger than for the manufacturer's range (0.12 versus 0.10 g/cm²). The combination of these two changes meant that the femoral neck BMD figure required to fulfil the WHO study group's definition of osteoporosis[29] (T-score < -2.5) was significantly reduced (0.558 versus 0.645 g/cm²).

As a consequence of the controversy over the accuracy of femur reference data, Hologic have recently issued revised system software that allows hip scans to be interpreted using the NHANES study data. Following the ICSBM committee recommendations on femur standardization[23] discussed below, the new software uses the total hip ROI as the default site for scan interpretation.

Longitudinal studies using femur BMD

The choice of the optimum BMD measurement site for longitudinal studies was discussed in Chapter 8 where PA and lateral spine, femur, forearm and total body sites were compared in terms of both treatment effect (defined as the difference between the percentage changes in BMD in the treatment and placebo groups) and the sensitivity to monitoring change (defined as

the ratio of treatment effect to long-term precision) (see Figures 8.4 and 8.5).

Preston et al.[30] have examined femur BMD data from a clinical trial of cyclical etidronate therapy in early postmenopausal women, including results for the central hip site described by Takada et al.[28] The findings (Figure 12.17) show that the largest treatment response is shown by Ward's triangle and the trochanter ROI. After normalizing the treatment effect to precision (Figure 12.17B), differences between the femur sites were not statistically significant. Within this limitation, however, both the trochanter and total hip ROIs performed well.

STANDARDIZED BMDS FOR FEMUR DXA SCANS

As discussed in Chapter 10 for the case of PA spine BMD, differences in bone-edge detection, ROI placement algorithms and scanner calibration lead to significant differences in BMD figures for the same patient measured on different manufacturers' DXA systems.

Following its earlier report recommending equations for the standardization of lumbar spine BMD,[31] the ICSBM has recently issued guidelines for the standardization of femur BMD.[23] Like the earlier report, the femur equations were based on an in vivo cross-calibration study of 100 healthy women published by the UCSF Osteoporosis Research Group.[32] However, the femur equations are different from the spine due to different effects of edge detection and the adoption of a more sophisticated statistical approach to comparing values from different systems.[33]

Femur standardization is based on the total hip ROI rather than the femoral neck ROI that, until recently, has been the conventional BMD measurement for interpreting femur BMD results. This choice was based on the relative ease of implementing a closely identical total hip ROI on different manufacturers' equipment, and also the recognized higher precision of measurements at this site.

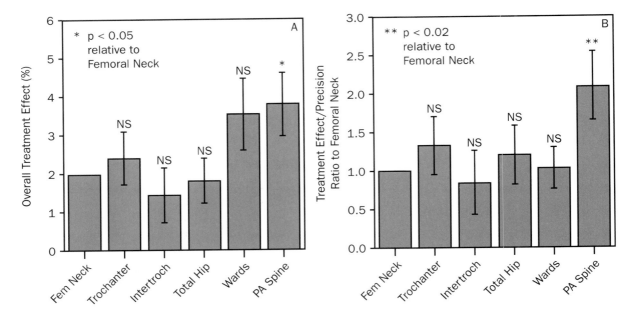

Figure 12.17 Comparison of BMD measurement sites in the proximal femur for monitoring response to treatment in early premenopausal women receiving placebo or cyclical etidronate therapy. (A) The total treatment effect, defined as the difference between the etidronate and placebo groups at 2 years; (B) sensitivity of the different sites to measuring longitudinal change calculated by dividing the total treatment effect by the long-term precision. Results are shown normalized to femoral neck BMD. (Data from Preston et al.[30])

Standardized femur BMD figures (denoted sBMD and expressed in units of mg/cm^2 to distinguish them clearly from the conventional manufacturer-specific BMD figures) are derived from the manufacturers' existing BMD results (expressed in units of g/cm^2) using the following conversion equations:[23]

For Hologic instruments:

$$sBMD = 1000(1.008 \times BMD_{Hologic} + 0.006)$$

For Lunar instruments:

$$sBMD = 1000 (0.979 \times BMD_{Lunar} - 0.031)$$

For Norland instruments:

$$sBMD = 1000 (1.012 \times BMD_{Norland} + 0.026)$$

The manufacturers have recently issued software giving users the option of scan reports using sBMD units. sBMD values obtained by scanning a patient on any one of the three manufacturers' instruments should agree within 3–6%.[23]

The ICSBM report on the standardization of femur BMD includes a recommendation for the use of standardized reference data, thereby making T- and Z-score figures derived from different manufacturers' equipment compatible. The recommended reference ranges are based on data collected during the NHANES III study conducted across the USA between 1988 and 1994 using mobile Hologic QDR-1000 densitometers.[25,27] The mean sBMD and standard deviation for the young adult reference range used to calculate T-score figures were 956 mg/cm^2 and 123 mg/cm^2 respectively based on 409 US white women aged 20–29 years.[23] The full age-specific reference data based on a total of 3251 US white women are listed in Table 12.4

ILLUSTRATIVE CASES

The following cases (Figures 12.18–12.41) are presented to familiarize technologists and clinicians with commonly encountered scan findings that deviate from the standard normal image and may require a special approach to patient positioning, scan analysis or scan interpretation. The images presented were all obtained with Hologic instruments. While some

Table 12.4 Standardized total femur reference data (sBMD) for white women derived from the NHANES III Study.[23]

Age (years)	Reference sBMD (mg/cm^2) for white women
20–29	956
30–39	944
40–49	920
50–59	876
60–69	809
70–79	740
80+	679

The population standard deviation is 123 mg/cm^2.

of the suggested solutions are specific for this make of equipment, the issues demonstrated in these examples need to be addressed regardless of the instrument used. Specific suggestions can be found in the manufacturers' manuals.

Unusual shapes and deformity of the proximal femur

k = 1.226 d0 = 118.4(1.000)[1]

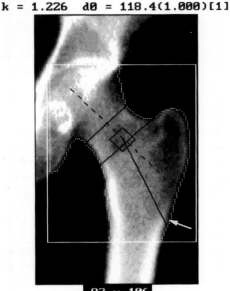

82 x 106

Hologic QDR 1000 (S/N 148)
Left Hip Version 4.03

Region	Area (cm2)	BMC (grams)	BMD (gms/cm2)
Neck	5.03	3.47	0.689
Troch	14.36	8.84	0.616
Inter	11.55	12.17	1.054
TOTAL	30.94	24.48	0.791
Ward's	1.07	0.60	0.558
Midline	(82,122)-(142, 60)		
Neck	-48 x	16 at [24, 12]	
Troch	-19 x	55 at [0, 0]	
Ward's	-11 x	11 at [5, 4]	

Figure 12.18 The smooth contour of the lateral edge of the greater trochanter lacks the usual point of inflection that triggers the search algorithm to set the inferior border of the trochanter ROI. The ROI illustrated extends almost into the shaft. In this case the mid-line would be an acceptable alternative for the inferior border and this can be sent manually. Note that the global ROI cuts into the femoral head and should be enlarged by a few pixels. (Reproduced with permission from the National Center for Health Statistics, NHANES III, 1988–94.)

k = 1.214 d0 = 107.5(1.000)[1]

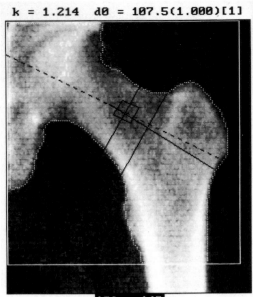

126 x 143

Hologic QDR 1000 (S/N 148)
Left Hip Version 4.20

Region	Area (cm2)	BMC (grams)	BMD (gms/cm2)
Neck	6.75	4.68	0.693
Troch	15.85	10.65	0.672
Inter	25.68	32.71	1.274
TOTAL	48.28	48.05	0.995
Ward's	0.72	0.33	0.456
Midline	(110,186)-(232,120)		
Neck	-61 x	16 at [25,-10]	
Troch	-7 x	69 at [0, 0]	
Ward's	-11 x	11 at [6, -5]	

Figure 12.19 An unusually long femoral neck. Note that the standard neck ROI width is 16 mm. In this case it covers less of the neck than usual. Despite this, the width of the ROI should not be extended beyond 16 mm. (Reproduced with permission from the National Center for Health Statistics, NHANES III, 1988–94.)

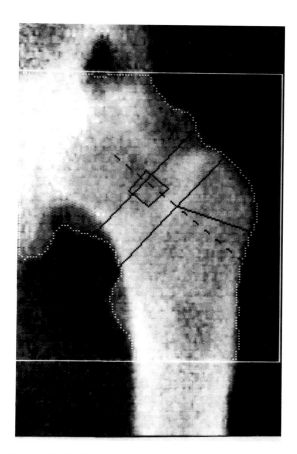

Figure 12.20 A congenital hip deformity. In this case diagnostically useful BMD data for osteoporosis work-up and fracture prediction are not obtainable. Another skeletal site should be selected. (Reproduced with permission from the National Center for Health Statistics, NHANES III, 1988–94.)

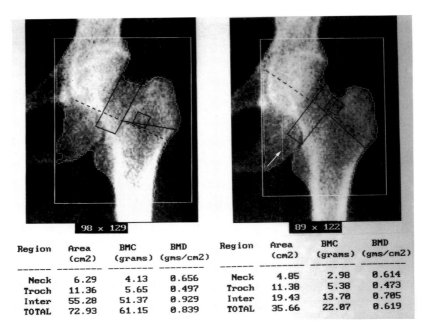

Region	Area (cm2)	BMC (grams)	BMD (gms/cm2)		Region	Area (cm2)	BMC (grams)	BMD (gms/cm2)
Neck	6.29	4.13	0.656		Neck	4.85	2.98	0.614
Troch	11.36	5.65	0.497		Troch	11.38	5.38	0.473
Inter	55.28	51.37	0.929		Inter	19.43	13.70	0.705
TOTAL	72.93	61.15	0.839		TOTAL	35.66	22.07	0.619

Figure 12.21 An ischio-femoral angle is not visualized (left). The patient was unable to abduct her leg. However, the software allows manual deletion of bone from the ischium to create a 'soft tissue' space for the femoral neck ROI (right). For research studies, this scan should be rejected or flagged. Scanning of the contralateral hip or another skeletal site is preferable to accepting this scan for clinical decision making.

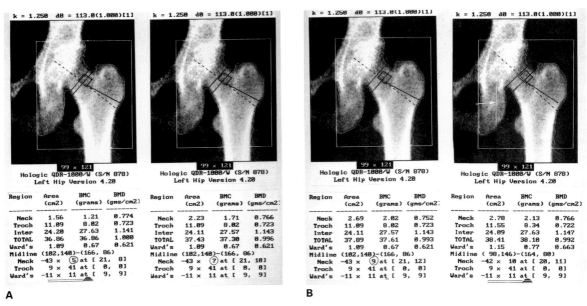

A

B

Figure 12.22 (A) In this patient a short neck combined with a small ischio-femoral angle is not sufficient to accommodate the standard femoral neck ROI of 16-mm-width. The width should not be reduced to less than 10 mm. The width of the neck ROI is encircled in the data printout below the images. (B) A femoral neck box of 10-mm-width can be fitted with manual deletion of bone from the ischium (right). The series of four images shows the effect of different femoral neck ROIs on BMD. Although the difference is not significant when a single clinical measurement is made, the precision of repeated measurements is significantly better if strict criteria are applied.

Focal abnormalities in or adjacent to bone in the proximal femur

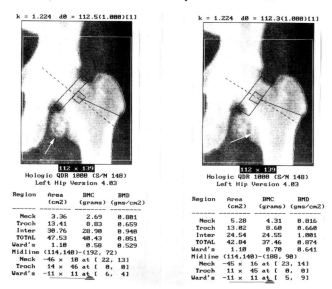

Figure 12.23 Calcification contiguous with the lesser trochanter. This is inside the global ROI, recognized by the algorithm as bone, and is therefore included within the bone contour. This creates difficulties in positioning the femoral neck ROI. In the left-hand image, a small femoral neck ROI positioned proximally to this calcification in the neck is seen. On the right, the excess bone has been manually deleted and a standard ROI used. The image on the right is the best way to analyse this scan. (Reproduced with permission from the National Center for Health Statistics, NHANES III, 1988–94.)

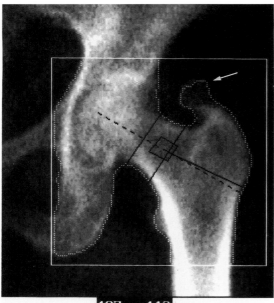

```
107 x 113
```

Hologic QDR 1000 (S/N 190)
Left Hip Version 4.26

Region	Area (cm2)	BMC (grams)	BMD (gms/cm2
Neck	4.67	3.19	0.683
Troch	11.61	7.02	0.604
Inter	20.84	19.32	0.927
TOTAL	37.13	29.52	0.795

Figure 12.24 Bone growth at the greater trochanter at the point of tendon insertion. Positioning of the femoral neck ROI is not affected. Trochanter BMD is low because a bone area with low bone mass is included in the ROI. Deletion of this extra bone to manually defining the bone edges is suggested.

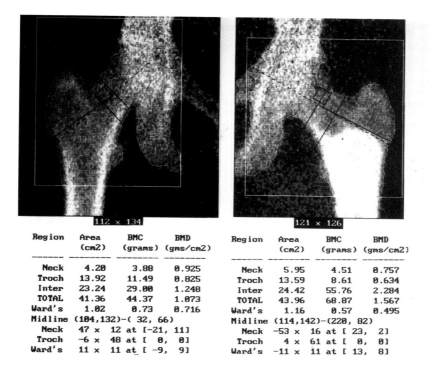

Region	Area (cm2)	BMC (grams)	BMD (gms/cm2)
Neck	4.20	3.88	0.925
Troch	13.92	11.49	0.825
Inter	23.24	29.00	1.248
TOTAL	41.36	44.37	1.073
Ward's	1.02	0.73	0.716

Midline (104,132)-(32, 66)

Neck	47 x	12 at [-21, 11]
Troch	-6 x	48 at [0, 0]
Ward's	11 x	11 at [-9, 9]

Region	Area (cm2)	BMC (grams)	BMD (gms/cm2)
Neck	5.95	4.51	0.757
Troch	13.59	8.61	0.634
Inter	24.42	55.76	2.284
TOTAL	43.96	68.87	1.567
Ward's	1.16	0.57	0.495

Midline (114,142)-(220, 82)

Neck	-53 x	16 at [23, 2]
Troch	4 x	61 at [0, 0]
Ward's	-11 x	11 at [13, 8]

Figure 12.25 The left femur (right panel) shows a sclerotic lesion in the proximal femoral shaft extending into the femoral neck. BMD measurements at the standard ROIs are not representative of skeletal bone mineral status since they measure abnormal bone. The right hip (left panel) shows significantly different BMD values. The difference is larger than usually seen in the right and left hips of normal and osteoporotic patients, and is due to the abnormal bone on the left.

Focal abnormalities in soft tissue surrounding the proximal femur

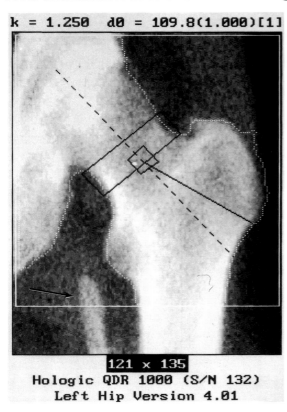

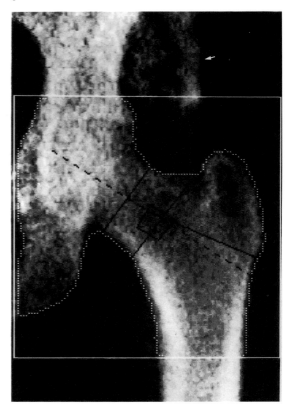

Figure 12.26 Artefact showing bone in the soft tissue space inside and outside the global ROI. There is no effect when the artefact is outside the global ROI. When inside, it may affect the baseline settings and thus change BMD. In this case, the density is lower than that of the femur or pelvis, and the size of the artefact inside the global ROI is small. There is no measurable effect on BMD when analysed as shown. Another option is to delete the artefact manually, which removes this area from the data matrix.

Figure 12.27 Large soft tissue calcification outside the global ROI. This does not affect the results. (Reproduced with permission from the National Center for Health Statistics, NHANES III, 1988–94.)

Unusual body composition and thickness

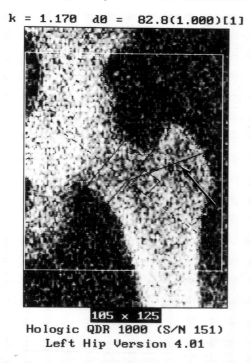

k = 1.170 d0 = 82.8(1.000)[1]

105 x 125

Hologic QDR 1000 (S/N 151)
Left Hip Version 4.01

Region	Area (cm2)	BMC (grams)	BMD (gms/cm2)
Neck	4.56	5.25	1.151
Troch	4.52	3.87	0.855
Inter	23.82	28.70	1.205
TOTAL	32.90	37.82	1.149
Ward's	1.16	1.20	1.038

Midline (108,102)-(186, 40)

Neck	-42 x	16 at [23,	15]
Troch	39 x	22 at [0,	0]
Ward's	-11 x	11 at [11,	-3]

A

Region	Area (cm2)	BMC (grams)	BMD (gms/cm2)
Neck	6.39	6.28	0.983
Troch	13.75	14.57	1.059
Inter	29.72	55.01	1.851
TOTAL	49.86	75.86	1.522
Ward's	1.10	0.68	0.622

B

Figure 12.28 (A) Unreliable measurements due to the effects of obesity. This is indicated by the noisy (grainy) image due to the effects of high soft tissue attenuation. This is confirmed by the relatively low value of the $d0$ number shown on the top of the image on Hologic instruments (in this case $d0$ = 82.8, compared with values of 110–120 in the preceding figures). Noise degrades the image quality and causes errors in soft tissue baseline calculations, from which BMD is determined. Weight 113 kg (250 lbs), age 56, female, height 1.68 m (5 feet, 6 inches), thickness of hip 25.3 cm. (Reproduced with permission from the National Center for Health Statistics, NHANES III, 1988–94.) (B) Obesity: 177 kg (390 lbs) body weight; height 1.88 m (6 feet, 2 inches); thickness at the hip 24.5 cm. Although the algorithm correctly placed the ROIs, the BMD values cannot be interpreted because of abnormal weight and poor precision due to high attenuation. Note that the weight exceeded the recommended weight limit for the imaging table of 300 lbs.

Problems related to difficulties in bone-edge detection

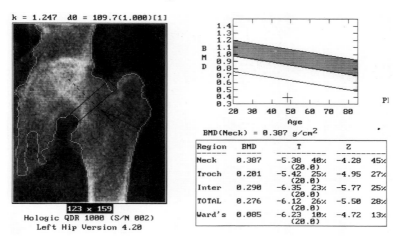

Figure 12.29 Very low bone mineral. Note the exceptionally low BMD for Ward's triangle and the enlarged global ROI needed to obtain a useful baseline.

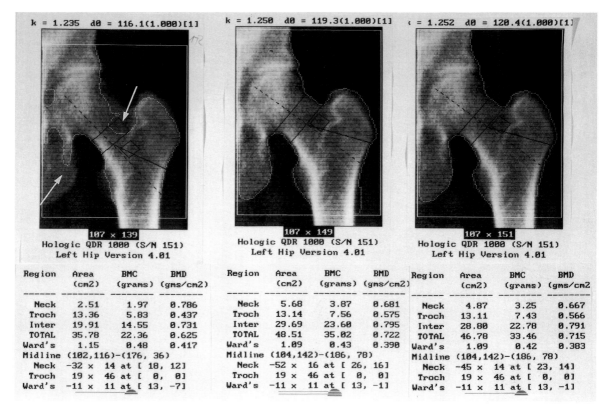

Figure 12.30 Setting of global ROI. ***Left panel:*** Standard global ROI shows a false mid-line, incomplete display of bone edges and specific ROIs are not properly displayed. ***Centre panel:*** Enlarging the ROI upwards (see the dimensions at the bottom of the scans) rectifies the error by including more soft tissue. ***Right panel:*** Further enlargement has no additional effect. (Reproduced with permission from the National Center for Health Statistics, NHANES III, 1988–94.)

k = 1.230 d0 = 111.6(1.000)[1]

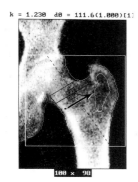

100 x 98

k = 1.234 d0 = 110.5(1.000)[1]

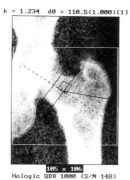

105 x 106

Hologic QDR 1000 (S/N 148)
Left Hip Version 4.07

Region	Area (cm2)	BMC (grams)	BMD (gms/cm2)
Neck	4.34	3.31	0.762
Troch	12.20	5.78	0.474
Inter	22.34	20.00	0.895
TOTAL	38.88	29.09	0.748
Ward's	1.04	0.50	0.483

Midline (100,114)-(182, 58)

Neck	-45 ×	14 at [	23, 12]
Troch	20 ×	42 at [	0, 0]
Ward's	-11 ×	11 at [	10, 6]

Figure 12.31 False positioning of the global ROI. ***Left panel***: The left margin of the global ROI is too close to the femoral head. Note the erroneous position of the femoral neck axis, the false femoral neck and trochanter ROIs and the exclusion of bone in the trochanter. ***Right panel***: Enlargement of the box (see dimensions in millimetres at base of image) results in proper position of all ROIs. (Reproduced with permission from the National Center for Health Statistics, NHANES III, 1988–94.)

Artefacts due to medical interventions

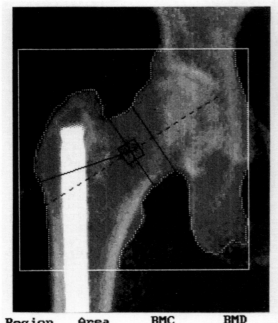

Region	Area (cm2)	BMC (grams)	BMD (gms/cm2)
Neck	5.25	2.56	0.488
Troch	13.49	25.36	1.880
Inter	23.77	48.05	2.022
TOTAL	42.50	75.98	1.788
Ward's	0.99	0.26	0.265

A

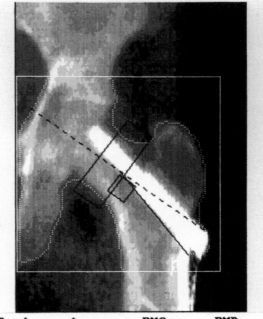

Region	Area (cm2)	BMC (grams)	BMD (gms/cm2)
Neck	5.08	10.79	2.123
Troch	17.57	47.55	2.706
Inter	10.19	11.98	1.176
TOTAL	32.84	70.33	2.141
Ward's	1.10	0.99	0.899

B

Figure 12.32 (A) Intramedullary rod in the global ROI interferes with BMD measurements in the trochanter, the intertrochanter and total hip ROI. (B) Nail fixation of femoral neck fracture.

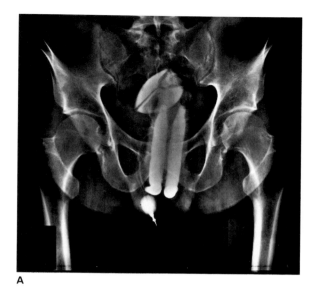

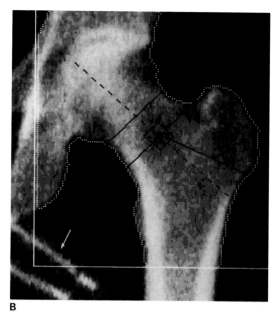

A

B

Figure 12.33 Artefact over soft tissue within the global ROI produced by a penile prosthesis. (A) Radiograph; (B) bone mineral scan. No effect on bone mineral results were noted.

Metal artefacts in soft tissue surrounding the proximal femur

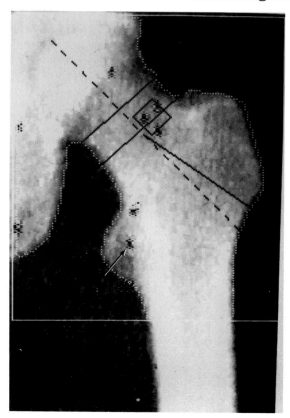

Figure 12.34 Scattered buckshot pellets in the hip area affect the specific ROIs. The scan is invalid for BMD assessment.

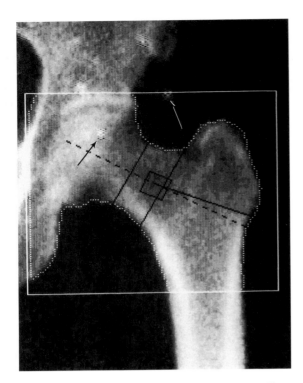

Figure 12.35 Buckshot pellets outside the specific ROIs do not influence results, particularly when over bone. (Reproduced with permission from the National Center for Health Statistics, NHANES III, 1988–94.)

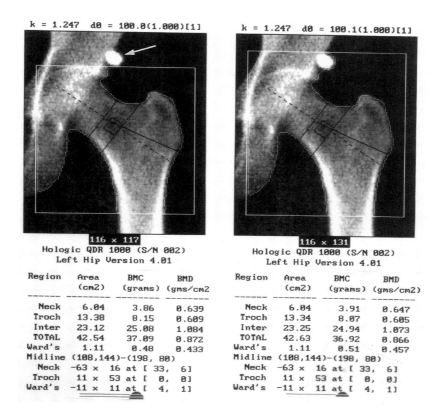

k = 1.247 d0 = 100.0(1.000)[1]

116 x 117
Hologic QDR 1000 (S/N 002)
Left Hip Version 4.01

Region	Area (cm2)	BMC (grams)	BMD (gms/cm2
Neck	6.04	3.86	0.639
Troch	13.38	8.15	0.609
Inter	23.12	25.08	1.084
TOTAL	42.54	37.09	0.872
Ward's	1.11	0.48	0.433

Midline (108,144)-(198, 80)

Neck	-63 x	16 at [33,	6]
Troch	11 x	53 at [0,	0]
Ward's	-11 x	11 at [4,	1]

k = 1.247 d0 = 100.1(1.000)[1]

116 x 131
Hologic QDR 1000 (S/N 002)
Left Hip Version 4.01

Region	Area (cm2)	BMC (grams)	BMD (gms/cm2
Neck	6.04	3.91	0.647
Troch	13.34	8.07	0.605
Inter	23.25	24.94	1.073
TOTAL	42.63	36.92	0.866
Ward's	1.11	0.51	0.457

Midline (108,144)-(198, 80)

Neck	-63 x	16 at [33,	6]
Troch	11 x	53 at [0,	0]
Ward's	-11 x	11 at [4,	1]

Figure 12.36 Shrapnel contiguous with bone outside (left) and inside (right) the global ROI. Because the artefact is registered as 'bone', but is outside the specific ROIs, it does not affect the results.

Artefacts originating at time of acquisition

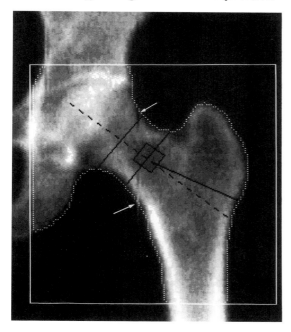

Figure 12.37 Motion artefact through femoral neck ROI and Ward's triangle. For scans performed on Hologic QDR-1000 instruments, motion artefacts are in the vertical direction reflecting the motion of the scanning arm. Instruments that scan across the femur show horizontal motion artefacts. When motion artefacts are detected, the scan should be repeated.

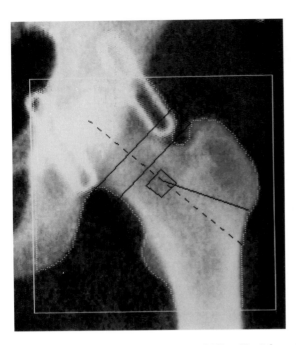

Figure 12.38 External artefact. Metal appliances with a truss worn for an inguinal hernia. When an external artefact is noted, the scan should be stopped and the artefact removed.

Issues related to the position of Ward's triangle

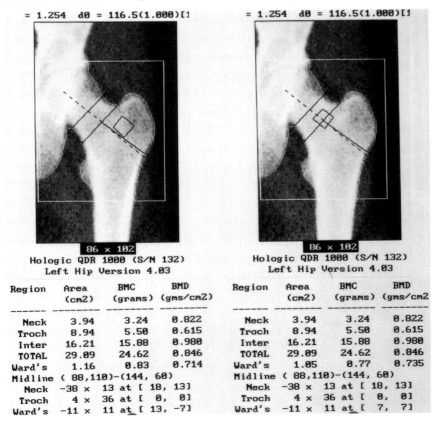

Figure 12.39 Off-site location of Ward's triangle ROI. Reprocessing after manually confining the search area of the Ward's triangle will result in a correct position. (Reproduced with permission from the National Center for Health Statistics, NHANES III, 1988–94.)

= 1.254 d0 = 116.5(1.000)[]   = 1.254 d0 = 116.5(1.000)[]

86 x 102   86 x 102

Hologic QDR 1000 (S/N 132)   Hologic QDR 1000 (S/N 132)
Left Hip Version 4.03   Left Hip Version 4.03

Region	Area (cm2)	BMC (grams)	BMD (gms/cm2)		Region	Area (cm2)	BMC (grams)	BMD (gms/cm2)
Neck	3.94	3.24	0.822		Neck	3.94	3.24	0.822
Troch	8.94	5.50	0.615		Troch	8.94	5.50	0.615
Inter	16.21	15.88	0.980		Inter	16.21	15.88	0.980
TOTAL	29.09	24.62	0.846		TOTAL	29.09	24.62	0.846
Ward's	1.16	0.83	0.714		Ward's	1.05	0.77	0.735

Midline (88,110)-(144, 60)   Midline (88,110)-(144, 60)

Neck	-38 x	13 at [18, 13]			Neck	-38 x	13 at [18, 13]	
Troch	4 x	36 at [0, 0]			Troch	4 x	36 at [0, 0]	
Ward's	-11 x	11 at [13, -7]			Ward's	-11 x	11 at [7, 7]	

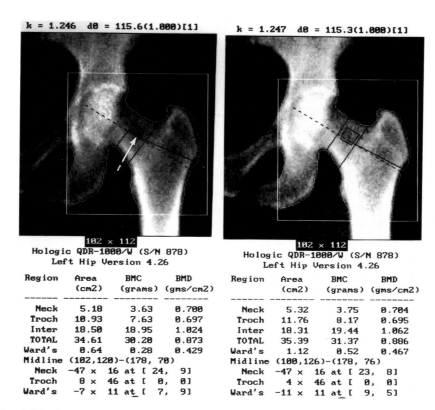

k = 1.246   d0 = 115.6(1.000)[1]   k = 1.247   d0 = 115.3(1.000)[1]

| 102 × 112 | | 102 × 112 |

Hologic QDR-1000/W (S/N 878)
Left Hip Version 4.26

Region	Area (cm2)	BMC (grams)	BMD (gms/cm2)
Neck	5.18	3.63	0.700
Troch	10.93	7.63	0.697
Inter	18.50	18.95	1.024
TOTAL	34.61	30.20	0.873
Ward's	0.64	0.28	0.429

Midline (102,120)-(178, 70)

Neck	-47 ×	16 at [24,	9]
Troch	8 ×	46 at [0,	0]
Ward's	-7 ×	11 at [7,	9]

Hologic QDR-1000/W (S/N 878)
Left Hip Version 4.26

Region	Area (cm2)	BMC (grams)	BMD (gms/cm2)
Neck	5.32	3.75	0.704
Troch	11.76	8.17	0.695
Inter	18.31	19.44	1.062
TOTAL	35.39	31.37	0.886
Ward's	1.12	0.52	0.467

Midline (100,126)-(178, 76)

Neck	-47 ×	16 at [23,	8]
Troch	4 ×	46 at [0,	0]
Ward's	-11 ×	11 at [9,	5]

Figure 12.40 Small Ward's triangle ROI due to an inadvertent operator error during processing. Repeating the scan analysis is all that is needed.

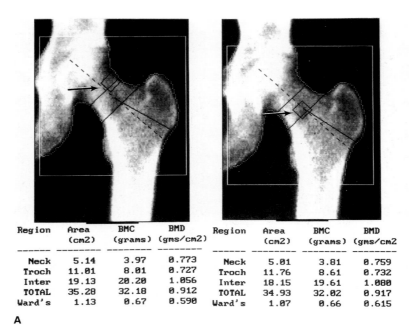

Region	Area (cm2)	BMC (grams)	BMD (gms/cm2)	Region	Area (cm2)	BMC (grams)	BMD (gms/cm2
Neck	5.14	3.97	0.773	Neck	5.01	3.81	0.759
Troch	11.01	8.01	0.727	Troch	11.76	8.61	0.732
Inter	19.13	20.20	1.056	Inter	18.15	19.61	1.080
TOTAL	35.28	32.18	0.912	TOTAL	34.93	32.02	0.917
Ward's	1.13	0.67	0.590	Ward's	1.07	0.66	0.615

A

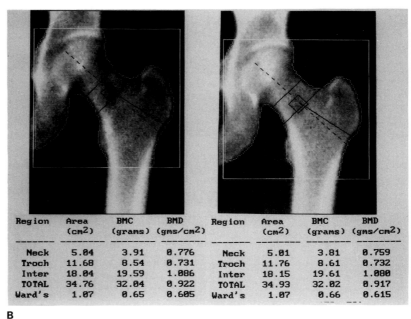

Region	Area (cm^2)	BMC (grams)	BMD (gms/cm^2)	Region	Area (cm^2)	BMC (grams)	BMD (gms/cm^2)
Neck	5.04	3.91	0.776	Neck	5.01	3.81	0.759
Troch	11.68	8.54	0.731	Troch	11.76	8.61	0.732
Inter	18.04	19.59	1.086	Inter	18.15	19.61	1.080
TOTAL	34.76	32.04	0.922	TOTAL	34.93	32.02	0.917
Ward's	1.07	0.65	0.605	Ward's	1.07	0.66	0.615

B

Figure 12.41 Two approaches for the placement of Ward's triangle in longitudinal studies shown in two scans acquired 1 year apart. (A) In early software versions the placement of the Ward's triangle ROI was allowed to shift between scans. In this case the location has shifted from a default position (left) to a standard position (right). (B) For Hologic software version 6.10 and later the placement on the follow-up scan matches that on the original scan. Changes in BMD in the Ward's triangle ROI should be interpreted with caution.

REFERENCES

1. Melton LJ, Thamer M, Ray NF et al. Fractures attributable to osteoporosis: report from the National Osteoporosis Foundation. *J Bone Miner Res* (1997) **12:** 16–23.
2. Ray NF, Chan JK, Thamer M, Melton LJ. Medical expenditures for the treatment of osteoporotic fractures in the United States in 1995: report from the National Osteoporosis Foundation. *J Bone Miner Res* (1997) **12:** 24–35.
3. Cummings SR, Black DM, Nevitt MC et al. Bone density at various sites for the prediction of hip fractures. *Lancet* (1993) **341:** 72–5.
4. Marshall D, Johnell O, Wedel H. Meta-analysis of how well measures of bone mineral density predict occurrence of osteoporotic fractures. *Br Med J* (1996) **312:** 1254–9.
5. Harty M. The calcar femorale and the femoral neck. *J Bone Joint Surg Am* (1957) **29:** 625–30.
6. Singh M, Nagrath AR, Maini PS. Changes in trabecular pattern of the upper end of the femur as an index of osteoporosis. *J Bone Joint Surg Am* (1970) **54:** 457–67.
7. Riggs BL, Wahner HW, Seeman E et al. Changes in bone mineral density of the proximal femur and spine with aging: differences between the postmenopausal and senile osteoporosis syndrome. *J Clin Invest* (1982) **70:** 716–23.
8. Pesch HJ, Henschke F, Siebold H. Einfluss von mechanik und alter auf den spongiosaumbau in lendenwirbelkorpern und im schenkelhals. *Virchows Arch Path Anat and Histol* (1977) **377:** 27–42.
9. Martens M, van Audekercke R, Delport P et al. The mechanical characteristics of cancellous bone at the upper femoral region. *J Biomech* (1983) **16:** 971–83.
10. Khairi MRA, Cronin JH, Robb JA et al. Femoral trabecular pattern index and bone mineral content measurement by photon absorption in senile osteoporosis. *J Bone Joint Surg Am* (1976) **58:** 221–6.
11. Kranendonk DH, Jurist JM, Lee HG. Femoral trabecular patterns and bone mineral content. *J Bone Joint Surg Am* (1972) **54:** 1472–8.
12. Singh M, Riggs BL, Beabout JW et al. Femoral trabecular pattern index for evaluation of spinal osteoporosis: a detailed methologic description. *Mayo Clinic Proc* (1973) **48:** 184–9.
13. Singh M, Riggs BL, Beabout JW et al. Femoral trabecular pattern index for evaluation of spinal osteoporosis. *Ann Intern Med* (1972) **77:** 63–7.
14. Wahner HW, Riggs BL, Beabout JW. Diagnosis of osteoporosis: usefulness of photon absorptiometry at the radius. *J Nucl Med* (1977) **18:** 432–7.
15. Dequeker J, Gantama K, Roh YS. Femoral trabecular patterns in asymptomatic spinal osteoporosis and femoral neck fracture. *Clin Radiol* (1976) **25:** 243–6.
16. Barnett E, Nordin BEC. The radiological diagnosis of osteoporosis: a new approach. *Clin Radiol* (1960) **11:** 166–74.
17. Fredensborg N, Nilsson BE. Cortical index of the femoral neck. *Acta Radiol Diag* (1977) **18:** 492–6.
18. Kerr R, Resnick D, Sartoris DJ et al. Computerized tomography of proximal femoral trabecular patterns. *J Orthop Res* (1986) **4:** 45–56.
19. Sartoris DJ, Andre M, Resnick C et al. Trabecular bone density in the proximal femur: quantitative CT assessment (work in progress). *Radiology* (1986) **160:** 707–12.
20. Glüer C-C, Genant HK. Quantitative computed tomography of the hip. In: Genant HK, ed. *Osteoporosis Update 1987* (Radiology Research Education and Foundation: San Francisco, 1987), 187–95.
21. Faulkner KG, Cummings SR, Glüer C-C et al. Simple measurement of femoral geometry predicts hip fracture: the study of osteoporotic fractures. *J Bone Miner Res* (1993) **8:** 1211–17.
22. Glüer C-C, Cummings SR, Pressman A et al. Prediction of hip fractures from pelvic radiographs: the study of osteoporotic fractures. *J Bone Miner Res* (1994) **9:** 671–7.
23. Hanson J. Standardization of femur BMD [letter]. *J Bone Miner Res* (1997) **12:** 1316–17.
24. Faulkner KG, Roberts LA, McClung MR. Discrepancies in normative data between Lunar and Hologic DXA systems. *Osteoporos Int* (1996) **6:** 432–6.
25. Looker AC, Wahner HW, Dunn WL et al. Proximal femur bone mineral levels of US adults. *Osteoporos Int* (1995) **5:** 389–409.
26. Wilson CR, Fogelman I, Blake G et al. The effect of positioning on dual energy x-ray bone densitometry of the proximal femur. *Bone Miner* (1991) **13:** 69–76.
27. Looker AC, Wahner HW, Dunn WL et al. Updated data on proximal femur bone mineral levels of US adults. *Osteoporos Int* (1998) (in press).
28. Takada M, Grampp S, Ouyang X et al. A new trabecular region of interest for femoral dual x-ray absorptiometry: short-term precision, age

related bone loss, and fracture discrimination compared with current femoral regions of interest. *J Bone Miner Res* (1997) **12:** 832–8.

29. Kanis JA, Melton LJ, Christiansen C et al. The diagnosis of osteoporosis. *J Bone Miner Res* (1994) **9:** 1137–41.

30. Preston NG, Blake GM, Patel R et al. Monitoring skeletal response to therapy using DXA: which site to measure in the femur? In: Ring EFJ, ed. *Current Research in Osteoporosis and Bone Mineral Measurement V: 1998* (British Institute of Radiology: London, 1998) 35–6.

31. Steiger P. Standardization of measurements for assessing BMD by DXA [letter]. *Calcif Tissue Int* (1995) **57:** 469.

32. Genant HK, Grampp S, Glüer C-C et al. Universal standardization of dual x-ray absorptiometry: patient and phantom cross-calibration data. *J Bone Miner Res* (1994) **9:** 1503–14.

33. Hui SL, Gao S, Zhou X-H et al. Universal standardization of bone density measurements: a method with optimal properties for calibration amongst several instruments. *J Bone Miner Res* (1997) **12:** 1463–70.

13

Measurement of Bone Density in the Distal Forearm

CHAPTER OVERVIEW

Instrumentation for measuring bone mineral in the forearm based on the principles of single photon absorptiometry (SPA) was the first type of commercial bone densitometry equipment to become widely used nearly 30 years ago. Because of its simplicity, compactness and low cost, recent years have seen a revival of interest in equipment dedicated to performing BMD measurements in the peripheral skeleton. However, the ^{125}I radionuclide source used in the first SPA systems has been superseded by the technology of dual-energy X-ray absorptiometry (DXA). A review of current commercial equipment for X-ray absorptiometry of the peripheral skeleton can be found in Chapter 5. The present chapter includes an account of the early development of SPA, particularly the choice of measurement sites, since an appreciation of this is relevant to many of the procedures adopted with modern equipment.

INTRODUCTION

The original technique for the measurement of forearm bone mineral by SPA was a simple, inexpensive test with a precision (CV) of 2–4% and an accuracy (SD) of 6%.[1–3] The SPA test is backed by years of experience and its value for predicting global fracture risk is well established.[4–7] Because the forearm is an easily accessible site and very convenient for the patient, interest in forearm measurements has never stopped. In recent years a large variety of innovative new equipment for making measurements in the peripheral skeleton has become available. Today, the ready acceptance of the new devices is largely based on three decades of experience with SPA.

Recent developments in bone mineral measurements in the forearm have centred on the use of DXA.[8–14] A review of modern equipment is given in Chapter 5 of this book. The accuracy of DXA measurements is about equal to that of SPA.[15] Because of the acquisition of a scan image to aid repositioning, precision is comparable with the best that could be achieved with SPA.[10] DXA-based instruments are preferred for both clinical and research use because they permit measurements of the skeleton at both axial and peripheral sites, and particularly the sites of frequent fractures. Compared with SPA, DXA is especially convenient because it eliminates the requirement of a water bath for the patient's arm and also avoids the need for frequent replacement of the ^{125}I radionuclide source. However, little in the way of new or different information can be expected from the replacement of SPA by DXA for forearm measurements. Both are planar absorptiometry methods, projecting the mineral content in the scanning beam into a reference area. The final result for both techniques depends on the bone geometry as well as on the bone mineral. Errors from the variable fat content in the marrow cavity of the radius or from fat surrounding the bone are comparable for both techniques.[9]

SINGLE PHOTON ABSORPTIOMETRY

In the original implementation of SPA, a collimated gamma-ray beam made a single traverse across the mid-radius. Subsequent improvements included multiple traverses of the scanning site, selection of the distal (and latterly the ultra-distal) sites where more trabecular bone could be measured, corrections for fat, and the investigation of other peripheral sites such as the calcaneus and phalanx. The physical principles of SPA measurements have been explained previously in Chapter 3. The present chapter emphasizes those aspects that aid the understanding and interpretation of forearm BMD measurements and are helpful in the appreciation of the techniques used in modern DXA equipment.

SINGLE TRAVERSE SPA INSTRUMENTS

The first commercially available instrument for SPA at the radius, based on a single scan line, was developed by Norland Medical Systems (Fort Atkinson, WI, USA). A number of other companies subsequently developed similar equipment. In this technique bone mineral is measured as the mass of hydroxyapatite in a 1-cm-long bone segment estimated from a single scan traverse across the bone (beam diameter 2 mm) (units: g/cm). Results can also be normalized for bone diameter by dividing bone mineral content (BMC) per unit length (g/cm)

by the diameter (cm) to give bone density in units of g/cm^2. For this purpose it is assumed that the bone is a cylinder with a diameter measured by the width of the scan line and with a uniform distribution of mineral within this piece of bone. This assumption is more accurate in the mid-radius than at the distal end, where the bone flares out and the trabecular to cortical bone ratio changes rapidly. Such single path instruments are no longer commercially available.

Multiple traverse SPA instruments

The scanning approach to SPA was introduced to improve the precision of the measurements. Several scan lines across the bone are acquired with increments of a few millimetres along the radius shaft, and measurements of BMC per unit length and diameter are averaged. Except for a better estimation of the average bone diameter of the 1 cm length of bone, the general approach to bone mineral estimation is the same as outlined for the single scan line approach. However, the multiple path approach improves precision (CV) from 2–4% (single path) to 1–2%.

Tissue fat surrounding the bone may modify the baseline resulting in errors in the measured BMC. Some commercial instruments report both a raw BMC value and a corrected value after allowing for varying amounts of fat in the subcutaneous tissue.[16] The correction may vary from nothing in lean patients to about 30% in very obese subjects. With this instrument, precision (CV) in normal premenopausal women was 1.5% for both raw and fat corrected data. Commonly used corrections made on SPA attenuation curves are explained in Figure 13.1.

Another improvement was the ability to measure sites in both the distal and proximal radius with one set-up of the patient.[16] By selecting a site where the gap between the radius and ulna was 8 mm, this instrument made four paths (2 mm apart) in a distal direction from the reference line, and four similar paths proximal to it. The resulting measurements are referred to as distal (25% trabecular

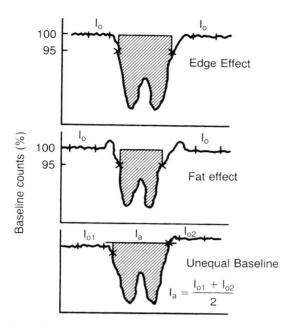

Figure 13.1 Commonly used corrections made on SPA attenuation curves.

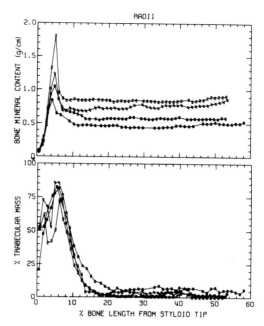

Figure 13.2 Bone mineral content and trabecular bone mass along the distal radius in four ashed bone studies. The position of the measuring point along the long axis of the radius is given in terms of per cent of total bone length measured from the styloid tip of the ulna. The same scale is used in positioning the scanning site in patients. (Reproduced with permission from Schlenker and Von-Seggen.[20])

bone) and proximal (7% trabecular bone) respectively.

Vogel and Anderson built a device for scanning the calcaneus.[17] Because of its high content of trabecular bone, the heel seemed particularly well suited as a skeletal sampling site with information on the status of the axial skeleton.[18] The successor of this instrument is still commercially available from Norland Medical Systems (see Chapter 5) and it has now been modified to measure calcaneus BMD using the principles of DXA. Because of variations in the trabecular bone distribution within the calcaneus, the entire posterior portion is scanned. Very recently an innovative new device for DXA studies in the calcaneus, the Lunar PIXI, has also become available.[19] It should be noted that mineral loss in the calcaneus is recognizable during prolonged bedrest and exceeds the losses at other skeletal sites. This suggests a particular dependence of calcaneal bone mineral density (BMD) on weight-bearing and exercise.

MEASUREMENT SITES IN THE DISTAL FOREARM

Studies of excised bones show that bone mass and bone composition (i.e. the percentage of compact and trabecular bone) show marked changes at the ends of long bones.[20] For the radius and ulna, this is illustrated in Figure 13.2. Forearm measurements made between 20% and 60% of ulna length (i.e. based on external measurements from the ulna styloid to the olecranon and projected onto the radius) show a rather constant distribution of compact and trabecular bone, and the BMC per unit length (units: g/cm) is relatively uniform along the bone axis. In contrast, measurements in the distal forearm show large variations in the percentage of trabecular and compact bone and give BMC values per unit length of just over a few millimetres of axial length. Accurate repositioning of a measurement region of interest (ROI) in this situation can be very difficult. Techniques for positioning measurement ROIs are largely designed to overcome this problem.

In the earlier methodology of SPA, early commercial instruments performed a scan at a single point in the forearm, usually at 10% of ulna length.[21] As demonstrated in Figure 13.2, at this site there is about 25% trabecular bone and the BMC per cm is just beginning to become more stable along the bone axis.

In the mid-1980s, three groups developed SPA scanning techniques to study the radius at a distal site where the percentage of trabecular bone is 50–60%, similar to that found in the lumbar spine. This site is referred to as the *ultra-distal radius*, since its location is further distal to the conventional distal radius site described above. The major difficulty in studying the ultra-distal radius is the large change in bone mineral content over a short distance, as shown in Figure 13.2. Methods that depend

upon palpation of bony landmarks, such as the ulna styloid process, do not allow sufficiently accurate relocation of the scanning site. Hence, Nilas et al.[16] scanned the distal forearm and used a computer-based edge-detection programme to determine the site at which the radius–ulna gap was 8 mm. From this point, four scans were made distally at 2 mm increments.

Awbrey et al.[22] also used the radius–ulna gap to achieve accurate repositioning, but made only one scan at the site where the radius–ulna gap was 5 mm.

Eastell et al.[23] selected a distal radius site to coincide with the site of Colles' fracture, i.e. the most distal 30 mm of the radius, where trabecular bone content as measured on cadaver bones was 60% by weight. Measurements were made by SPA using computer-assisted image processing. The area of interest was 10 mm wide, and the distal end of this area was 4 mm proximal to the medial edge of the distal end-plate of the radius. The end-plate is recognizable on scan images as a line of high bone density. A fat correction was applied. The location of this ROI and others is shown in Figure 13.3. Precision as determined by duplicate measurements in healthy women was 1.7%.[24]

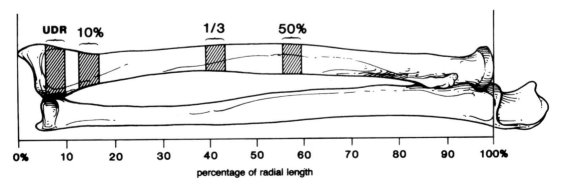

Figure 13.3 Tracing of a radiograph of forearm bone excised post mortem from a 94-year-old man. Sites marked '50%', '1/3' and '10%' are standard sites, and distances are related to ulna length. The ultra-distal (UD) site of Nilas et al.[16] begins where the radius–ulna gap is 8 mm and extends a distance of 8 mm distally. This site is at the distal end of the 10% ROI. The UD site of Awbrey et al.[22] is one measurement line where the radius–ulna gap is 5 mm. This site is at the proximal border of the ultra-distal radius (UDR) ROI in this illustration. UDR is the ROI used by Eastell et al.[23]

DXA SCANNING OF THE DISTAL FOREARM

Details of how to perform a DXA bone density scan of the distal forearm vary with the make of instrument. For axial systems designed for spine and femur studies, the patient's arm is placed on the imaging table, supported with a positioning device and scanned in air (Figure 13.4). In dedicated peripheral DXA systems a hand grip is usually provided (Figure 13.5) together with straps to keep the arm still during the scan. For many instruments a measurement of the length of the ulna from the styloid process to the olecranon is required. This figure is entered into the computer and aids the location of the measurement site. The wrist and distal forearm are usually scanned in pencil-beam mode with scan times of around 5 minutes. However, fan-beam DXA systems, such as the Lunar Expert-XL (Lunar Corp., Madison, WI, USA) and the Hologic QDR-4500 (Hologic Inc., Waltham, MA, USA), will perform equivalent scans in less than 30 seconds.

For all instruments, scan analysis includes two or more ROI, usually comprising a site with a high percentage of trabecular bone (usu-

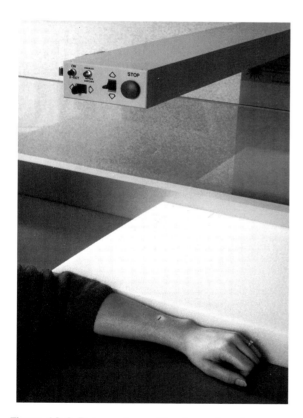

Figure 13.4 Forearm in position for performing a forearm DXA study on a Hologic QDR-1000 instrument. Note that only a simple position device is used (styrofoam block) and no water bath is needed. The patient is sitting at the side of the imaging table. The marker on the arm is used by the technician to position the laser beam.

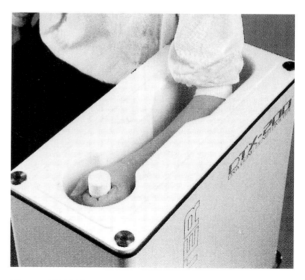

Figure 13.5 Forearm in position for a DXA scan on an Osteometer DTX-200 instrument. Note the handgrip for positioning the forearm and keeping it still.

ally called the ultra-distal or distal ROI), and a predominantly cortical site (usually the one-third radius ROI). The ROIs are positioned on the scan images using anatomical reference points together with the measurement of forearm length. An advantage of the DXA method of forearm densitometry compared with earlier techniques is the good quality image provided with the scan. However, even with this advantage, good repositioning is of crucial importance for obtaining high precision BMD measurements.

Scan analysis on Hologic QDR instruments

Examples of a forearm scan and data output from a Hologic QDR instrument are shown in Figure 13.6. In Hologic systems an outer box, the global ROI, defines the limits of the BMD analysis. Within this region the scan analysis software segments the image into air, soft tissue and bone. Inclusion of a sufficient area of air is important for scan analysis, since it is this region that establishes the baseline against which the attenuation due to soft tissue and bone is measured.

The line perpendicular to the axis of the forearm that defines the distal border of the global ROI is set by the operator to touch the tip of the styloid process of the ulna (Figure 13.6A). This line is marked '0 mm' and is the reference for locating the other ROI settings. Within the global ROI, the ultra-distal (UD) region is set by placing its distal border to touch the proximal edge of the radius end-plate. Frequently this means that the distal border of the UD ROI is set approximately 10 mm proximal to the reference line (Figure 13.6A). Since the UD ROI is 15 mm in length, its proximal border is usually 25 mm proximal to the reference line. However, it is important that the final location of the UD ROI is set by eye so that it does not include any of the denser bone of the radius end-plate.

The one-third radius ROI is 20 mm long and its mid-point is set at exactly one-third of the ulna length measurement entered by the operator proximal to the reference line (Figure

13.6A). The computer printout of the scan analysis (Figure 13.6B) also includes the mid-region (the ROI between the UD and one-third sites) and the total region, which is the area weighted mean of the UD, mid- and one-third BMDs. All four ROIs can be evaluated for either the radius or ulna separately, or both together. The mid-region is approximately equivalent to the distal site measured on some forearm instruments, and should not be confused with the mid-radius site formerly used in some SPA procedures.

Scan analysis on the Osteometer DTX-200

An example of a forearm scan and data output from an Osteometer DTX-200 instrument (Osteometer Meditech, Hoersholm, Denmark) is shown in Figure 13.7. The algorithm for finding the ROIs is fully automated. The software automatically identifies a reference line, which is defined as the first scan line starting from the proximal end of the scan at which the separation between the radius and ulna is equal to or less than 8 mm. The distal ROI is identified by the computer as the 24-mm-long section of the radius and ulna going in the proximal direction from the reference line. It typically consists of 87% cortical bone and 13% trabecular bone. The ultra-distal ROI covers the radius only and includes the area between the reference line and the proximal edge of the radius end-plate. It consists of 55% trabecular and 45% cortical bone. The system will also measure a quarter distal ROI, which is a 20-mm-long section covering both the radius and the ulna with its mid-line placed at a distance one-quarter of the length of the forearm from the distal end of the ulna. This site consists of 100% cortical bone.

In the most recent update of system software, the ultra-distal ROI has been replaced by a new ROI (nROI) based on a software-defined area distal to the reference line but excluding the end-plates and the cortical shell of the radius and ulna. This site is estimated to consist of 65% trabecular and 35% cortical bone and is included as a sensitive site for monitoring response to treatment.[25]

A

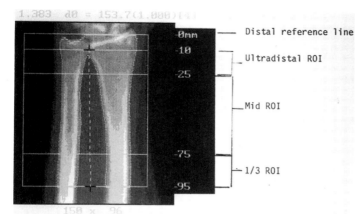

— Distal reference line

Ultradistal ROI

Mid ROI

1/3 ROI

Forearm Length 25.5 cm

Figure 13.6 (A) Definition of ROIs at the forearm. Data are from a Hologic QDR-1000 instrument. (B) Scan image and data output for distal forearm scan with DXA. Regions of interest are indicated. UD is the ultra-distal radius site, 15 mm axial length. The location is close to, but not identical to, the regions defined by Awbrey[22] and by Nilas,[16] but more proximal to the ROI used by Eastell.[23]

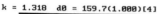
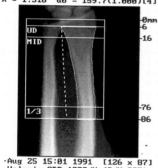

k = 1.318   dθ = 159.7(1.000)[4]

·Aug 25 15:01 1991 [126 x 87]
Hologic QDR-1000/W (S/N 907)
Left Forearm V5.41+

I.D.:   OSU Bone Lab   Sex: F
S.S.#:   000-00-0000 Ethnic: W
ZIP Code: 97330 Height:5' 3"
Scan Code: AWS Weight: 110
BirthDate: Age: 32
Physician:
Forearm Length: 24.5 cm
Image not for diagnostic use

        TOTAL BMD CV IS LESS THAN 1.0%
        C.F.   1.001   1.060   1.000

RADIUS	Area (cm2)	BMC (grams)	BMD (gms/cm2)
UD	2.57	1.13	0.439
MID	8.78	5.54	0.631
1/3	1.49	1.06	0.714
TOTAL	12.84	7.74	0.602

B

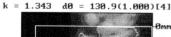
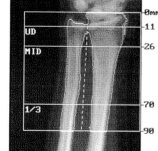

k = 1.343   dθ = 130.9(1.000)[4]

·24.Sep.1994 12:11 [172 x 91]
Hologic QDR-2000 (S/N 2611)
■Left Forearm V5.67

E09249412   Sat 24.Sep.1994 12:00
Name:
Comment:
I.D.:   Sex: F
S.S.#:   —   —   Ethnic: C
ZIPCode: Height: 162.30 cm
Operator: Weight: 54.80 kg
BirthDate: 02.May.46   Age: 48
Physician:
Forearm Length: 24.0 cm
Image not for diagnostic use

        TOTAL BMD CV IS LESS THAN 1.0%
        C.F.   1.003   1.058   1.000

RADIUS + ULNA	Area (cm2)	BMC (grams)	BMD (gms/cm2)
UD	5.67	1.80	0.318
MID	10.91	5.13	0.470
1/3	4.68	2.79	0.596
TOTAL	21.27	9.72	0.457

HOLOGIC

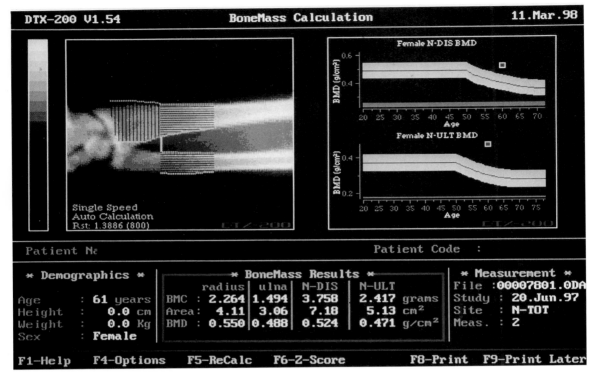

Figure 13.7 Example of a scan printout from a DXA forearm scan on a Osteometer DTX-200 instrument.

Guidelines for inspecting and interpreting forearm scans

The following points should be examined when interpreting forearm scans:

1) Verify proper positioning of forearm and scan analysis ROIs.
2) Compare patient data with the manufacturer's reference range and interpret scan using T- and Z-score figures.
3) All instruments include a phantom, which should be scanned daily when the equipment is in use. Results of these instrument quality control studies should be inspected regularly to ensure that instrument calibration remains within defined limits. The interpretation of follow-up scans in particular is sensitive to any instrumental drift.

Examples of scan printouts from the Osteometer and Hologic instruments discussed earlier are shown in Figures 13.7 and 13.8. Some care is needed with respect to the use of manufacturers' reference range data for forearm DXA. After the demonstration by Faulkner et al. of systematic differences between the spine and femur reference ranges provided for Lunar and Hologic DXA instruments,[26] and the demonstration of significant differences between the NHANES III study femur BMD data[27] and the Hologic's femur reference range,[28] it would be surprising if comparable anomalies do not exist for some other manufacturers' forearm data. Little independent information exists on this subject and further work is needed.

DXA is a precise and accurate technique for

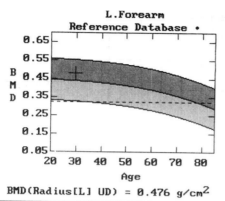

L.Forearm
Reference Database ·

$BMD(Radius[L] UD) = 0.476 \ g/cm^2$

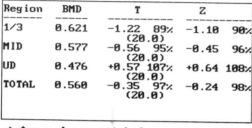

Region	BMD	T		Z	
1/3	0.621	−1.22	89%	−1.10	90%
		(20.0)			
MID	0.577	−0.56	95%	−0.45	96%
		(20.0)			
UD	0.476	+0.57	107%	+0.64	108%
		(20.0)			
TOTAL	0.560	−0.35	97%	−0.24	98%
		(20.0)			

✦ Age and sex matched
T = peak bone mass
Z = age matched   PS   10/25/91

Figure 13.8 Example of scan printout from a DXA forearm scan on a Hologic QDR-1000 instrument. Similar printouts are available for each of the different ROIs.

in vivo measurements of forearm bone mineral. The measurements are relatively insensitive to the potential limitations introduced by changes in forearm thickness, soft tissue composition and small deposits of fat over the distal radius.[15] Current DXA forearm software and bone images impart several advantages over SPA, including:

1) ROI selection based on anatomical rather than surface landmarks;
2) the ability to analyse retrospectively alternative regions;
3) recognition of unsuspected bone lesions that would otherwise contribute to inaccurate results;

4) measurement performance that is largely unaffected by clinical variables such as forearm thickness, localized fat deposits and increased fat subcutaneously;
5) shorter scanning times;
6) images of the forearm of excellent resolution, which enhances long-term precision in vivo.

These factors indicate that DXA is a clinically satisfactory alternative to SPA for forearm bone mineral measurement.

CLINICAL ASPECTS OF BONE MINERAL MEASUREMENTS AT THE FOREARM

Age-related bone loss

Age-related bone loss at peripheral skeleton sites has been the topic of many studies.[29-33] When measured at the mid-radius and one-tenth distal sites in normal women, area bone mineral density, expressed as BMD (g/cm²) or BMC (g/cm), reaches a peak at about 30–35 years of age. Significant bone diminution does not occur until 50 years of age, but is accelerated between 51 and 65 years of age and then decelerates. Overall bone diminution throughout life is 30% for the mid-radius and 39% for the one-tenth distal site.[30] The lifetime rate of loss at these forearm sites is less than seen in the spine or femur. For women aged between 51 and 65 years, rates of loss are about 1% per year for a 15-year period.[30] However, bone loss is not uniform throughout this period, but shows the highest values at the beginning of the menopause. In men, bone diminution in the radius is small. The decline is linear at about 0.3% per year at the distal one-tenth measuring point, and is insignificant in the mid-radius.

Unlike other long bones, such as the hip, the loss of bone mineral with age in the forearm does not seem to be accompanied by an increase in bone diameter due to periosteal bone aposition. In contrast with measuring sites in the spine and femur, where bone marrow fat increases slowly with age, bone marrow fat in the distal forearm plateaus in early adulthood. BMD in the dominant ultra-distal radius is about 3% higher than in the non-dominant measuring site.[24] Results in the literature vary from zero to 10%.

The decreased bone density is associated with a decrease in bone strength. In studies of cadaver bones, Horsman and Currey[34] showed a strong positive correlation between BMD and breaking strength in the distal 30 mm of the radius.

Do measurements of radius BMD predict bone mineral at other sites?

How do measurements made on the ultra-distal radius compare with lumbar spine and femur BMD? Nilas et al. reported a correlation coefficient of $r = 0.56$ between bone density at the ultra-distal radius and the lumbar spine.[16] From measurements made at the '5 mm' site in normal women, Awbrey et al. found a correlation coefficient of $r = 0.52$.[22] Using DXA measurements, Ryan et al. found correlation coefficients of $r = 0.67$ and $r = 0.57$ between ultra-distal BMD and spine and femoral neck BMD respectively.[10] The correlation coefficients with the one-third radius site were $r = 0.53$ and $r = 0.49$ respectively.

Although these correlation coefficients were highly statistically significant, in terms of predicting spine or femur BMD from ultra-distal radius BMD in an individual, the appropriate parameter is the 95% confidence interval. This is derived from the standard error of the estimate (SEE) of the linear regression line of 0.11 g/cm^2 for the spine and 0.08 g/cm^2 for femoral neck BMD.[10] The 95% confidence intervals of spine and femur BMD as predicted from the forearm measurement are equivalent to an error in T-score of approximately ± 2.0. Similar figures are obtained when predicting axial BMD from age alone.

These comments should not be interpreted as a criticism of the usefulness of forearm BMD measurements. Eastell et al. showed that women with Colles' fracture, but not spinal compression fractures, were better discriminated from age-matched normal women by ultra-distal radius measurements, while women with spinal fractures, but no radius fracture, were discriminated better by BMD measurements on the spine.[24] Both axial and peripheral measurements will correctly identify as 'at risk' only a certain proportion of patients who actually go on to experience an osteoporotic fracture. Other patients will be correctly identified by either one technique or the other, or will be missed by both. The odds ratio, as determined by prospective studies of incident fractures,[4-7] is the best basis for comparing the utility of different measurement sites.[35]

Local changes in BMD

Local changes in BMD, not reflecting changes in total skeletal mineralization, can be observed in joint diseases at the wrist, particularly rheumatoid arthritis, with immobility, and as the result of healing fractures. Finsen and Berum[36] found that 2–3 years after a healed fracture, patients showed an increase in BMD in the distal radius on the fractured side when compared with the uninjured side. However, no difference in BMD was noted in the radial shaft or metacarpal bones. Such local changes in bone mineral need to be kept in mind when a specific bone site is used to predict general skeletal mineralization and to assess the risk for osteoporotic fractures. Measurements on the fractured arm should be avoided, since local BMD changes may lead to erroneous interpretations.

REFERENCES

1. Cameron JR, Sorenson J. Measurement of bone mineral in vivo: an improved method. *Science* (1963) **142**: 230–2.
2. Sorenson J, Cameron JR. A reliable in vivo measurement of bone mineral content. *J Bone Joint Surg* (1967) **49A**: 481–97.
3. Cameron JR, Mazess RB, Sorenson MS. Precision and accuracy of bone mineral determination by direct photon absorptiometry. *Invest Radiol* (1968) **3**: 141–50.
4. Ross PO, Davis JW, Vogel JM et al. A critical review of bone mass and the risk of fractures in osteoporosis. *Calcif Tissue Int* (1990) **46**: 149–61.

5. Cummings SR, Black DM, Nevitt MC et al. Bone density at various sites for the prediction of hip fractures. *Lancet* (1993) **341:** 72–5.
6. Marshall D, Johnell O, Wedel H. Meta-analysis of how well measures of bone mineral density predict occurrence of osteoporotic fractures. *Br Med J* (1996) **312:** 1254–9.
7. Düppe H, Gärdell P, Nilsson B, Johnell O. A single bone density measurement can predict fractures over 25 years. *Calcif Tissue Int* (1997) **60:** 171–4.
8. Weinstein RS, New KD, Sappington LJ. Dual-energy X-ray absorptiometry *versus* single photon absorptiometry of the radius. *Calcif Tissue Int* (1991) **49:** 313–16.
9. Larcos G, Wahner HW. An evaluation of forearm bone mineral measurement with dual-energy absorptiometry. *J Nucl Med* (1991) **32:** 2101–6.
10. Ryan PJ, Blake GM, Fogelman I. Measurement of forearm bone mineral density in normal women by dual-energy X-ray absorptiometry. *Br J Radiol* (1992) **65:** 127–31.
11. Nelson D, Feingold M, Mascha E et al. Comparison of single-photon and dual-energy x-ray absorptiometry of the radius. *Bone Miner* (1992) **18:** 77–83.
12. LeBoff MS, El-Hajj A, Fuleihan G et al. Dual-energy x-ray absorptiometry of the forearm: reproducibility and correlation with single photon absorptiometry. *J Bone Miner Res* (1992) **7:** 841–6.
13. Faulkner KG, McClung MR, Schmeer MS et al. Densitometry of the radius using single and dual-energy absorptiometry. *Calcif Tissue Int* (1994) **54:** 208–11.
14. Genant HK, Engelke K, Fuerst T et al. Noninvasive assessment of bone mineral and structure: state of the art. *J Bone Miner Res* (1996) **11:** 707–30.
15. Svendsen OL, Hassager C, Skodt V, Christiansen C. Impact of soft tissue on *in vivo* accuracy of bone mineral measurements in the spine, hip, and forearm: a human cadaver study. *J Bone Miner Res* (1995) **10:** 868–73.
16. Nilas L, Borg J, Godfredsen A et al. Comparison of single and dual photon absorptiometry in post menopausal bone mineral loss. *J Nucl Med* (1985) **26:** 1257–62.
17. Vogel JM, Anderson JT. Rectilinear transmission scanning of irregular bones for quantification of mineral content. *J Nucl Med* (1973) **13:** 13.
18. Vogel JM, Wasnich RD, Ross PD. The clinical relevance of calcaneus bone mineral measurements: a review. *Bone Miner* (1988) **5:** 35–58.
19. Borg J, Mazess R, Hanson J. Peripheral instantaneous x-ray imager: the PIXI bone densitometer. *J Bone Miner Res* (1997) **12**(suppl 1): S258.
20. Schlenker RA, Von-Seggen WW. The distribution of cortical and trabecular bone mass along the lengths of the radius and ulna and the implications for in vivo bone mass measurements. *Calcif Tissue Res* (1976) **20:** 41–52.
21. Wahner HW, Eastell R, Riggs BL. Bone mineral density of the radius: where do we stand? *J Nucl Med* (1985) **26:** 1339–41.
22. Awbrey BJ, Jacobsen PC, Grubb SA et al. Bone density in women: a modified procedure for measurement of distal radius density. *J Orthop Res* (1984) **2:** 314–21.
23. Eastell R, Riggs BL, Wahner HW et al. Colles' fracture and bone density of the ultradistal radius. *J Bone Miner Res* (1989) **4:** 607–12.
24. Eastell R, Wahner HW, O'Fallon WM et al. Unequal decrease in bone density of lumbar spine and ultradistal radius in Colles' and vertebral fracture syndromes. *J Clin Invest* (1989) **83:** 168–74.
25. Christiansen C, Ravn P, Alexandersen P, Mollgaard A. A new region of interest (nROI) in the forearm for monitoring the effect of therapy. *J Bone Miner Res* (1997) **12**(suppl 1): S480.
26. Faulkner KG, Roberts LA, McClung MR. Discrepancies in normative data between Lunar and Hologic DXA systems. *Osteoporos Int* (1996) **6:** 432–6.
27. Looker AC, Wahner HW, Dunn WL et al. Proximal femur bone mineral levels of US adults. *Osteoporos Int* (1995) **5:** 389–409.
28. Steiger P, von Stetten E, Kelly TL, Stein JA. DXA reference data for the hip: making sense of WHO, NHANES, T-scores and standardization. *Osteoporos Int* (1997) **7:** 307.
29. Christiansen MS, Christiansen C, Nastoft J et al. Normalization of bone mineral content to height, weight, and lean body mass: implications for clinical use. *Calcif Tissue Int* (1981) **33:** 5–8.
30. Riggs BL, Wahner HW, Dunn WL et al. Differential changes in bone mineral density of the appendicular and axial skeleton with aging: relationship to spinal osteoporosis. *J Clin Invest* (1981) **67:** 328–35.
31. Wasnich RD, Vogel JM, Ross PD et al. Age-specific, longitudinal bone loss rates at multiple cortical and trabecular skeletal sites. *J Nucl Med* (1986) **27:** 885.
32. Bjarnason K, Hassager C, Ravn P, Christiansen C. Early postmenopausal diminution of forearm

and spinal bone mineral density: a cross-sectional study. *Osteoporos Int* (1995) **5:** 35–8.

33. Arlot ME, Sornay-Rendu E, Garnero P et al. Apparent pre- and postmenopausal bone loss evaluated by DXA at different skeletal sites in women: the OFELY cohort. *J Bone Miner Res* (1997) **12:** 683–90.

34. Horsman A, Currey JD. Estimation of mechanical properties of the distal radius from bone mineral content and cortical width. *Clin Orthop* (1983) **176:** 298–304.

35. Blake GM, Patel R, Fogelman I. Peripheral or axial bone density measurements. *J Clin Densitometry* (1998) **1:** 55–63.

36. Finsen V, Berum P. Regional bone mineral density changes after Colles' and forehand fractures. *J Hand Surg* (1986) **11B:** 357–9.

14

Total Body Bone Mineral and Body Composition by Absorptiometry

Guest chapter by Carmelo A Formica

CHAPTER OVERVIEW

This chapter gives an introduction to non-invasive in vivo measurements of gross body composition. To this end, body composition models and concepts relevant to the dual-energy X-ray absorptiometry (DXA) technique are presented and available measurement procedures which are used for validation and comparison are briefly discussed. The contributions of DPA (dual-energy photon absorptiometry) and DXA to the understanding of body composition are reviewed. As DPA has become an obsolete technology, this chapter will be concerned primarily with DXA. Examples of DXA instrument performance are given and potential clinical applications are discussed. The physical principles of DPA and DXA body composition studies are discussed in the Appendix to this chapter.

INTRODUCTION

Information on body composition is of interest for studies of energy expenditure, energy stores, protein mass, skeletal mineral status and for defining relative hydration. Beyond this there are applications in the assessment of nutrition, in studies of growth and development, in sports medicine, and for monitoring the impact of treatment regimens on body tissues. A wide range of different approaches are used in this field of research. Wang et al.[1] have proposed a five-level model to organize the approach to body composition research ranging from investigations at the atomic level to studies of the entire body as a unity.

DXA is a new procedure for the non-invasive assessment of body composition capable of separating fat, fat-free mass and bone mineral at a relatively low cost, and with good patient acceptance. Because of its wide use for bone mineral measurements in diagnosing osteoporosis, the technique is more readily available than other reference methods, and is often referred to as a new 'gold standard' for the assessment of gross body composition. However, considerable controversy exists as to whether DXA should be referred to as a *gold standard*. Although DXA has surpassed DPA as the latest technology of choice, a considerable literature based around DPA remains of interest. Furthermore, many of the

Table 14.1 Terms used in body composition analysis based on the separation of body tissues into fat mass and lean mass.

Body fat mass	Quantity of triglyceride fat in the body
Adipose tissue mass	Storage form of body fat (body fat mass) plus its supporting cellular and extracellular structures
Lean body mass	Non-adipose tissue body mass (may include or exclude skeletal mass)
Fat-free mass	Lean body mass plus non-fat components of adipose tissue
Non-fat tissue	Term often used to refer to either lean body mass or fat-free mass

technological issues affecting DXA are also pertinent to the assessment of body composition using DPA. Therefore, the main focus of this chapter will be DXA. However, where appropriate, separate sections will be included for DPA for historical perspectives.

In dealing with body composition measurements obtained with DXA, it is necessary to understand clearly the terminology used. Definitions of frequently used terms are summarized in Table 14.1. These will be explained in greater detail later.

The history of developments in body composition analysis is a story of finding a useful compromise between its inherent complexity on the one hand, and the requirements of a practical method on the other. Since early efforts in the laboratory of Behnke in the 1940s, continuing studies of body composition have provided an ever growing number of laboratory procedures and parameters of body composition that can be measured with increasing precision. Most of the techniques are restricted to specialized laboratories because of their complexity or because the results are of special interest only. The more widely utilized in vivo procedures designed to measure body composition have been reviewed.[2–6]

The general approach to this gross body composition analysis is to subdivide the body weight into conceptual compartments containing relevant chemical compounds, tissues or spaces that share physiological properties of interest to the investigator. A very useful and time honoured body composition model is that proposed by Moore,[2] which is based on physiologically relevant compartments. These are fat, extracellular water (ECW), intracellular water (ICW) and body cell mass (BCM). In this model, skeletal mass is calculated as a constant proportion of the body weight, ECW and ICW are directly determined by dilution techniques, and BCM by low-level total body counting of the naturally occurring radionuclide ^{40}K. DXA can contribute by direct measurements of fat and skeletal mass. All models require one measurement technique for each compartment. Determination of body weight by weighing on scales counts as one measurement. For example, a measurement of total body water and body weight allows the calculation of lean and fat mass of the body.

In addition to the search for simpler procedures and new relevant compartments, attempts are made to demonstrate constant proportionality between various components of the body so that the determination of one component would permit the inference of the amounts of another related component which may not be accessible to direct measurement. This approach necessitates certain assumptions which have to be validated under the measurement conditions. The prediction of muscle mass by total body ^{40}K (TBK) measurement in normal subjects is an example. The need for actual measurements of muscle mass is eliminated by assuming a constant relationship between muscle mass and TBK. This approach has been found acceptable in well defined, normal populations, but the assumption of compositional constancy is not acceptable when disease is present, and it may change with age and other factors. This has restricted the use of this approach of body composition analysis for clinical applications where abnormal states need to be evaluated.

Validation of a new technique is difficult in the living organism. Animal studies have a limited usefulness for proving assumptions of proportionality between compartments because chemical analysis of body tissue varies within mammalian species. They are, however, of value to study measurement accuracy if chemical analysis can be performed. Pigs are often used for such experiments. Heymsfield et al.[5] have suggested a hierarchy of methodologies that assists in selecting methods for validation and helps in the analysis of potential errors. This has been summarized in Table 14.2. New procedures should be calibrated against procedures from a level higher on the list. Errors due to inaccurate assumptions are propagated downward from one level to the next.

Thus, any new procedure, particularly if based on a different measurement technique, is of great interest for its potential contribution to understanding body composition, for validation of assumptions made in previously established methods, and as a potentially useful clinical test on its own. For these reasons, the use of more recent absorptiometric techniques of DPA and DXA for quantifying skeletal and soft tissue components of body mass in vivo are of interest to investigators and clinicians in the field of body composition analysis.

The contributions of CT, ultrasound and MRI to this field at present consist of an assessment of tissue composition in distinct anatomical compartments that are sampled with cross-sectional images of body sections such as in thickness measurements of subcutaneous and visceral fat in the abdomen.[6] By using multiple slices, smaller animals and humans have been completely scanned and three-dimensional reconstructions of the fat and muscle volume have been possible. These approaches will not be reviewed in the context of this discussion of gross total body composition analysis. For additional information, the reader is referred to references. [7–16]

METHODS FOR THE ASSESSMENT OF GROSS HUMAN BODY COMPOSITION: BODY COMPARTMENTS

The concept of the fat-free body as a component of total body composition was originally conceived by Dubois and Benedict in 1915. This concept postulates that the body consists of two theoretical compartments: (1) a homogeneous cellular mass responsible for energy exchange and chemical and mechanical work; and (2) the metabolically inactive fat mass for energy storage. These two chemically distinct compartments, fat (mainly ether-extractable triglycerides) and fat-free tissues (principally water, protein and mineral), together add up to the body weight. Based on measurements of body density by underwater weighing, Behnke[17,18] defined the lean body mass as the weight of the body less all except indispensable fat. The latter was assumed to represent 2% of the lean body mass.

Fat, or stored triglyceride, when contrasted with lean body mass is anhydrous, free of potassium and has a density of $0.9007 \, g/cm^3$ at 37°C. This figure is relatively constant. In contrast, the chemical composition of the fat-free body compartment is very heterogeneous, including metabolically relatively inert tissues such as bone, tendons and the corneal part of the skin, as well as metabolically active tissues such as muscle, liver, kidneys and endocrine glands. Water, protein, bone mineral and non-skeletal mineral are the major chemical components of this compartment. From measurements on excised tissue and cadaver analysis, a mean density of $1.1 \, g/cm^3$ was determined for this compartment in healthy subjects. The great

Table 14.2 Methods used in body composition analysis. They are grouped using a hierarchical classification of techniques as proposed by Heymsfield et al.[5] DXA is shown in categories II and III.

Hierarchy of methodology	Component of body composition measured	Measurement technique	Remarks
I. Chemical analysis of human tissues and cadavers			Only limited data available
II. Direct quantitation of body constituents in vivo	Total body Na, Ca, N	Neutron activation analysis	Only a few available facilities
	Total body K	Low level total body counting	Readily available
	Bone mineral	DPA, DXA	Available in nuclear medicine laboratories
III. Model approach to estimating body compartments in vivo	Total body water, exchangeable Na, K	Isotope dilution technique	
	Total body fat	DPA, DXA	Generally available
IV. Somatic physical property measured in vivo, calibrated against body constituent derived by techniques above	Skinfold	Subcutaneous fat thickness, body water	Special training required for reproducible and accurate data
	Bioimpedance		
	QCT, US, MRI	Local fat content and distribution	Available in special laboratories

QCT, quantitative computed tomography; US, ultrasound; MRI, magnetic resonance imaging.

variability of this latter figure was recognized early, particularly in subjects with disease.[2]

If the densities of fat and lean mass are assumed constant, the body density measured by underwater weighing can be used to calculate the proportion of the body weight that is lean mass and fat. There are two additional measurement techniques in use to separate the body into lean fat-free mass and fat. These are total body potassium by low-level total body counting of [40]K and total body water by non-radioactive isotope dilution using heavy water. Both methods estimate lean mass, and fat is derived by subtracting lean mass from body weight. The TBK method measures lean body mass by assuming a constant relationship with potassium, while total body water measures it by assuming a constant relationship with body water.

Results obtained with these three techniques and DPA and DXA show a good correlation, but the results are not identical, particularly in obese subjects. Wang,[19] Pierson[20] and Jensen et al.[21] suggest that the differences found between these three methods in obese subjects are not only due to inherent inaccuracies of the techniques, but are most likely related to differences in the compartments being measured. DXA-measured fat-free mass includes lean body mass measured by TBK plus non-fat components of adipose tissue (extracellular water, supportive tissue). The definitions listed in Table 14.1 address these differences. When total body water is measured using hydrogen-labelled isotopes, the potential exists for exchange of body water and hydrogen in addition to dilution.[22] Values of 2% and 5% for isotopic exchange have been assumed.

With the introduction of in vivo neutron activation analysis (IVNAA), isotope dilution techniques and DXA, subcompartments of the original lean body mass can be measured directly. One four compartment model measures water, protein, bone mineral and fat.[23] DXA alone measures mineral mass in bone (which could only be measured by IVNAA or was estimated as a constant proportion of body weight in older models), fat-free mass and body fat mass. Examples of models are shown in

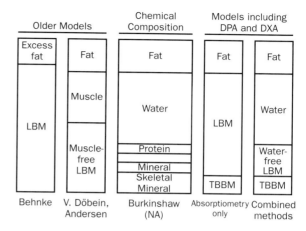

Figure 14.1 Examples of different models employed in body composition analysis. The centre panel contains a systematic summary of chemical compounds which constitute the body. Simple models are represented in the two panels to the left. Models that include DPA and DXA techniques are shown on the right. Additional models not shown in this figure have been proposed.

Figure 14.1. A summary of tests available for gross body composition analysis is given in Table 14.3.

Despite its recognized shortcomings, a gross body composition analysis based on fat and lean mass by total body water or DXA is a useful measurement for research and clinical studies, and is easy to perform and of low cost.

BODY COMPOSITION MEASUREMENTS WITH DPA

The principal approach used in dual photon absorptiometry for body composition analysis can be reduced to two parts. First, the body is considered to consist of bone mineral and soft tissue. This is the same approach as that used in bone mineral analysis as discussed previously in Chapter 3. Secondly, the soft tissue mass is

Table 14.3 Readily available methods for the estimation of body fat and obesity. Methods using IVNAA, CT and MRI are not included.

Method	Assumptions
Anthropometry: body mass index (BMI), skinfolds etc.	$BMI = \dfrac{weight\ (kg)}{[height\ (m)]^2}$
Underwater weighing: body density	Density: FFM = 1.10 g/cm^3 fat = 0.90 g/cm^3
Total body water: ^2H_2O	$LBM\ (kg) = \dfrac{TBW(l)}{0.732}$ (fat $\quad$ = BW − LBM)
Total body K: ^{40}K total body counting	FFM = 60 mmol K/kg (women) $\quad$ = 66 mmol K/kg (men) (fat = BW − FFM)
Absorptiometry: DPA, DXA	Soft tissue mass = body weight − skeletal mass Soft tissue has two compartments: fat and water-equivalent tissues

FFM, fat-free mass; LBM, lean body mass; BW, body weight.

partitioned into fat and lean body mass by a calibration procedure based on the ratio of the low- and high-energy attenuation by soft tissue pixels that do not include any bone. Detailed descriptions are given by Mazess et al.,[24,25] Heymsfield et al.,[4] Gotfredsen et al.[26] and Pietrobelli et al.[27] A brief review of the physical principles is given in the Appendix to this chapter and the reader is referred there for a discussion of the relationship between the measured R_{st} value (the ratio of the low-energy and high-energy soft tissue attenuation coefficients) and the estimated fat and lean mass. Heymsfield et al.[28] have proposed a chemical approach to measuring human body density in vivo by combining DPA with established methods. Using a four compartment model approach, they measured protein (by IVNAA), water (by ^2H_2O), skeletal mineral (by DPA) and fat (by DPA). The calculated lean body density of 1.096 ± 0.007 g/cm^3 agreed closely with three classic human cadaver studies (1.100 g/cm^3) used as a basis for density measurements by underwater weighing.

The accuracy of total body bone mass (TBBM) measured on isolated skeletons by DPA (expressed as 1 standard error of the estimate (SEE)) was 36 g (equal to 13 g of calcium), with a correlation coefficient of $r = 0.99$. The SEE is equal to 1–1.5% of TBBM in young adults and 2–2.5% in older women and women with osteoporosis.[24] When compared with measurements made by IVNAA, TBBM by DPA showed a high correlation ($r = 0.99$).[29] Comparisons with TBK measurements gave similar results ($r = 0.83$–0.90, SEE = 4–6% fat), although the correlation was not as good.[30] Heymsfield et al.[4] measured fat with four established methods in normal human subjects. Results were within 1.5% of each other and correlations were highly significant. This was not true in obese patients, as previously reviewed. Fat and lean mass agreed closely ($r = 0.86$–0.95) with indirect estimates made using anthropometric equations involving body weight, height and skin folds.[31]

BODY COMPOSITION MEASUREMENTS WITH DXA

Like DPA, DXA measures bone and partitions fat and lean by a calibration procedure. A detailed review of the principles behind DXA has been provided by Pietrobelli et al.[27] A brief explanation is included in the Appendix to this chapter. As previously discussed for bone mineral measurements, the use of an X-ray source improves image resolution resulting in improved bone and soft tissue edge detection. It also circumvents source strength related errors inherent in any radionuclide source and shortens the scanning time from 1 hour to 10–20 minutes, or as short as 3 minutes using fan-beam instruments. The sampling area (per cent of total body sampled) is increased with the potential of increasing precision and accuracy.

The development of the DXA technique for body composition measurements is still evolving. There is no standard approach to calibrating the instruments and each manufacturer proceeds independently. Thus, the results from the different commercial instruments may not exactly agree. Users of DXA body composition

software concerned about the accuracy of the algorithms should consult the manufacturer as well as the published literature. With the rapid development of software, many reported problems are quickly rectified.

Commercial instruments for body composition analysis are available from Hologic Inc., Lunar Corporation and Norland Medical Systems (see Chapter 4, Table 4.1). A single instrument can be used for regional bone mineral measurements, as used in osteoporosis work-up, as well as for body composition analysis. The Lunar and Norland instruments use a similar approach to that described for DPA in the Appendix, but have significant differences in hardware and software. This requires that different instrument are evaluated separately. Lunar instruments give a readout of the regional part-body and total body R_{st} values, which allows a certain insight and access to the calibration process. Hologic instruments use an internal calibration system (the reference wheel, see Chapter 3, Figure 3.14) and a step phantom with three lean tissue and three fat-equivalent steps of different thicknesses, which is scanned with every patient. More details of the principles involved are given in the Appendix.

INSTRUMENT EVALUATION AND LIMITATIONS

In general terms, evaluation of an instrument proceeds in four phases. The first step is the measurement of known samples of fat and water or equivalent pure chemical substances, alone and in mixtures, to prove linearity of the measurements (Figure 14.2A). Satisfactory standard curves have been shown for all three of the above instruments. The second step is a calibration with simple phantoms which have a uniform tissue composition such as meat blocks of known fat content (Figure 14.2B) or the Nord tissue phantom.[32] Again, data from all three instruments show good linearity of fat, lean and total weight measurements. For determination of per cent fat in such simple phantoms, an optimal performance is found between 10% and

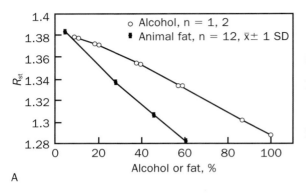

A

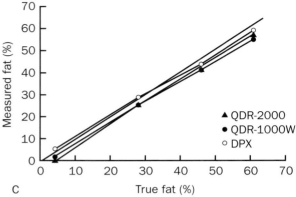

C

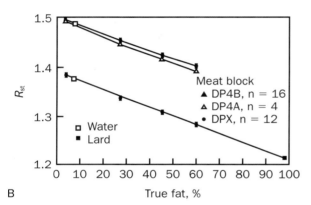

B

Figure 14.2 (A) Calibration curve for estimating body fat from measurement of the R-value (R_{st}) on an early DPX instrument. Note the difference between animal fat and ethanol. Ethanol is not a good substitute for fat for calibration purposes despite its similar absorption coefficient. (B) Standard curve for estimating fat and lean mass from the measured soft tissue absorption coefficient equivalent R_{st}, given on Lunar instruments. For R_{st}, see R-value in DPX data printout, as shown in Figure 14.5D. Meat blocks with known fat content were scanned. Values for R_{st} of tap water and lard are given. Using this standard curve, tap water reads 6% fat, lard 98% fat. (Wahner HW et al., unpublished data). (C) Calibration curve for three instruments obtained by scanning meat blocks of known fat content. The line of identity is given.

60% fat content with precision under 3% and accuracy about 4–8% (standard deviation) (Figure 14.2C). The third step uses complex phantoms (representing bone, fat and lean tissue at varying thicknesses) and animals, usually pigs, suitable for chemical analysis. The last step is a comparison of DXA results from human subjects with results from other methods. Such results are now more readily available for the different instruments, but results are not yet uniformly satisfactory.

Although DXA is primarily used to measure bone and soft tissue compartments, the full assessment of disease and nutritional status requires the understanding of changes in compartmental sizes, which may be a consequence or marker of disease. Several studies have demonstrated that changes in body weight can be measured accurately by DXA, and is reflected in the total mass and total soft tissue mass compartments.[33–35] However, changes in the individual soft tissue compartments, lean and fat mass, may not be accurately measured. These observations have been further supported by work using hydration and rehydration models.[36,37] These studies demonstrated that changes in body weight (1.5–1.8 kg) were accurately measured by total soft tissue mass, but less so by the lean mass. Appropriately there was no measured change in bone or fat masses.

When calculating bone mass, DXA simplifies the body into two compartments: bone and soft tissue. The attenuation in soft tissue can be resolved further to yield fat and lean tissue information, as fat and lean tissues have differing attenuation characteristics. The relationship between the R_{st} value and the per cent fat tissue has been determined in vitro.[24–27] Greater proportions of fat in tissue yield lower R_{st} values. This relationship is used to determine the relative amounts of fat and lean masses. If the R_{st} value is determined, the per cent fat can be inferred, and fat mass calculated in grams from the per cent fat of the total soft tissue mass. The bone-free lean mass is derived by subtracting the fat mass from the total soft tissue mass. The simplified two-compartment model of bone and soft tissue is now expanded to a three-compartment model: bone mineral, fat mass and bone-free lean mass. Since these three unknowns are being resolved by measurements at only two photon energies, there is an association between the fat and lean masses. Errors may propagate from one compartment to another, as the interdependent compartments are summed to derive total weight. When compartments are determined by subtraction, a given percentage error in the lean mass may cause a larger percentage error in the fat mass due to its usually smaller compartmental size.

The dependence of photon absorptiometry on subject thickness is another significant source of error. The dependence of bone mineral content on patient thickness has been shown to be negligible within a clinical range of 10–20 cm.[38,39] However, body composition studies are often concerned with measurements at both extremes of body weight. In addition, regional sites such as the arms and legs may be particularly prone to such errors. Mazess et al. demonstrated that there is an influence of patient thickness on measurements of fat mass such that fat mass may be underestimated in larger patients.[40] Furthermore, a wide variation in patient thickness accentuates technical issues such as beam hardening. The effect of patient

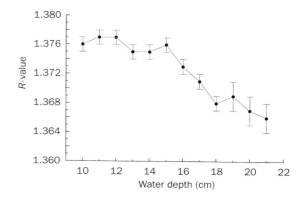

Figure 14.3 The effect of varying attenuator thickness (water) on the measured R-value using a Lunar DPX-L DXA system.

thickness on the R_{st} value can be simulated by measuring the R-value in water at different depths. Although the attenuating material is unchanged, the R-value decreases significantly with increasing thickness as shown in Figure 14.3. These results demonstrate that caution should be taken when measuring body composition at the extremes of body weight, and attention to the correct scan mode for subject thickness is critical to ensure accurate and reproducible measurements.

For Hologic instruments, Jebb et al.,[41] using an oil, water, aluminium phantom found a trend for overestimation of fat mass at water depths below 5 cm and above 25 cm. The 25-cm water depth was estimated to correspond with a body mass index of 45 kg/m^2 in patients. Within the 5–25-cm range, however, errors less than 3% were found for fat measurements. Similarly, Svendsen et al.,[42] using pigs, showed that in Lunar instruments the measured bone and fat mass may vary with absorber depth and the degree of adiposity outside an optimal measuring range. Within the optimal measuring range, the lines of regression of DXA-measured fat (%), fat tissue mass and lean body mass on actual fat content were not significantly different from the lines of identity. The standard errors were 2.9% for fat (%), 1.9 kg for fat mass and 2.7 kg for lean body mass. Added layers of lard to human subjects were accurately measured by DXA (99.5 ± 1.0%, mean ±1 SEM). The short-term precision of DXA in six adults was (CV%) 4.9% for fat (%), 4.6% for fat tissue mass and 1.5% for lean body mass.

Skeletal sites that have few pixels containing only soft tissue pose a particular problem in body composition analysis. The skull contains virtually no detectable soft tissue areas, and provides little additional information regarding soft tissue composition. Furthermore, DXA manufacturers make differing assumptions concerning the appropriate R_{st} value for the skull, therefore raising concern as to the comparability of skull measurements, or indeed the validity of skull measurements. Taylor et al.[43] have demonstrated, in a paediatric population, that subtotal BMD (total body BMD excluding the skull) was better predicted by age than total body BMD, possibly because of the use of an algorithm for head BMC developed and optimized for adults. Problems with the accurate measurement of skull BMD are not restricted to paediatric populations. In women with osteoporosis stabilized on hormone replacement therapy, an erroneous increase in total body BMD of about 3% over a 3-year period has been shown (Formica et al., unpublished data). When the skull was removed from the analysis no significant change was observed and the variability in the individuals' rates of change over the 3-year period was reduced. As the skull accounts for a significant proportion of total body calcium and mineral content, caution should be practised when interpreting changes in total body mineral.

The thorax also presents potential sources of error, the ribs being thin so that pixels containing only soft tissue cannot easily be separated from pixels containing bone. Likewise in the arms, where bone represents a large proportion of the total regional mass, measurements of soft tissue composition may be less accurate. The manufacturers of DXA equipment further complicate the assessment of body composition by introducing assumptions concerning the distri-

bution and composition of soft tissue for the derivation of tissue and bone masses. This in part explains why body composition assessed by one manufacturer cannot be directly compared with that of another manufacturer, and why cross-calibration phantoms between manufacturers may not yield completely consistent results. Tothill et al.[44] drew attention to the significant effect of large changes in weight on the projected area of bone in total body DXA studies, with consequent errors in total body BMC. BMD results were also affected, although to a lesser degree. The authors suggest caution in interpreting changes in total body BMC or BMD, particularly in the setting of significant weight change. Patel et al.[35] presented a similar analysis of the effect of weight change on total body DXA from data obtained during a clinical trial of bisphosphonate treatment. Although weight-change-dependent variations of total body BMC and BMD were found in the same sense as those reported by Tothill and colleagues,[44] the magnitude of the coefficients was considerably smaller and did not affect the interpretation of the clinical trial data.

DXA is an important method for body composition measurements based on its close agreement with reference methods such as underwater weighing and IVNAA. It should not, however, be considered a new reference method or 'gold standard'. Total mass and total soft tissue mass by DXA have been demonstrated to be accurate and precise measurements that reflect changes with sufficient sensitivity to be applied to serial studies. However, it is the size and changes in the various tissue compartments that are the basis of body compositional analysis. The inaccuracy of measuring individual compartments of body composition using DXA questions the validity of this methodology as a 'gold standard'. Other factors such as thickness dependence, variability with soft tissue mass and the assumptions about tissue distribution suggest that caution is needed when interpreting results. In particular, body composition analysis may be compromised in studies concerned with growth and development.

Total body measurements of bone and soft tissue masses can be performed using both pencil-beam and fan-beam DXA systems. The technical aspects of pencil- and fan-beam systems are discussed in Chapters 3 and 4 of this text. An explanation of the principles of the assessment of BMC and lean and tissue mass by DXA is simplest for pencil-beam instruments (see the Appendix). The use of fan-beam geometry for the assessment of body composition is made more complicated by the effects of differential magnification, which make results dependent on the thickness of the body and location. Using fan-beam geometry, the portion of the body that is closest to the source, and thus, furthest from the detector is magnified more than if the same region was closest to the detector. The effects of differential magnification due to position from the detector have been discussed by Griffiths and colleagues[45,46] and by Fuerst et al.[47] Other studies have also documented differences in body composition results between pencil- and fan-beam systems and using different software algorithms.[48–52] However, Kelly et al.[53] have recently described how the effects of differential magnification inherent in total body fan-beam DXA can be corrected using the known isocentric geometry of the fan-beam acquisition and the measurement of body thickness using the high-energy X-ray transmission factor. Fan-beam total body DXA using algorithms that correct for the effects of differential magnification are attractive because of the short scan times, improved image resolution and efficient sampling of the whole body.

Considerable care is needed when performing total body DXA scans for body composition analysis. Jewellery and outer clothing must be removed and the patient should wear a cotton gown. The standard imaging tables are suitable for patients up to 1.82 m (6 feet) in height and support patients up to 136 kg (300 lbs) in weight. When scanning very tall persons, accurate BMC measurements can be obtained with the knees slightly bent and the feet positioned with the toes straight up. However, the use of a pillow to support the knees may introduce errors (refer to Figure 14.16). For BMD measurements where the projected area is also critical, reproducible positioning is more important. In the average size subject, legs should be straight on the table and the feet should be taped together and either stretched as much as possible or held with the toes up. Care is also needed in positioning the hands which should be held with the palms down and fingers closed. For a constant projected area, a reproducible technique is essential. From the total area scanned, regions of interest can be selected for analysis. A magnified display of the image allows for detailed region of interest (ROI) selection (Figure 14.4).

Examples of the data output from body composition measurements made on different instruments are shown in Figure 14.5.

COMPARISON OF COMMERCIAL INSTRUMENT PERFORMANCE

Results from a comparison of two commercial DXA instruments (Hologic and Lunar) for body composition analysis are summarized in Tables 14.4A–C. In this study 25 normal women, aged 33–84 years (mean age 58.9 years), were scanned with Lunar DPX and Hologic QDR instruments on the same day in the Mayo Clinic laboratory. Both showed excellent correlation between estimated total body mass and body weight obtained by weighing (Figures 14.6A and B). Total body bone mineral density (TBBMD) was not significantly different between the two instruments. This is in contrast to BMD in the L-spine, where the Lunar instrument gives higher values by 8–10% when compared with the QDR-1000. Small differences were seen in the BMD of head, ribs and pelvis with no instrument being consistently higher or lower than the other. For lean mass, results were consistently lower on the QDR-1000 instrument and higher for fat in some part-body regions measured.

Considering the entire study population, the standard deviation for BMD for different ROIs was larger in the DPX instrument. ROIs could not be set with equal precision on the DPX. Software upgrades have since corrected this and equal results can be expected. Data on measurement precision for BMD in a torso phantom are given in Table 14.5A. The effect on BMD of changing tissue thickness is summa-

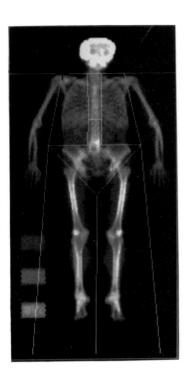
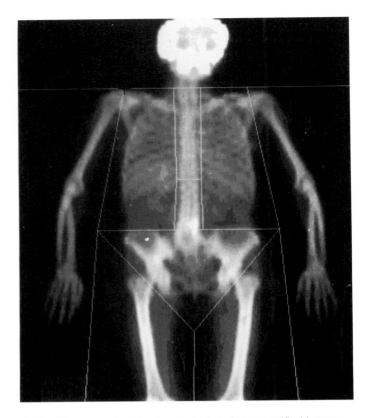

Figure 14.4 Scan image from total body scan (left) with a magnification image (right). The magnified image allows a better delineation of ROIs (image obtained with a QDR-1000W system).

rized in Table 14.5B. Long-term precision of the two instruments for bone and soft tissue measurements was tested by scanning a torso phantom bi-monthly for 11 months. Both instruments showed stable measurements over time, but systematic differences between the measurement results were noted (Table 14.6). These were not identical to those previously demonstrated in Table 14.4A–C, probably due to the limits of the phantom to represent measurements in patients.

Using newer technology (Hologic QDR-1500 and QDR-4500), significant differences between pencil- and fan-beam body composition methods have been reported. Using a variable composition phantom, (Formica et al.[54]) showed highly significant correlations between the expected per cent fat and the measured per cent fat ($r > 0.9$). However, when comparing pencil- and fan-beam instruments, despite the high correlations, significant differences in the intercepts and slopes were observed. Similar results were found in a sample of healthy volunteers studied in the author's laboratory (Helen Hayes Hospital, West Haverstraw, NY, USA) (Figure 14.7). In part, these differences reflect an upgrade in software to give better agreement with hydrodensitometry (T Kelly, personal communication), and in part the differences in X-ray beam geometry previously discussed. As indicated above, algorithms have now been developed to correct the latter, based on the known geometry of the fan-beam system.[53]

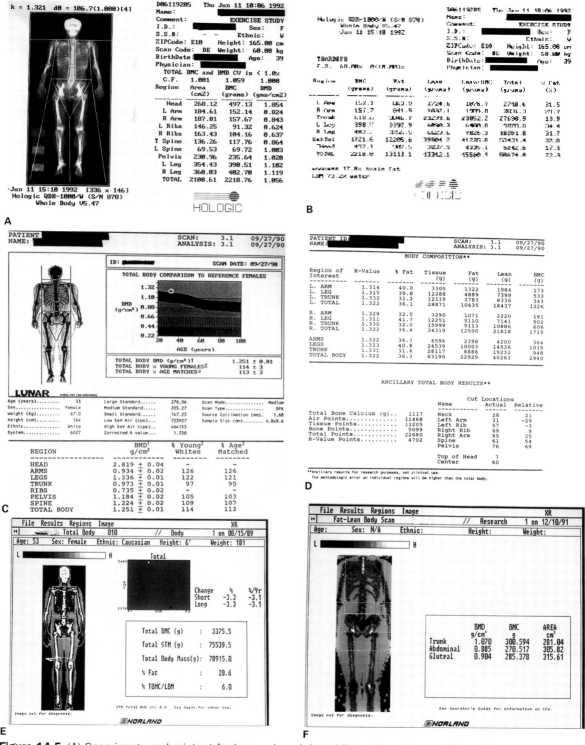

Figure 14.5 (A) Scan image and printout for bone mineral data, biography and essential quality control data (Hologic Inc., QDR-1000W). (B) Data summary from body composition analysis and patient biography (Hologic Inc., QDR-1000W). (C) Scan image, data display, quality control data and normal range for total body bone mineral analysis (Lunar Corp., DPX). (D) Display of body composition results (Lunar Corp., DPX). (E) Scan image and display of results for body composition analysis (Norland Medical Systems, XR-36). (F) Scan image and data summary for total body bone mineral analysis (Norland Medical Systems, XR-36).

Table 14.4 Comparison of two commercial DXA instruments (QDR-1000W, Hologic Inc.; DPX, Lunar Corp.); (A) BMD (g/cm²); (B) lean mass (g); and (C) estimated fat (% of body weight), for the entire skeleton and selected ROIs. All age groups (n = 25); mean age = 58.9 years; SD = 14.0 years. (Reproduced with permission from the Mayo Clinic Bone Mineral Laboratory.)

Region of interest	QDR Mean	Range	SD	DPX Mean	Range	SD	Sᵃ
A							
Arms—left	0.77	0.67–0.91	0.06	0.77	0.64–0.96	0.08	NS
right							
total							
Legs—left	1.08	0.89–1.32	0.10	1.07	0.86–1.34	0.11	NS
right							
total							
Head	2.20	1.64–2.90	0.33	2.29	1.73–2.82	0.29	S1
Ribs	0.60	0.54–0.69	0.04	0.63	0.51–0.81	0.07	S1
Pelvis	0.93	0.75–1.24	0.12	1.01	0.80–1.32	0.12	S1
Total	1.05	0.92–1.24	0.09	1.06	0.89–1.27	0.10	NS
B							
Arms—left	1 697.7	1 255.5–2 227.0	249.5	1 855.3	1 326–3 245	390.4	S1
right	1 787.1	1 322.4–2 316.6	231.3	1 977.8	1 515–2 658	306.7	S1
total	3 484.9	2 577.9–4 489.9	474.7	3 829.5	2 901–5 824	671.0	S1
Legs—left	5 223.1	3 836.6–6 603.7	653.6	6 735.4	5 386–8 781	842.8	S1
right	5 242.0	3 780.5–6 302.0	644.2	6 735.0	5 418–8 326	780.0	S1
total	10 465.1	7 617.1–12 768.6	1279.4	13 469.4	10 805–17 109	1591.6	S1
Trunk	20 737.5	16 392.3–25 085.6	2372.1	18 796.9	14 824–22 986	1981.3	S1
Total	37 803.8	29 284.3–45 744.3	4129.9	38 254.5	38 989–47 259	3995.9	S2

Table 14.4 Continued

C

Region of interest	QDR			DPX			
	Mean	Range	SD	Mean	Range	SD	S^a
Arms—left	46.2	35.5–58.4	6.3	45.0	26.1–65.1	9.3	NS
right	45.4	36.3–60.5	6.3	41.5	22.1–61.4	9.9	S1
total	45.8	36.2–58.4	6.2	43.4	24.5–63.3	9.4	S2
Legs—left	47.9	32.3–58.0	6.8	42.2	31.1–51.4	5.8	S1
right	48.3	35.4–59.5	6.9	42.9	31.1–52.4	6.0	S1
total	48.1	33.9–58.7	6.8	42.6	31.2–51.8	5.8	S1
Trunk	35.4	23.5–48.3	6.7	36.1	22.8–45.9	5.7	NS
Total	39.6	29.2–50.6	5.9	39.8	26.9–51.8	6.0	NS

[a] Significance (paired t-test): NS = not significant; S1 = $P < 0.01$; S2 = $P < 0.05$.

Table 14.5 Comparison of the same two instruments described in Table 14.4. (A) Precision of total body bone mineral (BMD) measurements. (B) Effect of increasing body fat and thickness. (Measurements were made with a torso phantom as described in the text.)

A	DPX		QDR		Difference: QDR per cent of DPX[a]
Site	Mean (g/cm²)	CV (%)	Mean (g/cm²)	CV (%)	
Total	0.870	0.52	0.856	0.38	98.4
T-spine	0.916	2.53	0.807	0.25	88.1
L-spine	0.956	4.60	0.855	1.89	89.4
Spine	0.931	3.37	0.831	0.98 (mean of L- and T-spine)	89.2
Pelvis	0.966	1.00	0.924	0.27	95.6
Ribs	0.695	1.67	0.674	0.62 (mean of left and right)	97.0

B	Experiment (configuration)	DPX: BMD (g/cm²), mean ± SD	QDR: BMD (g/cm²), mean ± SD
	4 in (10 cm) lard over abdomen	0.892 ± 1.69%	0.813 ± 0.49%
	2 in (5 cm) lard over abdomen	0.877 ± 0.93%	0.813 ± 0.07%
	1½ in (4 cm) lard over abdomen	0.847 ± 0.83%	0.814 ± 0.33%
	1 in (2.5 cm) lard over abdomen	0.847 ± 1.37%	0.822 ± 0.19%
	½ in (12 cm) lard over abdomen	0.860 ± 1.38%	0.830 ± 0.25%

[a] Measurements with the DPX were consistently higher.

EVALUATION OF A NEW INSTRUMENT

As a general rule, all commercial instruments are calibrated by the manufacturer to meet published performance standards. The user should not need to perform further tests when the instruments are used for the applications designed by the manufacturer. However, for those interested, an independent review of performance might include the following:

1) Proof of acceptable performance for regional bone mineral determination as outlined above (Table 14.5).

2) Precision and accuracy can be tested using a skeletal phantom such as that described by Nord.[32] In the Mayo Clinic laboratory, a measurement in triplicate is performed once a week. Results are plotted versus time as quality control for total body bone mineral measurements.

3) Precision and accuracy of soft tissue measurements can be tested by scanning a series of frozen meat blocks with known fat content. In the Mayo Clinic laboratory, such measurements are performed in triplicate every fortnight for quality control of soft

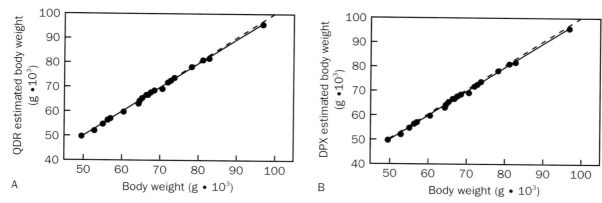

Figure 14.6 Comparison of estimated body mass (bone mass, fat mass, lean mass) and body weight by weighing from 25 normal women, aged 33–84 years. (A) Hologic QDR-1000W; r = 0.999, QDR (TBM) (g) = −845.29 + 1.003 × weight (g). (B) Lunar DPX; r = 0.998, DPX (TBM) (g) = −682.86 + 0.996 × weight (g). The line of identity is shown.

tissue measurements, whenever body composition studies are ongoing. Separate quality control graphs are kept for each specimen.

4) The effect of variation in soft tissue thickness on measured lean and fat masses can be tested by scanning stacked meat blocks.

This test may be relevant when measurements are performed on obese subjects.

5) The effect of changing soft tissue thickness on bone mineral results can be tested with the meat blocks positioned on top of the Lunar spine phantom. This study is relevant when small children or obese subjects

Table 14.6 Long-term precision of body composition measurements. Data were obtained from bi-monthly measurements of a torso phantom in the Mayo Clinic laboratory using a DPX (Lunar Corp.) and a QDR-1000W (Hologic Inc.). There were 22 measurements in 11 months.

	DPX[a]		QDR-1000W	
	Mean (kg)	CV (%)	Mean (kg)	CV (%)
Non-fat mass	46.0	1.3	47.4	0.5
Total body mass	55.1	0.6	54.1	0.4
Total fat mass	8.6	7.0	6.1	4.2
TBBM	0.75	1.9	0.619	0.6

[a] From Jensen et al.[21]

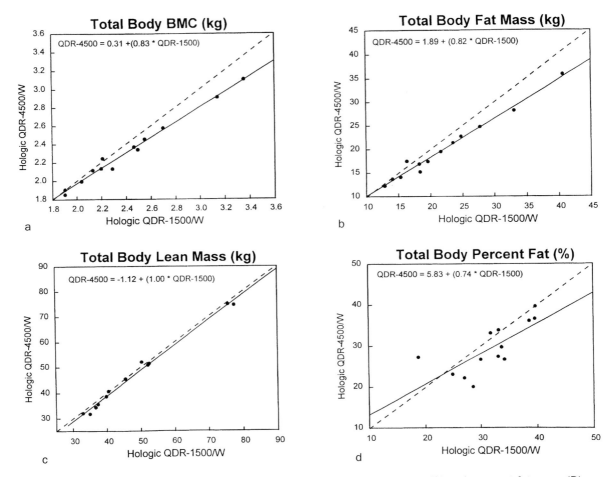

Figure 14.7 Correlation between total body BMC (A), fat mass (B), lean mass (C) and per cent fat mass (D), as measured using Hologic QDR-1500W pencil-beam and QDR-4500W fan-beam instruments (Formica CA et al., unpublished data). The line of identity is given. (Note that the QDR-4500W used a more recent software release designed to give closer agreement with hydrodensitometry.)

are scanned for bone mineral as well as body composition analysis.

CLINICAL USEFULNESS OF TOTAL BODY DXA STUDIES

The diagnostic utility of bone mass measurements is discussed in Chapter 16. However, it would appear an opportune time to discuss the discriminatory ability of total body bone mass measurements in patients with osteoporosis. While total body measurements are not routinely performed for osteoporosis diagnosis, it would nevertheless appear that total body bone mass and density are equally discriminatory of osteoporosis as are measurements at the conventional sites of the lumbar spine and proximal femur.[55–63] In many studies, ROC analysis or logistic regression have demonstrated

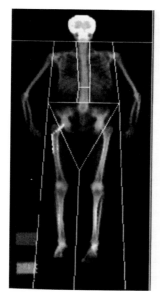

Region	Area (cm2)	BMC (grams)	BMD (gms/cm2)
Head	205.14	423.78	2.066
L Arm	150.25	99.75	0.664
R Arm	160.27	109.31	0.682
L Ribs	106.18	59.92	0.564
R Ribs	100.17	60.86	0.608
T Spine	122.60	84.40	0.688
L Spine	46.48	35.36	0.761
Pelvis	165.47	126.70	0.766
L Leg	344.57	297.20	0.863
R Leg	329.75	296.61	0.900
TOTAL	1730.87	1593.88	0.921

Figure 14.8 Total body bone mineral analysis. Note the right total hip arthroplasty and metal prosthesis. BMD and BMC in the legs are not significantly affected when compared with the contralateral side.

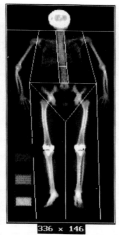

336 x 146

Region	Area (cm2)	BMC (grams)	BMD (gms/cm2)
Head	226.38	550.48	2.432
L Arm	224.37	189.89	0.846
R Arm	232.79	196.52	0.844
L Ribs	138.63	80.67	0.582
R Ribs	167.08	93.29	0.558
T Spine	159.06	149.31	0.939
L Spine	59.30	57.00	0.961
Pelvis	210.75	209.50	0.994
L Leg	467.57	714.14	1.527
R Leg	449.14	732.81	1.632
TOTAL	2335.07	2973.61	1.273

Figure 14.9 Bilateral total knee arthrodesis. Metal implants falsely raise BMC and BMD in the legs and affect TBBM.

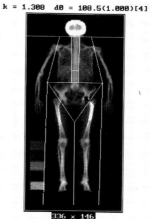

k = 1.308   d0 = 108.5(1.000)[4]

336 x 146
Hologic QDR-1000/W (S/N 878)
Whole Body Version 5.26

Region	Area (cm2)	BMC (grams)	BMD (gms/cm2)
Head	214.76	428.24	1.994
L Arm	149.45	101.47	0.679
R Arm	168.28	116.20	0.691
L Ribs	62.18	33.51	0.540
R Ribs	70.12	40.26	0.574
T Spine	135.83	99.23	0.731
L Spine	41.27	27.43	0.665
Pelvis	128.21	84.58	0.660
L Leg	304.91	314.50	1.031
R Leg	324.94	266.39	0.820
TOTAL	1599.85	1511.81	0.945

Figure 14.10 Left total hip arthrodesis. Note the falsely high BMD and BMC values in the femur.

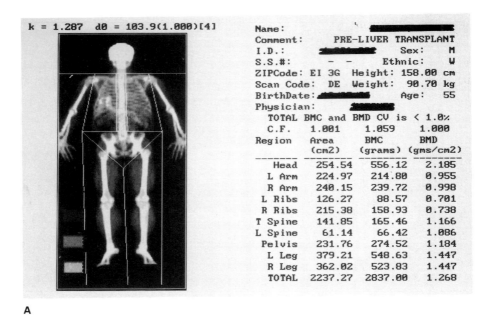

```
k = 1.287  d0 = 103.9(1.000)[4]
```

Name:			
Comment:	PRE-LIVER TRANSPLANT		
I.D.:		Sex:	M
S.S.#:	– –	Ethnic:	W
ZIPCode: EI 3G	Height:	158.00 cm	
Scan Code: DE	Weight:	90.70 kg	
BirthDate:		Age:	55
Physician:			

TOTAL BMC and BMD CV is < 1.0%

C.F.   1.001   1.059   1.000

Region	Area (cm2)	BMC (grams)	BMD (gms/cm2)
Head	254.54	556.12	2.185
L Arm	224.97	214.80	0.955
R Arm	240.15	239.72	0.998
L Ribs	126.27	88.57	0.701
R Ribs	215.38	158.93	0.738
T Spine	141.85	165.46	1.166
L Spine	61.14	66.42	1.086
Pelvis	231.76	274.52	1.184
L Leg	379.21	548.63	1.447
R Leg	362.02	523.83	1.447
TOTAL	2237.27	2837.00	1.268

A

greater fracture discriminatory ability using total body measurements compared with the regional sites.[55,56,59] Prospective longitudinal studies, however, are needed to corroborate the cross-sectional observations.

Likewise, limited studies have included total body bone measurements in multicentre therapeutic intervention studies.[64–69] Most have demonstrated therapeutic efficacy on total body bone mass. However, the change in total body measurements differed from those at the regional sites. For example, Kohrt and Birge,[64] in a small sample of subjects receiving conjugated oestrogens for 12 months showed an increase in total body bone density of 1.4%, compared with increases of 5% at the lumbar spine and 3% at the femoral neck. Liberman et al.[66] showed that women receiving 10 mg of alendronate daily had greater bone mass at most sites compared with those receiving placebo. However, the increase in total body BMD (2.5%) was less than the other regional sites (lumbar spine, 8.8%; femoral neck, 5.9%). Lindsay et al.[69] have shown that in women taking hormone replacement therapy and PTH(1–34), the total increase in vertebral bone mineral density was 13.0%, 2.7% at the hip and 8% in total body mineral compared with women taking hormone replacement therapy alone. The results concerning the association between total body bone mass and genomic allelic variation have been less convincing. Barger-Lux et al.[70] have reported that total body bone mineral content was significantly associated with *VDR* gene alleles. By contrast, Harris et al.[71] showed that there was no statistically significant interaction between race and *SCP* genotype in analyses of BMD at any skeletal site.

Regional body composition has been of growing interest because of its association with disease,[72,73] such as the relationship between intra-abdominal fat and diabetes,[74] cardiovascular disease,[74,75] overall mortality and the risk of falling with associated skeletal fracture.[72] In normal populations, with ageing there is a decline in lean tissue mass and an increase in fat tissue mass in both sexes.[76–78] A redistribution of fat with loss from the lower extremities and gains in the trunkal region occurs in men and women.[79,80] Seasonal changes in bone mineral,[81–84] total body fat and regional fat distribution have been described.[85] Associations between the level of physical activity, muscle strength and bone mass have been examined.[84] The role of total body fat mass and lean mass as

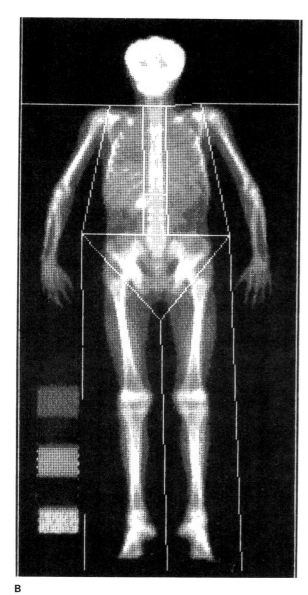

B

Figure 14.11 (A) Residual contrast material (barium sulphate) in the stomach and upper GI tract after a radiograph. BMC, and to a lesser degree BMD, reflect the additional absorptive material in the right upper abdomen. Note the delineation of the large muscle mass in the extremities. (B) Contrast material in the gallbladder. There was no measurable effect on soft tissue or bone. Occasionally the stomach is seen on scan images. A 2-hour fast prior to scanning for body composition analysis is good practice.

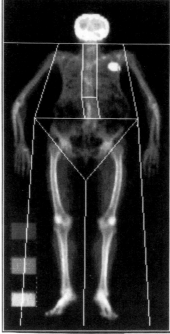

C.F. Region	1.001 Area (cm2)	1.077 BMC (grams)	1.000 BMD (gms/cm2)
Head	213.75	391.28	1.831
L Arm	188.98	123.39	0.653
R Arm	188.18	123.81	0.658
L Ribs	137.04	131.52	0.960
R Ribs	139.84	82.21	0.588
T Spine	147.03	108.61	0.739
L Spine	48.34	34.09	0.705
Pelvis	146.23	107.48	0.735
L Leg	395.54	363.83	0.920
R Leg	402.33	362.70	0.902
TOTAL	2007.24	1828.91	0.911

Figure 14.12 Pacemaker, left chest. Note error in BMC and BMD values of the left chest.

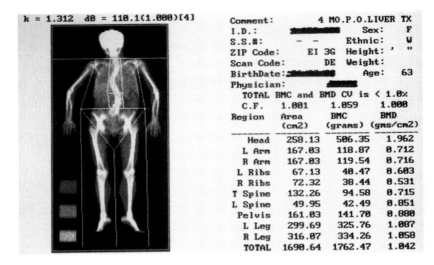

k = 1.312 d0 = 110.1(1.000)[4]

Comment:		4 MO.P.O.LIVER TX	

I.D.:		Sex:	F
S.S.#:	– –	Ethnic:	W
ZIP Code:	EI 3G	Height:	' "
Scan Code:	DE	Weight:	
BirthDate:		Age:	63
Physician:			

TOTAL BMC and BMD CV is < 1.0%

C.F.   1.001   1.059   1.000

Region	Area (cm2)	BMC (grams)	BMD (gms/cm2)
Head	258.13	506.35	1.962
L Arm	167.03	118.87	0.712
R Arm	167.03	119.54	0.716
L Ribs	67.13	40.47	0.603
R Ribs	72.32	38.44	0.531
T Spine	132.26	94.58	0.715
L Spine	49.95	42.49	0.851
Pelvis	161.03	141.70	0.880
L Leg	299.69	325.76	1.087
R Leg	316.07	334.26	1.058
TOTAL	1690.64	1762.47	1.042

Figure 14.13 Marked spinal scoliosis may interfere with ROI settings and patient positioning.

important independent predictors of BMD in pre- and postmenopausal women for both regional and the total skeleton is controversial.[86–88] There are differences in skeletal muscle, fat and bone mineral mass between black and white females.[89]

To date, nearly 20 years after its first evaluation and 15 years after practical clinical instruments based on DPA became available, body composition analysis has not moved out of the speciality laboratory. Its usefulness as a single test in general medical practice where decisions are made on individual patients is still being evaluated. This is due mainly to the fact that often the basic two- or three-compartment model approach gives little reliable additional information not already available from clinical examination, body weight and skinfold measurements. Together with other tests of body composition such as IVNAA, dilution techniques or bioimpedance, however, DXA may be more useful.

With respect to information on body compo-sition, clinical needs for body composition analysis can be grouped as follows:

1) In acutely ill patients in the intensive care unit, exact information on cell mass, nitrogen balance and fluid shifts from extracellular to intracellular compartments may be important. These patients are usually attached to life-support systems, are not easily transported and cannot co-operate. Bedside or hospital-based procedures are required. Data interpretation is very difficult owing to the frequent problem that assumptions made during calculations often do not apply. In these patients, fluid shifts between subcompartments of lean body mass are of decision-making importance (extra-intracellular water, protein, etc.) and cannot be supplied by absorptiometry methods. The bioimpedance method could be of help, perhaps in combination with absorptiometry. More aggressive measurement approaches using a combination

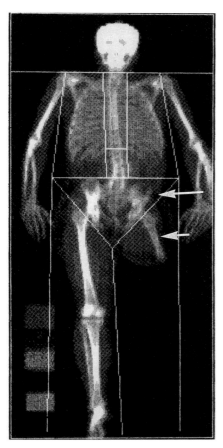

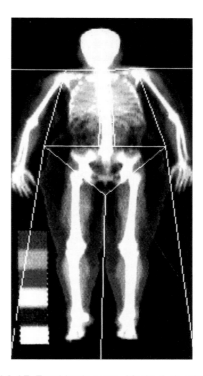

Figure 14.15 Total body scan. Marked obesity: weight 97 kg, height 157 cm. Note the distribution of bone, muscle mass and fat on the image.

Figure 14.14 Total body scan. Above the knee amputation of the left leg. Note the decrease in bone density in the remaining left femur and left hemipelvis due to disuse osteoporosis. In this case, reduced total bone mass does not suggest osteoporosis and correction for the missing limb is needed.

of tests including IVNAA have been proposed in critically ill patients but are not generally used.[90,91] More information on measurement accuracy is needed before the technique can be used on newborn and premature babies for monitoring lean mass and fat.

2) Chronically ill patients, who in general are co-operative and are able to travel to a laboratory outside a hospital if necessary, may need measurements of body composition such as cell mass, fat and energy requirements. It is here where absorptiometry together with other tests can have an impact. In the clinical management of chronic diseases such as cancer and obesity and in the evaluation of therapeutic regimens, body composition measurements by DXA offer an interesting alternative to the anthropometric, densitometric, dilution and body counting methods now used by nutrition specialists. DXA is simple to perform, less dependent on operator skills and experience, and highly reproducible.

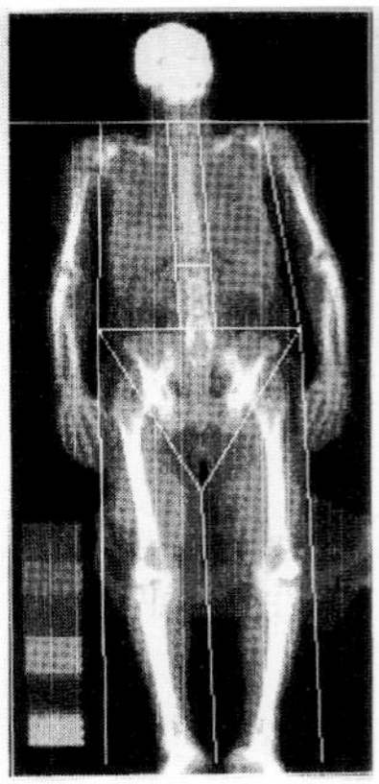

Region	BMC (grams)	Fat (grams)	Lean (grams)
L Arm	200.4	1295.7	3129.1
R Arm	208.0	1401.5	3264.9
Trunk	502.2	8450.1	35743.3
L Leg	571.6	3209.5	9357.1
R Leg	574.2	3139.9	9732.7
SubTot	2056.4	17496.8	61227.2
~Head	552.3	1241.4	4585.8
TOTAL	2608.7	18738.2	65812.9

Figure 14.16 A pillow used to support the knees interferes with soft tissue analysis. Patient was over 6 feet (1.82 m) in height. Note that the feet are cut off in the image.

3) Data collection in the framework of epidemiologic studies of defined population groups, performed at times in remote areas with limited technical facilities, requires non-invasive procedures with low risk and good subject acceptability. Usually, anthropometric and skinfold measurements are used. In this category, absorptiometry equipment may be applicable where technical facilities allow its operation.

4) Evaluation of the effects of therapeutic regimens and drugs on body compartments requires high precision. DXA-based body composition measurements may find application in this area.

ILLUSTRATIVE CASES

A few cases with technical artefacts or with conditions needing special considerations in data analysis are shown in Figures 14.8–14.17. Study of these cases may help in gaining an insight into the application and limits of DXA for gross body composition analysis.

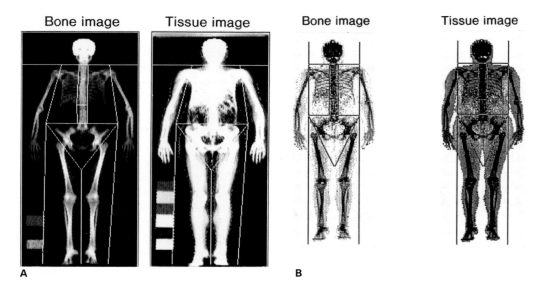

Figure 14.17 Bone and soft tissue images from different instruments: (A) Hologic QDR; (B) Lunar DPX.

APPENDIX: MATHEMATICAL BACKGROUND FOR BODY COMPOSITION STUDIES

By Glen M Blake

Body composition analysis by DPA

The following mathematical explanation of the approach to body composition analysis by DPA is developed from the explanation of bone density measurements by X-ray absorptiometry given in the Appendix to Chapter 3. As in Chapter 3, the equations will be simplified by writing J in place of the logarithmic transmission factor $-\ln(I/I_0)$. Also, as previously, primed variables denote the low-energy photon beam and unprimed variables denote the high-energy beam. The exponential transmission equations for the low- and high-energy beams therefore become:

$$J' = \mu'_s M_s + \mu'_b M_b \qquad (A1a)$$

$$J = \mu_s M_s + \mu_b M_b \qquad (A1b)$$

where μ denotes the mass attenuation coefficient and M the areal density (units: g/cm^2), and subscripts s and b denote soft tissue and bone respectively.

Equations A1a and A1b are two simultaneous equations that enable the areal densities of bone and soft tissue to be calculated from the logarithmic transmission factors, J' and J, measured at the two photon energies. Solving the two equations one obtains:

$$M_b = \frac{J' - (\mu'_s/\mu_s)J}{\mu'_b - (\mu'_s/\mu_s)\mu_b} \qquad (A2a)$$

$$M_s = \frac{(\mu'_b/\mu_b)J - J'}{(\mu'_b/\mu_b)\mu_s - \mu'_s} \qquad (A2b)$$

For total body DPA scans, equations A2a and A2b enable the areal densities of bone and soft tissue to be calculated for those pixels whose ray paths intersect bone. Because there are only two transmission equations to calculate two unknowns (bone and soft tissue mass), no derivation of body composition (i.e. the differentiation between lean and fat soft tissue mass) is possible for those pixels that include bone.

For pixels whose ray paths exclude bone, $M_b = 0$, and equations A1a and A1b reduce to:

$$M_s = J'/\mu'_s = J/\mu_s \qquad (A3)$$

Equation A3 can be rewritten to give:

$$J'_s/J_s = \mu'_s/\mu_s = R_{st} \qquad (A4)$$

where the parameter R_{st}, defined as the ratio of the logarithmic transmission factors for the low- and high-energy radiation through soft tissue, is also equal to the ratio of the respective mass attenuation coefficients. For body composition studies, the importance of R_{st} is that its value is a sensitive measure of the ratio of lean to fat tissue mass (see Figure 14.2). R_{st} values for fat and lean mass are established by calibration with phantoms equivalent to 100% fat and 100% lean mass. For the ^{153}Gd radionuclide source used in DPA systems, pure fat has an R_{st} value of 1.274, and pure lean tissue a value of 1.473. No universally acceptable standards are available, but similar R_{st} values can be obtained from scanning stearic acid (100% fat) and 0.6% saline solution (100% lean mass).

For pixels excluding bone, the total mass of soft tissue can be estimated from the high-energy transmission factor using equation A3 (there is a smaller difference between the μ values of fat and lean tissue for the high-energy photons than for the low-energy photons) and the soft tissue composition can be estimated from R_{st}. The principle is summarized in Figure 14.A1. Transmission measurements at any pixel excluding bone can be plotted, and total soft tissue areal density read from the horizontal axis and soft tissue composition from the vertical axis.

The following procedure can therefore be used to derive values for total body BMD, BMC and body composition:

1) Measure the unattenuated photon flux I_0 from scan pixels through air (e.g. from the first scan line above the patient's head).
2) Use equations A2a and A2b to measure M_b and M_s pixel by pixel over the scan image. Separate the measured points into pixels including bone and those excluding bone by applying a threshold.

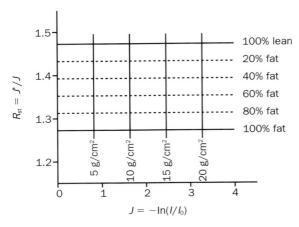

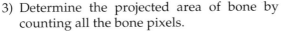

Figure 14.A1 Principle of body composition measurement in DPA. For each soft tissue pixel the high-energy logarithmic transmission factor, J, gives the areal density of total soft tissue. The ratio of low- to high-energy transmissions, $R_{st} = J'/J$, gives information on the percentage fat and percentage lean tissue.

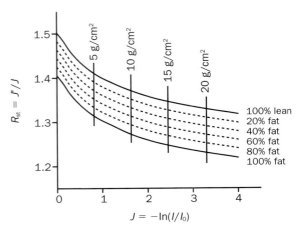

Figure 14.A2 Principle of body composition measurement in DXA. The rectilinear dependence of Figure 14.A1 is altered by beam hardening. In Hologic QDR systems the calibration curves are determined using measurements of a six-step phantom.

3) Determine the projected area of bone by counting all the bone pixels.
4) Determine mean total body BMD by averaging M_b values of all the individual bone pixels.
5) Calculate total body BMC by multiplying mean BMD by projected area.
6) For pixels excluding bone, use the measured values of R_{st} to partition M_s values into fat and lean areal densities using the body composition calibration (Figure 14.A1).
7) For pixels including bone, use the R_{st} values from adjacent soft tissue pixels to partition M_s values into fat and lean areal densities.
8) Determine the mean fat and lean components of M_s over all bone and non-bone pixels.
9) Sum all bone and non-bone pixels to determine the total projected area.
10) Calculate the lean and fat total body masses by multiplying the mean fat and lean components of M_s by the total projected area.

The sum of fat, lean and bone mass gives the body weight. The calculated body weight can be compared with the body weight obtained from scales as a measure of validation (Figure 14.6).

Body composition analysis by DXA

In body composition analysis by DXA the above explanation must be modified because of the effects of beam hardening. The most significant effect of beam hardening is that the relationship between R_{st} and soft tissue composition is no longer independent of total tissue thickness. The rectilinear calibration grid for lines of constant composition in the plot of R_{st} against J shown in Figure 14.A1 therefore becomes a series of curved lines (Figure 14.A2). In Hologic QDR systems, the body composition algorithm is calibrated using a six-step phantom with three thicknesses of lucite (representing 67% fat, 33% lean tissue) and three thicknesses of lucite and aluminium (representing 100% lean tissue). The thicknesses used correspond approximately to the arms, thighs and trunk. If R_{st} is plotted against log J instead of J, the curved lines of constant composition in Figure 14.A2 become quasi-linear. With this proviso, it can be shown that the three lean and three fat calibration points can be interpolated with sufficient accuracy for body composition studies (Rees A-M, Blake GM, unpublished data).

Normal values

Normal values for total bone mineral and body composition analysis performed by DXA on different instruments are included in Tables 14.A1–A3.

Table 14.A1 Normal values (total and regional BMD): Lunar instruments. (Reproduced with permission from J Hanson, Lunar Corp.)

Females (n = 1350)

Age (years)	n	Total body	Arms	Legs	Trunk	Pelvis	Spine
20–29	179	1.120	0.825	1.155	0.905	1.078	1.157
30–39	192	1.142	0.839	1.159	0.927	1.115	1.191
40–49	259	1.123	0.822	1.136	0.911	1.100	1.137
50–59	408	1.086	0.789	1.107	0.875	1.057	1.060
60–69	228	1.034	0.740	1.040	0.841	1.015	1.025
70–79	84	0.979	0.742	0.967	0.801	0.942	0.958
SD		0.08	0.08	0.09	0.07	0.10	0.14

Males (n = 395)

Age (years)	n	Total body	Arms	Legs	Trunk	Pelvis	Spine
20–29	35	1.234	0.976	1.401	1.002	1.218	1.160
30–39	64	1.215	0.984	1.345	0.986	1.204	1.146
40–49	83	1.210	0.995	1.339	0.990	1.196	1.166
50–59	86	1.232	1.000	1.351	1.001	1.196	1.179
60–69	69	1.205	0.977	1.332	0.996	1.164	1.203
70–79	58	1.160	0.937	1.306	0.974	1.126	1.182
SD		0.08	0.08	0.09	0.07	0.10	0.14

Table 14.A2 Normal values (TBBMD): Hologic instruments. (Reproduced with permission from P Steiger, Hologic Inc.)

Males			Females		
Age (years)	BMD (g/cm^2)	SD (g/cm^2)	Age (years)	BMD (g/cm^2)	SD (g/cm^2)
20	1.160	0.094	20	1.102	0.087
25	1.151	0.094	25	1.095	0.087
30	1.142	0.094	30	1.087	0.087
35	1.133	0.094	35	1.077	0.087
40	1.124	0.094	40	1.065	0.087
45	1.115	0.094	45	1.051	0.087
50	1.106	0.094	50	1.036	0.087
55	1.097	0.094	55	1.020	0.087
60	1.088	0.094	60	1.002	0.087
65	1.079	0.094	65	0.982	0.087
70	1.070	0.094	70	0.961	0.087
75	1.061	0.094	75	0.938	0.087
80	1.052	0.094	80	0.914	0.087
85	1.043	0.094	85	0.888	0.087

Table 14.A3 Representative body composition data illustrating age changes and differences between sexes. Data are pooled from studies in the USA and Great Britain. (Reproduced with permission from Howard S Barton, Lunar Corp.)

Females (n = 485)

Age (years)	n	TBBM (g)		Fat (g)		Lean		Non-fat[a]		Tissue[b] (g)		% Fat	
		Mean	SD	Mean	SD	Mean	SD	Mean	SD	Mean	SD	Mean	SD
20–29	111	2537	424	19 556	7836	39 506	4787	42 043	1312	59 062	12 457	31.3	10.4
30–39	94	2580	428	18 270	7951	39 538	4385	42 119	1914	57 771	9 758	30.6	8.6
40–49	60	2639	353	23 284	9353	40 120	3976	42 760	1340	63 404	10 385	35.6	9.2
50–59	143	2400	352	22 373	6932	38 057	4861	40 457	3868	60 468	10 181	36.4	6.6
60–69	52	2240	350	23 124	6581	38 549	4063	40 790	2144	61 673	9 210	36.9	5.9
70–79	25	2256	374	24 162	7369	38 082	4691	40 338	354	62 243	11 270	38.0	6.0

Males (n = 217)

Age (years)	n	TBBM (g)		Fat (g)		Lean		Non-fat[a]		Tissue[b] (g)		% Fat	
		Mean	SD	Mean	SD	Mean	SD	Mean	SD	Mean	SD	Mean	SD
20–29	6	2827	747	14 757	6986	56 954	5089	59 780	3851	71 711	11 918	19.7	6.6
30–39	33	3078	441	15 273	3755	56 036	5263	59 114	5583	71 300	7 121	21.3	4.2
40–49	53	3199	459	16 790	4516	57 007	6101	60 206	5537	73 796	8 760	22.5	4.5
50–59	59	3265	449	18 894	5011	58 150	6276	61 416	6168	77 045	9 929	24.2	4.0
60–69	42	3158	383	18 079	4849	57 473	5484	60 631	4023	75 552	8 533	23.7	4.5
70–79	24	3144	358	17 538	5310	55 255	4527	58 399	2722	72 792	8 445	23.7	5.2

[a] Lean mass + TBBM; [b] fat and lean mass excluding TBBM.

REFERENCES

1. Wang Z, Pierson RN, Heymsfield SB. The five level model: a new approach to organizing body-composition research. *Am J Clin Nutr* (1992) **56**: 19–28.
2. The body cell mass and its supporting environment. In: Moore, Olesen, McMurrey et al. eds. *Body Composition in Health and Disease* (WB Saunders: Philadelphia, London, 1963).
3. Lukaski HC. Methods for the assessment of human body composition: traditional and new. *Am J Clin Nutr* (1987) **46**: 537–56.
4. Heymsfield SB, Wang J, Heshka S et al. Dual photon absorptiometry: comparison of bone mineral and soft tissue mass measurements in vivo with established methods. *Am J Clin Nutr* (1989) **49**: 1283–9.
5. Heymsfield SB, Wang J, Lichtman S et al. Body composition in elderly subjects: a critical appraisal of clinical methodology. *Am J Clin Nutr* (1989) **50**: 1167–75.
6. Whitehead RG, Prentice A, eds. *New techniques in nutritional research* (Academic Press: Boston, 1991).
7. McNeill G, Fowler PA, Maughan RJ et al. Body fat in lean and overweight women estimated by six methods. *Br J Nutr* (1991) **65**: 95–103.
8. van der Kooy K, Seidell JC. Techniques for the measurement of visceral fat: a practical guide. *Int J Obes* (1993) **17**: 187–96.
9. Larson DE, Hesslink RL, Hrovat MI et al. Dietary effects of exercising muscle metabolism and performance by ^{31}P-MRS. *J Appl Physiol* (1994) **77**: 1108–15.
10. Ross R, Pedwell H, Rissanen J. Effects of energy restriction and exercise on skeletal muscle and adipose tissue in women as measured by magnetic resonance imaging. *Am J Clin Nutr* (1995) **61**: 1179–85.
11. Yanovski JA, Yanovski SZ, Filmer KM et al. Differences in body composition of black and white girls. *Am J Clin Nutr* (1996) **64**: 833–9.
12. Tothill P, Han TS, Avenell A et al. Comparisons between fat measurements by dual-energy X-ray absorptiometry, underwater weighing and magnetic resonance imaging in healthy women. *Eur J Clin Nutr* (1996) **50**: 747–52.
13. Abe T, Tanaka F, Kawakami Y et al. Total and segmental subcutaneous adipose tissue volume measured by ultrasound. *Med Sci Sports Exerc* (1996) **28**: 908–12.
14. Seidell JC, Bakker CJG, van der Kooy K. Imaging techniques for measuring adipose-tissue distribution – a comparison between computed tomography and 1.5-T magnetic resonance. *Am J Clin Nutr* (1990) **15**: 589–99.
15. Zamboni M, Armellini F, Milani MP et al. Evaluation of regional body fat distribution: comparison between W/H ratio and computed tomography in obese women. *J Intern Med* (1992) **232**: 341–7.
16. Ross RL, Leger L, Guardo R et al. Adipose tissue volume measured by magnetic resonance imaging and computerized tomography in rats. *J Appl Physiol* (1991) **70**: 2164–72.
17. Behnke AR. Physiologic studies pertaining to deep sea diving and aviation, especially in relation to the fat content and composition of the human body. *Harvey Lect* (1941–1942) **37**: 198–265.
18. Behnke AR, Feen BG, Welham WC. Specific gravity of healthy men. *JAMA* (1942) **118**: 495–8.
19. Wang J, Pierson RN Jr. Disparate hydration of adipose and lean tissue require a new model for body water distribution in man. *J Nutr* (1976) **106**: 1687–93.
20. Pierson RN Jr, Wang J. Body composition denominators for measurements of metabolism: what measurements can be believed? *Mayo Clinic Proc* (1988) **63**: 947–9.
21. Jensen MD, Kanaley JA, Roust LR et al. Body composition assessment using dual energy x-ray absorptiometry: evaluation and comparison with other methods. *Mayo Clinic Proc* (1993) **68**: 867–73.
22. Schoeller DA, van Santen E, Peterson DW et al. Total body water measurement in humans with ^{18}O and ^{2}H labelled water. *Am J Clin Nutr* (1980) **33**: 2686–93.
23. Burkinshaw L, Morgan DB, Silverton NP et al. Total body nitrogen and its relation to body potassium and fat free mass in healthy subjects. *Clin Sci* (1981) **61**: 457–62.
24. Peppler WW, Mazess RB. Total body bone mineral and lean body mass by dual photon absorptiometry. I. Theory and measurement procedure. *Calcif Tissue Int* (1981) **33**: 353–9.
25. Mazess RB, Peppler WW, Gibbons MS. Total body composition by dual photon (^{153}Gd) absorptiometry. *Am J Clin Nutr* (1984) **40**: 834–9.
26. Gotfredsen A, Jensen J, Borg J, Christiansen C. Measurement of lean body mass and total body fat using dual photon absorptiometry. *Metabolism* (1986) **35**: 88–93.
27. Pietrobelli A, Formica C, Wang Z, Heymsfield

SB. Dual-energy x-ray absorptiometry composition model: review of physical concepts. *Am J Physiol* (1996) **34:** E941–51.

28. Heymsfield SB, Wang J, Kehayias JJ et al. Chemical determination of human body density in vivo: relevance to hydrodensitometry. *Am J Clin Nutr* (1989) **50:** 1282–9.

29. Mazess RB, Peppler WW, Chesnut CH et al. Total body bone mineral and lean body mass by dual photon absorptiometry. II. Comparison with total body calcium by neutron activation analysis. *Calcif Tissue Int* (1981) **33:** 361–3.

30. Hassager C, Sorensen SS, Nielsen B et al. Body composition measurement by dual photon absorptiometry: comparison with body density and total body potassium measurements. *Clin Physiol* (1989) **9:** 353–60.

31. Hassager C, Gotfredsen A, Jensen J et al. Prediction of body composition by age, height, weight, and skin fold thickness in normal adults. *Metabolism* (1996) **35:** 1081–4.

32. Nord RH, Payne RK. Whole body phantom for DEXA performance evaluation. In: Ring EFJ ed. *Current Research in Osteoporosis and Bone Mineral Measurement.* (London: British Institute of Radiology, 1990), 28.

33. Koyama H, Nishizawa Y, Yamashita N et al. Measurement of composition changes using dual-photon absorptiometry in obese patients undergoing semistarvation. *Metabolism* (1990) **39:** 302–6.

34. Lands LC, Heigenhausser GJF, Gordon C et al. Accuracy of measurements of small changes in soft tissue mass by use of dual-photon absorptiometry. *J Appl Physiol* (1992) **71:** 698–702.

35. Patel R, Blake GM, Herd RJM, Fogelman I. The effect of weight change on DXA scans in a 2-year trial of etidronate therapy. *Calcif Tissue Int* (1997) **61:** 393–9.

36. Formica C, Atkinson MG, Nyulasi I et al. Changes in body composition following haemodialysis: studies using dual energy x-ray absorptiometry and bioelectrical impedance analysis. *Osteoporos Int* (1993) **3:** 192–7.

37. Going SB, Murano MP, Hall MC et al. Detection of small changes in body composition by dual energy x-ray absorptiometry. *Am J Clin Nutr* (1993) **57:** 845–50.

38. Blake GM, McKeeney DB, Chhaya SC et al. Dual energy x-ray absorptiometry: the effects of beam hardening on bone density measurements. *Med Phys* (1992) **19:** 459–65.

39. Johnson J, Dawson-Hughes B. Precision and stability of dual-energy x-ray absorptiometry measurements. *Calcif Tissue Int* (1991) **49:** 174–8.

40. Mazess RB, Barden HS, Bisek JP, Hansen J. Dual energy x-ray absorptiometry for total-body and regional bone mineral and soft tissue composition. *Am J Clin Nutr* (1990) **51:** 1106–12.

41. Jebb SA, Goldberg GR, Elia M. The effect of depth and composition on fat and bone measured by dual energy X-ray absorptiometry. International Symposium on In vivo Body Composition Studies, 10–12 November 1992, Houston, Texas (abstract 71).

42. Svendsen O, Haarbo J, Hassager C et al. Accuracy of measurements of body composition by dual energy X-ray absorptiometry in vivo. International Symposium on In vivo Body Composition Studies, 10–12 November 1992, Houston, Texas (abstract 78).

43. Taylor A, Konrad PT, Norman ME, Harcke HT. Total body bone mineral density in young children: influence of head bone mineral density. *J Bone Miner Res* (1997) **12:** 652–5.

44. Tothill P, Hannan WJ, Cowen S, Freeman CP. Anomalies in the measurement of changes in total-body bone mineral by dual-energy x-ray absorptiometry during weight change. *J Bone Miner Res* (1997) **12:** 1908–21.

45. Griffiths MR, Noakes KA, Pocock NA. Correcting the magnification error of fan beam densitometers. *J Bone Miner Res* (1997) **12:** 119–23.

46. Griffiths M, Noakes K, Pocock N. Errors in body composition using fan beam DXA due to variation in fat distribution. Annual Scientific Meeting of the Australian and New Zealand Bone and Mineral Society, Canberra, Australia, 1997 (abstract).

47. Fuerst T, Genant HK. Evaluation of body composition and total body bone mass with the Hologic QDR-4500. *Osteoporos Int* (1996) **6**(suppl 1): 203.

48. Blake GM, Parker JC, Buxton FMA, Fogelman I. Dual x-ray absorptiometry: a comparison between fan beam and pencil beam scans. *Br J Radiol* (1993) **66:** 902–6.

49. Eiken P, Kolthoff N, Bärenholdt O et al. Switching from DXA pencil-beam to fan-beam. II. Studies in vivo. *Bone* (1994) **15:** 671–6.

50. Abrahamsen B, Gram J, Hansen TB, Beck-Nielsen H. Cross calibration of QDR-2000 and QDR-1000 dual-energy x-ray densitometers for bone mineral and soft-tissue measurements. *Bone* (1995) **16:** 385–90.

51. Spector E, LeBlanc A, Shackelford L. Hologic QDR 2000 whole body scans: a comparison of three combinations of scan modes and analysis software. *Osteoporos Int* (1995) **5:** 440–5.

52. Clasey JL, Hartman ML, Kanaley J et al. Body composition by DEXA in older adults: accuracy and influence of scan mode. *Med Sci Sports Exerc* (1997) **29:** 560–7.

53. Kelly TL, Shepherd JA, Steiger P, Stein JA. Accurate body composition assessment using fan-beam DXA: technical and practical considerations. *J Bone Miner Res* (1997) **12**(suppl 1): S269.

54. Formica C, Nieves J, Dixon J et al. A body composition cross calibration phantom. *Osteoporos Int* (1997) **7:** 278.

55. Gotfredsen A, Podenphant J, Nilas L, Christiansen C. Discriminative ability of total body bone-mineral measured by dual photon absorptiometry. *Scand J Clin Lab Invest* (1989) **49:** 125–34.

56. Nuti R, Martini G. Measurements of bone mineral density by DXA total body absorptiometry in different skeletal sites in postmenopausal osteoporosis. *Bone* (1992) **13:** 173–8.

57. Nuti R, Martini G. Effects of age and menopause on bone density of entire skeleton in healthy and osteoporotic women. *Osteoporos Int* (1993) **3:** 59–65.

58. Bagur A, Vega E, Mautalen C. Discrimination of total body bone mineral density measured by DEXA in vertebral osteoporosis. *Calcif Tissue Int* (1995) **56:** 263–7.

59. Lau EMC, Chan HHL, Woo J et al. Body composition and bone mineral density of Chinese women with vertebral fracture. *Bone* (1996) **19:** 657–62.

60. Michaëlsson K, Bergström R, Mallmin H et al. Screening for osteopenia and osteoporosis: selection by body composition. *Osteoporos Int* (1996) **6:** 120–6.

61. Greenspan SL, Maitland-Ramsey L, Myers E. Classification of osteoporosis in the elderly is dependent on site-specific analysis. *Calcif Tissue Int* (1996) **58:** 409–14.

62. Nordin BEC, Chatterton BE, Schultz CG et al. Regional bone mineral density interrelationships in normal and osteoporotic postmenopausal women. *J Bone Miner Res* (1996) **11:** 849–56.

63. Revilla RM, Hernández ER, Villa LF et al. Total body bone measurements in spinal osteoporosis by dual-energy x-ray absorptiometry. *Calcif Tissue Int* (1997) **61:** 44–7.

64. Kohrt WM, Birge SJ Jr. Differential effects of estrogen treatment on bone mineral density of the spine, hip, wrist and total body in late postmenopausal women. *Osteoporos Int* (1995) **5:** 150–5.

65. Chesnut CH, McClung MR, Ensrud KE et al. Alendronate treatment of the postmenopausal osteoporotic woman: effect of multiple dosages on bone mass and bone remodeling. *Am J Med* (1995) **99:** 144–51.

66. Liberman UA, Weiss SR, Bröll J et al. Effect of oral alendronate on bone mineral density and the incidence of fractures in postmenopausal osteoporosis. *N Engl J Med* (1995) **333:** 1437–43.

67. Lloyd T, Martel JK, Rollings N et al. The effect of calcium supplementation and tanner stage on bone density, content and area in teenage women. *Osteoporos Int* (1996) **6:** 276–83.

68. Tucci JR, Tonino RP, Emkey RD et al. Effect of three years of oral alendronate treatment in postmenopausal women with osteoporosis. *Am J Med* (1996) **101:** 488–501.

69. Lindsay R, Nieves J, Formica C et al. Randomised controlled study of effect of parathyroid hormone on vertebral-bone mass and fracture incidence among postmenopausal women on oestrogen with osteoporosis. *Lancet* (1997) **350:** 550–5.

70. Barger-Lux MJ, Heaney RP, Hayes J et al. Vitamin D receptor gene polymorphism, bone mass, body size, and vitamin D receptor density. *Calcif Tissue Int* (1995) **57:** 161–2.

71. Harris SS, Eccleshall TR, Gross C et al. The vitamin D receptor start codon polymorphism (FokI) and bone mineral density in premenopausal American black and white women. *J Bone Miner Res* (1997) **12:** 1043–8.

72. Seidell JC, Oosterlee A, Deurenberg P et al. Abdominal fat depots measured with computed tomography: effects of degree of obesity, sex, and age. *Eur J Clin Nutr* (1988) **42:** 805–15.

73. Seidell JC, Deurenberg P, Hautvast JGAJ. Obesity and fat distribution in relationship to health – current insights and recommendations. *World Rev Nutr Diet* (1987) **52:** 51–87.

74. Kissebah AH, Vydelingum N, Murray R et al. Relation of body fat distribution to metabolic complications of obesity. *J Clin Endocrinol Metab* (1982) **54:** 254–60.

75. Larsson B, Svardsudd K, Welin L et al. Abdominal adipose tissue distribution, obesity, and risk of cardiovascular disease and death: a 13 year follow-up of participants in the study of men born in 1913. *Br Med J* (1984) **288:** 1401–4.

76. Cohn SH, Vaswani A, Zanzi I et al. Changes in body chemical composition with age measured by total-body neutron activation. *Metabolism* (1976) **25**: 85–95.

77. Flynn MA, Nolph GB, Baker AS et al. Total body potassium in aging humans: a longitudinal study. *Am J Clin Nutr* (1989) **50**: 713–17.

78. Forbes GB, Raina JC. Adult lean body mass declines with age: some longitudinal observations. *Metabolism* (1970) **19**: 653–63.

79. Shimokata H, Tobin JD, Muller DC et al. Studies in the distribution of body fat. I. Effects of age, sex, and obesity. *J Gerontol* (1989) **44**: 66–73.

80. Schwartz RS, Shuman WP, Bradbury VL et al. Body fat distribution in healthy young and older men. *J Gerontol* (1990) **45**: 181–5.

81. Aitken JM, Anderson JB, Horton PW. Seasonal variation in bone mineral content after the menopause. *Nature* (1973) **241**: 59–60.

82. Hyldstrup L, McNair P, Jensen GF et al. Seasonal variations in indices of bone formation precede appropriate bone mineral changes in normal men. *Bone* (1986) **7**: 167–70.

83. Krolner B. Seasonal variation of lumbar spine bone mineral content in normal women. *Calcif Tissue Int* (1983) **35**: 145–7.

84. Bergstrahl EJ, Sinaki M, Offord KP et al. Effect of season on physical activity score, back extensor muscle strength, and lumbar bone mineral density. *J Bone Miner Res* (1990) **5**: 371–7.

85. Dawson-Hughes B, Harris S. Regional changes in body composition by time of year in healthy postmenopausal women. *Am J Clin Nutr* (1992) **56**: 307–13.

86. Reid IR, Ames R, Evans MC et al. Determinants of total body and regional bone mineral density in normal postmenopausal women – a key role for fat mass. *J Clin Endocrinol Metab* (1992) **75**: 45–51.

87. Nishizawa Y, Koyama H, Shoji T et al. Obesity as a determinant of regional bone mineral density. *J Nutr Sci Vitaminol* (1991) **37**: S65–70.

88. Seeman E, Hopper JL, Young NR et al. Do genetic-factors explain associations between muscle strength, lean mass and bone-density – a twin study. *Am J Physiol* (1996) **33**: E320–7.

89. Adams WC, Deck-Cote K. Racial comparison of % body fat via dual energy x-ray absorptiometry and a hydrostatic weighing multicomponent model in young adult females. *Med Sci Sports Exerc* (1992) **24**: S117.

90. Beddoe AH, Streat SJ, Hill GL. Evaluation of an in vivo prompt gamma neutron activation facility for body composition studies in critically ill intensive care patients: results on 41 normals. *Metabolism* (1984) **33**: 270–80.

91. Beddoe AH, Streat SJ, Hill GL. Hydration of fat-free body in protein depleted patients. *Am J Physiol* (1985) **249**: E227–33

15

DXA in the Growing Skeleton

Guest chapter by H Theodore Harcke

CHAPTER OVERVIEW

The objective of this chapter is to review pertinent issues concerning the use of dual-energy X-ray absorptiometry (DXA) to measure the growing skeleton. Assumptions made in the development of algorithms for adults may not be valid in younger children. The detection of very low bone mineral density appears to require alteration of scan techniques established for adults. Normative data have been published for most age groups and the effects of puberty on bone mineral density (BMD) are evident. Some clinical reports attest to the potential for use of bone mineral measurements in diagnosis and management of paediatric disorders affecting the skeleton.

INTRODUCTION

Measurement of bone mass density in paediatric patients is not simply a matter of applying adult principles and methodology to a younger age group. The focus in adults is on osteoporosis, decreased bone mass with normal mineralization. In children, decreased bone mass should be considered osteopenia, a less specific description encompassing all classes of pathology involving reduced bone mass. The focus in adults has been with women's health, where a large segment of the population is at risk.

Specific attention has been given to identification of fracture risk in that population and, more recently, the use of osteotrophic treatments to lower this risk. Conversely, only small segments of the paediatric age group are the focus of BMD studies. Principally, these are targeted groups of children with conditions that have the potential for reducing bone mineral content. These include congenital and acquired skeletal and metabolic disorders, secondary effects of medical therapy and neuromuscular disorders that affect ambulation (mobility). As with adults, the study of bone mass is currently directed towards identifying children at risk and instituting interventions that lower the risk. While a short-term goal might be prevention of fracture, an equally important long-term goal is the achievement of an appropriate peak bone mass in early adult life as 'preparation' for the later adult decades. In this latter goal, it may be that attention will shift from targeted groups to the 'well' paediatric population also.

Fundamental to the use of bone densitometry in infants, children and adolescents is an understanding of normal patterns of mineralization in the growing skeleton. DXA studies of lumbar spine, whole body and specific regional sites have begun and are continuing. The advent of DXA with its good precision, faster scan time and low radiation dose has given new impetus to the acquisition of normal data, the study of factors that influence development of bone mass, and the identification of decreased bone mass in patients with specific paediatric disorders and therapies.

SPECIAL CONSIDERATIONS IN PAEDIATRIC BONE MINERAL MEASUREMENTS

The same controversies that exist in adult methodology have paediatric counterparts. Which is the best way to measure the 'health' of bone? Trabecular bone, as in adults, is considered more sensitive than cortical bone. What sites provide the best indication of bone 'health'? Whole body, lumbar spine and peripheral sites are being assessed. Peripheral measurements at the hip, wrist and calcaneus are potential indicators for whole body density and fracture risk but this probably depends upon the nature of the pathology. Considerable work is going to be required because assumptions from adult data on fracture risk may not necessarily be applicable to paediatrics.

Growth and development of the skeleton, occurring throughout the paediatric age range until skeletal maturity in adolescence, raise a number of fundamental questions about DXA measurements. Bone mineral measurements made by DXA are not independent of bone size. As bone mineral content (BMC) is measured with DXA, both bone mineralization and bone size influence the result. The calculation of bone mineral density (bone mineral content in grams/area in cm^2) can correct for changes in bone size in the scanning plane, but cannot account for changes in the thickness of the bones scanned. This has been a criticism of DXA by those who advocate the determination of density by quantitative computed tomography (QCT).

In small children, the physical size of the bones and relatively low levels of BMC have presented technical problems for equipment manufacturers. Adult algorithms utilize a soft tissue/bone threshold above the level required for young and profoundly osteopenic patients. This results in the reporting of zero values for BMC in regions of the skeleton such as the spine and extremities. It will result in the erro-

neous estimation of regional and total body BMD. If the area measure used for the calculation of BMD does not include all the bones, the calculation (BMC/area) will give a falsely elevated value (Figure 15.1). When interpreting children's DXA scans, particular attention should be paid to the clues that spurious values are being generated. Some manufacturers have developed software modifications that improve the ability to identify low-density bone. At present, such software can be used for regional scans (e.g. lumbar spine) but is not yet available for total body scanning (Figure 15.2).

The change in bone mineral composition with age in the developing skeleton could also introduce error. A changing absorption coefficient for bone would make measurements of BMD invalid since both changing bone mass and absorption coefficient would confuse the outcome of the measurement. It is assumed that changes in bone composition do not constitute a source of error for DXA measurements. Dunnill et al. suggest that bone composition shows no major changes throughout life.[1]

The growth plates of the growing skeleton are highly active metabolically and contain increased bone mineral content. Contributions of individual growth plates to regional or total body BMC could vary, depending upon the maturational state. These plates fuse at variable times during adolescence and introduce the potential for variability in measurements made in populations. In assessing a peripheral site such as the distal radius and hip, growth plate activity has the potential to influence longitudinal measurements made at that site. Region of interest selection that excludes the plate may be prudent in peripheral DXA studies.

The distribution of fat in bone marrow changes during childhood. Magnetic resonance imaging (MRI) has documented the pattern of change from red marrow to yellow marrow, but it is not clear if this has a significant effect on regional DXA measurements. It has been established in adults that fat falsely reduces mineral values. The percentage of fat in the bone marrow increases in bones such as the pelvis and appendicular skeleton throughout childhood and may produce an effect on BMD.

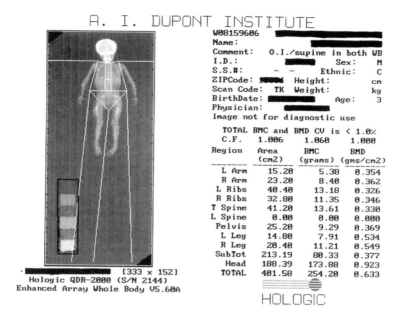

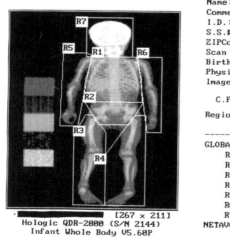
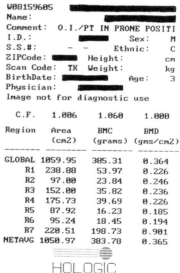

Figure 15.1 A 3-year-old female with osteogenesis imperfecta and healing fractures shows the effect of technique on measurement of BMC and BMD. (A) Whole body scan; enhanced array whole body (adult) software gives a zero value for the lumbar spine and highly variable area measures for the limbs. (B) Scanning with infant whole body software yields substantially different BMC, which may be more accurate but raises other concerns. This may underestimate the BMD if area measures include non-osseous tissue.

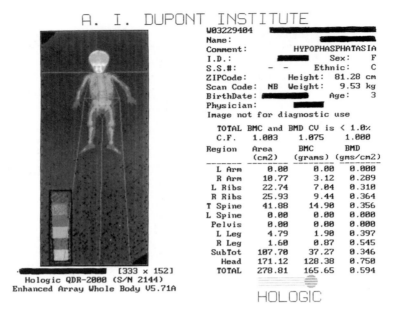

A

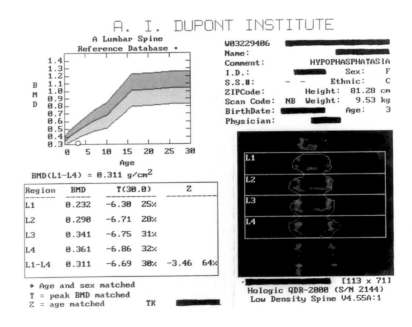

B

Figure 15.2 A 3-year-old female with hypophosphatasia. (A) The whole body scan overlooks bone below the detectable threshold of adult-based software (enhanced whole body array). This is manifest by regional zero values. (B) A lumbar spine scan with special low-density software identifies bone with density significantly below the normal range for age (Z = −3.46).

Changes in body dimensions that occur in the growing child may conflict with assumptions made for adults. Algorithms for calculating BMD in the axial and appendicular skeleton rely on separation of bone from soft tissue. The assumptions made for adults may not be valid in small children.

Similarly, the algorithm for total body imaging in adults makes assumptions for the skull that there has been reason to question. In correlating whole body measurements with age, it was found that subtotal BMD, all the bones of the skeleton except for the skull, correlated better with age than did total body BMD.[2] With the authors' equipment, the algorithm for determining skull bone mineral content was developed and optimized for adults. The algorithm for determining head BMC uses the body composition step phantom to determine the soft tissue baseline of the skull. This is necessary because there is insufficient soft tissue surrounding the calvarium to enable the same methodology employed for BMC determination in other regions. In clinical work, patients have been encountered with low subtotal and regional values of BMD whose total body BMD falls within the normal range (within 2 standard deviations (SD) of the age mean) because of the skull contribution. It is not known if it is clinically accurate to consider these studies 'normal' and call attention to the pattern in the report.

NORMAL VALUES IN PAEDIATRICS

The utility of DXA in clinical applications is dependent upon the existence of well constructed normative data. There is no disagreement with the need for separate tables by sex. In constructing tables for males and females, there is the option of separating the population by age, weight, height, body mass index or sexual development (Tanner score). It is most common to select age, as has been done with adults.[3–5]

The selection criteria for subjects used in developing normative tables generally exclude individuals with extremes of height and weight. In the authors' laboratory, any child falling below the 5th percentile or exceeding the 95th percentile for either height or weight was excluded.[2] Obviously, children with congenital, metabolic and system diseases must be excluded. The influence of chronically used medications would also be grounds for exclusion. Where it becomes more difficult to judge subjects, is in regard to diet and physical exercise. There is a wide range of variability and these questions are best dealt with by accumulating a large sample size with some socioeconomic heterogeneity. In selecting adolescents for normative studies, it would be important to exclude those who smoked and/or had a history of alcohol or drug consumption.

It is accepted that the onset of puberty will influence the normative data because of its influence on skeletal growth. It is well established that sexual maturity brings a significant rise in bone mineral content; however, the standard normative tables continue to use chronologic age for the population without regard to sexual maturity. In areas where genetic and/or environmental effects affect the onset of puberty, revised normal BMD values could be required.

The influence of geography is interesting to contemplate. Exposure to sunlight is known to affect circulating levels of vitamin D and this could influence bone mineralization. It could be argued that normative data obtained from subjects in temperate climates might differ from data obtained in tropical climates. Sheth et al. studied healthy Newfoundland adolescents and compared their lumbar spine BMD to a predicted value by age and gender for different areas of North America and Europe.[6] They concluded that lumbar spine BMD measurements in most healthy adolescent populations are comparable. Based upon their report, the requirement for specific normative data by region may not be necessary. Seasonal variation in BMD has not been studied; however, seasonable variability in circulating vitamin D levels would raise the possibility that a small variation in measurement could take place. It is probable that seasonal variation is of less significance than other factors; nevertheless an attempt was made to control for this in developing laboratory norms by studying children only in the spring and autumn months of the year.

Racial differences in bone mineral density have been found as might be expected. While the reasons for this are varied, Gilsanz et al. proposed that this is due to bone size and not BMD.[7] Their QCT study, which controlled for the morphologic characteristics of the bone, determined that black and white children had no actual differences in BMD. The apparent differences from DXA studies were due to the failure of the technique to compensate for volumetric differences in the bones of the black and white subjects.

Recognizing the combination of factors that have the potential to influence BMD, Boot et al. analysed the association of height, weight, pubertal stage, calcium intake and physical activity with BMD measurements in 500 subjects in the paediatric age range 4–12 years.[8] They analysed lumbar spine volumetric BMD, which was calculated to correct for bone size. While several variables were significantly associated with spinal BMD, the major independent determinate of BMD was the Tanner stage in girls and weight in boys.

Finally, the technique itself, used in the derivation of normal values, may influence the measurement. It was found that regression equations for total bone density with age as a predictor did not explain enough of the variance to warrant use for predicting total body BMD (TBMD). Subtotal bone mineral density, obtained by eliminating the head contribution to TBMD, was predicted better by age.[2] As explained in the previous section, this was attributed to the head algorithm used in determining BMC. In addition, skull size, in proportion to the body, is not constant in children as it is in adults. In children, 80% of adult skull volume is achieved by 3 years, whereas other body structures grow linearly.

Recognizing that a number of variables will influence the establishment of norms, DXA studies have been reported for most age groups and form the basis for comparison as individual laboratories acquire their own data. Before using norms established by equipment manufacturers or published literature, it is important for each laboratory to understand the basis for the construct of the data.

In 1992, Venkataraman and Ahluwalia published values for newborns based upon a study of 28 term infants.[9] Their total body bone mineral content correlated significantly with the bone mineral content as measured in the distal third of the radius by single photon absorptiometry. They also determined body composition and found that determinations of bone mineral content, fat and lean body mass fell within the ranges expected based upon values measured by chemical analysis of an infant cadaver.

Between newborn and 2 years of age, there is a paucity of normative DXA data. Naturally, this is due to the difficulty in examining normal subjects. Since sedation in this age group is virtually a necessity, there is an increased risk of participation in any study designed to obtain these values. Institutional review boards are reluctant to approve studies when sedation is incorporated with the procedure. The authors' laboratory has been successful in obtaining whole body data on only a few children under 4 years of age that have been scanned successfully while asleep. Infant whole body software may be required for accurate assessment, especially when osteopenia is present (Figure 15.3). Lumbar spine and peripheral measurements are available for this age group and are based on small sample sizes.

A number of studies have reported normative values for children and adolescents in the 2–20-year-old age range.[10] A large group of Canadian children aged 8–17 years are being studied longitudinally by Faulkner et al.[3,4] The sample size makes their findings credible and their observations reflect what predominates in the literature. While they initially reported total body bone mineral content and density with values for selected regions of interest,[3] the subsequent data continue tracking the total body data but focus on regional measurement on the proximal femur and antero-posterior lumbar spine.[4] Bone mineral content and density progressively increase during childhood and then

A. I. DUPONT INSTITUTE

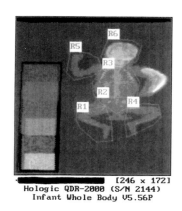

```
W08129306    ███████████████
Name:        █████████████
Comment:                  FX LT HUMRUS
I.D.:              ██████   Sex:     F
S.S.#:        -   -   Ethnic:        C
ZIPCode:           Height:   30.48 cm
Scan Code:   NB  Weight:    4.54 kg
BirthDate:   ████████   Age:      0
Physician:              ███
Image not for diagnostic use
```

```
   C.F.     1.003      1.075      1.000

 Region    Area       BMC        BMD
           (cm2)    (grams)   (gms/cm2)
------- --------- --------- ----------
 GLOBAL   427.36    137.84      0.323
     R1    28.81      4.64      0.161
     R2    19.35      2.62      0.136
     R3   121.73     23.26      0.191
     R4    35.91      6.45      0.180
     R5    13.89      1.69      0.122
     R6   118.75     51.86      0.437
 NETAVG   336.60     90.24      0.268
```

HOLOGIC

[246 x 172]
Hologic QDR-2000 (S/N 2144)
Infant Whole Body V5.56P

Figure 15.3 A 2-month-old female with osteopenia and a left humeral fracture (splinted). Note that the scan was performed with infant whole body software. The whole body density is well below the range reported for normal term newborns.[9]

increase at an accelerated rate with the onset of puberty during adolescence. Normal children aged 8 years and below were studied by the authors in order to overlap the data with Faulkner's values. These were consistent and form the basis for the laboratory's values (Figure 15.4).

CLINICAL UTILIZATION

Bone mineral measurement with DXA is becoming more widely utilized in the clinical evaluation of children with conditions that affect mineralization of the skeleton. The precision and accuracy of DXA have been documented and are deemed acceptable in the assessment of paediatric patients. When dealing with young children or older patients, who are

unable to co-operate, it may be necessary to use sedation. Duration required will depend upon extent of the scan. A whole body scan is influenced by the length of the patient and the procedure will be further extended if separate regional data such as the spine and/or hip are being acquired in addition to the whole body scan. Monitoring equipment, which is in standard use for other paediatric imaging techniques, will create artefacts and/or influence measurement if it is included in the scan area. It is also common to encounter current and/or past medical treatments which can potentially influence the performance of a whole body scan or regional scan. The effect of prior surgical procedures involving bone and soft tissue with and without metal instrumentation is an obvious issue. For acute cases, the presence of casts, splints, intravenous apparatus and monitoring

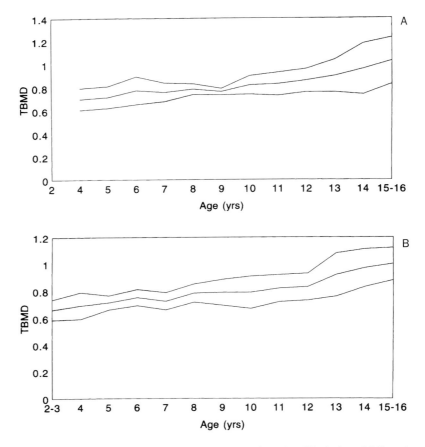

Figure 15.4 Normative values: total body BMD in males (A) and females (B) during childhood and adolescence. The curves with mean and range (±2 SD) represent a combination of data from Taylor[2] and Faulkner.[4] Note the gradual increase with age and the increase at puberty.

equipment must also be considered when planning a study and in interpreting the results.[11]

When patient co-operation and the present and past effects of the disease and/or treatment restrict the use of DXA, the question arises as to how reliably measurement of one region reflects other regions and/or the whole body measurement itself. For example, measurement of the lumbar spine may or may not be predictive of whole body measurement and/or measurement at the hip. Henderson[12] found correlation between the measurement of lum-

bar spine BMD and the proximal femur. On the other hand, Shore[13] found the correlation between the lumbar spine and forearm in children to be negligible. Care must be taken to infer that axial and appendicular measurements can be used interchangeably with whole body measurements and vice versa.

Another related question concerning regional measurements would be correlation between measurements of paired sites. Henderson compared the right and left proximal femur in a group of patients and found that measurements did not significantly differ in the absence of an obvious clinical situation. He stated, however, that sampling is best done from different regions such as the hip and spine rather than by sampling contralateral structures.[12]

While in adults it has become routine to use BMD in clinical practice, there are some that advocate expressing results as BMC.[14] This is done to overcome the potential problem of changing bone thickness in the growing child and adolescent. It also may negate the issue of positioning differences from scan to scan and the scanning of patients who cannot be in the anatomic whole body position because of musculoskeletal deformity.

An obviously confounding issue in the study of patients with disease is the use of BMD Z-scores. As noted above, it is common to relate BMD measurements of whole body and regional density to age-matched standard deviation (Z-score). It is interesting from a statistical viewpoint that ±2 SD is usually considered as the normal range. When outliers are encountered, there could be factors such as race, weight and pubertal status that account for value and alter the risk compared with the population measured. While the Z-score is quite useful in situations where growth and development have been appropriate for age and the clinical condition and/or intervention is relatively acute, the age-related Z-score for a handicapped child with profound developmental delay is more difficult to accept as relevant. One option is to use the patient as his or her own control and undertake longitudinal measurements. Another conceivable option is to utilize morphologic data such as length and weight to match a child with 'normals' of similar characteristics, irrespective of age. While this may be done for prepubertal children, it may be completely invalid in older children where pubertal effects play a role. Here, it might be more valid to compare patients based on sexual development (Tanner score) in addition to anthropometrics.

CLINICAL APPLICATIONS

The use of DXA in the clinical care of children is currently being defined. The basis for adult evaluation is risk of fracture. Currently, there are no established values for children but it is assumed that low bone mass constitutes a risk and it is prudent to minimize the risk. With the advent of pharmacologic agents, which have the potential for treatment of children with osteopenia, there is an increasing call for the clinical use of DXA to assess populations at risk. In the past, the principal approach to the diagnosis of decreased bone mineralization was made from skeletal radiographs and was suboptimal. Bone densitometry became the preferred technique. With DXA, it is possible to have more precise longitudinal measures (Figure 15.5). Experience to date suggests that BMD changes relatively slowly (over months as opposed to days/weeks) in the absence of catastrophic alteration of lifestyle. This has implications for the frequency of monitoring children at risk. Most longitudinal studies assess BMD on a semi-annual to annual basis. The more rapidly the clinical situation disrupts calcium homeostasis by mobilizing stores or preventing absorption, the more justifiable is short interval evaluation.

Some congenital forms of osteopenia, such as osteogenesis imperfecta, skeletal dysplasias, storage and metabolic disease, have clinical and radiographic features, which are used in diagnosis (Figure 15.6). There is interest in the use of DXA to establish diagnosis in milder forms of osteogenesis imperfecta, which may not be easily diagnosed. It is also felt that DXA might be helpful in assessing prognosis and in monitoring response to treatment.[15] It should be emphasized that the images produced by DXA are not of diagnostic quality and cannot be used as a substitute for skeletal radiographs.

Acquired forms of osteopenia are associated with conditions in which there is abnormal skeletal development because of an associated disease such as cerebral palsy or other neuromuscular deficiency. Henderson[16] and Wilmshurst[17] have established the importance of ambulatory status to BMD in children and

A

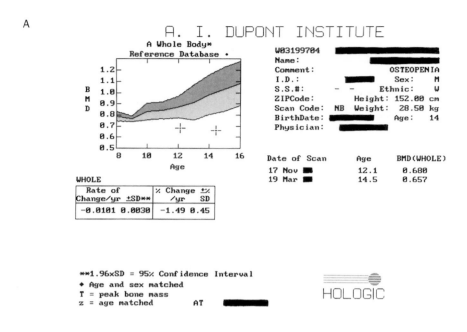

B

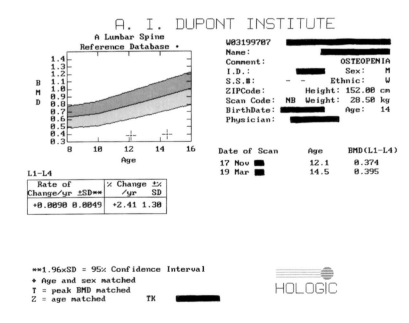

Figure 15.5 A 14-year-old male with osteopenia of undetermined aetiology. Serial DXA measurements of both whole body (A) and lumbar spine (B) reflect no improvement over a 2-year interval. While the rate and per cent change is in the opposite direction, these values are not felt to be significant with just two measurements and small differences.

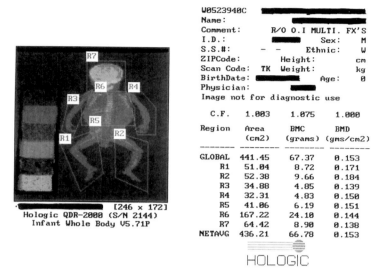

Figure 15.6 A 4-month-old male with multiple fractures and clinical features of osteogenesis imperfecta. Scanning with infant whole body software reveals severely decreased density throughout the skeleton. Note that region R2, the left lower extremity, with healing fractures, has higher BMC and BMD than the right lower extremity (R1).

adolescents with cerebral palsy (CP). Because of physical deformity and prior surgical procedures, it may be impossible to study these patients with whole body, spine or hip techniques. The authors' laboratory has found that scanning the lateral femur is a practical alternative.[18] While lumbar spinal BMD was found to fall further below normal with increasing age in the CP population, there were other factors that were better predictors of fracture risk.[19] This study points out the technical difficulty in studying CP patients and the inherent limitation of using one regional measurement to predict fracture risk in another region.

Decreased bone mineralization can also occur with any condition that results in malnutrition,[20] vitamin deficiency and/or endocrinopathy.[21] Many of the children with low bone mineral density will have this as a result

of treatment for acquired disease. Steroids and anti-metabolites are commonly used for both systemic and neoplastic conditions. Hopp et al. showed no pubertal increase in BMD of the total body and spine in adolescent girls receiving steroids for juvenile rheumatoid arthritis (JRA).[22] Spinal BMD was also reduced in children treated for severe juvenile polyarthritis.[23] A mechanism for the observed decrease in BMD in JRA patients under treatment is suggested by Pepmueller et al. who found lower than normal bone formation.[24] An expected consequence of studies such as these is that DXA will become part of the periodic evaluation of patients whose therapies could lower BMD significantly. For example, the authors are evaluating the DXA monitoring of patients receiving treatment with anti-convulsants that could negatively effect BMD (Figure 15.7).

A

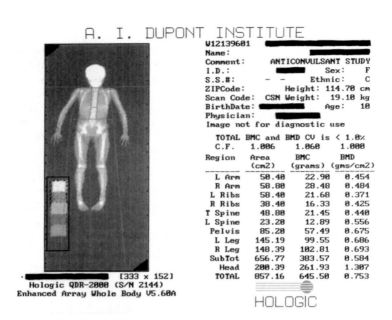

B

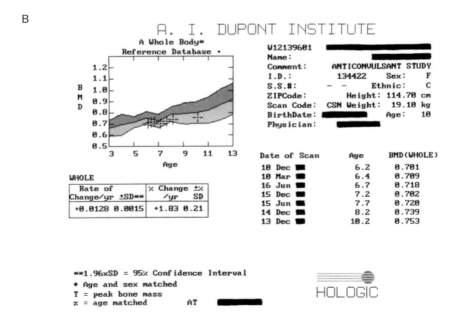

Figure 15.7 A 10-year-old female on long-term anti-convulsant therapy maintained a normal total body density during 4 years of monitoring for drug-induced osteoporosis. (A) Most recent study. (B) Serial measurements. Note rate and per cent change/year.

BMD evaluation is being used to further the understanding of recognized disorders, particularly those in which there is a genetically determined effect on the growth, modelling and/or remodelling of the skeleton and a risk of fracture. Through these studies, the potential is available to learn about the mechanism of the disease and at the same time to learn about the complex biological processes that influence normal bone development prior to skeletal maturity. Finally, if it is correct to assume that optimal peak bone mass in adults requires accumulation of strong bone during childhood and adolescence,[25] then consideration could be given to population screening. This introduces an array of difficult questions ranging from who would be screened, how it should be done and when (age) to do it. A cost justification for any screening plan is an obvious and difficult determination. While the long-term cost/benefit is one aspect, a short-term benefit might be the reduction in fracture risk prior to skeletal maturity. Goulding et al. found that low bone density throughout the skeleton was more common in girls aged 3–15 years than in age- and gender-matched controls that had never broken a bone.[26] It is not inconceivable that simple, inexpensive mass screening techniques could achieve a sensitivity and specificity that justified their use. It would be their role to identify those individuals requiring a more definitive evaluation such as DXA.

REFERENCES

1. Dunnill MS, Anderson JA, Whitehead R. Quantitative histological studies on age changes in bone. *J Pathol Bacteriol* (1967) **94**: 275–91.
2. Taylor A, Konrad PT, Norman ME et al. Total body bone mineral density in young children: influence of head bone mineral density. *J Bone Miner Res* (1997) **12**: 652–5.
3. Faulkner RA, Bailey DA, Drinkwater DT et al. Regional and total body bone mineral content, bone mineral density, and total body tissue composition in children 8–16 years of age. *Calcif Tissue Int* (1993) **53**: 7–12.
4. Faulkner RA, Bailey DA, Drinkwater DT et al. Bone densitometry in Canadian children 8–17 years of age. *Calcif Tissue Int* (1996) **59**: 344–51.
5. Ogle GD, Allen JR, Humphries IRJ et al. Body composition assessment by dual-energy x-ray absorptiometry in subjects aged 4–26y. *Am J Clin Nutr* (1995) **61**: 746–53.
6. Sheth RD, Hobbs GR, Riggs JE et al. Mineral density in geographically diverse adolescent populations. *Pediatrics* (1996) **98**: 948–51.
7. Gilsanz V, Kovanlikaya A, Costin G et al. Differential effect of gender on the sizes of the bones in the axial and appendicular skeleton. *J Clin Endocrinol Metab* (1997) **82**: 1603–7.
8. Boot AM, Ridder MAJ, Pols HAP et al. Bone mineral density in children and adolescents: relation to puberty, calcium intake, and physical activity. *J Clin Endocrinol Metab* (1997) **82**: 57–62.
9. Venkataraman PS, Ahluwalia BW. Total bone mineral content and body composition by X-ray densitometry in newborns. *Pediatrics* (1992) **90**: 767–70.
10. Zanchetta JR, Plotkin H, Alvarez-Filgueira ML. Bone mass in children: normative values for the 2–20 year old population. *Bone* (1995) **16**: 393–95.
11. Koo WWK, Walters J, Bush AJ. Technical considerations of dual-energy X-ray absorptiometry-based bone mineral measurements for pediatric studies. *J Bone Miner Res* (1995) **10**: 1998–2004.
12. Henderson RC. The correlation between dual-energy X-ray absorptiometry measurements of bone density in the proximal femur and lumbar spine of children. *Skeletal Radiol* (1997) **26**: 544–7.
13. Shore RM, Langman CB, Donovan JM et al. Bone mineral disorders in children: evaluation with dual X-ray absorptiometry. *Radiology* (1995) **196**: 535–40.
14. Ponder SW. Clinical use of bone densitometry in children: are we ready yet? *Clin Pediatr* (1995) **34**: 237–40.
15. Zionts LE, Nash JP, Rude R et al. Bone mineral density in children with mild osteogenesis imperfecta. *Br J Bone Joint Surg* (1995) **77B**: 143–7.
16. Henderson RC, Lin PP, Greene WB. Bone-mineral density in children and adolescents who have spastic cerebral palsy. *Am J Bone Joint Surg* (1995) **77A**: 1671–81.
17. Wilmshurst S, Ward K, Adams JE et al. Mobility status and bone mineral density in cerebral palsy. *Arch Dis Child* (1996) **75**: 164–5.
18. Harcke HT, Taylor A, Bachrach S, Miller F, Henderson RC. The lateral femoral scan: an alternative method for assessing bone mineral density in children with cerebral palsy. *Pediatr Radiol* (1998) (in press).

19. Henderson RC. Bone density and other possible predictors of fracture risk in children and adolescents with spastic quadriplegia. *Dev Med Child Neurol* (1997) **39:** 224–7.

20. Stallings VA, Oddleifson NW, Negrini BY et al. Bone mineral content and dietary calcium intake in children prescribed a low-lactose diet. *J Pediatr Gastroenterol Nutr* (1994) **18:** 440–5.

21. Gussinye M, Carrascosa A, Potau N et al. Bone mineral density in prepubertal and in adolescent and young adult patients with salt-wasting form of congenital adrenal hyperplasia. *Pediatrics* (1997) **100:** 671–4.

22. Hopp R, Degan J, Gallagher JC et al. Estimation of bone mineral density in children with juvenile rheumatoid arthritis. *J Rheumatol* (1991) **18:** 1235–9.

23. Kotaniemi A, Savolainen A, Kautiainen H et al. Estimation of central osteopenia in children with chronic polyarthritis treated with glucocorticoids. *Pediatrics* (1993) **91:** 1127–30.

24. Pepmueller PH, Cassidy JT, Allen SH et al. Bone mineralization and bone mineral metabolism in children with juvenile rheumatoid arthritis. *Arthritis Rheum* (1996) **39:** 746–57.

25. Fassler A-LC, Bonjour J-P. Osteoporosis as a pediatric problem. *Pediatr Clin North Am* (1995) **42:** 811–24.

26. Goulding A, Cannan R, Williams SM et al. Bone mineral density in girls with forearm fractures. *J Bone Miner Res* (1998) **13:** 143–8.

16

Clinical Interpretation of Bone Density Scans

CONTENTS • Chapter overview • Introduction • Bone density and bone strength • Estimation of fracture risk • The accuracy of reference data • Clinical indications for bone density measurements • Interpretation of bone density measurements • Screening for osteoporosis • Choice of measurement site • Clinical use of bone densitometry • Male osteoporosis

CHAPTER OVERVIEW

Over the past decade bone density measurements have entered routine clinical practice as the basis for the diagnosis of osteoporosis, for making decisions over treatment, and for monitoring patients' responses. This chapter discusses the clinical interpretation of bone mineral density (BMD) measurements undertaken for these three purposes. Many aspects that have already been mentioned in the preceding chapters are summarized and emphasized here. The clinical indications for the diagnostic use of bone densitometry and recommendations for treatment based on the findings are areas of continuing debate; recent important reviews have been published by the European Foundation for Osteoporosis (EFFO)[1] and the United States National Osteoporosis Foundation (NOF).[2] Other areas of debate include the choice of technology (axial DXA, peripheral DXA or quantitative ultrasound), the accuracy of reference ranges and the question of which skeletal site to measure. A discussion is also included of osteoporosis in males, which is an important but relatively neglected area of study.

INTRODUCTION

The term *osteoporosis* is often used without any clear indication of its meaning. Thus, osteoporosis is used to describe both the clinical outcome (a low trauma fracture) and the changes in bone tissue that precede a fracture. The most helpful and inclusive definition of osteoporosis is that given by the Consensus Development Conferences in 1991 and 1993,[3,4] since it embraces the combination of skeletal and other factors that are the cause of fractures:

> *A disease characterised by low bone mass and microarchitectural deterioration of bone tissue, leading to enhanced bone fragility and a consequent increase in fracture risk.*

This definition of osteoporosis encompasses the important concept that patients with increased fracture risk can be identified on the basis of a non-invasive measurement of either bone mass or the integrity of bone microarchitecture. In practice, patients at increased risk of fracture are identified exclusively by the determination of bone mass (usually based on a measurement of BMD) rather than bone microarchitecture. Although the variables measured by quantitative ultrasound (QUS) can be related to bone architecture,[5,6] in practice QUS parameters such as broadband ultrasonic attenuation (BUA) and speed of sound (SOS) correlate closely with BMD.[7] For the purposes of this chapter, therefore, a QUS measurement will be regarded as a substitute for BMD. Although high-resolution peripheral quantitative computed tomography (pQCT) may in future allow the direct non-invasive measurement of bone architecture in vivo,[8,9] there is at present no routine radiological method for the diagnosis of osteoporosis based on the measurement of bone structure. This chapter will therefore concentrate on the investigation of osteoporosis based on the interpretation of BMD measurements.

The introduction of dual-energy X-ray absorptiometry (DXA) has had a decisive influence on the clinical use of bone densitometry because it made available for the first time a technique that allows rapid, convenient, accurate and precise measurements of BMD to be obtained routinely with stable and reliable equipment in the setting of a speciality bone clinic, a physician's office or a screening programme. However, the use and interpretation of bone densitometry measurements to diagnose osteoporosis and make decisions over treatment is a subject that continues to generate controversy. Debate on these issues is far from being concluded.[1,2] Indeed, it has become more complicated following the introduction of a new generation of devices for X-ray absorptiometry of the peripheral skeleton (pDXA), as well as a variety of devices for QUS measurements at the calcaneus and other sites. Controversies about how to use these procedures in everyday patient management, and whether these measurements should be reimbursed through medical insurance are still ongoing in the USA and Europe.

Within the general setting of the measurement of BMD or QUS variables, several approaches have been used to define osteoporosis and interpret scan findings. Usually, to interpret a scan it is necessary to compare the patient's measurements with an appropriate reference range matched for sex and race. This comparison may be made using either normal young adults or healthy age-matched subjects. The former group is intended to represent the mean and population standard deviation (SD) at *peak bone mass*, i.e. the maximum BMD achieved in adult life. The comparison is made using the *T-score* parameter, which is the result of the patient's BMD less the mean BMD for the young adult population in units of the young adult population SD. A patient's T-score result is defined by the equation:

$$T \text{ score} = \frac{\text{Measured BMD} - \text{Young adult mean BMD}}{\text{Young adult SD}}$$

The *Z-score* is similar in concept to the T-score except that the mean BMD and SD for a healthy age-matched population is used instead of the young adult group as the reference population. A patient's Z-score result is defined by the equation:

$$Z\text{-score} = \frac{\text{Measured BMD} - \text{Age-matched mean BMD}}{\text{Age-matched SD}}$$

Debate continues about the relative merits of T-score and Z-score figures for the interpretation of bone densitometry investigations. However, T-scores have assumed an important status and have been the main focus of attention since the publication of the report from the World Health Organization (WHO) Study Group,[10,11] which categorized patients' skeletal status by dividing them into four groups on the basis of T-score results as follows (Figure 16.1):

Normal: The BMD result is not more than 1 SD below the young adult mean value (T-score > −1.0).

Osteopenia: The BMD result is between 1.0 and 2.5 SD below the young adult mean (−1.0 > T-score > −2.5).

Osteoporosis: The BMD result is more than 2.5 SD below the young adult mean (T-score < −2.5).

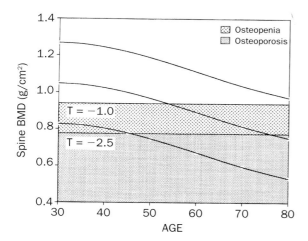

Figure 16.1 Reference curve for PA lumbar spine BMD in normal white female subjects measured on a Hologic DXA bone densitometer. The curves have been plotted to include the World Health Organization Study Group definitions of osteopenia and osteoporosis.[10,11] The lighter stippled area denotes osteopenia (−1.0 > T-score > −2.5) and the darker shaded area denotes osteoporosis (T-score < −2.5). (Reproduced with permission from Blake et al.[55])

Established osteoporosis: The BMD result is more than 2.5 SD below the young adult mean (T-score < −2.5) and the patient has one or more fragility fractures.

Throughout the rest of this chapter the terms *normal, osteopenia, osteoporosis* and *established osteoporosis* will be used according to their WHO definitions. With this terminology, a patient with osteopenia is at a moderately increased risk and a patient with osteoporosis is at a significantly increased risk of fracture compared with normal subjects (Figure 16.2). However, not all individuals with low BMD will actually sustain a fracture. Conversely, a normal BMD does not exclude the possibility of fracture. Osteoporotic fractures are analogous to diseases such as coronary heart disease and hypertension, where risk factors such as hypercholesterolaemia and high blood pressure pre-

dispose patients to myocardial infarction and stroke respectively.

Apart from the debate over the use of T-scores and Z-scores, there are other potential areas of contention, such as which technology to use (axial DXA, pDXA or QUS), the accuracy of reference data and which site to measure in the skeleton. While the clinically most important fractures occur in the spine and femur, bone density measurements at most sites throughout the skeleton correlate reasonably well. Therefore, if mass screening is being advocated, peripheral measurements might be preferred if they can be obtained more simply and cheaply. Even when the spine and femur are measured, osteoporosis may be diagnosed on the basis of low BMD results at one site but not the other (Figure 16.3). Does this indicate localized abnormal bone loss? If not, are results from one site to be preferred to another? Such issues continue to cause controversy, especially when peripheral measurements are compared with axial measurements.

BONE DENSITY AND BONE STRENGTH

The organic matrix of bone is impregnated with mineral salts that confer upon the skeleton properties of hardness and rigidity. Bone mineral measurements have shown a high correlation with tensile strength of bone in numerous studies on excised human and animal bones.[12-18] In addition, both prospective and cross-sectional epidemiology studies have shown a strong association between BMD and fracture risk.[19-31] In bones where there is a complex structural relationship between cortical and trabecular bone, such as in the spine or hip, it is not clear whether the trabecular or cortical component contributes more to bone strength. This may vary with skeletal site, and may be important for future attempts to increase the sensitivity of bone mineral measurements for fracture prediction, since cortical and trabecular bone can be measured separately by some techniques. While any individual can sustain a fracture depending on the severity of the trauma (e.g. a skiing accident), and while in individuals

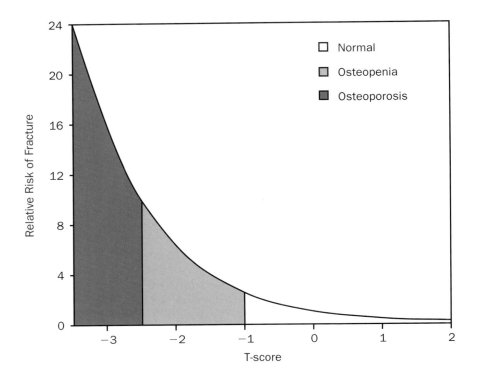

Figure 16.2 Relationship between femoral neck bone density and hip fracture risk. Bone density is shown in T-score units. The plot includes the World Health Organization Study Group thresholds for the definitions of osteopenia (−1.0 > T-score > −2.5) and osteoporosis (T-score < −2.5).[10,11] For every unit decrease in T-score, fracture risk increases by a factor of 2.5.[27]

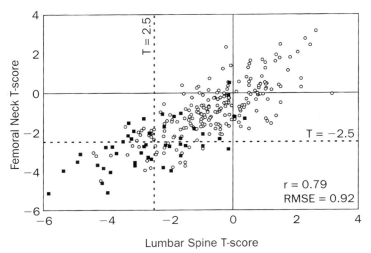

Figure 16.3 Scatter plot between the T-scores for lumbar spine and femoral neck bone density in 219 normal white women (open circles) and 48 women with vertebral fracture (black squares). Dashed lines show the World Health Organization Study Group threshold for the definition of osteoporosis (T-score < −2.5).[10,11] (Data reproduced with permission from Ms M Frost.)

with low BMD other factors, such as frequency of falls, may be important, the amount of bone present is the single most important factor determining the likelihood of fracture.

ESTIMATION OF FRACTURE RISK

As explained above, by using BMD measurements it has become possible to move away from the definition of osteoporosis in terms of the occurrence of one or more fragility fractures, and instead define osteoporosis as the state of increased fracture risk associated with low bone mass. Efforts have therefore been directed at finding BMD values below which fracture risk is significantly increased. Today, the WHO criterion of a T-score, <-2.5, is the widely accepted definition of osteoporosis.[11] However, before the publication of the WHO Study Group report,[10] several authors had developed the concept of *fracture threshold*. This

was first proposed on the basis of histomorphometric data by Meunier et al.[32] in 1981. They showed that 95% of 106 women with at least one crushed vertebra had an iliac trabecular bone volume value lower than 14% (Figure 16.4). Analogous fracture threshold values were also derived for BMD values,[33-35] while Nordin suggested a bone mineral threshold 2 SD below the mean value of young normal subjects.[36] However, a limitation of setting any particular threshold BMD for increased fracture risk is that there is a continuous gradient of increasing fracture risk with decreasing bone mass (Figure 16.2).[19] As explained in the Appendix to Chapter 2, this relationship between BMD and fracture incidence makes it appropriate to analyse prospective and cross-sectional studies of osteoporotic fractures using logistic regression models. The results are conveniently expressed as the increased fracture risk for each 1 SD decrease in the BMD value.

Methods of interpreting BMD values for frac-

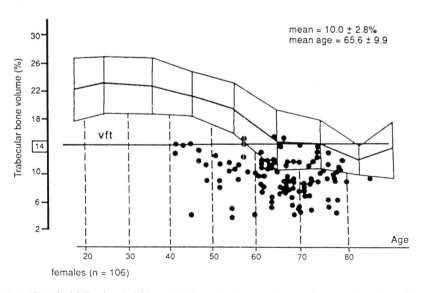

Figure 16.4 Fracture threshold (horizontal line at trabecular bone volume of 14%) defined as the trabecular bone volume below which 95% of all fracture cases occur. Normal range (mean ± 1 SD) is given. Dots represent trabecular bone volume in 106 women with osteoporosis defined by the presence of vertebral compression fractures. (Reproduced with permission from Meunier et al.[32])

ture risk prediction have developed over the years. Initial expectations of finding a test to separate subjects with osteoporosis clearly from normals proved to be over-optimistic. It is now apparent that a specific test for the occurrence of osteoporotic fractures cannot be expected from bone mineral measurements. Many studies comparing older women with and without fragility fractures show that there is no clear separation between these groups on the basis of BMD. This is well illustrated in Figure 16.3, which shows lumbar spine and femoral neck BMD measurements in a group of healthy pre- and postmenopausal women and a second group of women with vertebral compression fractures. Any chosen threshold, be it the WHO criterion of a T-score <-2.5 or any other, will correctly identify only a certain percentage of subjects in the fracture group. Some fracture patients are identified by the spine BMD measurement, but not by the hip measurement, and vice versa; some patients are missed by both BMD measurements. Conversely, it is evident from Figure 16.1 that at about 75 years of age the mean BMD value for normal white women passes through the -2.5 T-score threshold. However, not all these women will experience a low trauma fracture. Thus, a BMD measurement can only provide a guide to fracture risk and cannot predict with certainty which individuals will or will not sustain fragility fractures.

An important issue raised by Figure 16.3 is the choice of BMD measurement site for the optimum prediction of fracture risk. A key variable for evaluating different measurement sites is the *risk ratio* (RR) or *odds ratio* (OR) derived from the proportional hazards or logistic regression model used to analyse fracture studies (see the Appendix to Chapter 2). The importance of these ratios can be demonstrated by dividing patients' BMD results into four quartiles and plotting the percentage of future fracture cases expected in each quartile (Figure 16.5, see also Table 2.A2 in the Appendix to Chapter 2). If a given measurement has no predictive power (RR or OR = 1.0), then 25% of all fracture cases will occur in each quartile and no useful information is provided. However, as the

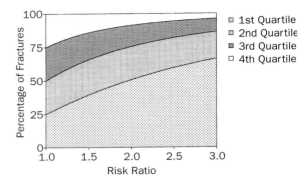

Figure 16.5 Plot of the percentage of fractures expected to occur in each of the four quartiles of bone density as the risk ratio varies from 1.0 to 3.0. The risk ratio expresses the increased risk of fracture for each 1 SD decrease in the BMD measurement. If a methodology has no predictive power (RR = 1.0), then 25% of all fractures occur in each quartile. As the risk ratio becomes larger, an increasing percentage of fractures will occur in the lowest quartile and a decreasing percentage in the highest quartile. (Reproduced with permission from Blake et al.[92])

RR or OR ratio becomes larger, a steadily higher percentage of future fractures will occur in patients in the lowest quartile and a dwindling percentage in the highest quartile. A detailed review of clinical studies relating bone density measurements to fracture risk together with tabulated results for RR or OR values is given in Chapter 2. There is considerable evidence, especially for hip fracture, that for a given fracture site the most reliable risk assessment is provided by a BMD measurement at that site.[27,29,37] However, if *all* types of skeletal fractures are considered regardless of site, then the choice of measurement site has little influence on fracture risk prediction (see, for example, Figure 2.3).[29]

There are now a large number of prospective studies confirming that bone mass measurements can predict fractures.[19–30] As discussed above, results of studies are usually presented in terms of the increased fracture risk for a 1 SD decrease in BMD. However, as indicated in Figure 16.5, an alternative and perhaps more intuitive presentation is to express the results in terms of the variation in fracture incidence in the four quartiles of BMD of the study population. One of the most influential studies is the Study of Osteoporotic Fractures (SOF) reported by Cummings et al.[27] in which 8134 women aged 65 years or over were enrolled from four centres in the USA. BMD was measured in the proximal femur, the spine, the radius and the calcaneus. During a mean follow-up period of 1.8 years, 65 women had hip fractures. The authors found that women in the lowest quartile of femoral neck BMD were 8.5 times more likely to sustain a hip fracture than women in the highest quartile. Each 1 SD decrease in femoral neck BMD increased the risk of hip fracture 2.6 times (95% confidence interval: 1.9–3.6). Femoral neck BMD was a better predictor of hip fracture risk than BMD measurements of the spine ($p < 0.0001$) or radius ($p < 0.002$), and moderately better than the calcaneus ($p = 0.10$). This study provides some of the most convincing evidence that a measurement of femur BMD is the optimum site for predicting hip fracture. However, at present, the statistical limitations arising from the limited follow-up available continue to restrict conclusions concerning the relative merits of different measurement sites (see Figure 12.8).

It is important to recognize that BMD or QUS measurements provide only an estimate of patients' fracture risks. Clinicians should be aware of the limitations of the information provided, and scan findings should be interpreted alongside other risk factors such as age, history of prior fragility fracture in adult life, low body weight, cigarette smoking or family history of osteoporosis.[2] At the present time, studies of the prediction of fracture risk over significant periods of time are only available for single photon absorptiometry (SPA) measurements of the forearm.[30] Long-term follow-up of axial DXA and QUS measurements over periods up to 25 years are needed to explore fully the predictive value of different technologies and dif-

ferent skeletal sites for the prediction of fracture risk.

THE ACCURACY OF REFERENCE DATA

As discussed above, bone mineral measurements cannot be used to make a definite prediction that a patient will sustain a fragility fracture. However, by comparing the measured bone density with an appropriate reference population, the presence of osteopenia or osteoporosis can be established and BMD can be interpreted in terms of fracture risk. The accuracy of reference data is therefore fundamental to the reliable interpretation of bone densitometry investigations using either T-score or Z-score findings. Since many centres issue clinical reports based on reference data provided by the equipment manufacturers, the accuracy of such data is an issue that continues to generate controversy. As discussed in Chapter 12, one of the most influential analyses of reference data is the study by Faulkner et al.[38] comparing T-score results based on the Lunar and Hologic manufacturers' ranges (see Figure 12.16). Scans obtained on Lunar DPX (Lunar Corp., Madison, WI, USA) and Hologic QDR-1000/W (Hologic Inc., Waltham, MA, USA) systems showed mean differences in T-score (Hologic − Lunar) of −0.05 ($p = 0.02$) for PA spine BMD and −0.93 ($p < 0.001$) for femoral neck BMD. The difference for the spine is too small to have clinical significance, but that for the hip indicated a major discrepancy in scan interpretation between the two manufacturers' systems.

That such discrepancies exist is not surprising. Manufacturers' databases are frequently pooled from several sites. It is often unclear what degree of vetting has been used and to what extent these individuals represent an unbiased cross-section of the population. There may be selection effects, in as much as they were individuals who were interested in having their bone density measured, hospital volunteers, etc. Often, different and incompatible methods of smoothing BMD results are employed. Thus, data can be interpreted by fitting polynomial functions of age over a broad age range,[39] or by fitting a number of shorter sections of linear or exponential change to represent premenopausal, early postmenopausal and later postmenopausal phases. There may or may not be any smoothing of the population SD. The standard deviation is particularly difficult to measure because of the large numbers of subjects required for statistical accuracy. Moreover, when T-scores are used for scan interpretation, any inaccuracy in the measurement of standard deviation is multiplied 2.5 times in setting the threshold for the definition of osteoporosis.

Few independent studies provide an adequately large body of data for comparison with the manufacturers' databases.[40–43] However, one especially influential study has been the recently completed third National Health and Nutrition Survey (NHANES III), which included a DXA examination of the proximal femur conducted using mobile Hologic QDR-1000 densitometers.[44] The combined phase 1 and phase 2 data from this study include a nationally representative sample of 14 646 men and women aged 20 years and older.[45,46] Unlike many previous studies that were limited to white Caucasian subjects, NHANES III includes approximately equal numbers of non-Hispanic white, non-Hispanic black and Mexican Americans. The survey included 3251 non-Hispanic white women. In the youngest group (age 20–29 years, $n = 409$), mean femoral neck BMD was lower than the manufacturer's young adult figure (0.858 versus 0.895 g/cm²), while the population SD was larger than in the manufacturer's range (0.12 versus 0.10 g/cm²). The combination of these two changes meant that the femoral neck BMD value required to fulfil the WHO definition of osteoporosis (T-score < −2.5) was significantly reduced (0.558 versus 0.645 g/cm²).

Owing to its large size, nationally representative character, and clear inclusion and exclusion criteria, the NHANES study is now being widely adopted as reference range data for femur DXA studies.[47]

CLINICAL INDICATIONS FOR BONE DENSITY MEASUREMENTS

Over the years, many studies have identified factors that may affect bone mass or fracture risk,[48–51] and that may be used as indicators for the use of bone mineral measurements. For many of these indications taken individually, the routine clinical use of BMD measurements may not be justified since the correlations are either too weak or the results are unlikely to influence patient or physician behaviour or lead to distinct diagnostic decisions. However, when several risk factors are present significant relationships with fracture risk can be demonstrated (Figure 16.6).[51]

Table 16.1 lists clinical risk factors providing indications for the diagnostic use of bone densitometry as recommended by the European

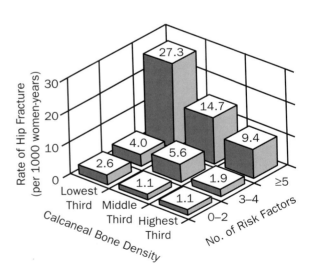

Figure 16.6 Annual risk of hip fracture according to the number of risk factors and the age-specific calcaneal bone density. Results are from the Study of Osteoporotic Fractures (SOF).[51] The list of 16 risk factors, besides bone density, against which subjects were assessed is given in Table 16.3. (Reproduced with permission from Cummings et al.[51])

Table 16.1 Clinical risk factors providing indications for the diagnostic use of bone densitometry. (Data from Kanis et al.[1])

1) Presence of strong risk factors

    Oestrogen deficiency

        Premature menopause (<45 years)

        Prolonged secondary amenorrhoea (>1 year)

        Primary hypogonadism

    Corticosteroid therapy (>7.5 mg/day for 1 year or more)

    Maternal family history of hip fracture

    Low body mass index (<19 kg/m^2)

    Other disorders associated with osteoporosis

        Anorexia nervosa

        Malabsorption

        Primary hyperparathyroidism

        Post-transplantation

        Chronic renal failure

        Hyperthyroidism

        Prolonged immobilization

        Cushing's syndrome

2) Radiographic evidence of osteopenia and/or vertebral deformity

3) Previous fragility fracture, particularly of the hip, spine or wrist

4) Loss of height, thoracic kyphosis

Foundation for Osteoporosis.[1] These include the presence of strong risk factors such as early menopause, amenorrhoea, long-term corticosteroid therapy, or maternal hip fracture. Other indications are radiographic evidence of osteopenia or vertebral deformity and previous fragility fracture, especially in the hip, spine or wrist. In their report for the National

Osteoporosis Foundation, Eddy et al.[2] identified four risk factors for fracture in addition to BMD, which are useful in a clinical setting because they are readily evaluable and relatively common (Table 16.2). On the basis of cost–benefit analysis, the authors provide nomograms from which using information on the patient's age, history of prior fracture, and the number of other risk factors present, a decision can be made on whether to request a bone densitometry scan.

One of the most detailed analyses of risk factors for hip fracture was the report of Cummings et al.[51] based on 9516 white women aged 65 years or older enrolled in the SOF study. During an average of 4.1 years of follow-up, 192 women had fragility fractures of the hip. The analysis identified 16 independent risk factors for hip fracture besides bone density (Table 16.3). Taken with calcaneal BMD, an individual's aggregated score of risk factors was highly predictive of the annual risk of hip fracture (Figure 16.6).

INTERPRETATION OF BONE DENSITY MEASUREMENTS

The diagnosis of osteoporosis

At the present time there is an overwhelming consensus that the diagnosis of osteoporosis should be based on the WHO Study Group report recommendation of a T-score < −2.5. Indeed, failure to interpret bone densitometry studies according to the WHO criteria might have serious medico-legal implications. There are, however, a number of difficult issues surrounding the use of T-scores that require discussion.

First, as discussed above, the BMD value equivalent to the T-score threshold of −2.5 is sensitive to errors in reference range data, thus opening the way for significant inconsistencies among measurements on different manufacturers' equipment or for measurements on the same type of equipment using different reference ranges. The effect of the introduction of reference ranges for femoral neck BMD based on the NHANES study[44–46] has been discussed

Table 16.2 Risk factors for osteoporosis including prevalence and relative risks. (Data from Eddy et al.[2])

Risk factor	Prevalence (%)	Relative risk[a]
History of fracture after age 40	37	1.80
History of hip, wrist or vertebra fracture in first-degree relative	7	1.40
Being in the lowest quartile in weight (<57.8 kg)	25	1.90
Current cigarette smoking	10	1.70

[a]Relative risk with versus without risk factor assuming BMD is unknown.

earlier. Such changes can have a significant effect on the percentage of patients diagnosed as osteoporotic. Thus, Abrahamsen et al. reported a study of 2005 perimenopausal women recruited by direct mailing to a random sample of 45- to 58-year-old Danish women who had scans on four Hologic DXA densitometers.[52] Results for the percentage of subjects with T-score < −2.5 at the femoral neck were 7.9% using the manufacturer's reference range, but only 0.7% using the NHANES values (Table 16.4). Many clinicians issuing DXA scan reports have changed to using the NHANES reference data for the femur because of the large size of the study, the representative cross-section of the population sampled, and concerns about the possible overdiagnosis of osteoporosis. However, it is important to emphasize that the difficulty in determining reference peaks, means and standard deviations is a significant weakness of the T-score approach.[53] Thus, even in a study as large as NHANES, some surprisingly large differences (up to 23%) in the population SD values of the non-Hispanic white young adult group were reported between the phase 1 and phase 2 halves of the study.[46]

Another issue affecting the use of T-score results to diagnose osteoporosis is the choice of BMD measurement site. Even given compatible reference ranges, different rates of age- and menopause-related losses at different sites will lead to systematically different findings when results are expressed in T-scores (Figure 16.7). Thus, in the study of Abrahamsen and colleagues described above,[52] 4.3% of perimenopausal women were diagnosed as osteoporotic on the basis of the lumbar spine T-score compared with 0.7% for the femoral neck using the NHANES reference range, (Table 16.4) which reflects the larger and earlier menopause-related losses from the spine. Related issues arise with the use of multiple sites. Clearly, the more sites scanned the more likely that at least one will be found that meets the WHO criteria. Thus, if osteoporosis is diagnosed in the event that any spine, femur or forearm site has a T-score < −2.5, then 6.9% of women in the Abrahamsen study were classified as osteoporotic (Table 16.4).

Finally, it is unclear at present how QUS

Table 16.3 Risk factors for hip fracture and relative risks with and without adjustment for history of previous fracture and calcaneal BMD. (Data from Cummings et al.[51])

Risk factor (comparison or unit)	Relative risk[a] (95% confidence interval)	
	Base model	Add fracture history and BMD
Age (per 5 years)	1.5 (1.3–1.7)	1.4 (1.2–1.6)
Maternal hip fracture (vs none)	2.0 (1.4–2.9)	1.8 (1.2–2.7)
Weight increase since age 25 (per 20%)	0.6 (0.5–0.7)	0.8 (0.6–0.9)
Height at age 25 (per 6 cm)	1.2 (1.1–1.4)	1.3 (1.1–1.5)
Self-rated health (per 1-point decrease)[b]	1.7 (1.3–2.2)	1.6 (1.2–2.1)
Previous hyperthyroidism (vs none)	1.8 (1.2–2.6)	1.7 (1.2–2.5)
Current use of long-acting benzodiazepines (vs no current use)	1.6 (1.1–2.4)	1.6 (1.1–2.4)
Current use of anti-convulsant drugs (vs no current use)	2.8 (1.2–6.3)	2.0 (0.8–4.9)
Current caffeine intake (per 190 mg/day)	1.3 (1.0–1.5)	1.2 (1.0–1.5)
Walking for exercise (vs not walking for exercise)	0.7 (0.5–0.9)	0.7 (0.5–1.0)
On feet <4 h/day (vs > 4 h/day)	1.7 (1.2–2.4)	1.7 (1.2–2.4)
Inability to rise from chair (vs no inability)	2.1 (1.3–3.2)	1.7 (1.1–2.7)
Lowest quartile for depth perception (vs other three)	1.5 (1.1–2.0)	1.4 (2.0–1.9)
Low-frequency contrast sensitivity (per 1 SD decrease)	1.2 (1.0–1.5)	1.2 (1.0–1.5)
Resting pulse rate > 80/min (vs <80/min)	1.8 (1.3–2.5)	1.7 (1.2–2.4)
Any fracture since age 50 (vs none)		1.5 (1.1–2.0)
Calcaneal BMD (per 1 SD decrease)		1.6 (1.3–1.9)

[a]For continuous variables relative risks are expressed as change in risk for each specified change in risk factor.
[b]Health was rated as poor (1 point), fair (2 points) or good (3 points).

Table 16.4 Proportion of healthy perimenopausal and postmenopausal women fulfilling the WHO Study Group criteria for osteoporosis (T-score < −2.5).[a] (Data from Abrahamsen et al.[52])

BMD measurement site		Percentage with T-score < −2.5
Individual anatomical regions:		
Lumbar spine (L2–L4)		4.3
Femur	Total hip	1.2
	Femoral neck	7.9 (0.7)[b]
	Trochanter	1.5
	Any femur site	8.6 (2.6)[b]
Forearm	One-third	2.9
	Ultra-distal	1.4
Combination of regions:		
Spine and total hip		5.0
Spine, total hip and ultra-distal forearm		5.9
Spine and any femur site		10.9 (6.1)[b]
Any of the above regions		12.5 (6.9)[b]

[a]Calculations are based on the manufacturer's reference range.
[b]Numbers in brackets indicate percentages obtained if the NHANES reference range[44-46] is used for femoral neck BMD.

measurements should be incorporated into the WHO classification scheme. Because QUS was largely a research tool at the time of the WHO Study Group report, no advice was given on the interpretation of bone ultrasound measurements. Because the relationship between age-, menopause- and osteoporosis-related changes and the population SD may be different for QUS compared with DXA, a different threshold for defining osteoporosis may be appropriate. Further studies comparing QUS and DXA measurements in representative population samples should clarify this issue in the near future.

The treatment of osteoporosis and osteopenia

Although there is general agreement that a T-score < −2.5 should be the basis of the diagnosis of osteoporosis, it is clear that this criterion should not be the sole basis of treatment in all age groups irrespective of other considerations. Other factors such as age, previous fractures, family history and body weight are equally important in the assessment of the individual patient (Table 16.2). A previous fragility fracture is an important indicator that the

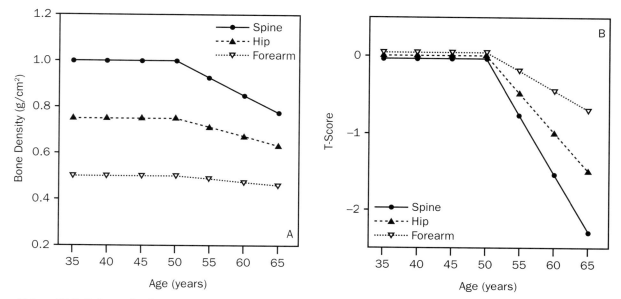

Figure 16.7 Schematic diagram of the changes in bone density before and after the menopause as measured at the spine, hip and forearm: (A) changes plotted showing BMD varying as a function of age; (B) changes plotted showing T-score varying as a function of age.

patient is at high risk of a further fracture independent of BMD,[2,21,26] and most clinicians would treat such patients irrespective of the findings of the DXA scan. Age is also an important independent indicator of fracture risk with many prospective studies confirming that risk approximately doubles for each decade increase in age.[20,27,31] When considering lifetime fracture risk, age variation is relatively slow (Figure 16.8A). However, when considering the risk of fracture in the subsequent 5 years there is a marked dependence on age such that a typical 50-year-old woman has an approximately 20-fold lower risk of hip fracture and an eight-

fold lower risk of a vertebral fracture compared with an 80-year-old woman (Figure 16.8B).

Table 16.5 lists diagnostic categories based on bone density and treatment recommendations within each category as set out in the position paper of the European Foundation for Osteoporosis.[1] Decisions about the need for treatment depend not only on establishing a diagnosis, but also on the age of the patient, as well as the efficacy, costs and side effects of treatment. The decision to treat osteoporosis may differ between a 50-year-old and an 80-year-old patient (Table 16.5). Osteoporosis in the latter is found in more than 50% of individ-

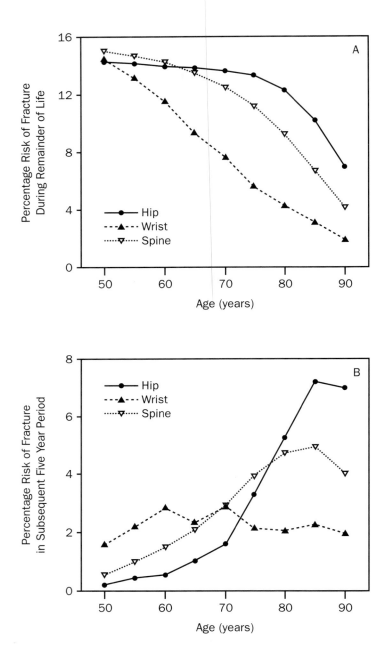

Figure 16.8 The probabilities of spine, hip and wrist fractures for average-risk white women of various ages: (A) probabilities during the remainder of life (lifetime fracture risk); (B) probabilities during the next 5 years. (Data from Eddy et al.[2])

Table 16.5 Diagnostic categories based on bone mineral density and treatment recommendations within each category. (Recommendations from Kanis et al.[1])

Diagnostic category	Risk of fracture	Action
Normal	Low	No intervention
Osteopenia	Medium	Consider prevention in perimenopausal women or assess bone loss. Consider treatment in more elderly patients with history of fragility fractures
Osteoporosis	High	Exclude contributing causes, particularly if young. Intervention recommended, particularly if less than 75 years of age
Established osteoporosis	Very high	Exclude contributing causes. Intervention strongly indicated

uals (Figure 16.1), but life expectancy is short. Up to the age of 75 years the −2.5 T-score cut-off point of BMD to diagnose osteoporosis is an appropriate threshold for treatment. However, after the age of 75 years the lifetime risk of fracture decreases (Figure 16.8A). In the authors' view it may be more appropriate to base treatment decisions in the elderly on the Z-score rather than the T-score finding. A decision to treat patients on the basis of a spine or femur Z-score < −1.0 results in about 25% of patients

receiving treatment, i.e. the lowest quartile of the population, and better matches the proportion of patients being treated to the actual incidence of fragility fractures. One advantage of the use of Z-scores is that they allow for the different age-related losses at different skeletal sites and do not result in differences in the numbers of patients identified as osteoporotic on the basis of different measurement sites (cf. Table 16.4).

In one of the most careful analyses of the

cost-effectiveness of treatments for osteoporosis, Eddy and colleagues[2] present nomograms for treatment decisions based on BMD, age, history of previous fracture, and the number of other evaluable risk factors (Table 16.2). For women without previous fracture, T-score thresholds for instigating oestrogen replacement therapy vary from −2.5 at 50 years to −1.9 at 80 years of age. Equivalent figures for treatment with a bisphosphonate are −2.9 at 50 years to −2.2 at 80 years of age, and differ from the thresholds for oestrogen treatment because of differences in the costs and estimated benefits. Much higher thresholds are recommended in patients with a previous fracture because of the importance of this as a risk factor for future fractures.

Treatment of osteopenia as opposed to osteoporosis is more controversial, since a T-score threshold of −1.0 includes a large percentage of all postmenopausal women (Figure 16.1).[52] In the authors' view, a Z-score threshold of −1.0 in the spine or femur may be a more appropriate threshold for recommending treatment since, as argued above in the case of elderly osteoporotic women, it results in treatment of the lowest quartile, and therefore matches the percentage of women offered treatment with lifetime fracture risk (Figure 16.8A).

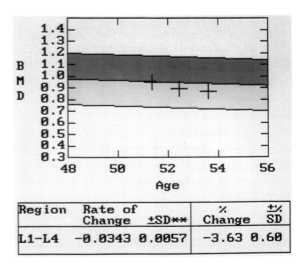

Region	Rate of Change	±SD**	% Change	±% SD
L1–L4	−0.0343	0.0057	−3.63	0.60

Figure 16.9 Bone mineral data from a 54-year-old white woman who had three annual bone mineral measurements beginning the year after onset of menopause. Data are plotted superimposed on a normal range. Rate of loss is illustrated in terms of per cent change per year from baseline measurement. Two standard deviations define the confidence limit that should be used.

Monitoring response to treatment

The use of repeated BMD measurements to monitor the rate of bone loss or the response of patients commencing treatment needs careful consideration.[54–56] As discussed in Chapter 8, the sensitivity of bone densitometry measurements for these purposes is limited by the natural slow rates of gain or loss of bone mass and the long-term precision error of the technique (see Figure 8.3). The optimum DXA measurement site for this purpose is the PA spine scan. For a woman in the early postmenopausal years, losing bone at the average rate (≈1.5%/year), BMD measurements are required over 3 years (see Chapter 8, equation 8.16) to determine whether an individual has successfully responded to treatment (i.e. BMD is no longer falling), or is losing bone at twice the average rate (i.e. could be considered a 'fast loser'). Only larger rates of gain or loss can be detected in a shorter time period (Figure 16.9), a factor that limits the value of repeating scans in a shorter time interval.

An alternative method of monitoring response to treatment is the use of biochemical markers of bone formation and bone resorption (Table 16.6), which show large changes on timescales of weeks to months following the start of treatment (Figure 16.10). However, biochemical markers vary from day to day, and several measurements are necessary both before and during treatment if they are to be useful in monitoring treatment response.[56] The poor precision of biochemical markers means that their use is still under investigation.

Table 16.6 Biochemical markers of bone turnover. (Data from Eastell.[56])

Bone formation
  Serum alkaline phosphatase (bone
    isoenzyme)
  Serum osteocalcin
  Serum C- and N-propeptides of type I
    collagen

Bone resorption
  Urinary excretion of pyridinium cross-links of
    collagen
    (e.g. deoxypyridinoline)
  Urinary excretion of C- and N-telopeptides of
    collagen
  Urinary excretion of galactosyl hydroxylysine
  Urinary excretion of hydroxyproline
  Serum tartrate-resistant acid phosphatase

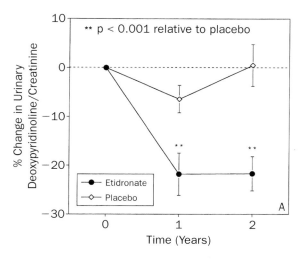

Figure 16.10 Mean percentage change from baseline of urinary deoxypyridinoline to creatinine ratio in placebo and etidronate-treated subjects in a clinical trial to prevent bone loss in early postmenopausal women. (Reproduced with permission from Herd et al.[75])

SCREENING FOR OSTEOPOROSIS

Osteoporosis is a major healthcare issue. Although the average life expectancy of individuals is increasing, the age of women at the menopause has remained essentially static at about 51 years. Thus, the women of the twenty-first century will spend a longer period in the postmenopausal part of their lives than any previous generation. Unless prophylactic measures are introduced, the incidence of osteoporotic fractures will continue to rise and the need for therapeutic measures will increase.

It is likely that future advances in the healthcare of postmenopausal women will relate to the prevention of fractures rather than the treatment of patients who have already sustained an osteoporotic fracture. Established disease is difficult to treat, while prevention of the bone loss that precedes a fragility fracture may be practical. Population-based approaches should be considered and, through education (e.g. relating to exercise and diet), it is possible that major benefits could be achieved. However, these measures, while sensible, are not of proven benefit, since long-term studies are not yet available. Problems may also arise in altering the lifestyles of teenagers. This is an important aspect, since if these measures are to be successful, then it is likely that they would have their greatest impact on the growing skeleton.

An alternative approach is selective screening, that is, targeting those individuals who are at greatest risk of developing osteoporosis in later life. The risk factors recommended in the most recent NOF study[2] have already been discussed (Table 16.2). The introduction of DXA has made available a technique that permits routine and reliable measurements of BMD, and one of the most important applications of bone densitometry measurements is to identify peri- and postmenopausal women with low bone density who can be advised to take preventive therapy. Since such patients may receive follow-up scans after 2 or 3 years to monitor their response, it is important that measurements are performed at a site where response can be reliably measured after a short time interval.

With regard to screening, osteoporosis seems an ideal candidate since it has high prevalence, significant morbidity, and can be identified at an early stage using a test that is safe, quick to perform, and accurate and acceptable to patients. There are treatments (oestrogen, bisphosphonates, selective oestrogen receptor modulators (SERMs)) that are effective in preventing bone loss and that can significantly reduce fracture incidence.[56,57] However, the concept of screening for osteoporosis remains contentious. There are concerns about the more widespread use of long-term oestrogen therapy,[58] and it is apparent that, in addition to bone mass, other factors such as the frequency of falls, contribute to the overall risk of fracture. Thus, even if all women who are perceived to be at risk were to receive long-term oestrogen therapy, it is likely that the reduction of fracture incidence would only be of the order of 50%. When other factors such as side effects of treatment and drug compliance are taken into account, it may be that a realistic goal is 30%.[59] A key issue with regard to screening relates to the cost–benefit analysis. Many assumptions are required in any such analysis, such as the prevalence of fracture, the efficacy of treatment in preventing fracture, patient compliance and the savings that might be achieved. On balance it seems probable that any screening programme for osteoporosis would incur some net costs, and decisions will therefore have to be made regarding whether such costs are justified on the basis of improved health.

CHOICE OF MEASUREMENT SITE

Clinical investigation of patients

The controversy on which site in the skeleton is most appropriate for measurement has already been mentioned. It is important to separate measurements used for the clinical investigation of patients from measurements used for screening. It might be argued that since peripheral measurements are simpler and cheaper to perform and correlate reasonably well ($r \approx 0.7$) with axial measurements, then peripheral mea-

surements are adequate for clinical investigations. However, while such relationships are reasonably good in normal subjects, the correlation can fall off dramatically when osteoporotic patients are studied.[60] The situation becomes further complicated if longitudinal studies are considered. Perimenopausal bone loss and the effect of different diseases and drugs can be different at various sites throughout the skeleton. A dramatic example is the rare osteoporosis of pregnancy. As shown in Figure 16.11, there may be a loss of over 50% of spinal bone density, although femoral density is normal. A peripheral measurement would fail to identify the magnitude of the problem in this case.

Since trabecular bone is more metabolically active than cortical bone, it responds more rapidly to stimuli, and it is not surprising that different patterns of loss are noted at different sites. For an individual, measurement of bone mass at one site does not accurately predict that at another, although they may well be correlated. Considering the individual with suspected osteoporosis, several sites may have to be measured. In general, the lumbar spine (compression fractures) and proximal femur (hip fractures) are clinically the most valuable sampling sites. In elderly patients, deformity, degenerative disease or aortic calcification may make the lumbar spine scan difficult to interpret. In this case, the hip, radius or calcaneus must be used as an alternative sampling site to predict fracture risk.

Screening

The issue of the choice of measurement site is more complicated if mass screening is considered. A rapid, simple and inexpensive test is desirable to measure large numbers of patients. DXA scanning of the axial skeleton is unlikely to meet this need since the cost is high and resources are limited. In this situation, a peripheral measurement site such as the forearm, hand or calcaneus is adequate for stratifying risk in large populations. The introduction of many innovative new peripheral X-ray absorptiometry devices, as described in Chapter 5, has

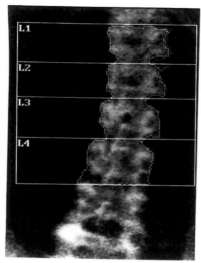

Region	Area (cm²)	BMC (grams)	BMD (gms/cm²)
L1	8.24	3.74	0.454
L2	7.81	3.96	0.507
L3	9.24	5.17	0.560
L4	12.48	6.95	0.557
TOTAL	37.77	19.81	0.525

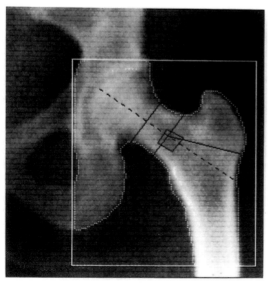

Region	Area (cm²)	BMC (grams)	BMD (gms/cm²)
Neck	3.95	3.35	0.847
Troch	9.33	6.87	0.736
Inter	23.02	25.20	1.095
TOTAL	36.30	35.42	0.976
Ward's	1.06	0.60	0.569

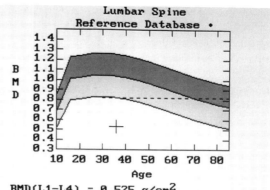

$BMD(L1-L4) = 0.525$ g/cm²

Region	BMD	T(30.0)		Z	
L1	0.454	-4.28	49%	-4.21	50%
L2	0.507	-4.74	49%	-4.65	50%
L3	0.560	-4.77	52%	-4.67	52%
L4	0.557	-5.08	50%	-4.99	50%
L1-L4	0.525	-4.75	50%	-4.66	51%

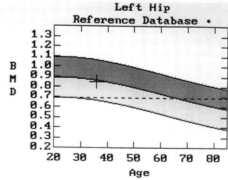

$BMD(Neck[L]) = 0.847$ g/cm²

Region	BMD	T		Z	
Neck	0.847	-0.47 (22.0)	95%	-0.19	98%
Troch	0.736	+0.15 (30.0)	102%	+0.22	103%
Inter	1.095	-0.37 (29.0)	95%	-0.31	96%
TOTAL	0.976	+0.01 (28.0)	100%	+0.09	101%
Ward's	0.569	-2.07 (20.0)	71%	-1.37	79%

Figure 16.11 Spine and hip scans and data printout from a woman with osteoporosis of pregnancy, showing preferential bone loss in the lumbar spine.

overcome many of the disadvantages of the old technology of SPA. For mass screening, QUS measurements of the calcaneus are of interest since they avoid altogether concerns about exposure to ionizing radiation. The QUS technique is simple, rapid to perform, mobile and inexpensive, and now that the first devices have received approval by the Food and Drug Administration, is clearly set for a major expansion in clinical use.

CLINICAL USE OF BONE DENSITOMETRY

Radiological identification of osteopenia

Back pain is a common symptom, and when persistent may lead to an X-ray being requested. The report may then include a statement such as the following: 'No significant abnormality seen, but bones appear osteopenic'. This may cause concern for patients requesting more information regarding their skeleton and risk of fracture. This seems to be an increasingly common reason for referral for bone density measurements. Another situation that may lead to referral is where an individual sustains an unexpected fracture and wishes clarification on whether this is an isolated incident related to trauma or attributable to the more general problem of osteoporosis. In one such referral to the authors' clinic, a woman had sustained a rib fracture while having sex with her husband. Patients have also been referred after being told by their dentists that they have osteopenia based on the findings of dental X-rays.

The evaluation of drug effects on the skeleton

It is well recognized that certain drugs may have significant effects on the skeleton, but it is only now, with ready access to BMD measurements, that these effects can be investigated. The most widely recognized drug effect is with corticosteroids.[61–62] These agents cause progressive bone loss that is dose-related and is most marked in the first 6 months of treatment.[63] The critical level is thought to be 7.5 mg/day of prednisolone or equivalent.[64] The effect is greater in trabecular than cortical bone. While steroids can be extremely damaging to the skeleton, response may vary, with some individuals being relatively resistant. Physicians are now giving greater consideration to the possible damaging effects on the skeleton when steroid use is being considered. Baseline bone density measurements to monitor the effects on the skeleton are now readily available. Further, prophylactic measures, such as combining steroids with bisphosphonates or other anti-resorptive agents are possible, and are increasingly being used.[65] Further discussion of secondary osteoporosis associated with steroid use can be found in Chapter 18.

With BMD measurements it is possible to evaluate the drug effects throughout the whole skeleton. Oestrogen has been shown to have a protective effect against bone loss, not only in the peripheral skeleton, but also in the spine and femoral neck,[66,67] and in addition is able to preserve total body calcium.[68] However, while fluoride has been found to increase spinal bone mass,[69] appendicular bone mass has not been shown to increase, and there is even the suggestion that there may be loss at that site, with an increased incidence of peripheral fracture at certain dose levels.[70,71] Nasal calcitonin has been shown to prevent spinal bone loss, but not loss from the peripheral skeleton and total body.[72] This may simply be a dose-related phenomenon, but, by increasing dosage, there is likely to be an increased incidence of side effects. In contrast, bisphosphonates have been shown to increase BMD in the spine, femur, forearm and total body.[73–75]

Gonadotrophin agonists are increasingly being used in clinical practice, and by inducing hypo-oestrogenism may cause bone loss.[76] As many of the conditions being treated are benign, such as endometriosis and fibroids, the duration of the drug use will be limited by its skeletal effects. It would appear that with treatments of up to 6 months bone loss is largely reversible. However, for regimes combining gonadotrophin agonists with anti-resorptive

Table 16.7 The effect of alendronate on risk of fracture in women with existing vertebral fractures. (Data from the Fracture Intervention Trial.[57])

Fracture site	Relative risk (95% confidence interval)
Morphometric vertebral fractures	0.53 (0.41–0.68)
Clinically apparent vertebral fractures	0.45 (0.27–0.72)
Any clinical fracture	0.72 (0.58–0.90)
Hip fracture	0.49 (0.23–0.99)
Wrist fracture	0.52 (0.31–0.87)

agents bone mass measurements are critical to their evaluation. Long-term heparin therapy is associated with osteoporosis. Although the mechanism is uncertain, the effect is dose-related and may be reversible when treatment is stopped.[77] There is some controversy about the effect of the combined contraceptive pill on the skeleton. Most recent data suggest that it does not influence bone density, and part of the apparent conflict may reflect the higher oestrogen dosage that was formerly used.[78] To reiterate, such issues are open to investigation now that BMD can be readily measured.

Occasionally, surprises do arise. Tamoxifen is widely used in the treatment of breast cancer and, since it is an anti-oestrogen, there was some concern that it could lead to bone loss. However, the drug itself has some oestrogenic properties, and studies to date have shown that it is in fact protective with regard to the skeleton in postmenopausal women.[79,80] A related compound, raloxifine,[81] is a member of a class of drugs called SERMs, compounds that have the potential ability to mimic the beneficial effects of oestrogen on osteoporosis and cardiovascular disease while antagonizing the effects on the breast and uterus. This agent is already

licensed for use in the USA, and is expected to become available in Europe during 1998.

Bone densitometry measurements have had an important role in the evaluation of new treatments for osteoporosis in controlled clinical trials.[73,75,82,83] Verifying that these treatments actually reduce fracture incidence is of fundamental importance and studies such as the Fracture Intervention Trial (FIT) have shown that fracture incidence in the highest risk groups can be reduced by 50% (Table 16.7).[57] Cummings et al. have drawn attention to the fact that in the FIT study and other recent trials, the increase in BMD in the treatment group could explain only 40% of the reduction in fracture incidence.[84] Similar studies of other new treatments, including other bisphosphonates and SERMs are nearing completion. If the large reduction in fracture incidence in elderly subjects is confirmed, the success of anti-resorptive therapy is likely to have a significant influence on perceptions of how to prevent osteoporosis and on which populations should be targeted for treatment.

Clinical decision making

Even when osteoporosis is diagnosed according to the WHO criteria, patients may have reservations about commencing treatment such as hormone replacement therapy (HRT). Clearly, all the therapeutic options will have been discussed with these individuals, and they will have weighed up the possible advantages and disadvantages. It may be that a decision is reached to take long-term oestrogen therapy simply because of a low bone density result. Although it is probably not essential with HRT, follow-up scans are often performed to check a patient's response to treatment. A good case can be made for at least one further BMD measurement after 2–3 years of treatment. In this situation, it is reassuring for both the patient and the physician to know that treatment is indeed preventing further bone loss. Another situation where serial measurements may be of value is at the time of initial consultation when results are equivocal and the patient wishes to avoid treatment if at all possible. Repeat measurements over the next few years, depending on the clinical situation, would enable a final decision to be reached, since in addition to baseline results there would also be an assessment of the rate of bone loss.

There are many clinical situations where BMD measurements may help in reaching decisions regarding therapy, such as primary hyperparathyroidism, where it may be difficult to decide whether to continue with conservative management or advise surgery. If significant bone loss is occurring then this would clearly influence a decision towards surgery. Other conditions where BMD measurements may influence management include anorexia nervosa and rheumatoid arthritis. Osteoporosis of pregnancy has been mentioned previously. This condition is rare and incompletely understood. However, affected women will often ask how severe the skeletal involvement is and should they have further pregnancies? These are difficult questions to answer, but at least the severity of disease can be assessed and, since there is often spontaneous improvement, this can be documented with serial measurements.

Bone mineral measurements in the elderly

It has been shown that in older women also, bisphosphonate and other drugs can retard bone loss and even restore some bone mass. This makes it important not to exclude the older patient from bone mineral measurements. There are, however, a few caveats to be considered. With advancing age, coexisting degenerative changes in the lumbar spine become more frequent. In the authors' clinic about one-third of women over the age of 70 years that are seen for bone mineral measurements because of a clinical suspicion of osteoporosis, have significant degenerative changes in the lumbar spine, which may prevent this site being used for fracture risk prediction. In addition, in this age group 50% or more of women may have a T-score below −2.5. As discussed above, in older women it may be best to interpret BMD results using Z-score results.

MALE OSTEOPOROSIS

Although osteoporosis is predominantly a disease of women, it is apparent that significant numbers of men are affected with up to 30% of hip fractures and 20% of vertebral fractures occurring in this population. Further, while the mortality associated with hip fracture is around 18% in the UK, men have an approximately threefold higher likelihood of death after hip fractures than women.[85] In addition, there seems to be an increasing incidence of osteoporotic fractures in men, which may be due to increased life expectancy, reduced physical activity, and perhaps smoking and alcohol consumption. In men with symptomatic vertebral fractures, secondary causes of osteoporosis are more common and involve about 50% of cases compared with 35% in women. The most important factors in men include hypogonadism, alcoholism, steroid therapy and hyperthyroidism. In the majority of cases no underlying pathology is found. However, in the experience of the authors a significant minority have low–normal testosterone levels with no evidence of organ failure, in as much as gonadotrophins are normal. It is still to be shown whether testosterone supplementation will prove to be effective in such cases.

With the increasing availability of bone density measurements, there is a marked rise in the number of males who are found to have osteopenia or osteoporosis. It is important to realize that the WHO criteria for the diagnosis of osteoporosis relate specifically to Caucasian women. However, several studies have related bone density in men to the risk of fracture and, in general, low BMD in the spine or hip is associated with greater fracture risk.[86–89] On the basis of the data available from Europe, the fracture risk increases approximately twofold for every 1 SD reduction in BMD, which is similar to the risk found in women.[90] It may well be, therefore, that the WHO criteria are appropriate in men, but further research is required. Also, less attention has been paid to the accuracy of manufacturer reference ranges in men, and these need to be validated in clinical practice. For the femur, however, the NHANES study included approximately equal numbers of men and women.[44,46]

As stated above, a large number of men are now being diagnosed as having osteopenia and management of these cases is problematic since they are often otherwise healthy and relatively young. In general, the use of BMD measurements for clinical decision making relating to therapy in men remains contentious and data are awaited that such intervention may lead to a reduction in fracture risk. Management of male osteoporosis is a complex topic, but one that is attracting growing interest, including a recent extensive review by a UK Consensus Group.[91]

REFERENCES

1. Kanis JA, Delmas P, Burckhardt P et al. Guidelines for the diagnosis and management of osteoporosis. *Osteoporos Int* (1997) **7:** 390–406.
2. Eddy DM, Johnston CC, Cummings SR et al. Osteoporosis: cost effectiveness analysis and review of the evidence for prevention, diagnosis and treatment: the basis for a guideline for the medical management of osteoporosis. *Osteoporos Int* (1998) (in press).
3. Consensus development conference: diagnosis, prophylaxis and treatment of osteoporosis. *Am J Med* (1991) **90:** 107–10.
4. Consensus development conference: diagnosis, prophylaxis and treatment of osteoporosis. *Am J Med* (1993) **94:** 646–50.
5. Glüer C-C, Wu Y, Jergas M et al. Three quantitative ultrasound parameters reflect bone structure. *Calcif Tissue Int* (1994) **55:** 46–52.
6. Glüer C-C. Quantitative ultrasound techniques for the assessment of osteoporosis: expert agreement on current status. *J Bone Miner Res* (1997) **12:** 1280–8.
7. Laugier P, Droin P, Laval-Jeantet AM et al. In-vitro assessment of the relationship between acoustic properties and bone mass density of the calcaneus by comparison of ultrasound parametric imaging and quantitative computed tomography. *Bone* (1997) **20:** 157–65.
8. Genant HK, Engelke K, Fuerst T et al. Noninvasive measurement of bone mineral and structure: state of the art. *J Bone Miner Res* (1996) **11:** 707–30.
9. Glüer C-C, Jergas M, Hans D. Peripheral measurement techniques for the assessment of osteoporosis. *Semin Nucl Med* (1997) **27:** 229–47.
10. World Health Organization. Assessment of fracture risk and its application to screening for postmenopausal osteoporosis. WHO Technical Report Series 843 (WHO: Geneva, 1994).
11. Kanis JA, Melton LJ, Christiansen C et al. The diagnosis of osteoporosis. *J Bone Miner Res* (1994) **9:** 1137–41.
12. Rockoff SD, Sweet E, Bleustein J. The relative contribution of trabecular and cortical bone to the strength of human lumbar vertebrae. *Calcif Tissue Res* (1969) **3:** 163–75.
13. Dalen N, Hellstrom LG, Jacobsen B. Bone mineral content and mechanical strength of the femoral neck. *Acta Orthop Scand* (1976) **47:** 503–8.
14. Hansson T, Roos B, Nachemson A. The bone mineral content and ultimate compressive strength of lumbar vertebrae. *Spine* (1980) **5:** 46–55.
15. Horsman A, Currey JD. Estimation of mechanical properties of the distal radius from bone mineral content and cortical width. *Clin Orthop* (1983) **A6:** 298–304.
16. Myers BS, Arbogast KB, Lobaugh B et al. Improved assessment of lumbar vertebral body strength using supine lateral dual-energy x-ray

absorptiometry. *J Bone Miner Res* (1994) **9:** 687–93.

17. Moro M, Hecker AT, Bouxsein ML, Myers ER. Failure load of thoracic vertebrae correlates with lumbar bone mineral density measured by DXA. *Calcif Tissue Int* (1995) **56:** 206–9.

18. Bjarnason K, Hassager C, Svendesen OL et al. Anteroposterior and lateral spinal DXA for the assessment of vertebral body strength: comparison with hip and forearm measurements. *Osteoporos Int* (1996) **6:** 37–42.

19. Melton LJ, Kan SH, Wahner HW et al. Lifetime fracture risk: an approach to hip fracture risk assessment based on bone mineral density and age. *J Clin Epidemiol* (1988) **41:** 985–94.

20. Hui SL, Slemenda CW, Johnston CC. Age and bone mass as predictors of fractures in a prospective study. *J Clin Invest* (1988) **81:** 1804–9.

21. Ross PD, Davis JW, Epstein RS et al. Pre-existing fractures and bone mass predict vertebral fracture incidence in women. *Ann Intern Med* (1991) **114:** 919–23.

22. Seeley DG, Browner WS, Nevitt MC et al. Which fractures are associated with low appendicular bone mass in elderly women? *Ann Intern Med* (1991) **115:** 837–42.

23. Black D, Cummings SR, Genant HK et al. Axial and appendicular bone density predict fractures in older women. *J Bone Miner Res* (1992) **7:** 633–8.

24. Black D, Cummings SR, Melton LJ. Appendicular bone mineral and a woman's lifetime risk of hip fracture. *J Bone Miner Res* (1992) **7:** 639–46.

25. Suman VJ, Atkinson EJ, Black DM et al. A nomogram for predicting lifetime hip fracture risk from radius bone mineral density and age. *Bone* (1993) **14:** 843–6.

26. Ross PD, Genant HK, Davis JW et al. Predicting vertebral fracture incidence from prevalent fractures and bone density among non-black osteoporotic women. *Osteoporos Int* (1993) **3:** 120–6.

27. Cummings SR, Black DM, Nevitt MC et al. Bone density at various sites for prediction of hip fractures. *Lancet* (1993) **341:** 72–5.

28. Hui SL, Slemenda CW, Carey MA et al. Choosing between predictors of fractures. *J Bone Miner Res* (1995) **10:** 1816–22.

29. Marshall D, Johnell O, Wedel H. Meta-analysis of how well measures of bone mineral density predict occurrence of osteoporotic fractures. *Br Med J* (1996) **312:** 1254–9.

30. Düppe H, Gärdsell P, Nilsson B, Johnell O. A single bone density measurement can predict fractures over 25 years. *Calcif Tissue Int* (1997) **60:** 171–4.

31. Melton LJ, Thamer M, Ray NF et al. Fractures attributable to osteoporosis: report from the National Osteoporosis Foundation. *J Bone Miner Res* (1997) **12:** 16–23.

32. Meunier PJ, Sellami S, Briancon D et al. Histological heterogeneity of apparently idiopathic osteoporosis. In: DeLuca H, Frost J, Jee WSS et al., eds, *Osteoporosis* (University Park Press: Baltimore, 1981), 321.

33. Riggs BL, Wahner HW, Seeman E et al. Changes in bone mineral density of the proximal femur and spine with aging. Differences between the postmenopausal and senile osteoporotic syndromes. *J Clin Invest* (1982) **70:** 716–23.

34. Mazess RB. Bone density in diagnosis of osteoporosis: thresholds and breakpoints. *Calcif Tissue Int* (1987) **41:** 117–18.

35. Ryan PJ, Blake GM, Herd R et al. Spine and femur BMD by DXA in patients with varying severity of spinal osteoporosis. *Calcif Tissue Int* (1993) **52:** 263–8.

36. Nordin BEC. The definition and diagnosis of osteoporosis. *Calcif Tissue Int* (1987) **40:** 57.

37. Eastell R, Wahner HW, O'Fallon WM et al. Unequal decrease in bone density of lumbar spine and ultradistal radius in Colles and vertebral fracture syndromes. *J Clin Invest* (1989) **83:** 168–74.

38. Faulkner KG, Roberts LA, McClung MR. Discrepancies in normative data between Lunar and Hologic DXA systems. *Osteoporos Int* (1996) **6:** 432–6.

39. Kelly TL. Bone mineral density reference databases for American men and women. *J Bone Miner Res* (1990) **5**(suppl 1): S249.

40. Steiger P, Cummings SR, Black DM et al. Age-related decrements in bone mineral density in women over 65. *J Bone Miner Res* (1992) **7:** 625–32.

41. Petley GW, Cotton AM, Murrills AJ et al. Reference ranges of bone mineral density in southern England: the impact of local data on the diagnosis of osteoporosis. *Br J Radiol* (1996) **69:** 655–60.

42. Ahmed AIH, Blake GM, Rymer JM, Fogelman I. Screening for osteopenia and osteoporosis: do the accepted normal ranges lead to overdiagnosis? *Osteoporos Int* (1997) **7:** 432–8.

43. Truscott JG, Simpson DS, Fordham JN. A suggested methodology for the construction of national bone densitometry reference ranges:

1372 caucasian women from four UK sites. *Br J Radiol* (1997) **70:** 1245–51.

44. Looker AC, Wahner HW, Dunn WL et al. Proximal femur bone mineral levels of US adults. *Osteoporos Int* (1995) **5:** 389–409.

45. Looker AC, Orwoll ES, Johnston CC et al. Prevalence of low femoral bone density in older US adults from NHANES III. *J Bone Miner Res* (1997) **12:** 1761–8.

46. Looker AC, Wahner HW, Dunn WL et al. Updated data on proximal femur bone mineral levels of US adults. *Osteoporos Int* (1998) (in press).

47. Hanson J. Standardization of femur BMD [letter]. *J Bone Miner Res* (1997) **12:** 1316–17.

48. Aloia JF, Cohn SH, Vaswani A et al. Risk factors for postmenopausal osteoporosis. *Am J Med* (1985) **78:** 95–100.

49. Elders PJ, Netelenbos JC, Lips P et al. Perimenopausal bone mass and risk factors. *Bone Miner* (1989) **7:** 289–99.

50. Slemenda CW, Hui SL, Longcope C et al. Predictors of bone mass in perimenopausal women. *Ann Intern Med* (1990) **112:** 96–101.

51. Cummings SR, Nevitt MC, Browner WS et al. Risk factors for hip fractures in white women. *N Engl J Med* (1995) **332:** 767–73.

52. Abrahamsen B, Hansen TB, Bjorn Jenson L et al. Site of osteodensitometry in perimenopausal women: correlation and limits of agreement between anatomic regions. *J Bone Miner Res* (1997) **12:** 1471–9.

53. Black DM, Palermo L, Genant HK, Cummings SR. Four reasons to avoid the use of BMD T-scores in treatment decisions for osteoporosis. *J Bone Miner Res* (1996) **11**(suppl 1): S118.

54. Eastell R. Assessment of bone density and bone loss. *Osteoporos Int* (1996) **6**(suppl 2): S3–S5.

55. Blake GM, Fogelman I. Interpretation of bone densitometry studies. *Semin Nucl Med* (1997) **27:** 248–60.

56. Eastell R. Treatment of postmenopausal osteoporosis. *N Engl J Med* (1998) **338:** 736–46.

57. Black DM, Cummings SR, Karpf DB et al. Randomised trial of effect of alendronate on risk of fracture in women with existing vertebral fractures. *Lancet* (1996) **348:** 1535–41.

58. Collaborative Group on Hormonal Factors in Breast Cancer. Breast cancer and hormone replacement therapy: collaborative reanalysis of data from 51 epidemiological studies of 52,705 women with breast cancer and 108,411 women without breast cancer. *Lancet* (1997) **350:** 1047–59.

59. Ross PD, Wasnich RD, MacLean CJ et al. A model for estimating the potential costs and savings of osteoporosis prevention strategies. *Bone* (1988) **9:** 337–47.

60. Mazess RB, Peppler WW, Chesney RW et al. Does bone measurement on the radius indicate skeletal status? Concise communication. *J Nucl Med* (1984) **25:** 281–8.

61. American College of Rheumatology Task Force on Osteoporosis Guidelines. Recommendations for the prevention and treatment of glucocorticoid-induced osteoporosis. *Arthritis Rheum* (1996) **39:** 1791–801.

62. Eastell R, Reid DM, Compston J et al. UK Consensus Group on management of glucocorticoid-induced osteoporosis: an update. *J Internal Med* (1998) (in press).

63. LoCascio V, Bonucci E, Imbimbo B et al. Bone loss in response to long-term glucocorticoid therapy. *Bone Miner* (1990) **8:** 39–51.

64. Lukert BP, Raisz LG. Glucocorticoid-induced osteoporosis: pathogenesis and management. *Ann Intern Med* (1990) **112:** 352–64.

65. Reid IR. Preventing glucocorticoid-induced osteoporosis. *N Engl J Med* (1997) **337:** 420–1.

66. Savvas M, Studd JW, Fogelman I et al. Skeletal effects of oral oestrogen compared with subcutaneous oestrogen and testosterone in postmenopausal women. *Br Med J* (1988) **297:** 331–3.

67. Al-Azzawi F, Hart DM, Lindsay R. Long term effect of oestrogen replacement therapy on bone mass as measured by dual photon absorptiometry. *Br Med J* (1987) **294:** 1261–2.

68. Riis B, Thomsen K, Christiansen C. Does calcium supplementation prevent postmenopausal bone loss? *N Engl J Med* (1987) **316:** 173–7.

69. Riggs BL, Seeman E, Hodgson SF et al. Effect of the fluoride–calcium regime on vertebral fracture occurrence in postmenopausal osteoporosis. *N Engl J Med* (1982) **306:** 446–50.

70. Inkovaara J, Heikinheimo R, Jarvinen K et al. Prophylactic fluoride treatment and aged bones. *Br Med J* (1975) **286:** 1283–8.

71. Riggs BL, Hodgson SF, O'Fallon WM et al. Effect of fluoride treatment on the fracture rate in postmenopausal women with osteoporosis. *N Engl J Med* (1990) **322:** 820–9.

72. Overgaard K, Riis BJ, Christiansen C et al. Effect of salcatonin given intranasally on early postmenopausal bone loss. *Br Med J* (1989) **299:** 477–9.

73. Libermann UA, Weiss SR, Bröll J et al. Effect of oral alendronate on bone mineral density and

the incidence of fractures in postmenopausal osteoporosis. *N Engl J Med* (1995) **333:** 1437–43.

74. Faulkner KG, McClung MR, Ravn P et al. Monitoring skeletal response to therapy in early postmenopausal women: which bone to measure? *J Bone Miner Res* (1996) **11**(suppl 1): S96.

75. Herd RJM, Balena R, Blake GM et al. The prevention of early postmenopausal bone loss by cyclical etidronate therapy: a 2-year double-blind placebo-controlled study. *Am J Med* (1997) **103:** 92–9.

76. Fogelman I. Gonadotrophin-releasing hormone agonists and the skeleton. *Fertil Steril* (1982) **57:** 715–24.

77. Avioli LV. Heparin-induced osteopenia: an appraisal. *Adv Exp Med Biol* (1975) **52:** 375–87.

78. Rodin A, Chapman M, Fogelman I. Bone density in users of combined oral contraception. *Br J Family Planning* (1991) **16:** 125–8.

79. Fentiman IS, Caleffi M, Rodin A et al. Bone mineral content of women receiving tamoxifen for mastalgia. *Br J Cancer* (1989) **60:** 262–6.

80. Fentiman IS, Saad Z, Caleffi M et al. Tamoxifen protects against steroid-induced bone loss. *Eur J Cancer* (1992) **28:** 684–5.

81. Delmas PD, Bjarnason NH, Mitlak BH et al. Effects of raloxifene on bone mineral density, serum cholesterol concentrations, and uterine endometrium in postmenopausal women. *N Engl J Med* (1997) **337:** 1641–7.

82. Storm T, Thamsborg G, Steiniche T et al. Effect of intermittent cyclical etidronate therapy on bone mass and fracture rate in women with postmenopausal osteoporosis. *N Engl J Med* (1990) **322:** 1265–71.

83. Watts NB, Harris ST, Genant HK et al. Intermittent cyclical etidronate treatment of postmenopausal osteoporosis. *N Engl J Med* (1990) **323:** 73–9.

84. Cummings SR, Black DM, Vogt TM. Changes in BMD substantially underestimate the antifracture effects of alendronate and other antiresorptive drugs. *J Bone Miner Res* (1996) **11**(suppl 1): S102.

85. Todd CJ, Freeman CJ, Camilleri-Ferrante C et al. Differences in mortality after fracture of hip: the East Anglian audit. *Br Med J* (1995) **310:** 904–8.

86. Gärdsell P, Johnell O, Nilsson BE. The predictive value of forearm bone mineral content measurements in men. *Bone* (1990) **11:** 229–32.

87. Chevallay T, Rizzoli R, Nydegger V et al. Preferential low bone mineral density of the femoral neck in patients with a recent fracture of the proximal femur. *Osteoporos Int* (1991) **1:** 146–54.

88. Karlsson MK, Johnell O, Nilsson BE et al. Bone mineral mass in hip fracture patients. *Bone* (1993) **14:** 161–5.

89. Resch A, Schneider B, Bernecker P et al. Risk of vertebral fractures in men: relationship to mineral density of the vertebral body. *Am J Roentgenol* (1995) **164:** 1447–50.

90. Lunt M, Felsenberg D, Adams J et al. Population-based geographic variations in DXA bone density in Europe: the EVOS study. *Osteoporos Int* (1997) **7:** 175–89.

91. Eastell R, Boyle IT, Compston J et al. Management of male osteoporosis: report of the UK Consensus Group. *QJM* (1998) **91:** 71–92.

92. Blake GM, Patel R, Fogelman I. Peripheral or axial bone density measurements? *J Clin Densitometry* (1998) **1:** 55–63.

17

The Use of Bone Densitometry in Clinical Trials

Guest chapter by Colin G Miller

CONTENTS • **Chapter overview** • **Introduction** • **Precision and discrimination** • **Reliability** • **Relevance and acceptability** • **Expense** • **Safety and ethical implications** • **Quality control in clinical trials** • **Conclusion**

CHAPTER OVERVIEW

The increased recognition of the scale of morbidity and mortality attributable to osteoporosis has led to a major effort by the pharmaceutical industry to develop new therapeutic strategies for fracture prevention. Bone densitometry measurements have played an important role in clinical trials to verify the efficacy and safety of these new treatments. Dual-energy X-ray absorptiometry (DXA) in particular, with its high precision, low radiation dose and long-term stability of calibration, has been widely used in trials of new pharmaceuticals to prevent bone loss or treat osteoporosis. This chapter discusses the requirements for instrumentation suitable for use in these studies. The benefits in terms of staff training and increased awareness of the requirements of instrumental quality control to centres participating in large international studies are also emphasized.

INTRODUCTION

Standards and requirements for physical measurements in clinical trials of new pharmaceuticals are ultimately defined by the acceptance of data by regulatory authorities. Currently, the accepted standard for the measurement of changes in bone mass is DXA of the lumbar spine and proximal femur, and optionally the total body and distal forearm.[1-4] The techniques of dual photon absorptiometry (DPA) and single photon absorptiometry (SPA), while accepted methods of measuring bone density, have now been superseded by DXA. As discussed in Chapter 5, newer peripheral instruments are being introduced, which add to the choices available.

Bone mass measurements are regarded as a surrogate endpoint for fractures of the spine, hip or forearm. However, with the widespread adoption of the guidelines published by the World Health Organization (WHO) Study Group,[5,6] osteoporosis has been redefined as a bone mineral density (BMD) more than 2.5 standard deviations (SD) below peak bone mass. Therefore, fractures are now regarded as a symptom of the disease of low bone mass. Some regulatory authorities, particularly the American Food and Drug Administration (FDA), question the use of DXA alone and require supporting evidence that bone quality is not being compromised by therapeutic intervention. This is particularly the case for non-oestrogenic compounds. Many other agencies have accepted bone mass as a surrogate end-point of efficacy, but this is changing. Therefore, the pharmaceutical industry is continually reviewing new methodologies that may have an important role in assessing skeletal status.

The general parameters that should be evaluated for instruments used in clinical trials are as follows:[7]

- Precision
- Discrimination (clinical range)
- Reliability (dependability)
- Relevance (measures a pertinent parameter)
- Acceptance by regulatory agencies
- Expense
- Safety

Due to the problems associated with the frequent replacement of the radionuclide source and the poorer precision of measurements compared with DXA, DPA was superseded by DXA in 1987[8] and is now regarded as being obsolete.[9] Quantitative computed tomography (QCT) has limited utility due to the high patient radiation dose, its cost and the limited number of sites where the technology is available. With the advent of software to perform forearm scans with axial DXA scanners, SPA instruments have also been superseded. More recently, new devices dedicated to studies of the peripheral skeleton and based on the principles of dual-energy X-ray absorptiometry have been developed.[10] This type of technology will be referred to as peripheral DXA (pDXA). Peripheral QCT (pQCT) instruments which allow the measurement of forearm trabecular and cortical bone have also gained popularity in some countries, notably Germany.[10] The new forearm instruments have reopened the debate on the potential usefulness of peripheral measurements. However, most experts agree that a BMD measurement at the specific site of interest provides the most reliable way of predicting fracture risk at that site.[11] Recent studies suggest that, if a single measurement is to be made,

then the proximal femur is probably the optimum site.[12] However, with the latest developments in axial DXA instruments, scan times are now so short that there is no reason why the clinician should not obtain measurements at both the spine and hip. The optimum peripheral site is probably the calcaneus.[11]

Quantitative ultrasound (QUS) measurement of bone, although not yet approved by regulatory agencies for use in clinical trials, is rapidly becoming an accepted methodology for the prediction of fracture risk.[13] The measurement of broadband ultrasonic attenuation (BUA), speed of sound (SOS), and a combination of the two termed Stiffness, or Quantitative Ultrasound Index (QUI), offers new assessments whose application in clinical trials has only recently started to be explored.[13] A majority of commercial QUS instruments measure the calcaneus, although instruments measuring other skeletal sites are now being assessed (see Chapter 7). Most published studies using ultrasonometry are cross sectional, comparing results to the recognized standards of SPA, QCT or DXA without therapeutic intervention;[14,15] or they are prospective studies designed to assess the applicability of ultrasound to predict fracture risk.[16-18] These latter have provided important evidence that QUS measurements at the calcaneus have a role in assessing skeletal status, since they demonstrate that ultrasound has a similar predictive capability for fracture as has DXA. Ultrasonometry methodologies for other sites are still awaiting the completion of prospective studies.

In general, peripheral devices measure either the calcaneus or the forearm, although there are now devices that measure the phalanges, or other sites such as the tibia. However, there are many new peripheral instruments becoming available, with new data being published continually, and it is outside the scope of this chapter to evaluate them all. The aim instead is to provide generic assessments that the trialist can use to evaluate the different modalities. New devices evaluating other anatomical sites will have to withstand the same rigours of judgement prior to gaining widespread acceptance as did existing modalities, particularly in the evaluation of predictive capabilities for determining fracture risk.

PRECISION AND DISCRIMINATION

Precision is a measure of the repeatability of a measurement, and is normally expressed by the coefficient of variation (CV), which is calculated as the standard deviation (SD) of repeated measurements divided by the mean (CV = (SD/mean) × 100). Discrimination is the ability of an instrument to distinguish normal from abnormal, or, in this instance, an osteoporotic from a non-osteoporotic individual. For clinical trials, and whenever serial measurements are being made, the two parameters should be considered together. The clinically useful precision of a device depends not only on the CV, but also the range of values obtained with the instrument in clinical studies. This latter will be referred to as the *clinical range* of the instrument. If two instruments have a similar CV, the device with the wider clinical range relative to the mean will have the better clinical precision.

To allow for this factor, a better comparison of instruments is obtained using the standardized coefficient of variation (SCV), which is calculated as the standard deviation of repeated measurements divided by the clinical range (SCV = (SD/clinical range) × 100). Originally, the clinical range was defined as the 5th to 95th percentiles of the population under assessment.[19] For the sake of this discussion, however, the clinical range will be defined as the difference between the mean for healthy young normal adults and that for healthy individuals aged 70 years or over. This definition makes the inherent assumption that diseased individuals demonstrate a similar pattern of bone loss as the age-related losses in the elderly population.

A comparison of precision and discrimination of DXA and ultrasound is presented in Table 17.1. For spine DXA measurements, the CV of 1.0% and clinical range (on Lunar densitometers) of 0.9–1.2 g/cm^2 gives an SCV of 4.0%

Table 17.1 A comparison of precision and discrimination of DXA and ultrasound measurements.

	DXA spine (g/cm^2)	DXA hip (g/cm^2)	BUA calcaneus (dB/MHz)	SOS calcaneus (m/s)	Stiffness or QUI (No units)
Range of values (osteoporotic – normal)	0.9–1.2	0.7–1.0	100–125	1500–1560	67–100
Precision (CV)	1.0%	1.2%	1.5%	0.3%	1.8%
Discrimination as SCV	4.0%	4.0%	7.5%	7.8%	5.4%

CV, (SD/mean) × 100; SCV, (SD/clinical range) × 100; CV = coefficient of variation; SD = standard deviation; SCV = standardized coefficient of variation.

(Lunar Corp., Madison, WI, USA). With the better precision of hip DXA measurements offered by the total femur site, the SCV for a hip BMD scan is now comparable to the spine. SCV is particularly useful for comparing QUS and DXA measurements. Stiffness or QUI, which combines information from BUA and SOS, has been demonstrated to have an SCV comparable or even slightly superior to DXA. DXA measurements of the spine and hip, and all other instrumental evaluations using density, have probably reached their optimum precision due to the problems of accurate repositioning for repeated measurements.

In the clinical trial setting, the precision determines the length of time required to see a statistically significant change in the measurements. The time obviously depends on the type of therapy. This is explained more fully in Table 17.2. For example, if a therapeutic intervention is expected to produce an increase of 1% per year in BMD or stiffness, and a 2% measurement precision is anticipated, it would take 5.5 years to see a significant change from baseline, based at the 95% confidence interval. If an 80% confidence level was selected, then the difference could be observed in 3.6 years. Alternatively, a therapeutic intervention causing an increase of 5% per year would require only 0.7 years or 1.1 years at the 80% and 95% levels of confidence respectively.

RELIABILITY

Table 17.3 gives details of the other important characteristics for instruments used for clinical trials. The reliability of an instrument is a mark of its stability in performance over time. For DXA this is assessed by daily measurements of phantoms. Axial DXA instruments have a proven record of reliability,[20-22] and methods have been developed for identifying and correcting problems should they occur (see Chapter 9). Peripheral DXA systems, due to their similarities with axial DXA instruments, are also likely to prove reliable. For QUS instruments there is currently no recognized calibra-

Table 17.2 Instrument precision: the effect on length of study and statistically significant changes for instruments used in clinical trials.

Precision of measurement	Confidence level	Statistically significant BMD change	Time (in years) required to see significant change in BMD		
			Expected 1% change per year	Expected 2% change per year	Expected 5% change per year
1%	80%	±1.8%	1.8	0.9	0.4
	95%	±2.8%	2.8	1.4	0.6
2%	80%	±3.6%	3.6	1.8	0.7
	95%	±5.5%	5.5	2.8	1.1
3%	80%	±5.4%	5.4	2.7	1.1
	95%	±8.5%	8.3	4.2	1.7

Table 17.3 A comparison of reliability, relevance, acceptance by regulatory agencies and expense of axial DXA, peripheral DXA and ultrasound equipment in the clinical trial setting.

	Peripheral DXA	Spine DXA	Hip DXA	BUA	SOS	Stiffness or QUI
Safe	Yes	Yes	Yes	Yes	Yes	Yes
Reliable	Yes	Yes	Yes	Yes	Yes	Yes
Relevant	Yes	Yes	Yes	Yes	Yes	Yes
Accepted by regulatory agencies	Yes	Yes	Yes	Yes/no[a]	Yes/no[a]	Yes/no[a]
Expensive	No	Yes	Yes	No	No	No

[a] While ultrasound instruments are now accepted for patient assessment, their use is not yet accepted by regulatory authorities for measurements in clinical trials.

tion standard although, as with DXA, each manufacturer has developed its own independent phantom. A phantom for the measurement of SOS is not a major difficulty since there are quoted values in reference books for various materials.[23] However, the development of a phantom for the assessment of BUA, or the parameters of Stiffness and QUI that combine BUA and SOS, has proved to be more difficult to develop due to the need to represent properly the varying structural components of the bone.

RELEVANCE AND ACCEPTABILITY

There is no consensus at present that DXA, pDXA or QCT measurements alone are acceptable surrogates for the structural integrity of bone. However, DXA measurements are the currently accepted standard for the measurement of bone density. It has been argued that for the highest clinical reliability, measurements should be made at the site of fracture. For this reason, forearm measurements are accepted. However, although the calcaneus is not a com-

mon site of osteoporotic fracture, instruments utilizing the calcaneus may actually be assessing one of the best locations for predicting fragility fractures at other sites in the skeleton.[11] Since QUS utilizes a different technology from the other methodologies described above, the FDA has required a considerable amount of data to accept the benefit of this modality. However, there are now more published data on QUS than when DXA was introduced onto the market.

EXPENSE

The expense of equipment is not a major consideration until Phase III and Phase IV studies are undertaken. Phase II studies are usually very specialized, and the sites where these studies are conducted are normally centres of excellence where the most up-to-date equipment and techniques are usually available, or can be purchased as part of a research grant. QCT may be utilized for its ability to identify changes in trabecular bone alone. However, the limitations of expense, radiation dose and precision mean that QCT has not been used in many clinical trials.

The cost of equipment plays an important role in planning by pharmaceutical companies attempting either to expand market size or increase market share by ensuring that the widest possible range of suitable patients has access to treatment. This is factored into the planning of Phase III and Phase IIIb studies with the inclusion of the relevant instrumentation in such trials. The new peripheral instruments are now being assessed more thoroughly to evaluate their role in making bone density measurements more widely available, and ensuring that the optimum market size is available for new pharmaceutical products reaching the market.

SAFETY AND ETHICAL IMPLICATIONS

The final requirement for instruments used in clinical trials must relate to the safety and ethical implications of undertaking repetitive measurements of bone density. As discussed in Chapter 8, the radiation exposure from DXA, pDXA and pQCT measurements is almost negligible, and the perception of ethical problems is greater than their reality. Nevertheless, QUS is radiation free, and therefore the risk to the patient is non-existent. Thus QUS assessments have the potential to be ideal from the ethical stand-point in the clinical trial setting. QCT measurements involve a significantly higher level of radiation exposure than the other modalities, and therefore care has to be taken with respect to the number of repeated measurements being undertaken, particularly if patients are required to have additional planar radiographs.

QUALITY CONTROL IN CLINICAL TRIALS

The large number of clinical trials involving bone densitometry which have been initiated in the past 10 years have made an important contribution to the efforts of the pharmaceutical industry in developing new therapeutic strat-

---

Table 17.4 Components of DXA operator training programmes for clinical trials.[7]

1) *Trial requirements*
   Patient entry criteria with respect to DXA measurements

2) *Consistency of patient measurements*
   Patient positioning
   Scan analysis

3) *Ensuring daily instrument quality control check*

4) *Requirement for sponsor to review and perform instrument quality control* (particularly in multicentre trials)

5) *Troubleshooting*
   Whom to contact regarding trial patients if problems arise

---

egies for treating and preventing osteoporosis. At the same time, a significant additional benefit has been the opportunity for technologists to gain further training in the operation of equipment and the requirements of instrument quality control.

In large multicentre clinical trials it is now usual for an experienced centre to co-ordinate quality assurance for bone densitometry studies.[21,22] Protocol training is given to technologists (Table 17.4),[7] and scans are analysed at a central laboratory. This ensures a consistent approach to analysis and ensures that both patient and doctor remain blinded to whether the subject is taking active drug or placebo. A set of master phantoms is passed between participating centres to cross calibrate DXA systems. Results from cross calibration are evaluated to assess the homogeneity of the study population. Results of daily phantom quality control scans at individual sites are reviewed regularly to verify that systems are functioning within specifications, and may be used to correct scan data in the event of drifts in system calibration. Requirements for regular preventive maintenance of equipment can be established, and cross-calibration studies can be used to derive corrections if old instruments are replaced by new.

CONCLUSION

The key to the use of physical measurements in clinical trials is to ensure the consistency of the data for each patient. For DXA measurements, an important element of consistency is to ensure that the same anatomical region is scanned in exactly the same position each time the patient attends for a measurement. Following this, the scan must be analysed in the same manner, selecting an identical region of interest. Other parameters to review include: the projected area of the anatomical region under investigation; technical specifications of certain parameters (e.g. R_{st}-value, $d0$-value); and changes in BMC and BMD that are greater than those expected with or without therapeutic intervention.

For any trial, be it for osteoporosis or any other therapeutic area, careful consideration of instrumentation is required. In the field of BMD measurements, as new instruments come onto the market, it is important that they are evaluated appropriately for use in clinical trials.

In conclusion, spine and femur DXA is the accepted standard for bone density measurements in clinical trials. QCT of the vertebral bodies and spine is used mainly in Phase II trials, or perhaps in subsets of Phase III populations, but its use is limited due to prohibitive costs and relatively high radiation exposure. Ultrasonometry, while not at present an accepted methodology for use in clinical trials, is being actively evaluated. With the approval by regulatory agencies of ultrasonometry for the assessment of fracture risk, it is likely that this modality will find large-scale application in clinical trials in the near future, although prob- ably in conjunction with DXA measurements in Phase III and Phase IIIb studies.

REFERENCES

1. Kanis JA, Geusens P, Christiansen C, on behalf of the Working Party of the European Foundation for Osteoporosis and Bone Disease. Guidelines for clinical trials in osteoporosis. *Osteoporos Int* (1991) **1:** 182–8.
2. Notes for guidance on involutional osteoporosis in women, CPMP/EWP/552/95 (European Agency for the Evaluation of Medicinal Products, Human Evaluations Unit: London, 1996).
3. Reginster JY, on behalf of the Group for the Respect of Ethics and Excellence in Science (GREES). Recommendations for the registration of new chemical entities used in the prevention and treatment of osteoporosis. *Calcif Tissue Int* (1995) **57:** 247–50.
4. Kanis JA, Delmas P, Meunier P et al. The GREES recommendations for the registration of new drugs in the prevention and treatment of osteoporosis. *Calcif Tissue Int* (1996) **59:** 410–11.
5. WHO. Assessment of fracture risk and its application to screening for postmenopausal osteoporosis. *Technical Report Series no. 843* (World Health Organization: Geneva, 1994).
6. Kanis JA, Melton LJ, Christiansen C et al. The diagnosis of osteoporosis. *J Bone Miner Res* (1994) **9:** 1137–41.
7. Miller CG. Bone densitometry in clinical trials: the challenge of ensuring optimal data. *Br J Clin Res* (1993) **4:** 113–20.
8. Wahner HW, Dunn WL, Brown ML et al. Comparison of dual-energy x-ray absorptiometry and dual photon absorptiometry for bone mineral measurements of the lumbar spine. *Mayo Clin Proc* (1988) **63:** 1075–84.
9. Genant HK, Engelke K, Fuerst T et al. Noninvasive assessment of bone mineral and structure: state of the art. *J Bone Miner Res* (1996) **11:** 707–30.
10. Glüer C-C, Jergas M, Hans D. Peripheral measurement techniques for the assessment of osteoporosis. *Semin Nucl Med* (1997) **27:** 229–47.
11. Marshall D, Johnell O, Wedel H. Meta-analysis of how well measures of bone mineral density predict occurrence of osteoporotic fractures. *Br Med J* (1996) **312:** 1254–9.

12. Cummings SR, Black DM, Nevitt MC. Bone density at various sites for prediction of hip fractures. *Lancet* (1993) **341:** 72–5.

13. Glüer C-C. Quantitative ultrasound techniques for the assessment of osteoporosis — expert agreement on current status. *J Bone Miner Res* (1997) **12:** 1280–8.

14. Njeh CF, Boivin CM, Langton CM. The role of ultrasound in the assessment of osteoporosis: a review. *Osteoporos Int* (1997) **7:** 7–22.

15. Gregg EW, Kriska AM, Salamone LM et al. The epidemiology of quantitative ultrasound: a review of the relationships with bone mass, osteoporosis and fracture risk. *Osteoporos Int* (1997) **7:** 89–99.

16. Porter RW, Miller CG, Grainger D, Palmer SB. Prediction of hip fracture in elderly women: a prospective study. *Br Med J* (1990) **301:** 638–41.

17. Hans D, Dargent-Molina P, Schott AM et al. Ultrasonographic heel measurements to predict hip fracture in elderly women: the EPIDOS prospective study. *Lancet* (1996) **348:** 511–14.

18. Bauer DC, Glüer C-C, Cauley JA et al. Broadband ultrasonic attenuation predicts fracture strongly and independently of densitometry in older women. *Arch Intern Med* (1997) **157:** 629–34.

19. Miller CG, Herd RJM, Ramalingam T et al. Ultrasonic velocity measurements through the calcaneus: which velocity should be measured? *Osteoporos Int* (1993) **3:** 31–5.

20. Orwoll ES, Oviatt SK. Longitudinal precision of dual-energy x-ray absorptiometry in a multicentre study. *J Bone Miner Res* (1991) **6:** 191–7.

21. Glüer C-C, Faulkner KG, Estilo MJ et al. Quality assurance for bone densitometry research studies: concept and impact. *Osteoporos Int* (1993) **3:** 227–35.

22. Faulkner KG, McClung MR. Quality control of DXA instruments in multicentre trials. *Osteoporos Int* (1995) **5:** 218–27.

23. Wells PNT. *Biomedical Ultrasonics* (Academic Press: New York, 1977).

18

Bone Densitometry in Secondary Osteoporosis

CONTENTS • Steroid osteoporosis • Bone disease with chronic renal failure, dialysis and renal transplantation • Post-transplantation bone disease

STEROID OSTEOPOROSIS

Use of bone mineral measurements

The most common secondary form of osteoporosis is that induced by glucocorticoid treatment. Bone loss is diffuse, affecting both cortical and axial skeleton, although axial bone loss appears more substantial.[1,2] Vertebral and other fractures have been documented.[3–8] Steroid-induced osteoporosis occurs at any age, but is particularly worrisome in older patients who are already at risk of having reduced bone mass,[9] and in children because of retardation of skeletal growth.[10] The magnitude of bone loss with a given dose of steroids is not predictable in a given patient, and some patients show little or no effect at generally used therapeutic doses. Sanbrook et al.[11] have shown that chronic low-dose corticosteroid treatment has no bone lowering effect in patients with rheumatoid arthritis. Steroid-induced bone loss is most pronounced initially (in the first 3–6 months) and levels off later. In one study, measurements of bone density by photon absorptiometry at the radius (SPA) showed normal bone density at the mid-radius, but a decrease at the distal measuring site.[8] Bone loss has also been demonstra-ted in the lumbar spine with dual photon absorptiometry (DPA)[2,8,11,12] and quantitative computed tomography (QCT).[13] Lukert et al.[14] have reviewed bone mineral results obtained from different skeletal sites.

It is unlikely that lost bone can be completely restored when steroid therapy is stopped. However, at least partial bone restoration is suggested by the observation that bone is gained after surgical therapy of Cushing's disease.[15,16] Patients with a liver transplant usually gain bone after high doses of steroids are reduced to maintenance levels.[17] In these patients, however, an improvement of hepatic osteodystrophy may also play a role.

The Scientific Advisory Board of the National Osteoporosis Foundation has designated chronic steroid use to be an indication for the implementation of bone mineral measurements in patients.[18] According to these recommendations, measurements on spine (or appendicular bones) are indicated in a subgroup of patients placed on long-term (more than 1 month) glucocorticoid treatment at a dose of 7.5 mg or more of prednisone a day or an equivalent dose of another steroid. In the management of such cases it is important to reduce the dose of steroids wherever possible or consider substituting prednisone with another agent (e.g. deflazacort[19]) which may have a less detrimental effect on the skeleton. In some cases specific anti-resorptive therapy will be necessary to prevent or reduce the side effects of steroids on bone and options include bisphosphonates,[20] calcitonin,[21] NaF[22,23] or vitamin D,[24] and bone mineral measurements are indicated to assist management. A low bone mineral density (BMD) may trigger these treatment options. It should be noted that the normal relationship between bone density and fracture risk, i.e. an approximate doubling of fracture risk with every 1 standard deviation (SD) reduction in bone density,[25] may not be appropriate for patients being treated with steroids. There is some evidence to suggest that in this situation fractures may occur at bone density values higher than in postmenopausal osteoporosis.[26,27] Figure 18.1 provides some possible guidelines for the use of bone mineral measurements in chronic steroid therapy. However, the interested reader should refer also to the sets of guidelines recently produced by the American College of Rheumatology Task Force on Osteoporosis[28] and by a UK Consensus Group.[29]

Steroid effect on bone

The effect of steroids is complex and not completely understood. Effects are on bone, the kidneys and the gastrointestinal tract. In bone, the normally occurring cyclic process of resorption and formation (which takes 90–150 days per cycle) is uncoupled. There is increased osteoclastic bone resorption and a decrease in osteoblastic bone formation, with decreased production of osteoblasts from precursor cells. Onset of the steroid effect is immediate, although a measurable decrease in BMD manifests itself after only a few months to a year. Serum osteocalcin levels, a marker for bone formation, are reduced almost immediately. A single dose of 10 mg prednisone given to a normal subject reduces serum osteocalcin levels by 50–80% for 24 hours.[30] A 5-day course of 60 mg prednisone daily to normal subjects causes a 68% decrease in osteocalcin levels from baseline lasting 4 days.[31] At 6 months, after 10–25 mg prednisone daily, bone biopsy studies have shown a 27% reduction in trabecular bone volume.[32] One-third of these patients showed no further bone loss after 18 months.

Detailed discussions of the complex mechanism of steroid effects on bone, kidney, gastrointestinal tract and parathyroid glands are available in the recent literature. [14,33] Radiographs in patients with steroid-induced osteoporosis show a typical translucent appearance of the vertebrae (in contrast with the 'corduroy stripe' appearance in idiopathic osteoporosis), abundant pseudocallus formation, osteonecrosis and fractures.[34]

At the level of the *gastrointestinal tract*, glucocorticoids reduce vitamin D-dependent calcium absorption. Also, phosphate absorption is decreased. The reduced intestinal calcium absorption then results in secondary hyperparathyroidism. While PTH levels are not always elevated in steroid-induced hyperparathyroidism, nephrogenous cyclic AMP in urine is generally higher than normal.

At the level of the *kidneys*, steroids induce hypercalciuria and hyperphosphataemia.

BONE DISEASE WITH CHRONIC RENAL FAILURE, DIALYSIS AND RENAL TRANSPLANTATION

Bone disease in chronic renal failure

There are a variety of skeletal abnormalities that may complicate the clinical course of the patient with chronic renal failure and end-stage renal disease. These, and the additional skeletal abnormalities that are side effects from treatment of renal failure, are collectively known as renal osteodystrophy.[35] By the time patients with progressive renal failure start dialysis, the majority have abnormalities on bone biopsy, while only 10% have clinical symptoms.[36] Abnormalities in circulating parathyroid hormone levels and of vitamin D metabolism predominate in the pathophysiology, leading to

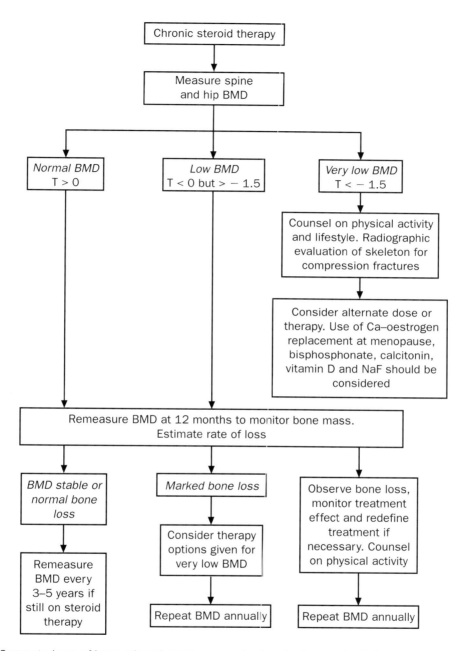

Figure 18.1 Suggested use of bone mineral measurement in chronic glucocorticoid therapy.

Table 18.1 Potential indications for bone mineral measurements in renal bone disease.

A) *Individual patient management*

1) Quantitating the degree of osteopenia (regardless of cause) at time of first diagnosis to estimate the fracture risk. Radiographic correlation is needed because of non-uniformity of bone involvement

2) Baseline study prior to the use of large doses of oral steroids (renal transplantation), with follow-up studies 6 and 12 months later

3) Routine (6 or 12 months) measurements during the course of dialysis and after transplantation to monitor the impact of the treatment regimen on the skeleton. Radiographic correlation is needed for interpretation

B) *Studies of groups of patients*

1) Epidemiological surveys of bone density in patients with renal failure, on dialysis or with renal transplants

2) Monitoring bone mineral in treatment trials in the evaluation of new drugs

---

renal osteodystrophy, although other factors may also play a role. Low levels of calcium and phosphate by themselves can affect bone by inhibiting mineralization of osteoid. Acidosis impairs osteoid mineralization in normal subjects. Magnesium abnormalities may interfere with tissue response to PTH, and uraemia itself inhibits many cellular processes.

The radiographic bone changes of chronic renal disease are osteomalacia, osteitis fibrosa, osteoporosis and extraskeletal calcifications. A number of patients have osteosclerosis, which has an unknown biochemical basis. The skeletal involvement is often regional and focal at times, in contrast with involutional osteoporosis, where – at least in the later stages – the skeleton is uniformly involved. Bone density values vary with the stage of the disease. Potential indications for bone mineral measurements in renal bone disease are given in Table 18.1.

The diagnosis of renal osteodystrophy is made by histological examination of bone biopsy after the administration of two labels of tetracycline 2–3 weeks apart. Based on this examination, five different bone diseases are seen:

1) mild bone disease;
2) hyperparathyroid bone disease;
3) mixed renal osteodystrophy (1 and 2 above);
4) osteomalacia;
5) low-turnover bone disease or aplastic bone disease.

About two thirds of patients have hyperparathyroid bone disease. Of the remaining one-third, 70% have osteomalacia and 30% low-turnover bone disease. Pure osteomalacia and aplastic bone disease are rare. A schematic outline of the progression of bone disease is given in Table 18.2.

Hyperparathyroid bone disease occurs primarily as a result of malabsorption of calcium from the intestine, and is a form of secondary hyperparathyroidism. In a chain of events, hyperphosphataemia occurs owing to the inability of

Table 18.2 Development of renal osteodystrophy.

Glomerular filtration rate	Bone disease
Decrease by 50%	Mild hyperparathyroid bone disease
Decrease to 20% of normal	Mineralization defect
Dialysis	Mixed uraemic osteodystrophy in moderate to advanced renal failure on maintenance dialysis progresses to hyperparathyroid bone disease, osteitis fibrosa or low bone turnover osteomalacia

the failing nephrons to excrete phosphate. This in turn decreases the synthesis of 1,25-dihydroxyvitamin D_3, which leads to a decrease in calcium absorption and hypocalcaemia. PTH increases and leads to bone disease and, with time, hyperplasia of the parathyroid glands. Clinical features include bone pain, myalgia and arthralgia. Fractures generally do not occur, and bone mineral in the spine is generally normal and sometimes even increased.[1]

Osteitis fibrosa shows marrow fibrosis, immature woven bone, and subperiosteal, subchondral and endosteal bone resorption, and is regional in its distribution. An altered amount of collagen or bone marrow fat, as seen with metabolic bone disease and with medullary fibrosis, may introduce errors in bone density measurements by QCT and, to a lesser extent, by dual-energy X-ray absorptiometry (DXA).[37] As the disease progresses, or treatment is instituted, redistribution of bone mineral within the skeleton may occur, leading to regional changes in bone mineral.

Osteomalacia is characterized by excessive osteoid and reduced mineralization. The origin of the mineralization defect is not clear, although aluminium and uraemic toxins have been implicated as possible causes. Clinical features are myopathy, bone pain, and rib, pelvis and other bone fractures. Diabetes mellitus, the

post-parathyroidectomy state, steroid use and the anephric state predispose to its development. Bone mineral in the spine is low to low normal.

Mixed bone disease patients generally do not have fractures and bone mineral is generally normal to low normal. With predominance of the osteomalacic feature, lower bone mineral can be expected.

Low-turnover bone disease shows poor osteoblastic and osteoclastic activity. There is impaired mineralization and aluminium stains may be positive. Low bone mineral values are seen.

Osteoporosis is rarely seen in chronic renal failure prior to dialysis treatment, but may coexist with osteosclerosis. Osteoporosis results in low bone mineral values.

Osteosclerosis presents with thickening of trabeculi, and affects the spine, long bones and pelvis, and is often associated with periosteal new bone formation. Bone mineral measurements are again unreliable except for regional information, because of the regional nature of bone involvement. Compared with normal bone, bone mineral is often high in the areas of osteosclerosis.

Soft tissue calcifications can be seen on routine bone mineral scans. If included in the region of interest, these focal calcium deposits can interfere with measurements of bone mineral in adjacent bones (see the discussions on artefacts in Chapters 10 and 12). Total body or local bone mineral scans can be used to quantify soft tissue deposits and follow the effects of therapy on them.

Bone disease in dialysis patients

When dialysis is instituted, blood urea nitrogen (BUN) and other biochemical factors may improve, but in a high proportion of patients the osteodystrophy is not affected and may even become more complex. Another set of factors may now be superimposed on the initial renal osteodystrophy. Heparin can induce osteopenia when given continuously. Oral alkali and acetate given as substitutes for bicarbonate may interfere with normal mineralization. High circulating aluminium levels in the blood from aluminium given orally as a phosphate binder suppress bone formation, although nowadays this is much less common. Radiographic bone changes developing during dialysis include vascular and soft tissue calcification, osteomyelitis and increasing bone mineral loss. The incidence of fracture rises with the length of haemodialysis. Monitoring patients on long-term haemodialysis with bone mineral measurements has been proposed, and may be particularly useful in centres where dialysis bone disease is frequent. Axial and probably also peripheral skeletal sites should be monitored.

Bone disease in renal transplantation

Renal transplantation is the only method of curing the morphological uraemic bone lesions as demonstrated by serial bone biopsy.[38] In well functioning renal transplants this occurs within 10–12 months. Improvement of tubular function leads to increased renal excretion of phosphate. The hyperfunctioning parathyroid glands recover their normal functional equilibrium somewhat more slowly, and the trans-

planted kidney again normally produces 1,25-dihydroxyvitamin D_3. Persistent hyperparathyroidism occasionally occurs. Despite the improvement of uraemic bone lesions, histoquantitative analysis of trabecular bone from the iliac crest shows a continuing reduction of total bone volume that is osteopenia. This is reflected in decreasing BMD at the spine[39] and radius.[40] Because of necessary therapeutic interventions, transplantation confers additional problems. Corticosteroids can induce significant bone loss, particularly in the early months after high doses of prednisone. The mechanism is discussed elsewhere in this chapter. An immunosuppressive drug regimen may also lead to the reduction of osteoblast and osteoclast activity. Radiographical skeletal changes arising de novo following transplantation are focal avascular necrosis, probably due to steroid medication, osteopenia and bone fractures, delayed skeletal maturity in children, and bone and joint infection.

Clinical use of bone density measurements

Bone mineral measurements have limited usefulness in the specific diagnosis of renal osteodystrophy or related bone disorders. Diagnosis is made on the basis of skeletal radiographs, biochemical tests on blood and bone biopsy. However, since radiographs are insensitive and not useful in quantitating bone loss, bone mineral measurements are used to:

1) assess the magnitude of osteopenia and possibly the fracture risk at the time of diagnosis;
2) monitor patients for progressive osteopenia prior to and during renal dialysis, and prior to and after renal transplantation; and
3) follow patients on treatment programmes.[41]

Bone mineral measurements have an established position in evaluations during new drug trials. Patients with significant osteopenia who have a high fracture risk may need counselling on physical activities and changing the treatment regimen, and treatment with bisphosphonates or calcitonin may be considered. Because of the complex and more focal nature of renal osteodystrophy, data on fracture risk from studies of involutional osteoporosis may have limited application for clinical fracture risk prediction in this group of patients. The heterogeneous changes of normal bone structure in renal osteodystrophy and the presence of woven bone both result in a different relationship between bone strength and bone mineral compared with that seen in normal or osteoporotic bone. When repeated bone mineral measurements are performed in these patients, possible changes in a patient's weight (oedema), abdominal diameter (girth) due to ascites and significant changes in body composition (fat–lean mass) or of the bone itself may influence bone mineral measurements. Combinations of reduction in bone mineral content at the radius with gain or stabilization of BMD in spine and either response in the hip are frequently seen in haemodialysis patients when renal hyperparathyroidism is successfully treated. This reflects a redistribution of bone mineral and a differential response of cortical and trabecular bone with treatment. It points to the importance of bone density measurements at multiple skeletal sites.[42]

Over the last 25 years, many studies on the radius by SPA have evaluated bone mineral measurements in patients on haemodialysis with symptomatic and non-symptomatic bone disease. An early study of bone mineral content (BMC) at the one-third radius (cortical bone) in 303 patients with renal failure covering every stage of the disease (including 123 renal transplants), showed that there was loss of bone mineral (BMC) with prolonged azotaemia and continuing gradual loss of BMC with dialysis. Parathyroidectomy slowed down this loss, but did not reverse it. Transplantation slowed down the bone loss or stopped it, but there was no increase in BMC.[40] Rickers et al.[43] showed that patients on prolonged haemodialysis as a group have a decline in BMC values in the radius over time, but with considerable variation. Of these patients, 42% lost over 10% of BMC in the radius in 3 years (rapid loss), while 39% had either no bone loss or less than 5%. Biochemical tests were more abnormal in the rapid loss group. About 20% of the patients showed an increase in BMC over the 3-year period. It was not possible to predict future bone loss by means of sex, age or initial BMC, which again reinforces the need for repeated BMD measurements in the spine or femur.[42] The degree of BMC loss at onset of dialysis varied with the type of underlying renal disease.[43]

General comments on bone density interpretation

The complex nature and non-uniform occurrence of bone abnormalities associated with chronic renal disease, dialysis and transplantation make clinically useful interpretations of radius, spine, hip or total body BMD measurements complex. When used as the sole test, BMD values are potentially misleading in this group of diseases, since the skeleton shows heterogeneous changes, and results from one region are not necessarily representative of another.[44–46] Interpretation of a baseline bone density result should only be attempted with knowledge of the findings of the skeletal radiograph and biochemical tests.

Even within a small region such as L1–L4, which is frequently used in bone mineral assessments, marked variations in BMD between individual vertebra are often present. This becomes apparent when reviewing the bone mineral images from DXA instruments for the BMD results of individual vertebrae. Ito et al.[46] attempted to use a vertebral density distribution pattern based on CT images, rather than QCT density information. In patients on haemodialysis, they described five patterns (Figure 18.2). These patterns illustrate the heterogeneous bone mineral distribution and the limitations of regional or total body bone mineral measurements for diagnosis or follow-up studies in this disease.

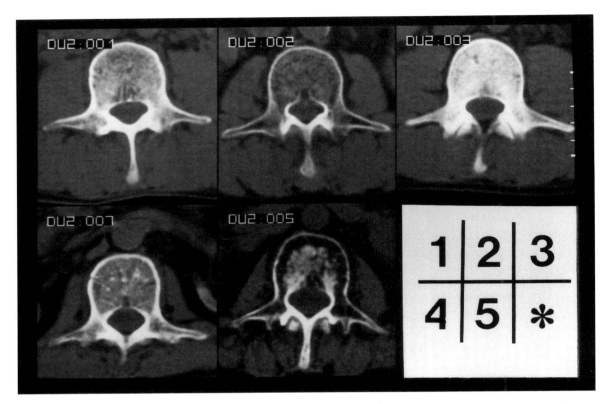

Figure 18.2 Vertebral density pattern with CT in patients on maintenance hemodialysis, demonstrating the heterogeneous bone distribution in renal bone disease: Type 1 = normal; Type 2 = osteopenia (aluminium osteopathy); Type 3 = diffuse osteosclerosis; Type 4 = spotty osteosclerosis; Type 5 = central osteosclerosis (secondary hyperparathyroidism). (From Ito et al.[44] with permission of the authors.)

Illustrative cases

Figures 18.3–18.6 illustrate how bone mineral measurements can give useful information in the diagnosis and management of patients with chronic renal failure, dialysis and transplantation. However, these cases also demonstrate that BMD measurements alone generally give insufficient information for clinical decision making.

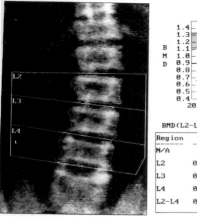

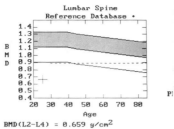

Lumbar Spine
Reference Database •

BMD(L2-L4) = 0.659 g/cm²

Region	BMD	T(30.0)		Z	
N/A					
L2	0.622	-4.29	57%	-4.29	57%
L3	0.647	-4.15	59%	-4.15	59%
L4	0.698	-4.06	61%	-4.06	61%
L2-L4	0.659	-4.15	59%	-4.15	59%

A

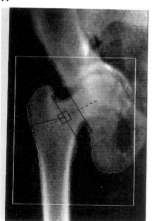

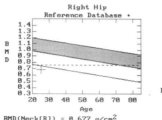

Right Hip
Reference Database •

BMD(Neck[R]) = 0.677 g/cm²

Region	BMD	T		Z	
Neck	0.677	-2.75 (20.0)	69%	-2.54	71%
Troch	0.439	-3.26 (20.0)	55%	-3.17	56%
Inter	0.592	-4.34 (20.0)	48%	-4.23	48%
TOTAL	0.571	-3.85 (20.0)	53%	-3.74	54%
Ward's	0.602	-1.92 (20.0)	72%	-1.64	75%

* Age and sex matched
T = peak bone mass
Z = age matched   TK   10/25/91

B

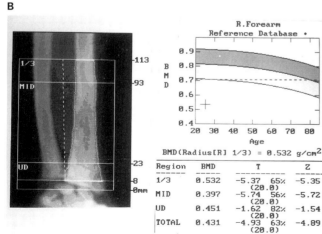

R.Forearm
Reference Database •

BMD(Radius[R] 1/3) = 0.532 g/cm²

Region	BMD	T		Z	
1/3	0.532	-5.37 (20.0)	65%	-5.35	65%
MID	0.397	-5.74 (20.0)	56%	-5.72	56%
UD	0.451	-1.62 (20.0)	82%	-1.54	83%
TOTAL	0.431	-4.93 (20.0)	63%	-4.89	63%

C

Figure 18.3 Bone mineral analysis of a 25-year-old black male on renal dialysis after three failed renal transplants: (A) lumbar spine; (B) proximal femur; (C) distal radius. BUN 52 mg/dl, creatinine 19 mg/dl, sodium 142 mmol/l, potassium 4.6 mmol/l, chloride 113 mmol/l, bicarbonate 14 mmol/l, calcium 8.2 mg/dl. Note that the lowest values were seen at the radius, as indicated by the Z-score. Radiographs showed osteopenia and compression fractures T5, T6, with deformity. Pelvis: insufficiency fractures in the right acetabular region and the superior pubic ramus; bones have appearance consistent with renal osteodystrophy. Left shoulder: extensive metastatic calcification in the axilla; prominent periosteal erosion on the metaphyseal region of the proximal humerus, consistent with hyperparathyroidism. Bone mineral measurements demonstrate low bone mass in axial and appendicular skeletal sites. A high risk for future fractures should be considered in any future management decision. Follow-up BMD measurements are indicated to monitor treatment effect on bone. (Courtesy of Professor Eva Dubovsky, University of Alabama, Birmingham.)

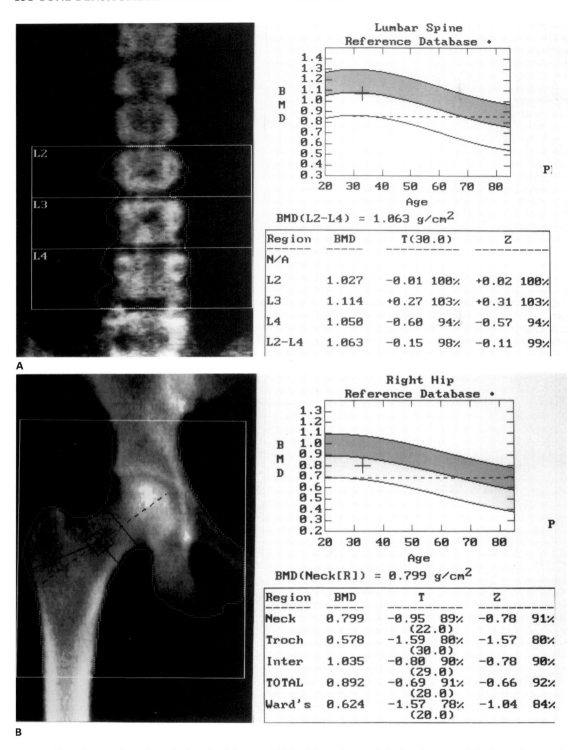

Lumbar Spine
Reference Database •

BMD(L2-L4) = 1.063 g/cm^2

Region	BMD	T(30.0)		Z	
N/A					
L2	1.027	-0.01	100%	+0.02	100%
L3	1.114	+0.27	103%	+0.31	103%
L4	1.050	-0.60	94%	-0.57	94%
L2-L4	1.063	-0.15	98%	-0.11	99%

A

Right Hip
Reference Database •

BMD(Neck[R]) = 0.799 g/cm^2

Region	BMD	T		Z	
Neck	0.799	-0.95 (22.0)	89%	-0.78	91%
Troch	0.578	-1.59 (30.0)	80%	-1.57	80%
Inter	1.035	-0.80 (29.0)	90%	-0.78	90%
TOTAL	0.892	-0.69 (28.0)	91%	-0.66	92%
Ward's	0.624	-1.57 (20.0)	78%	-1.04	84%

B

Figure 18.4 Bone mineral analysis of a 33-year-old black female on dialysis after one failed renal transplant: (A) spine; (B) hip. BUN 68 mg/dl, creatinine 18.7 mg/dl, potassium 4.8 mmol/l, calcium 8.5 mg/dl, phosphorus 7.4 mg/dl, PTH 967 pg/ml, alkaline phosphatase 84 u/l, albumin 4.1 g/dl. Radiographs of both hands showed no evidence of renal osteodystrophy. In this case, normal BMD measurements support the radiograph findings and show that bone mass is well within the normal range and fracture risk is low. (Courtesy of Professor Eva Dubovsky, University of Alabama, Birmingham.)

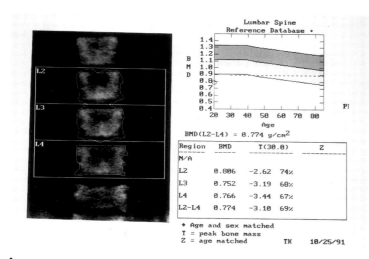

A

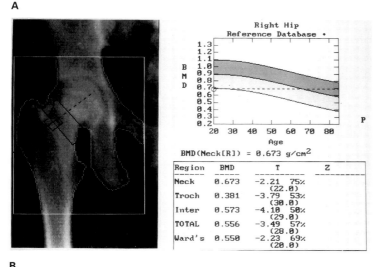

B

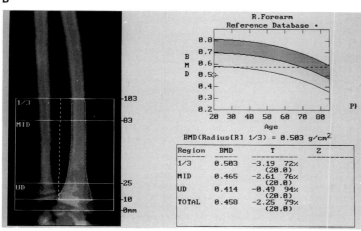

C

Figure 18.5 Bone mineral analysis of an 18-year-old white male with end-stage renal disease due to polycystic kidney disease who has been on dialysis three times a week for six years; he received an LRD renal transplant two weeks before this scan was made: (A) spine; (B) hip; (C) radius. Before transplantation, laboratory tests gave sodium 137 mmol/l, potassium 4.1 mmol/l, glucose 80 mg/dl, BUN 65 mg/dl, creatinine 10.4 mg/dl, alkaline phosphatase 679 u/l, phosphorus 6.9 mg/dl, calcium 9.2 mg/dl. At the time of the bone mineral analysis, the values were sodium 138 mmol/l, potassium 4.0 mmol/l, BUN 12 mg/dl, creatinine 1.1 mg/dl, phosphorus 1.4 mg/dl, calcium 9.1 mg/dl, protein 7.2 mg/dl, albumin 4.5 g/dl, alkaline phosphatase 527 u/l, cyclosporin 173 ng/ml. Daily medications: prednisone 30 mg, cyclosporin 650 mg, acyclovir 200 mg, azathioprine 75 mg, phosphosoda 5 ml. BMD values in the spine are outside the normal range. Radiographs of the AP pelvis showed diffuse osteoporosis, suggesting hyperparathyroidism. Chest: diffuse osteoporosis with marked resorption of the clavicles and classic rugger jersey spine in upper and lower thorax. AP both hands: marked resorption of all tufts as well as radial and ulnar cortices of the phalanges. Bone age was 15 years ± 14 months, which represents skeletal growth retardation. BMD results show the patient's bone density to be at the fracture threshold (spine 0.85 g/cm²) and that further bone loss will significantly increase his fracture risk. In this case of a young male, T- and Z-scores are identical, since he is at the age of maximal bone mass, the reference age for T-scores. Note that the margins of the L4 body and the ischium were below the instrument's threshold, and were drawn manually. (Courtesy of Professor Eva Dubovsky, University of Alabama, Birmingham.)

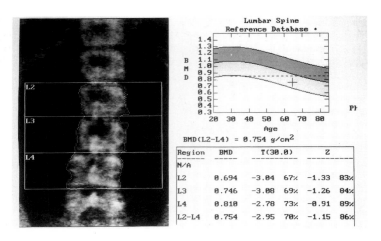

A

BMD(L2-L4) = 0.754 g/cm²

Region	BMD	T(30.0)		Z	
N/A					
L2	0.694	-3.04	67%	-1.33	83%
L3	0.746	-3.08	69%	-1.26	84%
L4	0.810	-2.78	73%	-0.91	89%
L2-L4	0.754	-2.95	70%	-1.15	86%

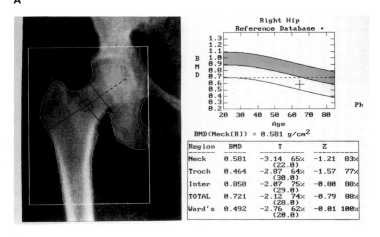

B

BMD(Neck[R]) = 0.581 g/cm²

Region	BMD	T		Z	
Neck	0.581	-3.14 (22.0)	65%	-1.21	83%
Troch	0.464	-2.87 (30.0)	64%	-1.57	77%
Inter	0.858	-2.07 (29.0)	75%	-0.80	88%
TOTAL	0.721	-2.12 (28.0)	74%	-0.79	88%
Ward's	0.492	-2.76 (20.0)	62%	-0.01	100%

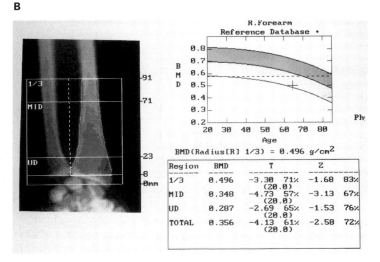

C

BMD(Radius[R] 1/3) = 0.496 g/cm²

Region	BMD	T		Z	
1/3	0.496	-3.30 (20.0)	71%	-1.68	83%
MID	0.348	-4.73 (20.0)	57%	-3.13	67%
UD	0.287	-2.69 (20.0)	65%	-1.53	76%
TOTAL	0.356	-4.13 (20.0)	61%	-2.58	72%

Figure 18.6 Bone mineral analysis of a 64-year-old white female on hemodialysis (three times a week) for several years for end-stage renal disease secondary to focal sclerosis: (A) spine; (B) hip; (C) radius. Biochemistry on day of BMD measurement: sodium 140 mmol/l, potassium 4.5 mmol/l, glucose 93 mg/dl, creatinine 2.1 mg/dl, BUN 40 mg/dl, phosphorus 2.4 mg/dl, calcium 10.6 mg/dl, alkaline phosphatase 131 u/L. Daily medications: cyclosporin 350 mg, prednisone 10 mg, immuran 100 mg. Radiographs: AP both hands. Thinning of the cortes of the tuberosity of the distal phalanx of the left second and third digits, consistent with early evidence of renal osteodystrophy. BMD data show that bone density is below the fracture threshold in all skeletal sites. Risk for fracture is high and will increase markedly with any further bone loss. (Courtesy of Professor Eva Dubovsky, University of Alabama, Birmingham.)

POST-TRANSPLANTATION BONE DISEASE

General comments

Bone disease in patients with organ transplants is recognized as a serious complication as new surgical procedures make organ transplantation more successful and prolong lives. There are sufficient similarities in bone diseases arising after transplantation of heart,[47–50] liver,[51–53] bone marrow,[54] pancreas or kidney that these can be considered together as post-transplantation bone disease.[55]

As previously discussed for renal osteodystrophy in more detail, post-transplantation bone disease may consist of components of a specific bone disease associated with the underlying organ disease together with skeletal changes associated with its treatment. A short summary of bone diseases associated with diseases of different organs that may be considered for transplantation is given in Table 18.3. Organ transplantation may improve the underlying bone disease, but also superimpose additional skeletal changes. Bone mineral measurements and radiographs of the spine prior to any organ transplantation are routinely performed in many transplant centres to establish a baseline measurement (Figure 18.7).

Table 18.3 Bone disease associated with diseases of organs that may be considered for transplantation.

Disease category	Mechanism of bone disease	Type of bone disease
Cholestatic liver disease: primary biliary cirrhosis, primary sclerosing cholangitis	Low levels of 25-hydroxyvitamin D, reduced production of fat-soluble vitamins	Osteoporosis
Chronic liver disease	Iron overload haemochromatosis	Osteoporosis
Hepatolenticular degeneration (Wilson's disease)	Copper overload	Osteoporosis
Long-term total parenteral nutrition	Aluminium deposition	Osteomalacia
Chronic heart disease	Prolonged loop diuretic therapy, inactivity, cachexia, poor nutrition	Osteoporosis
Diabetes (pancreas)	Poor nutrition and non-specific causes[a]	Osteoporosis (osteomalacia)

[a]Non-specific causes are inactivity, poor nutrition and drug effects.

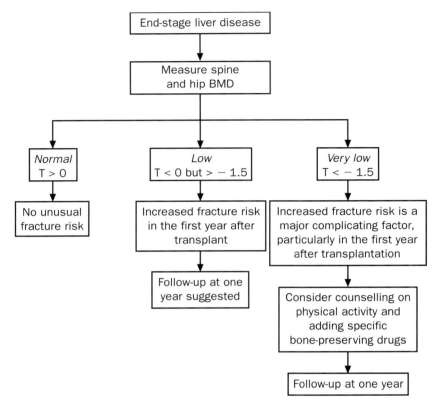

Figure 18.7 Suggested use of bone mineral measurements in patients undergoing orthotopic liver transplantation.

The transplant-induced changes are mainly due to the use of high doses of steroids and immunosuppressive drugs, notably cyclosporin A, azathioprine and methotrexate, either alone or in combination.

As discussed for renal transplants, bone loss in the lumbar spine is most pronounced in the first 6 months after transplantation, when steroid and immunosuppressive therapy is given in highest dosage.[56] After this initial period, there may be a gain in bone density to reach pretransplant levels in 1 or 2 years, as with liver transplants,[17] or there may be chronic bone loss for years following transplantation.[55]

Monitoring areas with a high percentage of trabecular bone (lumbar spine, femoral neck) for repeated bone mineral measurements and (if indicated) with serum bone markers is recommended for the detection of bone disease prior to fracture. The specific diagnosis of the bone disease is then made by biochemical tests and bone biopsy. To reduce bone loss bisphosphonates, calcitonin, lower steroid doses and the use of bone-sparing combinations of steroids and immunosuppressive drugs are being evaluated. Again, bone mineral measurements have a role in monitoring the effectiveness of such treatment.

Hepatic osteodystrophy

While bone loss with heart, bone marrow and pancreas transplants has only recently been described, bone loss and atraumatic fractures have been recognized for many years as serious complications of cholestatic liver disease.[57–60] Bone loss has been documented in skeletal sites composed mainly of trabecular bone, such as the iliac crest,[61–65] as well as at sites of compact bone, such as metacarpals and radius.[61,66–70] Using histomorphometry, osteoporosis was the only type of bone disease noted in primary biliary cirrhosis prior to and following transplantation.[71,72] Eastell et al.[17] showed that mean BMD measured in the lumbar spine in 210 ambulatory women with primary biliary cirrhosis was 7% lower than that of 139 age-matched controls. BMD was inversely related to the risk score index of liver disease severity. The mean rate of bone loss was 2–4%/year, twice as great as in normal women of equal age. Bone mineral density decreased during the first 3 months after transplantation, but then increased. The pretransplantation level was reached 12 months after transplantation, and at 2 years was 5% above it.

The initial bone loss and atraumatic fractures after transplantation are best explained by the initial high steroid doses, and perhaps in part also by the effects of cyclosporin A. The steroid effect is partly reversible when the drug is withdrawn, and an increase in BMD over the baseline level may result from elimination of the hepatic factor that had caused the bone loss.

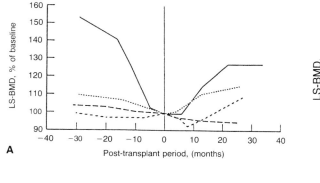

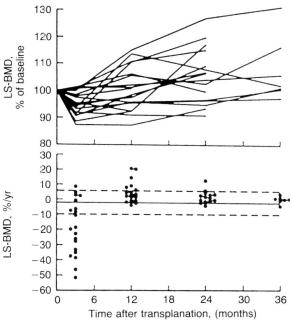

Figure 18.8 (A) Lumbar spine bone mineral (BMD) in four patients with end-stage PBC who had a liver transplant (time zero on abscissa). BMD is expressed as percent of BMD value at time of transplant. Note the bone loss with end-stage disease prior to transplantation and the recovery in the post-transplant period. (B) Change in lumbar spine BMD after orthotopic liver transplantation in 20 women with primary biliary cirrhosis (PBC). **Upper plot:** change in BMD expressed as per cent of the baseline value. **Lower plot:** rate of change in BMD (%/year) in 105 women with PBC after liver transplantation. The horizontal lines represent mean ± 95% confidence intervals for the rate of change. (From Eastell et al[17] by permission of authors and publisher.)

Illustrative cases

Figures 18.8–18.12 demonstrate how BMD measurements are used in the follow-up of ortho-topic liver transplants. Cases with ascites and postoperative artefacts in patients with liver transplants are shown in Chapter 10.

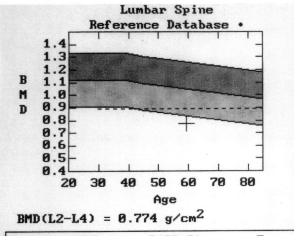

BMD(L2-L4) = 0.774 g/cm^2

Region	BMD	T(30.0)		Z	
N/A					
L2	0.796	-2.71	73%	-2.09	78%
L3	0.687	-3.78	62%	-3.16	66%
L4	0.834	-2.83	73%	-2.20	78%
L2-L4	0.774	-3.10	69%	-2.48	74%

A

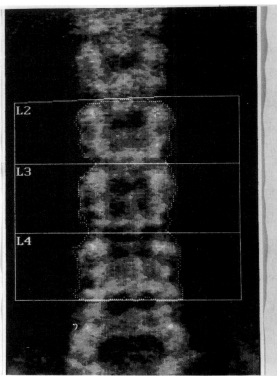

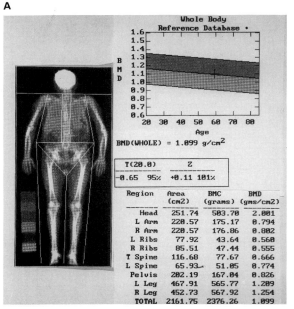

BMD(WHOLE) = 1.099 g/cm^2

T(20.0)		Z	
-0.65	95%	+0.11	101%

Region	Area (cm2)	BMC (grams)	BMD (gms/cm2)
Head	251.74	503.70	2.001
L Arm	220.57	175.17	0.794
R Arm	220.57	176.86	0.802
L Ribs	77.92	43.64	0.560
R Ribs	85.51	47.44	0.555
T Spine	116.68	77.67	0.666
L Spine	65.93	51.05	0.774
Pelvis	202.19	167.04	0.826
L Leg	467.91	565.77	1.209
R Leg	452.73	567.92	1.254
TOTAL	2161.75	2376.26	1.099

B

Figure 18.9 A 50-year-old white male 6 months after orthotopic liver transplantation for PBC. Note the low levels of BMD in the L-spine (mostly trabecular bone) (A) and normal values for total body BMD (80% cortical bone) (B).

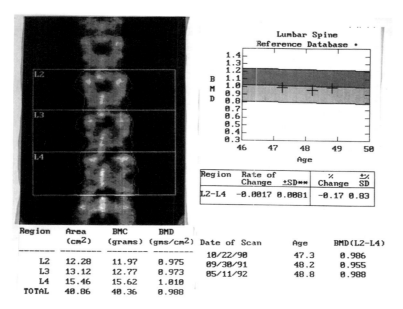

Region	Area (cm2)	BMC (grams)	BMD (gms/cm2)
L2	12.28	11.97	0.975
L3	13.12	12.77	0.973
L4	15.46	15.62	1.010
TOTAL	40.86	40.36	0.988

Date of Scan	Age	BMD(L2-L4)
10/22/90	47.3	0.986
09/30/91	48.2	0.955
05/11/92	48.8	0.988

Figure 18.10 A 48-year-old white female one year after orthotopic liver transplantation. BMD values are prior to 3 months and 12 months after transplantation. There were normal baseline BMD values and a decrease 3 months after transplantation. These are typical BMD changes.

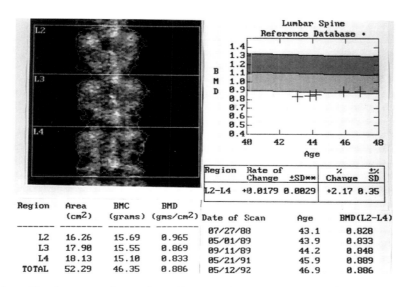

Region	Area (cm2)	BMC (grams)	BMD (gms/cm2)
L2	16.26	15.69	0.965
L3	17.90	15.55	0.869
L4	18.13	15.10	0.833
TOTAL	52.29	46.35	0.886

Date of Scan	Age	BMD(L2-L4)
07/27/88	43.1	0.828
05/01/89	43.9	0.833
09/11/89	44.2	0.848
05/21/91	45.9	0.889
05/12/92	46.9	0.886

Figure 18.11 Series of L-spine scans 3 months to 5 years after liver transplantation for PBC in a 46-year-old white male. There was a typical increase in BMD following the initial decrease at 3 to 6 months (baseline not shown here). *Left:* Last scan performed. *Right:* Data on rate of change.

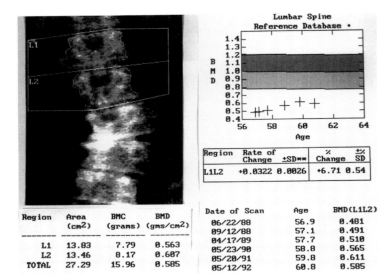

Region	Area (cm2)	BMC (grams)	BMD (gms/cm2)
L1	13.83	7.79	0.563
L2	13.46	8.17	0.607
TOTAL	27.29	15.96	0.585

Lumbar Spine
Reference Database •

Region	Rate of Change	±SD**	% Change	±% SD
L1L2	+0.0322	0.0026	+6.71	0.54

Date of Scan	Age	BMD(L1L2)
06/22/88	56.9	0.481
09/12/88	57.1	0.491
04/17/89	57.7	0.510
05/23/90	58.8	0.565
05/28/91	59.8	0.611
05/12/92	60.8	0.585

Figure 18.12 Series of L-spine scans on a 60-year-old white male 4 years after liver transplantation for PBC. *Left:* Last scan, showing deformity and compression. Reduced size ROI of L1 and L2. *Right:* Plot of results from present and previous scans performed 3 months to 4 years after transplantation. Because of the smaller ROI and spinal abnormalities, the 95% confidence limit of the rate of change is larger than usual. The patient was not on specific bone-stimulating treatment. The increase in bone density resulted from reversal of the initial steroid effect and perhaps healing of hepatic osteodystrophy. That this occurred even at this low level of baseline BMD is noteworthy.

REFERENCES

1. Seeman E, Wahner HW, Offord KP et al. Differential effects of endocrine dysfunction on the axial and the appendicular skeleton. *J Clin Invest* (1982) **69:** 1302–9.

2. Schaadt O, Bohr O. Loss of bone mineral in axial and peripheral skeleton in aging, prednisone treatment and osteoporosis. In: Dequeker J, Johnston CC, eds. *Noninvasive Bone Measurements: Methodological Problems* (IRL Press: Oxford and Washington, DC, 1982), 207–14.

3. Peck W, Gennari C, Raisz L et al. Corticosteroids and bone: round table discussion. *Calcif Tissue Int* (1984) **36:** 4–7.

4. Gennari C. Glucocorticoids and bone. In: Peck WA, ed. *Bone and Mineral Research/3* (Elsevier: Amsterdam, 1985), 213–32.

5. Baylink DJ. Glucocorticoid-induced osteoporosis. *N Engl J Med* (1983) **309:** 306–8.

6. Richardson ML, Pozzi-Mucelli RS, Kanter AS et al. Bone mineral changes in primary hyperparathyroidism. *Skeletal Radiol* (1986) **15:** 85–95.

7. Adinoff AD, Hollister JR. Steroid-induced fractures in patients with asthma. *N Engl J Med* (1983) **309:** 265–8.

8. Hahn TJ, Boisseau C, Avioli LV. Effect of chronic corticosteroid administration on diaphyseal and metaphyseal bone mass. *J Clin Endocrinol Metab* (1974) **39:** 274–82.

9. Seville PD, Kharmosh O. Osteoporosis of rheumatoid arthritis: influence of age, sex and corticosteroids. *Arthritis Rheum* (1967) **10:** 423–30.

10. Chesney RW, Mazess RB, Rose P et al. Effect of prednisone on growth and bone mineral content in childhood glomerular disease. *Am J Dis Child* (1978) **132:** 768–72.

11. Sambrook PN, Eisman JA, Yeates MG et al. Osteoporosis in rheumatoid arthritis: safety of low dose cortico-steroids. *Ann Rheum Dis* (1986) **45:** 950–3.

12. Verstraeten A, Dequeker J. Vertebral and peripheral bone mineral content and fracture incidence in postmenopausal patients with rheumatoid arthritis: effect of low dose corticosteroids. *Ann Rheum Dis* (1986) **45:** 852–7.

13. Ruegsegger P, Medici TC, Anliker M. Corticosteroid-induced bone loss, a longitudinal study of alternate day therapy in patients with bronchial asthma using quantitative computed tomography. *Eur J Clin Pharmacol* (1983) **25:** 615–20.

14. Lukert BP, Raisz LG. Glucocorticoid-induced osteoporosis: pathogenesis and management. *Ann Intern Med* (1990) **112:** 352–64.

15. Pocock NA, Eismon JA, Dunstan CR et al. Recovery from steroid-induced osteoporosis. *Ann Intern Med* (1982) **107:** 319–23.

16. Lufkin EG, Wahner HW, Bergstralh EJ. Reversibility of steroid-induced osteoporosis. *Am J Med* (1988) **85:** 887–9.

17. Eastell R, Dickson ER, Hodgson SF et al. Rates of vertebral bone loss before and after liver transplantation in women with primary biliary cirrhosis. *Hepatology* (1991) **14:** 296–300.

18. Johnston CC, Melton LJ, Lindsay R et al. Clinical indications for bone mass measurements. *J Bone Miner Res* (1989) **4**(suppl 2): 1–28.

19. Devogelaer JP, Huaux JP, Dufour JP et al. Bone-sparing action of deflazacort versus equipotent doses of prednisone: a double-blind study in males with rheumatoid arthritis. In: Christiansen C, Johansen JS, Riis BJ, eds. *Osteoporosis 1987* (Osteopress: Copenhagen, 1987), 1014–15.

20. Adachi JD, Bensen WG, Brown J et al. Intermittent etidronate therapy to prevent corticosteroid-induced osteoporosis. *N Engl J Med* (1997) **337:** 382–7.

21. Sambrook P, Birmingham J, Kelly P et al. Prevention of corticosteroid osteoporosis – a comparison of calcium, calcitriol and calcitonin. *N Engl J Med* (1993) **328:** 1747–52.

22. Lems WF, Jacobs WG, Bijlsma JWJ et al. Effect of sodium fluoride on the prevention of corticosteroid-induced osteoporosis. *Osteoporos Int* (1997) **7:** 575–82.

23. Rizzoli R, Chevalley T, Slosman DO, Bonjour J-P. Sodium monofluorophosphate increases vertebral bone mineral density in patients with corticosteroid-induced osteoporosis. *Osteoporos Int* (1995) **5:** 39–46.

24. Adachi JD, Bensen WG, Bianchi F et al. Vitamin D and calcium in the prevention of corticosteroid induced osteoporosis: a 3 year follow-up. *J Rheumatol* (1996) **23:** 995–1000.

25. Marshall D, Johnell O, Wedel H. Meta-analysis of how well measures of bone density predict occurrence of osteoporotic fractures. *Br Med J* (1996) **312:** 1254–9.

26. Luengo M, Picado C, Rio LD et al. Vertebral fractures in steroid dependent asthma and involutional osteoporosis: a comparative study. *Thorax* (1991) **46:** 803–6.

27. Peel NFA, Moore DJ, Barrington NA et al. Risk of vertebral fracture and relationship to bone mineral density in steroid treated rheumatoid arthritis. *Ann Rheum Dis* (1995) **54:** 801–6.

28. American College of Rheumatology Task Force on Osteoporosis Guidelines. Recommendations for the prevention and treatment of glucocorticoid-induced osteoporosis. *Arthritis Rheum* (1996) **39:** 1791–801.

29. Eastell R, Reid DM, Compston J et al. UK Consensus Group on management of glucocorticoid-induced osteoporosis: an update. *J Internal Med* (1998) (in press).

30. Nielsen HK, Charles P, Mosekilde L. Effect of single oral doses of prednisone on the circadian rhythm of serum osteocalcin in normal subjects. *J Clin Endocrinol Metab* (1988) **67:** 1025–30.

31. Godschalk MF, Downs RW. Effect of short-term glucocorticoids on serum osteocalcin in healthy young men. *J Bone Miner Res* (1988) **3:** 113–15.

32. LoCascio V, Bonucci E, Imbimbo B et al. Bone loss in response to long-term glucocorticoid therapy. *Bone Miner* (1990) **8:** 39–51.

33. Mitchel DR, Lyles KW. Glucocorticoid induced osteoporosis: mechanism for bone loss; evaluation of strategies for prevention. *J Gerontol* (1990) **45:** 153–8.

34. Maldague B, Malghem J, de Ceuxchaisnes C. Radiologic aspects of glucocorticoid-induced bone disease. *Adv Exp Med Biol* (1984) **171:** 155–90.

35. Coburn JW, Slatopolsky E. Vitamin D, parathyroid hormone and renal osteodystrophy. In: Brenner BM, Rector FC, eds. *The Kidney*, 2nd edition (WB Saunders: Philadelphia, 1981), 2213–305.

36. Kanis JA. Renal bone disease. *Nephrology* (1983) **18:** 136–43.

37. Goodsilt HMM, Kilkoyne RF, Gutchek RA et al. Effect of collagen on bone mineral analysis with CT. *Radiology* (1988) **167:** 787–91.

38. Bonomini V, Bortolotti G-C, Feletti C et al. Serial histomorphometric and histochemical bone biopsy studies in dialysis and transplantation. *J d'Urologie et de Nephrologie* (1975) **12:** 941–50.

39. Eeckhout E, Verbeelen D, Sennesael J et al. Monitoring of bone mineral content in patients on regular hemodialysis. *Nephron* (1989) **52:** 158–61.

40. Griffiths HJ, Zimmerman RE, Bailey G et al. The use of photon absorptiometry in the diagnosis of renal osteodystrophy. *Radiology* (1973) **109:** 277–81.

41. Madsen S, Olgard K, Ladefoget J. Bone mineral content in chronic renal failure during long term treatment with 1-hydroxycholecalciferol. *Acta Med Scand* (1978) **203:** 385–9.

42. Eisenberg B, Tzamaloukas AH, Murata GH et al. Factors affecting bone mineral density in elderly men receiving chronic in-center hemodialysis. *Clin Nucl Med* (1991) **16:** 30–6.

43. Rickers H, Christensen M, Rodbro P. Bone mineral content in patients on prolonged maintenance hemodialysis: a three year follow-up study. *Clin Nephrol* (1983) **20:** 302–7.

44. Ito M, Hayashi K. Vertebral density distribution patterns: CT classification of patients undergoing maintenance hemodialysis. *Radiology* (1991) **180:** 253–7.

45. Ito M. CT evaluation of trabecular and cortical bone mineral density of lumbar spine in patients on hemodialysis. *Nippon Acta Radiol* (1989) **49:** 1382–9.

46. Ito M, Hayashi K, Yamada N. Evaluation of bone mineral density with dual energy quantitative computed tomography (DEQCT). *Nippon Acta Radiol* (1989) **49:** 999–1008.

47. Muchmore JS, Cooper DK, Ye Y et al. Prevention of loss of vertebral bone density in heart transplant patients. *J Heart Lung Transplant* (1992) **11:** 959–63.

48. Muchmore JS, Cooper DKC, Ye Y et al. Loss of vertebral bone density in heart transplant patients. *Transplant Proc* (1991) **23:** 1184–5.

49. Rich BM, Mudge G, LeBoff MS. Cyclosporin A associated osteoporosis in cardiac transplant patients. *J Bone Miner Res* (1990) **5**(suppl 2): 435.

50. Rivas C, Silverberg SJ, Kim T et al. Osteopenia in cardiac transplant recipients. *J Bone Miner Res* (1991) **6**(suppl 1): 93.

51. Porayko MK, Wiesner RH, Hay JE et al. Bone disease in liver transplant recipients: incidence, timing and risk factors. *Transplant Proc* (1991) **23:** 1462–5.

52. Maddrey WC. Bone disease in patients with primary biliary cirrhosis. *Prog Liver Dis* (1990) **9:** 537–54.

53. Diamond T, Pojer R, Stiel D et al. Does iron affect osteoblast function? Studies in vitro and in patients with chronic liver disease. *Calcif Tissue Int* (1991) **48:** 373–9.

54. Kelly PJ, Atkinson K, Ward RL et al. Reduced bone mineral density in men and women with allogeneic bone marrow transplantation. *Transplantation* (1990) **50:** 881–3.

55. Katz IA, Epstein S. Perspectives: post transplantation bone disease. *J Bone Miner Res* (1992) **7:** 123–6.

56. Julian BA, Laskow DA, Dubovsky J et al. Rapid loss of vertebral mineral density after renal transplantation. *N Engl J Med* (1991) **325:** 544–50.

57. Ahrens EH, Payne MA, Kunkel HG et al. Primary biliary cirrhosis. *Medicine* (1950) **29:** 299–364.

58. Atkinson M, Nordin BEC, Sherlock S. Malabsorption and bone disease in prolonged obstructive jaundice. *Q J Med* (1955) **99:** 299–312.

59. Kehayoglou AK, Holdsworth CD, Agnew JE et al. Bone disease and calcium absorption in primary biliary cirrhosis. *Lancet* (1968) **i:** 715–19.

60. Compston JE, Crowe JP, Wells IP et al. Vitamin D prophylaxis and osteomalacia in chronic cholestatic liver disease. *Dig Dis* (1980) **25:** 28–32.

61. Herlong HF, Recker RR, Maddrey WC. Bone disease in primary biliary cirrhosis: histologic features and response to 25-hydroxyvitamin D. *Gastroenterology* (1982) **83:** 103–8.

62. Matloff DS, Kaplan MM, Neer RM et al. Osteoporosis in primary biliary cirrhosis: effects of 25-hydroxyvitamin D_3 treatment. *Gastroenterology* (1982) **83:** 97–102.

63. Cuthbert JA, Pak CYC, Zerwekh JE et al. Bone disease in primary biliary cirrhosis: increased bone resorption and turnover in the absence of osteoporosis or osteomalacia. *Hepatology* (1984) **4:** 1–8.

64. Recker R, Maddrey W, Herlong F et al. Primary biliary cirrhosis and alcoholic cirrhosis as examples of chronic liver disease associated with bone disease. In: Frame B, Potts JT, eds. *Clinical Disorders of Bone and Mineral Metabolism* (Excerpta Medica: Amsterdam, 1983), 227–31.

65. Stellon AJ, Webb A, Compston J et al. Lack of osteomalacia in chronic cholestatic liver disease. *Bone* (1986) **7:** 181–5.

66. Paterson CR, Losowsky MS. The bones in chronic liver disease. *Scand J Gastroenterol* (1967) **2:** 293–300.

67. Kato Y, Epstein O, Dick R et al. Radiological patterns of cortical bone modelling in women with chronic liver disease. *Clin Radiol* (1982) **33:** 313–17.

68. Stellon AJ, Davies A, Compston JE et al. Osteoporosis in chronic cholestatic liver disease. *Q J Med* (1985) **57:** 783–90.

69. Wagonfelt JV, Nemchausky BA, Bolt M et al. Comparison of vitamin D and 25-hydroxyvitamin in the therapy of primary biliary cirrhosis. *Lancet* (1976) **ii:** 391–4.

70. Vassilopoulou-Sellin R, Rey-Bear N, Oyedeji CO. Bilirubin as an inhibitor of cartilage metabolism: effect on avian chondrocyte proliferation in cell culture. *J Bone Miner Res* (1990) **5:** 769–74.

71. Hodgson SF, Dickson ER, Wahner HW et al. Bone loss and reduced osteoblast function in primary biliary cirrhosis. *Ann Intern Med* (1985) **103:** 855–60.

72. Hodgson SF, Eastell R, Dickson ER et al. Bone balance and turnover characteristics in osteopenia of primary biliary cirrhosis. *Clin Res* (1987) **35:** 861A.

19

Quantitation of Bone Density at Sites of Metal Implants

Guest chapter by John A Shepherd and Miroslaw Jablonski

CHAPTER OVERVIEW

This chapter presents the technique of monitoring bone density around metal joint prostheses and spinal implants, and refers to possible applications of this method in clinical practice. The chapter's primary focus is on total hip arthroplasty (THA). Total knee arthroplasty (TKA), spinal fusions and other prosthesis sites are covered in dedicated sections. A discussion on the utility of the periprosthetic bone density measurements will be followed by a review of radiographic techniques and how they compare to dual-energy X-ray absorptiometry (DXA). The unique aspects of periprosthetic DXA will then be discussed, followed by a survey of clinical investigations.

INTRODUCTION

Abnormal bone remodelling in the vicinity of metallic implants has long been recognized.[1] The stress shielding bone loss in the proximal femur with a prosthesis and osteoporosis of the anterior femoral condyles in total knee replacement is particularly striking.[2-6] Periprosthetic

bone atrophy is important from the clinical point of view since this kind of osteoporosis may be responsible for pain, loss of implant support, implant subsidence and, in extreme cases, fracture of the implant or surrounding bone.[7] Yet, the current criteria for the evaluation of arthroplasties are based on subjective clinical and radiographical findings as defined by the Knee Society[8,9] or the Harris hip score.[10] These criteria do not include an evaluation of the bone quality surrounding the prosthesis owing to the lack of a clinically meaningful interpretation of bone mineral density (BMD) and its changes during follow-up assessments. However, progress has been made in the past few years in utilizing bone density measurements to manage effectively individual arthroplasty patients. For instance, the measurement of bone loss has been instrumental in the design of prostheses in an attempt to minimize complications resulting from mechanical incompetence of bone stock in patient populations. Furthermore, if anti-resorptive drug therapy is shown to be effective in either reversing or reducing periprosthetic osteoporosis or osteolysis,[11] it is reasonable to consider the state and changes in periprosthetic bone density during therapy and when deciding to revise an arthroplasty. Currently, pain and some dramatic features of radiographic evaluation are the primary criteria for revision.[12,13] Clinically monitoring bone density in patients with various implants may therefore become a standard of care.

METHODS FOR EVALUATING BONE DENSITY

Visual inspection of standard single-energy radiographs has been used for many years to evaluate quantitatively bone geometry such as calcar atrophy, cortical atrophy, cancellous hypertrophy and endosteal new bone formation[14] as well as qualitative evaluation of bone loss.[14–17] The patient is radiographed pre- and post-surgery and periodically over the next several years. Radiographic findings include increased formation of subcortical cancellous bone at the bone–metal interphase, circumferentially complete or incomplete radiolucencies, subsidence, cortical thickening and calcar resorption. These reflect unwarranted interactions of the prosthetic material with bone tissue and vary with the prosthetic material used.[18] Although the method can precisely monitor these geometric qualities in the bone, bone mass changes of less than approximately 30% are difficult to visualize.[7]

Attempts have been made to make single-energy radiographs more sensitive. Scanning bone reference materials, such as an aluminium step-wedge[17,19,20] and digitizing the film became known as videodensitometry. Videodensitometry has been used to evaluate two-dimensional projected density from in vivo radiographs of THAs and also to map the three-dimensional loss patterns from harvested cadaveric femurs. In the three-dimensional method, the soft tissue is removed and the femur is sliced in a series of thin cross sections. Bone density can be determined and bone loss patterns imaged. Videodensitometry has been shown to be highly correlated to aluminium and potassium-phosphate density standards ($r > 0.99$).[19] However, Engh et al.[17] point out that severe problems are present when using videodensitometry as an in vivo method due to the single-energy nature of radiographs, including variability of the film response characteristics and film development, and hardening of the X-ray spectrum due to variable tissue thickness.

Bobyn et al. found that DXA could measure significant in vivo changes in BMD of 5–15% over a 2-year period.[7] In the same study, changes were not evident on serial radiographs until the BMD had decreased from 20% to 50%. A limitation to DXA is its two-dimensional projection of the three-dimensional bone loss process. However, DXA has been shown to be highly correlated to the volume density of calibrated videodensitometry ($r = 0.89$). Thus, for this and the reasons given in the next sections, in vivo monitoring of periprosthetic bone density is now done almost exclusively using DXA techniques.

MEASUREMENT OF BONE DENSITY BY DXA

Dual-energy X-ray absorptiometry has been shown to be an accurate and precise method of measuring the bone density of a variety of skeletal sites such as the hip, lumbar spine, forearm, heel and whole body. In its most ideal form, the assumption is made that the patient area being scanned contains only bone and soft tissue. The unanticipated presence of metal, plastic and other foreign materials can either bias the BMD results or make the algorithm fail. For example, metal typically looks like bone to the DXA algorithm. Thick metals of high atomic number can attenuate the X-rays to such an extent that all signal is lost and the metal may appear as soft tissue. Polyethylene looks like body fat, while urethane looks like very lean muscle. When these materials are present as a homogeneous superposition on the entire image field and are present in all scans of the subject, such as the examination table, foam pad, etc., they can be accounted for and pose no problem. However, the unexpected heterogeneous presence of an appreciable mass in comparison with the bone mass of these materials can bias BMD results. Thus, foreign materials must always be accounted for with special algorithms or shown empirically through experimentation not to affect bone density accuracy or precision.

Metal removal analysis algorithms are available for Hologic Inc., Lunar Corp. and Norland Medical Systems instruments and are currently implemented at over 1000 clinical sites worldwide. The DXA scan of sites containing metal is taken in a similar fashion to scans of other bone sites. Because the bone dimensions, such as the cortical shell, are considerably smaller than the equivalent spine or hip regions, higher spatial resolution is needed. The manufacturers apply proprietary algorithms first to remove the metal from the tissue analysis, then discriminate the bone from the soft tissue. This is necessary since better precision results if the computer algorithm is allowed to define the edges of the bone or metal regions compared with manual exclusion.[21] Once the metal-excluded bone region has been defined, the 'bone map' is broken into regions small enough to be sensitive to local bone adaptation but large enough to have adequate precision (i.e. typically larger than 1 cm^2).

DXA SCANNING PROTOCOL

For patient comfort and to maximize the projection of bone area, prosthetic hips are typically scanned in the neutral position, with the foot perpendicular to the image plane. Although there are exceptions,[22] change in BMD and BMC with respect to position angle seems to be minimized for most analysis zones around the neutral position.[23] This differs from DXA scanning of healthy hips in which a rotation of approximately 25° with respect to the image plane is recommended to maximize the projection of the femoral neck. The scan times for pencil-beam systems are typically over 10 minutes. Fan-beam scan modes on the Hologic QDR-4500 and the Lunar Expert have reduced scan times to less than 1 minute.

THA ANALYSIS METHODS

There is no one region of interest (ROI) analysis protocol that is universally accepted. The most popular are the Gruen zones, originally defined for radiographic assessment of bone quality.[24] Gruen divided the bone surrounding a femoral stem into seven regions to describe better the locations where stem loosening can occur (Figure 19.1). These seven regions are typically thought to be good compromises between precision and sensitivity. That is, smaller regions

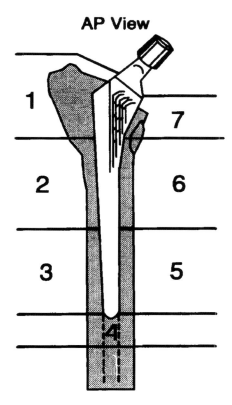

Figure 19.1 Schematic drawing of Gruen zones modified for DXA analysis. Note that the dividing line between zones 1–2 and zones 6–7 is the mid-line of the lesser trochanter. The dividing line between regions 3–4 and 4–5 is at the tip of the prosthesis. The cortical regions 2, 3, 5 and 6 are all the same height.

(A)

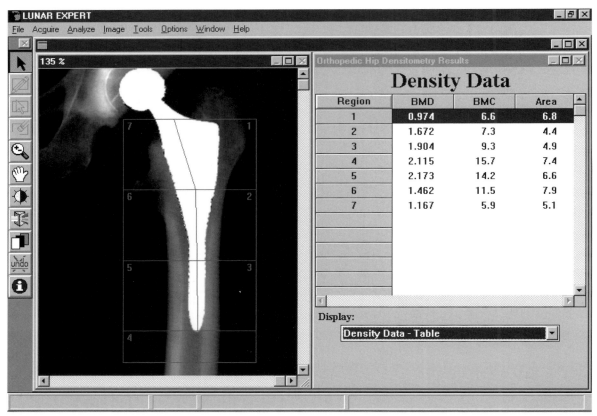

Figure 19.2 Bone density images using Gruen zone analysis for (A) Lunar, and (B) Hologic scan analysis software.

will have lower precision but higher sensitivity. Close approximations to these regions have become the most popular method of evaluating periprosthetic bone density.[25–27] The zones are defined by the stem size and readily adjust to different femur sizes.

The scan analysis software for Lunar DPX systems provides an automated Gruen zone analysis (Figure 19.2A).[5,28] Although other regional analyses exist,[29,30] no comparative investigations of precision or sensitivity are available. Hologic and Norland software includes a general region of interest analysis that allows the user to create ROIs of arbitrary size and location, including the Gruen zones (Figure 19.2B). Hologic also provides Gruen zone ROI templates for use with their COMPARE feature for different length

prostheses. Lunar and Hologic software also allows for the mirror image of the analysis zones to be superimposed onto the contralateral femur. These algorithms are most commonly used to analyse the periprosthetic bone surrounding hip and knee arthroplasties and spine fusions. For a more comprehensive review of analysis protocols, see Trevisan and Ortolani's review of the topic.[31]

CAPABILITIES AND LIMITATIONS OF DXA

Absolute accuracy

The accuracy of periprosthetic BMD measurements could be degraded due to a change in

(B)

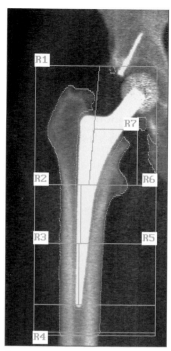

Region	Area (cm2)	BMC (grams)	BMD (gms/cm2)
GLOBAL	49.90	72.41	1.451
R1	14.87	14.16	0.952
R2	5.54	9.56	1.727
R3	5.62	10.72	1.909
R4	6.80	12.95	1.903
R5	5.46	10.53	1.929
R6	5.37	8.20	1.526
R7	4.10	4.97	1.213
NETAVG	46.83	69.59	1.486

scatter conditions related to the type and quantity of metal in the prosthesis. However, this has not been shown to be a problem. In experiments with human cadaver femurs on Hologic QDR-1000 systems with and without cementless titanium implants, the BMD of the Gruen zones changed on average by 0.6%.[27] In an experiment using hydroxyapatite phantoms ranging from 0.3 to 0.9 g/cm² , Hyman et al. found less than a 0.4% shift in all zones. Similar in vitro results have been reported for the Lunar DPX.[5]

However, absolute accuracy of projected BMD values is not generally relevant because interpatient comparisons are difficult to interpret. The bone quality at the time of surgery differs due to the diverse underlying bone pathology of the patients that elect for a THA (i.e. osteoporosis, osteonecrosis of the femoral head, fractures, etc.). Secondly, the sizes and styles of prostheses vary dramatically. Finally, pre- and post-surgical BMD values do not usually correlate well due to the compaction and removal of trabecular bone surrounding the implant.[32] Thus, the most common measure of interest is that of per cent change in BMD which is insensitive to absolute accuracy. Bone cement may affect accuracy as well but is treated separately below.

Correlation between manufacturers

The Hologic QDR-1000 has been compared with the Lunar DPX-L in an in vivo study using 24 subjects that had recently undergone THA. Using Gruen zone analysis, Cohen et al. showed that the Hologic QDR-1000 and the Lunar DPX-L were highly correlated.[33] Correlation coefficients ranged from $r = 0.78$ to $r = 0.99$ depending on the ROI. The following relationship was found for the regions *in toto*:

$$BMD_{Hologic} = 0.84 \times BMD_{Lunar} + 0.09$$

and

$$BMD_{Lunar} = 1.06 \times BMD_{Hologic} + 0.05$$

with a strong correlation of $r = 0.95$. The mean difference was approximately 11% and is similar to the differences seen between Lunar and Hologic devices on measurements of the proximal femur and lumbar spine.[34,35] Thus, while there is good correlation between the two instruments, they may not be used interchangeably.

Effects of cement

Barium is a common contrast agent added to bone cement (e.g. polymethacrylate or PMMA) to make the cement radiopaque. Using Gruen zone analysis, Hyman found the BMD of cadaveric THA femurs increased on average by 29% when the femurs were reseated with cement. The precision was unaffected. Thus, cement can add an offset to the BMC such that the true change in bone mass is underestimated. As an example, for a BMC of 10 g and a cement content that adds 3 g to the measured BMC, a true decrease of 10% in the BMC would measure as approximately 8%. Lunar has included an optional cement exclusion boundary layer to aid in removing the effects of cement around prostheses.[32] However, this type of algorithm does not guarantee exclusion and can cause a false confidence in measurement accuracy. Cement is often radiographically apparent deep in the greater trochanter, in the distal medullary canal and infused into the cortex. Thus, even with boundary-layer cement exclusion algorithms, accuracy similar to that of cementless prostheses cannot be assumed. For further discussion, see Maloney et al.[36]

An alternative analysis method for a cemented prosthesis is to use small regions of interest manually placed on the cortex in which exclusion of the cement can be assured.[6,37] Elvins et al. compared the precision of ROIs manually placed to exclude cement versus standard Gruen zone analysis including the cement. They found that the precision was approximately two times worse with the manual analysis.[21] Thus, the possible benefit of increased sensitivity might be negated by poor precision. Further work on this subject is necessary.

Rotation errors

Patient positioning limits precision in all in vivo measurement sites. One source of positioning error occurs when the femur is rotated such that the projected bone image changes in area and local BMC distribution. Rotation errors are potentially worse in periprosthetic measurements than in healthy femur scans since a large fraction of the bone is obscured by the prosthesis, especially in the anatomically asymmetric calcar region (Gruen 7). Kiratli et al. investigated the effects of rotation of the THA hip using the Lunar four-ROI analysis[5] and found

an error of approximately 5% attributable to rotation through angles of $\pm5°$ using six cadaveric femurs. Mortimer et al. found similar results using Gruen zones on nine cadaveric femurs, with 5% variation between $\pm15°$ of rotation.[23] Bouxsein et al.[38] reported changes of less than 5% for rotations of $\pm10°$ for all regions except the Gruen 7. Both Bouxsein et al. and Cohen and Rushton[39] reported large changes of up to 20% in the calcar region with rotations more than 10°. All the in vitro experiments were performed with femurs in a homogeneous soft tissue surrounding (i.e. water, rice, etc.) and may underestimate the total error. However, in one of the few in vivo rotation studies, Kröger et al. found up to a 5% variation between neutral and 30° (external rotation) measurements.[32]

Precision

A quantified precision is necessary to have confidence in the accuracy of the measurement and to determine the significance of change between baseline and follow-up measurements. To have 95% confidence that a follow-up bone density has changed from the baseline measurement, a difference of approximately 2.8 times the standard deviation of the measurement must be observed. This assumes the two measurements have the same standard deviation and that the errors are random and non-correlated. In vitro precision measurements are useful to characterize the precision limit due to dose, bone area and bone contrast. The precision on the QDR-1000 and QDR-2000 has been shown to be less than 2% precision at all Gruen zones using cadaveric femurs implanted with prostheses.[27,39] In vivo precision using Gruen zone analysis has been reported by many studies and varies from zone to zone, by prosthesis type and by manufacturer.[21,22,32,39,40] Precision has also been reported for the four-zone analysis used on Lunar machines.[41] BMD precision is lower around THAs because the bone areas are small when compared with healthy hip analysis, especially in the calcar region (zone 7). In general, the precision for zones 1–6 is <3% and <4% in the calcar, with 95% confidence of being able to determine changes of 8–12% using single scans on individual patients. To have confidence in the precision of a THA measurement in a clinical setting, it is advisable to determine the precision using a subset of the patient population. There are several appropriate references,[42,43] including Chapter 8 in this book.

CLINICAL USE OF BONE DENSITY MEASUREMENTS

As the bulk of the hip and knee osteoarthritis patient population consists of postmenopausal women, so do the patients with replaced joints. Another risk factor for augmented bone loss in this group is often prolonged bed rest after the operation and frequently sedentary lifestyle induced by malfunction of the motor system. A clinical approach considering both general and local osteoporosis in this group seems to be fully justified.

Osteolysis around total hip components has long been recognized. It can result in so-called aseptic loosening of the components and avulsion fractures of the greater trochanter. Both pose a serious clinical problem.[44] Zicat and colleagues[45] examined bone loss adjacent to hip prosthesis and reported the more frequent occurrence of osteolysis in younger patients. This finding stresses the clinical importance of monitoring osteolysis. The possible prevention of wear debris induced osteolysis by the administration of alendronate was demonstrated in a canine total hip arthroplasty model.[46] This drug is registered by the FDA for treatment of osteoporosis and nowadays is extensively used.[47] The monitoring of bone loss after THA merits special attention since the DXA technique potentially offers a unique method of detecting the early stages of local bone loss and initiating prevention with anti-resorptive therapy, thus enhancing the chances of longer survival of the THA.

Stiffness versus BMD

There is much debate on stiff versus elastic stems. Stiff stems are thought to produce proximal cortical atrophy and distal cortical hypertrophy. Comparing flexible versus stiff femoral stems in a canine model, Bobyn et al.[7] showed greater bone mass retention and more uniform normal cortical bone strain patterns. Similar clinical results were found by Niinimaki and Jalovaara.[48] However, there is the fear, as pointed out by Huiskes et al.,[2] that increased flexibility may cause premature joint loosening and failure. Ang and colleagues evaluated the difference in BMD between a stiff collarless titanium stem and a flexible isoelastic stem and found that both medial and lateral bone retention was higher in the isoelastic stem versus the stiff-stem controls the year following surgery. The short-term revision and loosening history of the prostheses were comparable.[30] In contrast, comparisons of similarly shaped cementless, collarless stems of titanium and cobalt-chromium (titanium has a Young's modulus of elasticity of approximately half that of cobalt-chromium) showed similar bone loss characteristics.[49]

Loss patterns and rates of loss

Typical loss patterns around specific types of prosthesis have been described.[22,37,41,50] Rates of loss have also been described for a variety of stems and stem coatings.[51–53] When determining rates of change, it is important to use a postoperative scan as a baseline versus a preoperative scan with the same ROI because of the erroneous difference due to cement, bone compaction or aggressive bone removal.[32,54] Also, stress-shielding losses may be overestimated if global limb-loading of the ipsilateral and contralateral femurs is not taken into account. Based on comparative measurements of these bone sites, unaffected by local periprosthetic stress shielding (distal femur and proximal tibia), Bryan et al. noted asymmetries between the ipsilateral and contralateral limbs in the region of 15%.[27] If this global limb-loading

A

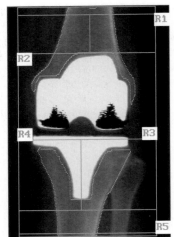

B

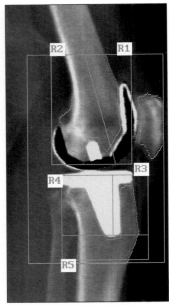

Region	Area (cm2)	BMC (grams)	BMD (gms/cm2)
GLOBAL	36.94	21.56	0.584
R1	5.44	3.13	0.575
R2	6.12	3.10	0.507
R3	7.32	4.68	0.639
R4	6.53	3.15	0.482
R5	5.50	4.08	0.741
NETAVG	30.33	17.78	0.586

Region	Area (cm2)	BMC (grams)	BMD (gms/cm2)
GLOBAL	46.36	35.48	0.765
R1	8.88	5.60	0.631
R2	14.39	13.54	0.941
R3	4.16	1.97	0.474
R4	4.62	4.19	0.907
R5	7.32	5.06	0.691
NETAVG	38.81	29.99	0.773

Figure 19.3 Examples of TKA DXA analysis using regions of analysis outlined by Marinoni et al.[64] (A) PA scan of right TKA; (B) lateral view and analysis. Note the necessary manual exclusion of the fibula. Scans were performed on a Hologic QDR-4500A.

effect had not been normalized out from the periprosthetic BMD losses, then the magnitude of the local stress-shielding bone loss would have been overestimated by approximately 50%.

Cemented versus uncemented THA

Orthopaedic surgeons widely accept the thesis that good bone quality is one of the prerequisites for long-lasting good clinical results of THA. In osteoporotic patients requiring a THA, prostheses are typically fixed with the use of

bone cement. In contrast, in younger subjects with stronger bones, uncemented hip replacements are usually performed. A natural question that arises is at what bone density should one discriminate between these two types of prosthesis? Similar questions arise for acetabular components, and for hybrid prostheses in which the stem is fixed with bone cement and the cup without. Prospective longitudinal studies with DXA with reference to clinical and standard radiological results should at least partially answer these questions.

Dysplastic hip and revision arthroplasty

Hip dysplasty and revision arthoplasty usually require massive auto- or allografting of the acetabular roof or proximal end of the femur in order to reconstruct the anatomical and biomechanical parameters of the hip.[55–57] Grafted bone material lasts for several years and the graft lifetime depends on several often unpredictable host- and graft-related factors. Although not as yet extensively utilized, DXA offers a precise method of monitoring bone density of the grafted material and of relating the results to clinical outcome.

KNEE MEASUREMENTS

The bone density surrounding total knee arthroplasty (TKA) (Figure 19.3) and its longitudinal changes have also been described.[58–65] Lateral and PA scans are necessary to describe the bone loss characteristics of both the distal femur (lateral) and proximal tibia (PA). The knee DXA scan is more technically challenging than that of the hip due to the limited amount and homogeneity of soft tissue surrounding the knee. Special precautions have to be taken to ensure the exclusion of air from the analysis region. The only comprehensive studies of precision and accuracy known to the authors were performed by Robertson et al.[62] and Bigoni et al.[65] In a cadaveric study of the distal femur fitted with a condial prosthesis, Robertson and colleagues found that the accuracy changes less than 4% in the presence of the prosthesis, and measurement precision in the lateral projection was on average 1.2% (QDR-1000). Comparisons with radiographs (visual inspection and digitized) were also reported. Bigoni et al. measured AP and lateral in vivo precision in 10 subjects who underwent uncemented TKA without patella replacement.[65] The precision ranged from 0.9% to 4.7%. Studies of tibial bone density loss over periods less than 3.5 years have shown that bone density is relatively stable and without significant loss.[58–61] Using a dual photon absorptiometry (DPA) device, Levitz et al. also reported insignificant losses in tibia BMD over

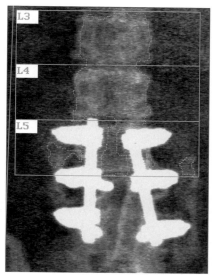

Region	Area (cm2)	BMC (grams)	BMD (gms/cm2)
L3	12.44	9.30	0.748
L4	14.08	12.08	0.858
L5	6.67	4.23	0.634
TOTAL	33.19	25.61	0.771

Figure 19.4 PA spine DXA scan and analysis of L3 and L4 from a patient with a L5–S1 spinal fusion. Note the fusion bone mass lateral to the metal instrument.

the first year, but a drop of 35% on an 8-year follow-up DXA measurement.[60] It should be noted that no cross calibration was performed between the DPA and DXA devices, which makes the accuracy of this change unknown. However, Petersen et al. reported losses of up to 44% in the distal femur after 1 year.[63] Bigoni et al.[65] also reported a 15% loss in the distal femur on longitudinal data at 6 months after surgery and less in the other regions. Thus, the magnitude and characteristics of loss have yet to be comprehensively described.

SPINE AND SHOULDER IMPLANT MEASUREMENTS

Little has been published on the in vivo effects of spinal fusion on spinal bone density (Figure

19.4). The long-term effects on vertebral body
BMD with respect to internal fixation and
changes in biomechanical loading of adjacent
vertebral bodies are unknown. The only DXA
study known to the authors was by Bogdanffy
et al.[66] In a 6-month prospective study of 15
subjects, significant decreases were found in the
L2 and L3 vertebrae above L4–S1 fusions. Both
AP and lateral projections of L2 and L3 were
measured. The precision of the AP measurements were 1.4% and 2% respectively, while the
lateral precision was 6% and 4.8%. A 10%
decrease was found in both the L2 and L3 AP
measurements at 6 months.

In a unique study of the proximal humerus
after shoulder surgery and immobilization,
Marchetti et al. observed statistically significant
BMD changes in the proximal humerus 6 weeks
after surgery.[67]

CONCLUSIONS

This chapter has described how DXA can be
used to monitor osteoporosis and osteolysis
around metal joint prostheses. The high accuracy and precision of the technique have been
demonstrated by many research groups, and on
a variety of makes and models. The ability to
monitor change accurately over time has also
been established. Even though DXA is at least
three times more sensitive than plain film radiographs and, furthermore, that metal removal
algorithms are available on over a thousand
scanners world-wide, its clinical use for individual patient management has not yet become
common practice for several reasons. First, the
ROIs presently used cannot distinguish
between osteoporosis due to stress shielding
and osteolysis. Secondly, until recently there
was no clinical intervention based on bone density. However, this may change since anti-
resorptive drugs with DXA monitoring may
soon be commonplace to treat osteolysis and
osteoporosis around joint implants. Using DXA
scans to distinguish between osteolysis and
osteoporosis is still a challenge for the future.

REFERENCES

1. Perren SM, Cordey J, Rahn BA et al. Early temporary porosis of bone induced by internal fixation implants. A reaction to necrosis, not to stress protection? *Clin Orthop* (1988) **232:** 139–51.
2. Huiskes R, Weinans H, van Rietbergen B. The relationship between stress shielding and bone resorption around total hip stems and the effects of flexible materials. *Clin Orthop* (1992) **274:** 124–34.
3. Cameron HU, Cameron G. Stress-relief osteo-porosis of the anterior femoral condyles in total knee replacement. *Orthopod Review* (1987) **16:** 449–56.
4. Mintzer CM, Robertson DD, Rackemann S et al. Bone loss in the distal anterior femur after total knee arthroplasty. *Clin Orthop* (1990) **260:** 135–43.
5. Kiratli BJ, Heiner JP, McBeath AA et al. Determination of bone mineral density by dual x-ray absorptiometry in patients with unce-mented total hip arthroplasty. *J Orthop Res* (1992) **10:** 836–44.
6. McCarthy CK, Steinberg GG, Agren M et al. Quantifying bone loss from the proximal femur after total hip arthroplasty. *J Bone Joint Surg Br* (1991) **73:** 774–8.
7. Bobyn JD, Mortimer ES, Glassman AH et al. Producing and avoiding stress shielding: labora-tory and clinical observations of noncemented total hip arthroplasty. *Clin Orthop* (1992) **274:** 79–96.
8. Ewald FC. The Knee Society total knee arthro-plasty roentgenographic evaluation and scoring system. *Clin Orthop* (1989) **248:** 9–12.
9. Insall JN, Dorr LD, Scott RD et al. Rationale of the Knee Society clinical rating system. *Clin Orthop* (1989) **248:** 13–14.
10. Harris WH. Traumatic arthritis of the hip after dislocation and acetabular fractures: treatment by mold arthroplasty: an end-result study using a new method of result evaluation. *J Bone Joint Surg Am* (1969) **51:** 737–55.
11. Crozier K. Alendronate protects against bone loss following THR. *Orthoped Today* (1997) **17:** 24–5.
12. Harris WH, McGann WA. Loosening of the femoral component after use of the medullary-plug cementing technique: follow-up note with a minimum five-year follow-up. *J Bone Joint Surg Am* (1986) **68:** 1064–6.

13. Pellicci PM, Salvati EA, Robinson HJ. Mechanical failures in total hip replacement requiring re-operation. *J Bone Joint Surg Am* (1979) **61**: 28–36.

14. Bobyn JD, Pilliar RM, Binnington AG et al. The effect of proximally and fully porous-coated canine hip stem design on bone modelling. *J Orthop Res* (1987) **5**: 393–408.

15. Capello WN. Technical aspects of cementless total hip arthroplasty. *Clin Orthop* (1990) **261**: 102–6.

16. Engh CA, Bobyn JD. The influence of stem size and extent of porous coating on femoral bone resorption after primary cementless hip arthroplasty. *Clin Orthop* (1998) **231**: 7–28.

17. Engh CA, McGovern TF, Schmidt LM. Roentgenographic densitometry of bone adjacent to a femoral prosthesis. *Clin Orthop* (1993) **292**: 177–90.

18. D'Antonio JA, Capello WN, Crothers OD et al. Early clinical experience with hydroxyapatite-coated femoral implants. *J Bone Joint Surg Am* (1992) **74**: 995–1008.

19. Martin RB, Papamichos T, Dannucci GA. Linear calibration of radiographic mineral density using video-digitizing methods. *Calcif Tissue Int* (1990) **47**: 82–91.

20. McGovern TF, Engh CA, Zettl-Schaffer K et al. Cortical bone density of the proximal femur following cementless total hip arthroplasty. *Clin Orthop* (1994) **306**: 145–54.

21. Elvins DM, Ring EFJ, Hueting JE et al. Precision study of DXA THR metal exclusion. *Osteoporos Int* (1997) **7**: 287.

22. Sabo D, Reiter A, Simank HG et al. Periprosthetic mineralization around cementless total hip endoprosthesis: longitudinal study and cross-sectional study on titanium threaded acetabular cup and cementless Spotorno stem with DEXA. *Calcif Tissue Int* (1998) **62**: 177–82.

23. Mortimer ES, Rosenthall L, Paterson I et al. Effect of rotation on periprosthetic bone mineral measurements in a hip phantom. *Clin Orthop* (1996) **324**: 269–74.

24. Gruen TA, McNeice GM, Amstutz HC. Modes of failure of cemented stem-type femoral components. *Clin Orthop* (1979) **141**: 17–27.

25. Nishii T, Sugano N, Masuhara K et al. Longitudinal evaluation of time related bone remodelling after cementless total hip arthroplasty. *Clin Orthop* (1997) **339**: 121–31.

26. Hyman JE, Bouxsein ML, Reilly DT et al. Dual energy X-ray absorptiometry precisely measures bone mineral density around uncemented and cemented proximal femoral prostheses in vitro. *J Bone Miner Res* (1993) **8**: S350.

27. Bryan JM, Sumner DR, Hurwitz DE et al. Altered load history affects periprosthetic bone loss following cementless total hip arthroplasty. *J Orthop Res* (1996) **14**: 762–8.

28. Kiratli BJ, Checovich MM, McBeath AA et al. Measurement of bone mineral density by dual-energy x-ray absorptiometry in patients with the Wisconsin hip, an uncemented femoral stem. *J Arthroplasty* (1996) **11**: 184–93.

29. Korovessis P, Piperos G, Michael A et al. Changes in bone mineral density around a stable uncemented total hip arthroplasty. *Int Orthop* (1997) **21**: 30–4.

30. Ang KC, Das De S, Goh JC et al. Periprosthetic bone remodelling after cementless total hip replacement: a prospective comparison of two different implant designs. *J Bone Joint Surg Br* (1997) **79**: 675–9.

31. Trevisan C, Ortolani S. Periprosthetic bone mineral density and other orthopedic applications. In: Genant HK, Guglielmi G, Jergas M, eds. *Bone density and osteoporosis* (Springer: Berlin, 1998), 541–82.

32. Kröger H, Miettinen H, Arnala I et al. Evaluation of periprosthetic bone using dual-energy x-ray absorptiometry: precision of the method and effect of operation on bone mineral density. *J Bone Miner Res* (1996) **11**: 1526–30.

33. Cohen B, Rushton N. A comparative study of peri-prosthetic bone mineral density measurement using two different dual-energy X-ray absorptiometry systems. *Br J Radiol* (1994) **67**: 852–5.

34. Laskey MA, Flaxman ME, Barber RW et al. Comparative performance in vitro and in vivo of Lunar DPX and Hologic QDR-1000 dual energy X-ray absorptiometers. *Br J Radiol* (1991) **64**: 1023–9.

35. Gundry CR, Miller CW, Ramos E et al. Dual-energy radiographic absorptiometry of the lumbar spine: clinical experience with two different systems. *Radiology* (1990) **174**: 539–41.

36. Maloney WJ, Sychterz C, Bragdon C et al. Skeletal response to well fixed femoral components inserted with and without cement. *Clin Orthop* (1996) **333**: 15–26.

37. Marchetti ME, Steinberg GG, Greene JM et al. A prospective study of proximal femur bone mass following cemented and uncemented hip arthroplasty. *J Bone Miner Res* (1996) **11**: 1033–9.

38. Bouxsein ML, Hyman JE, Reilly DT et al. Report:

assessment of peri-prosthetic bone mineral using the Hologic QDR-2000 densitometer: in vitro accuracy and precision. Orthopedics Biomechanics Laboratory, Beth Israel Hospital, October, 1993.

39. Cohen B, Rushton N. Accuracy of DEXA measurement of bone mineral density after total hip arthroplasty. *J Bone Joint Surg Br* (1995) **77:** 479–83.

40. Smart RC, Barbagallo S, Slater GL et al. Measurement of periprosthetic bone density in hip arthroplasty using dual-energy x-ray absorptiometry: reproducibility of measurements. *J Arthroplasty* (1996) **11:** 445–52.

41. Kilgus DJ, Shimaoka EE, Tipton JS et al. Dual-energy x-ray absorptiometry measurement of bone mineral density around porous-coated cementless femoral implants: methods and preliminary results. *J Bone Joint Surg Br* (1993) **75:** 279–87.

42. Glüer C-C, Blake G, Lu Y et al. Accurate assessment of precision errors: how to measure the reproducibility of bone density techniques. *Osteoporos Int* (1995) **5:** 262–70.

43. Blunt B, Kiratli J. Calculation of short term patient precision. *Scan:* the official newsletter of the International Society of Clinical Densitometry (1997) **IV**(5): 2–3.

44. Brown IW, Ring PA. Osteolytic changes in the upper femoral shaft following porous-coated hip replacement. *J Bone Joint Surg Br* (1985) **67:** 218–21.

45. Zicat B, Engh CA, Gokcen E. Patterns of osteolysis around total hip components inserted with and without cement. *J Bone Joint Surg Am* (1995) **77:** 432–9.

46. Shanbhag AS, Hasselman CT, Rubash HE. The John Charnley award, Inhibition of wear debris mediated osteolysis in a canine total hip arthroplasty model. *Clin Orthop* (1997) **344:** 33–43.

47. Black DM, Cummings SR, Karpf DB et al. Randomised trial of effect of alendronate on risk of fracture in women with existing vertebral fractures. *Lancet* (1996) **348:** 1535–41.

48. Niinimaki T, Jalovaara P. Bone loss from the proximal femur after arthroplasty with an iso-elastic femoral stem: BMD measurements in 25 patients after 9 years. *Acta Orthop Scand* (1995) **66:** 347–51.

49. Hughes SS, Furia JP, Smith P et al. Atrophy of the proximal part of the femur after total hip arthroplasty without cement: a quantitative comparison of cobalt-chromium and titanium

50. Mazurkiewicz H, Gusta A, Kwas A. Densitometric evaluation of the proximal femur after cemented hip prosthesis. *Chir Narzadow Ruchu Ortop Pol* (1995) **60:** 385–91.

femoral stems with use of dual x-ray absorptiometry. *J Bone Joint Surg Am* (1995) **77:** 231–9.

51. Engh CA, Hooten JP, Zettl-Schaffer KF et al. Porous-coated total hip replacement. *Clin Orthop* (1994) **298:** 89–96.

52. Trevisan C, Bigoni M, Randelli G et al. Periprosthetic bone density around fully hydroxy-apatite coated femoral stem. *Clin Orthop* (1997) **340:** 109–17.

53. Huiskes R, van Rietbergen B. Preclinical testing of total hip stems: the effects of coating placement. *Clin Orthop* (1995) **319:** 64–76.

54. Kroger H, Vanninen E, Overmyer M et al. Periprosthetic bone loss and regional bone turnover in uncemented total hip arthroplasty: a prospective study using high resolution single photon emission tomography and dual-energy X-ray absorptiometry. *J Bone Miner Res* (1997) **12:** 487–92.

55. Head WC, Emerson RH, Malinin TI. Chapter 15. In: Pritchard DJ, ed. *Instructional course lectures,* Vol 45 (American Society of Orthopedic Surgeons: Rosemont, IL, 1996), 131–4.

56. Gross AE, Garbuz D, Morsi ES. Chapter 16. In: Pritchard DJ, ed. *Instructional course lectures,* Vol 45 (American Society of Orthopedic Surgeons: Rosemont, IL, 1996), 135–41.

57. Paprosky WG, Bradford MS, Jablonsky WS. Chapter 18. In: Pritchard DJ, ed. *Instructional course lectures,* Vol 45 (American Society of Orthopedic Surgeons: Rosemont, IL, 1996), 149–59.

58. Bohr HH, Schaadt O. Mineral content of upper tibia assessed by dual photon densitometry. *Acta Orthop Scand* (1987) **58:** 557–9.

59. Bohr HH, Lund B. Bone mineral density of the proximal tibia following uncemented arthroplasty. *J Arthroplasty* (1987) **2:** 309–12.

60. Levitz CL, Lotke PA, Karp JS. Long-term changes in bone mineral density following total knee replacement. *Clin Orthop* (1995) **321:** 68–72.

61. Seitz P, Ruegsegger P, Gschwend N et al. Changes in local bone density after knee arthroplasty. The use of quantitative computed tomography. *J Bone Joint Surg Br* (1987) **69:** 407–11.

62. Robertson DD, Mintzer CM, Weissman BN et al. Distal loss of femoral bone following total knee arthroplasty: measurement with visual and computer-processing of roentgenograms and

dual-energy x-ray absorptiometry. *J Bone Joint Surg Am* (1994) **76:** 66–76.

63. Petersen MB, Kolthoff N, Eiken P. Bone mineral density around femoral stems, DXA measurements in 22 porous-coated implants after 5 years. *Acta Orthop Scand* (1995) **66:** 432–4.

64. Marinoni EC, Trevisan C, Bigoni M et al. Metodiche di valutazione strumentatle nel follow-up delle prostesi totali di ginocchio. In: Monteleone V, ed. *International Meeting Knee Prostheses* (Scuola Medica Ospedaliera Napoletana: Napoli, Italy, 1994).

65. Bigoni M, Trevisan C, Colombo L et al. Dual energy x-ray absorptiometry for the assessment of bone density after total knee prosthesis. *Osteoporos Int* (1996) **6:** 90.

66. Bogdanffy GM, Ohnmeiss DD, Guyer RD. Early changes in bone mineral density above a combined anteroposterior L4–S1 lumbar spinal fusion: a clinical investigation. *Spine* (1995) **20:** 1674–8.

67. Marchetti ME, Houde JP, Steinberg GG et al. Humeral bone density losses after shoulder surgery and immobilization. *J Shoulder Elbow Surg* (1996) **5:** 471–6.

20

Vertebral Morphometry Studies Using Dual X-ray Absorptiometry

By Glen M Blake, Jacqueline A Rea, Ignac Fogelman

CHAPTER OVERVIEW

This chapter reviews the potential for lateral dual X-ray absorptiometry (DXA) imaging of the spine to identify patients with vertebral fractures, a technique often referred to as morphometric X-ray absorptiometry (MXA). In addition to age and bone mineral density, a pre-existing vertebral fracture is one of the principal risk factors for identifying patients likely to suffer future osteoporotic fractures. The ability of fan-beam DXA systems to produce high-resolution digitized images of the lateral spine has the potential to provide an inexpensive and widely available low-dose procedure for vertebral morphometry that may approach or equal conventional radiography in accuracy and precision. This chapter first reviews the various published methodologies for performing vertebral morphometry studies on radiographs, since familiarity with these techniques is essential for understanding the analysis and output of MXA studies. The strengths and limitations of MXA and radi-ographic morphometry are compared. MXA has yet to be properly evaluated in a large clinical study, but one early conclusion is that a proper interpretation of MXA studies requires reference data generated from MXA images rather than from lateral radiographs. Some guidance on point placement in MXA scan analysis is provided in the Appendix to this chapter.

INTRODUCTION

The two most common manifestations of osteoporosis are fractures of the vertebral body and the hip.[1-4] Over the past decade both types of fracture have been extensively investigated in epidemiological studies[5,6] that have examined their prevalence and incidence in different populations.[7-11] These studies have also identified predictors of fracture risk such as X-ray absorptiometry measurements of bone mineral density (BMD)[12,13] and quantitative ultrasound measurements of broadband ultrasonic attenuation (BUA)[14,15] and speed of sound (SOS) in bone.[14]

Such non-invasive measurements are regarded as having an essential role in diagnosing osteoporosis and aiding decisions on treatment.

A further motive for the study of osteoporotic fractures is the large number of international, multicentre clinical trials of new treatments for osteoporosis that are currently in progress. Rather than simply demonstrating a favourable change in BMD, the primary objective of these studies is to obtain evidence of a statistically significant reduction in fracture incidence.[16–18] A recent study of the aminobisphosphonate alendronate in a group of women with at least one vertebral fracture at recruitment showed a 50% reduction in the incidence of further vertebral fractures during a 3-year follow-up period.[19] To achieve statistical significance, such trials require the recruitment and monitoring of several thousand subjects. It is of great importance for the reliability of these studies that all fractures are accurately and objectively verified.

Apart from epidemiological studies and clinical trials, the ability to identify and document fractures also plays an important role in the routine evaluation and treatment of patients with suspected osteoporosis. As well as BMD, age and prevalent fractures are important factors in assessing future fracture risk. While hip fractures may be identified unambiguously on radiographs, there are no comparable reliable criteria for identifying osteoporotic fractures in the spine.[20] The situation is complicated by the fact that half of all vertebral fractures are asymptomatic and may not present to medical attention.[21] The conventional practice is for radiologists to diagnose vertebral fractures by reading lateral radiographs of the lumbar and thoracic spine. A fracture is identified by observing an alteration in the normally rectangular shape of the vertebral body (Figure 20.1A and B). However, careful attention to detail is required to interpret correctly the X-ray films. One elegant method of confirming a recent fracture is to perform a technetium-99m methylene diphosphonate (^{99m}Tc-MDP) bone scan (Figure 20.1C). However, few clinicians would perform a radionuclide scan solely for this purpose. In practice, therefore, it is often difficult to dis-

criminate between an osteoporotic fracture and normal variation in vertebral shape or a vertebral deformation or fracture that may have occurred a long time ago following trauma or for some other reason. The range of possible causes of vertebral deformities and the lack of clearly defined criteria for vertebral fractures are the main reasons for the variability in the visual diagnosis of vertebral fractures.[20,22,23]

Over recent years considerable literature has developed describing different quantitative and semi-quantitative criteria to assist the radiologist in the identification of vertebral fractures.[24–33] Although presently there are no universally accepted criteria for the diagnosis of vertebral fractures, the importance of including the quantification of vertebral body shape as part of the evaluation of vertebral fracture is widely accepted.[34] The current debate centres on what type and degree of abnormality should be classified as a significant fracture.

VERTEBRAL MORPHOMETRY STUDIES USING SPINAL RADIOGRAPHS

Vertebral morphometry is the quantification of vertebral body shape from measurements performed on lateral radiographs of the lumbar and thoracic spine.[34,35] The purpose is to quantify the type and degree of deformity of the vertebral body (Figure 20.2). The method requires digitizing conventional radiographs obtained under carefully standardized conditions.[36] Films are acquired using a fixed focal spot to film distance (usually standardized between 100 and 120 cm) to ensure a constant magnification error. The patient must be carefully positioned on their side with the knees and hips flexed. Two radiographs are obtained, one of the thoracic spine centred over T7 and the second of the lumbar spine centred over L3 (Figure 20.1). After processing, the film is reviewed by an experienced radiologist and between six and ten points are marked on each vertebra to define its shape (Figure 20.3).[35] The film is then placed on a back-lit digitizing table and the co-ordinates of each point read into a computer for data analysis. Alternatively, the

A

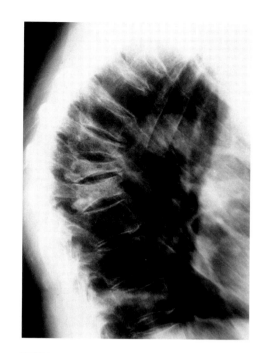

B

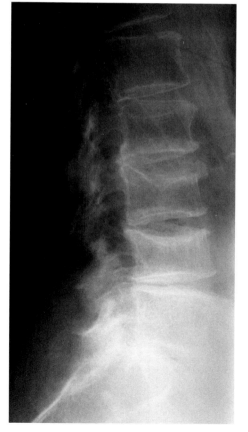

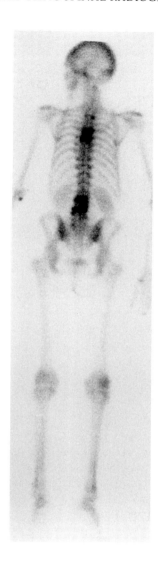

C

Figure 20.1 (A) Thoracic, and (B) lumbar lateral spinal radiographs in a patient with vertebral fractures in T6, T7, T8, L3 and L4. (C) Recent vertebral fractures such as those seen on the radiograph show clearly on a ^{99m}Tc-MDP radionuclide bone scan. (Reproduced with permission from Blake et al.[54])

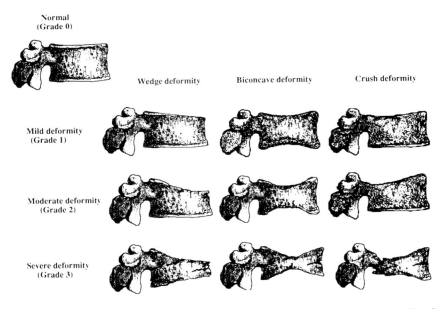

Figure 20.2 A graphic representation of wedge, biconcave and crush vertebral deformities. The figure illustrates the semi-quantitative visual grading system of Genant. (Reproduced with permission from Genant et al.[32])

entire film may be digitized and subject to an automated or semi-automated analysis to define the points.[37,38]

The points placed to characterize the shape of the vertebral body are used to determine the anterior (H_a), mid-vertebral (H_m) and posterior (H_p) heights of each vertebra (Figure 20.3). Generally, three types of deformities are recognized: anterior wedge (or wedge) (decreased ratio of H_a/H_p), mid-wedge (or biconcavity) (decreased ratio of H_m/H_p), and crush (or compression) (decreased ratio of posterior height compared with adjacent upper ($H_p(i)/H_p(i + 1)$) or lower ($H_p(i)/H_p(i - 1)$) vertebrae. Deviations from an exact rectangular shape are usually present and reflect the normal curvature of the spine. Some degree of anterior wedging (kyphosis, $H_a/H_p < 1$) is normally present in the thoracic spine and is replaced by a degree of posterior wedging (lordosis, $H_a/H_p > 1$) below L3.[35]

Vertebral height measurements may differ between patients depending on stature. Therefore, methods for interpreting these measurements usually adopt a convention to normalize the results to the patient's own spine. This may be done either by reference to a chosen vertebra (usually T4)[27] or by restricting analysis to the ratios of heights such as the anterior wedge, mid-wedge and crush ratios described above.[28] As well as normalizing for stature, the use of ratios of vertebral heights also corrects for any variation in the magnification factor for the radiograph.

CONVENTIONS FOR INTERPRETING RADIOGRAPHIC VERTEBRAL MORPHOMETRY MEASUREMENTS

In recent years a number of schemes have been published for interpreting vertebral morphometry measurements. The aim of these is to help

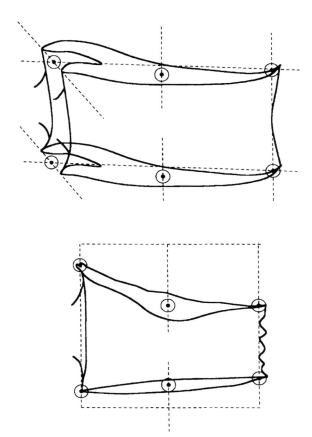

Figure 20.3 Schematic depiction of the placement of six points for the measurement of vertebral dimensions. The mid-points should be placed in the middle of the superior and inferior end-plates.

quantify the degree of vertebral lesions in patients with osteoporosis and to assess progress during follow-up. The principles behind some of the more widely used schemes are reviewed here.

The Minne method

One of the first studies to quantify vertebral deformation in an objective manner was that of Minne et al. who developed a measure called the spinal deformity index (SDI).[27] The basis of the Minne method is to normalize each anterior, middle and posterior height between T5 and L5 to the corresponding height measure in T4. T4 was chosen for the practical reason that it was unfractured in all but one of the osteoporotic subjects studied. Radiographs in 108 women and 38 men judged normal or exhibiting only minimal degenerative disease were used to develop normal range plots for the normalized anterior, middle and posterior vertebral heights from T5 to L5.[20] For each height measurement on the patient's radiograph the difference between the normalized height and the respective lower limit of the normal range is calculated in units of T4 height. Heights found to be below the lower limit of the normal range are classified as deformities (Figure 20.4). At each level the sum of any differences below the lower limit of normal for the three heights measured is defined as the vertebral deformity index (VDI) for that vertebra. The SDI is the sum of all the VDI values between T5 and L5.

The Eastell method

Eastell et al. developed morphometric algorithms to define vertebral fracture using lateral and antero-posterior radiographs for 195 subjects recruited from an age-stratified random sample of postmenopausal women from Rochester, Minnesota, USA.[28] Their classification recognizes three types of deformity (wedge, biconcavity and compression) that are quantified as explained in Table 20.1 and illustrated in Figure 20.5. In Eastell's definition, a vertebra is considered to be fractured if any one of the three ratios is more than 3 standard deviations (SD) below the normal mean for that vertebra (Table 20.1). Fractures between 3 SD and 4 SD are classified as grade 1, and those more than 4 SD as grade 2 (Figure 20.5). The grading system can be helpful when correlating the results of morphometry with clinical findings.

The Black method

Black et al. presented vertebral reference data derived from 2992 women aged 65–70 years

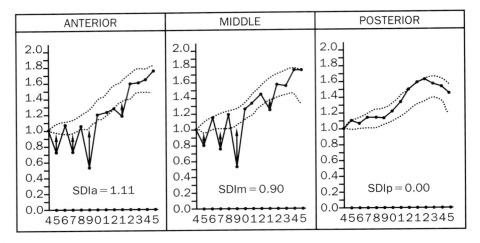

Figure 20.4 Principle of the calculation of Minne's spinal deformity index (SDI).[27] For each height measurement the difference between the normalized height and the lower limit of normal is calculated in T4 units and the results summed for all heights below the lower limit of normal. (Reproduced with permission from Leidig-Bruckner and Minne.[20])

from the Study of Osteoporotic Fractures.[29] Normative values were derived at each vertebral level for the wedge, biconcavity and compression ratios developed by Eastell et al.[28] Since the reference population included subjects with existing vertebral deformities, it was necessary to trim the most extreme values at either end of the distribution on the assumption that most fractured vertebrae lay in the tails of the curves. A truncated Gaussian distribution was fitted to the remaining data to derive the mean and population SD values at each vertebral level. Fractures were defined as values more than 3 SD below the mean (Figure 20.6).

Table 20.1 Classification of vertebral compression fractures from lateral spinal radiographs. (Reproduced from Eastell et al.[28])

Type of deformity	Wedge	$(H_p - H_a)/H_p \times 100$
	Biconcavity	$(H_p - H_m)/H_p \times 100$
	Compression	$(H_p^1 - H_p)/H_p^1 \times 100$
Degree of deformity	Normal	Mean $\pm$ 3 SD
	Fracture grade 1	>3 SD but <4 SD below mean
	Fracture grade 2	>4 SD below mean

H_p, posterior height of vertebral body (mm); H_a, anterior height (mm); H_m, height at mid-portion (mm); H_p^1, posterior height of adjacent normal vertebra (mm).

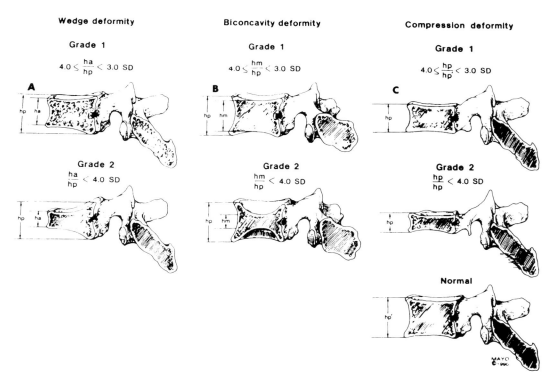

Figure 20.5 Principles of Eastell's method of classifying vertebral fractures by type and grade. (Reproduced with permission from Eastell et al.[28])

The Melton method

In a similar study to Black, Melton et al. examined the prevalence and incidence of vertebral deformities in 762 women aged 50 years or over from Rochester, Minnesota, USA.[30] However, instead of fitting a truncated Gaussian curve to the core of the distribution function, Melton used a non-parametric method to trim the extreme ratios on the assumption that these values represent deformed vertebrae. In this method the 25th percentile (Q1) and 75th percentile (Q3) of the distribution are found and the interquartile range (IQR = Q3 − Q1) calculated. Any observed ratios in the distribution function more than 1.5 IQR above Q3 or below Q1 are removed and then Q1, Q3 and the IQR recalculated for the remaining values. The

process is repeated until no more ratios lie outside the calculated limits. The method converges rapidly and is quick and simple to apply. For a Gaussian distribution the trimming limits correspond to ±2.7 SD. The trimmed data are used to derive the reference data in terms of the mean and SD of the final data set.

The McCloskey method

McCloskey et al. addressed the potential for vertebral morphometry studies to generate a significant proportion of false positive results simply due to the large number of measurements in each subject. When four parameters (wedge, biconcavity and two compression ratios) are measured in each of 14 vertebrae

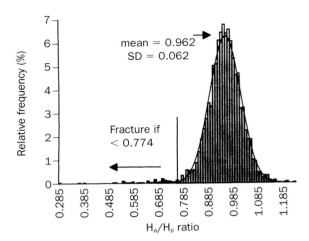

Figure 20.6 Principles of Black's method of defining a vertebral deformity. The curve shows the Gaussian fit to the distribution of H_a/H_p ratios measured in L1 in 2992 women. The vertical line indicates how a wedge fracture would be defined by setting a threshold value 3 SD below the mean. (Reproduced with permission from Black et al.[29])

(T4–L5), a total of 56 values per patient are generated. With a probability of any one ratio meeting the 3 SD criterion of 0.135%, the apparent prevalence of vertebral deformity would be 7% simply due to the statistical properties of the normal distribution. To reduce the problem of false positive results, the McCloskey method requires the fulfilment of two criteria for deformity rather than the single criterion usually adopted (Table 20.2).[31] The second criterion is generated by calculating a predicted posterior height at each vertebral level from up to four adjacent normal vertebrae. Thus, to identify an abnormal wedge ratio, both the ratio of measured anterior to measured posterior height and the ratio of measured anterior to predicted posterior height must be more than 3 SD below the normal mean. The normative data required to implement the method were derived from 100 women aged 45–50 selected randomly from a

Table 20.2 The McCloskey classification of vertebral deformities and the criteria that need to be fulfilled for each.[31]

Type of deformity	Criteria
Central collapse	C/P and C/PP < (mean C/P − 3 SD)
Anterior wedge	A/P and A/PP < (mean A/P − 3 SD)
Posterior wedge	P/PP < (mean P/PP − 3 SD) and A/P > (mean A/P + 3 SD)
Crush	P/PP < (mean P/PP − 3 SD) and A/PP < (mean A/P − 3 SD)

A, anterior height; C, central height; P, posterior height; PP, predicted posterior height of the vertebra under examination.
Note that two criteria must be fulfilled for each type of deformity.

general practice population with no history of back pain or osteoporotic fracture. Unlike some methods[27,28] there was no trimming of extreme values since it was assumed that in a young, healthy population all subjects should have normal vertebrae.

The Genant semi-quantitative method

None of the methods of quantitative morphometry outlined above can discriminate between vertebral fractures and other causes of vertebral deformity. For the radiologist viewing the X-ray films there is a long list of potential differential diagnoses for vertebral deformities and the correct classification can only be obtained by visual inspection and expert interpretation of the radiograph. This viewpoint is the basis of the semi-quantitative technique of Genant et al.[32,33] In the Genant method each vertebra from T4 to L4 is assessed visually without any direct vertebral measurement and graded as: normal (grade 0), mildly deformed (grade 1, reduction of 20–25% in anterior, middle or posterior height); moderately deformed (grade 2, reduction of 25–40% in any height); or severely deformed (grade 3, reduction of >40% in any height) (Table 20.3 and Figure 20.2). Borderline vertebrae are given a grade of 0.5. Following visual assessment a spinal fracture index (SFI) is calculated as the sum of all grades divided by the number of evaluable vertebrae. The advantage of this method is that it makes the trained human observer the basis of interpretation while also providing a quantitative index that allows for meaningful interpretation of changes on follow-up films.

REFERENCE DATA FOR RADIOGRAPHIC VERTEBRAL MORPHOMETRY

Table 20.4 summarizes details of some studies that have provided reference data for vertebral morphometry based on spinal radiographs. Several different strategies for subject recruitment and statistical analysis have been adopted. Black,[29] Melton[30] and O'Neill[39] all used population listings to recruit a large number of subjects. The subjects were not screened and the data set for each vertebral height ratio was trimmed (each study using a different trimming algorithm) to exclude deformed vertebrae from the reference range calculations. However, the trimming of the data set can have a significant effect on the calculated population SD, to the extent that significant errors might arise from some of the eliminated subjects actually being normal individuals in a non-Gaussian tail to the true population distribution.

In the McCloskey study,[31] a group of 100 younger women were recruited who were pre-screened for back pain and history of vertebral or other osteoporotic fracture. The prevalance of vertebral deformity was assumed to be zero. Uncertainties in this approach arise from the relatively small number of subjects included in the study, which generates random statistical errors in the population SD similar to those generated by the trimming methods described above.

Other studies have relied on qualitative reading by a clinician to identify deformed vertebrae for exclusion from reference range calculations,[20,27] or a combination of this approach and patient screening.[1]

ADVANTAGES AND DISADVANTAGES OF CONVENTIONAL RADIOGRAPHS FOR PERFORMING QUANTITATIVE VERTEBRAL MORPHOMETRY

The principal advantage of performing vertebral morphometry studies with conventional radiographs is the high resolution of the images (Table 20.5). Radiographs give excellent definition of the end-plates and the other edges of the vertebral body, which aids correct point placement even in patients with a significant degree of osteopenia, degenerative disease or scoliosis.

The limitations of the technique are associated with patient positioning, image geometry and radiation dose (Table 20.5). Films of the lateral spine are usually performed with the patient lying on his or her side in the decubitus position. This method is prone to differences in

Table 20.3 Classification of vertebral compression from anterior and posterior height measurements and inspection of lateral spinal radiographs. (Reproduced from Genant et al.[32])

Grade	Description	Fracture grade	Anterior to posterior height relationship
1/2	Minimal compression	No fracture	15–20%
1	Anterior wedging	Mild fracture	20–25%
2	Anterior wedging (with and without posterior wedging), mid-height deformity	Moderate fracture	>25%
3	Marked deformity (over 40% of volume loss compared with adjacent normal vertebrae)	Severe fracture	
Sum of grades for T4–L5		Spinal fracture index	

positioning, especially if performed by different radiographers. It is also difficult to ensure complete consistency on follow-up films. Care is necessary to ensure that a fixed focus to film distance is used. Separate films of the thoracic and lumbar spine are required and may lead to discontinuities in measured parameters across the boundary of the two films. Distortions due to the cone beam geometry may introduce errors of accuracy and precision. The radiation exposure of the patient is relatively high and results in an effective dose[40] of around 800 μSv.[36,41] Repeat films may be required to improve either the positioning or exposure factors, and this further increases patient dose.

VERTEBRAL MORPHOMETRY STUDIES USING DXA SCANNERS

In the past 5 years technical advances in DXA scanners have improved image quality to the extent that it is now realistic to consider the use of DXA images for vertebral morphometry studies.[42–44]

Improvements in DXA technology

When first introduced, DXA scanners such as the Hologic QDR-1000 and Lunar DPX used a pencil-beam scanning geometry with a pinhole collimator coupled to a single detector in the scanning arm. Lateral scans could only be per-

Table 20.4 Summary of reference range studies for radiographic vertebral morphometry.

Study	Number of subjects	Age (years)	Radiographs Tube-to-film (cm)	Centred on	Health exclusions	Data trimmed	Source country
Black et al.[29]	2992	65–70	101.6	T8/L3	No	Yes	USA
McCloskey et al.[31]	100	45–50	105	T9/L3	Yes	No	UK
Minne et al.[27]	73	42 < 50, 31 > 50	105	T9/L3	Yes	No	Germany
Melton et al.[1]	52	N/A	105	N/A	Yes	No	USA
O'Neill et al.[39]	819	50–89	120	T7/L2	No	Yes	Sweden, France and Austria

Centred on, vertebrae lateral thoracic and lumbar radiographs were centred on.
Health exclusions, subjects excluded for health reasons, e.g. metabolic bone disease or diagnosed vertebral fractures.
Data trimmed, data set trimmed to exclude possible deformed vertebrae.
N/A, data not available.

Table 20.5 Advantages and disadvantages of dual X-ray absorptiometry and conventional radiography for vertebral morphometry.

	Conventional radiography	Dual X-ray absorptiometry
Advantages	High definition images Point placement easier than DXA in patients with degenerative disease or scoliosis Exposure factors can be adjusted to help with obese patients	Patient positioning highly standardized Entire spine imaged in single scan Fixed image magnification factor No geometrical distortion of image Low radiation dose Digital image acquisition Semi-automated analysis Simplified image archiving and retrieval
Disadvantages	Difficult to reproduce patient positioning Requires separate films of lumbar and thoracic spine Image distortion from cone beam geometry Relatively high radiation dose Suboptimal exposures leading to repeat films are relatively common	Poorer image definition Limited control over exposure factors Images poor in obese patients Point placement may be difficult in patients with degenerative disease or scoliosis Automated analysis may be too readily accepted by operator

formed with the patient turned on his or her side. Patient positioning was difficult, scan times were long and image resolution poor.[45,46] Since then three significant advances in technology have improved the capability of DXA systems to acquire lateral scans of sufficient quality to permit vertebral morphometry.

The rotating C-arm

The use of a rotating C-arm to support the source and detectors enables the patient to be scanned in the supine position. This gives a significant advantage in reproducible patient positioning. The C-arm enables the lateral scan to be preceded by a postero-anterior (PA) projection scan from which the operator can check that the patient's spine is straight, assess the degree of any scoliosis and choose the correct starting point for the lateral scan. The PA scan also determines the centre line of the vertebral column. When the C-arm is rotated through 90° to acquire the lateral image, the scanning arm tracks the centre line and ensures that the X-ray tube and detectors are maintained at a fixed distance from the centre of the spine, thus eliminating errors due to variable magnification.

Fan-beam geometry

In fan-beam DXA scanners, a slit collimator generates a fan-beam coupled to a linear array of detectors. Details of the scanning geometry are discussed in Chapter 3. A study is acquired by the scanning arm performing a single sweep along the spine compared with the two-dimensional raster scan required by first generation pencil-beam systems. The result is greatly shortened scan times enabling vertebral morphometry studies to be acquired in times as short as 10 seconds. This arrangement enables the entire spine from L4 to T4 to be imaged with a single scan without any geometrical distortion in the cranio-caudal direction.

Improved image resolution

Use of a solid-state detector constructed in the form of a multi-element linear array has improved image resolution compared with first generation DXA systems. Although resolution still does not approach that of radiographs, the improvement is sufficient to aid significantly accurate point placement. However, it remains the case that the poorer resolution of DXA images compared with radiographs makes point placement more difficult and therefore errors are more likely to occur, especially in patients with scoliosis or degenerative disease.[43]

Image formation in DXA vertebral morphometry

The conventional use of DXA scanners is to quantify BMD. The image that is presented to the operator is formed by taking the low-energy attenuation map over the scanning field and subtracting a factor of the high-energy map. In this way the effects of soft tissue are eliminated and the final image represents the BMD map over the scanning field. The advantage for vertebral morphometry studies is that confusing structures in the image due to soft tissue features are removed. However, a less desirable consequence is that pixel noise is increased and the final image may appear noisy to the detriment of image resolution.

An alternative option that may be more suitable for vertebral morphometry applications is to use the DXA system to acquire a single-energy rather than a dual-energy image (Figure 20.7A and B). A single-energy image will show lower pixel noise and superior image definition, but at the cost of significant confusion of vertebral structure by soft tissue features around and above the diaphragm. This effect can be modified by use of a high-pass filter, which will reduce large-scale features while retaining the fine details such as the vertebral body endplates required for accurate point placement.

VERTEBRAL MORPHOMETRY ON COMMERCIAL DXA SYSTEMS

Two manufacturers of DXA scanners, Hologic Inc. (Waltham, MA, USA) and Lunar Corp. (Madison, WI, USA), presently offer commercial systems with software for vertebral

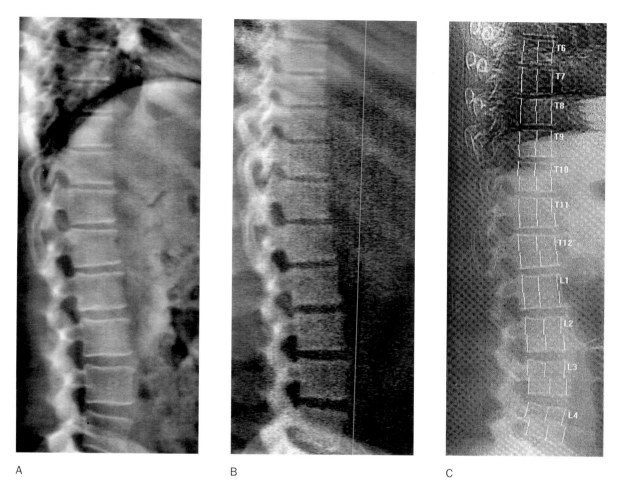

Figure 20.7 Three MXA scan images acquired on the same subject. (A) A single-energy scan and (B) a dual-energy scan performed on a Hologic QDR-4500A system. (C) Scan performed on a Lunar Expert-XL.

morphometry. Each manufacturer's equipment will be discussed in turn.

The Hologic QDR-4500A: choice of scan mode

The QDR-4500A (Figure 20.8A) continues the vertebral morphometry application first developed for the QDR-2000[42] and QDR-2000*plus*. At the start of a study, a PA pro-jection scan is performed to determine the centre line of the vertebral column. After the C-arm is rotated a choice of four scan modes is available for acquiring the lateral image. One mode performs a single-energy (SE) scan, while the other three perform dual-energy scans with a choice of scan speed and collimator widths. The three dual-energy (DE) scan modes are referred to as fast (F), array (A) and high-definition (HD) modes respectively. Examples of all four modes performed on the same subject are shown in

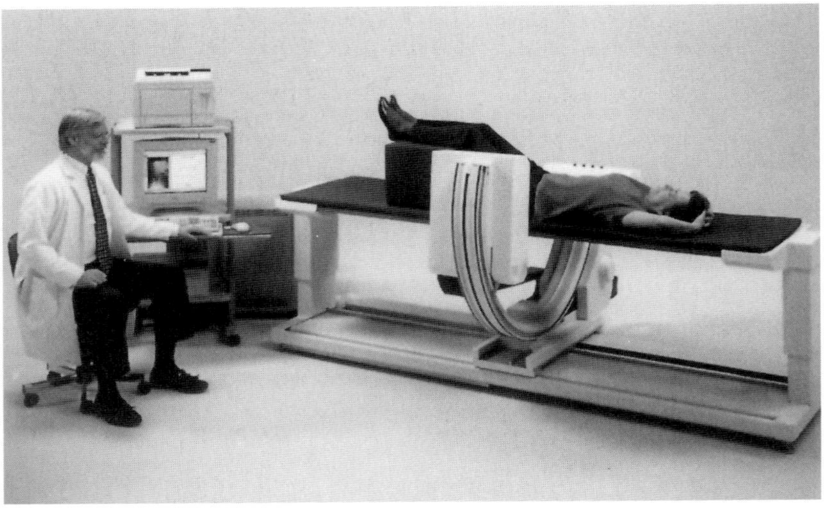

Figure 20.8 Two commercial DXA systems that offer vertebral morphometry facilities. (A) The Hologic QDR-4500A and (B) the Lunar Expert-XL. (Reproduced with permission from the manufacturers.)

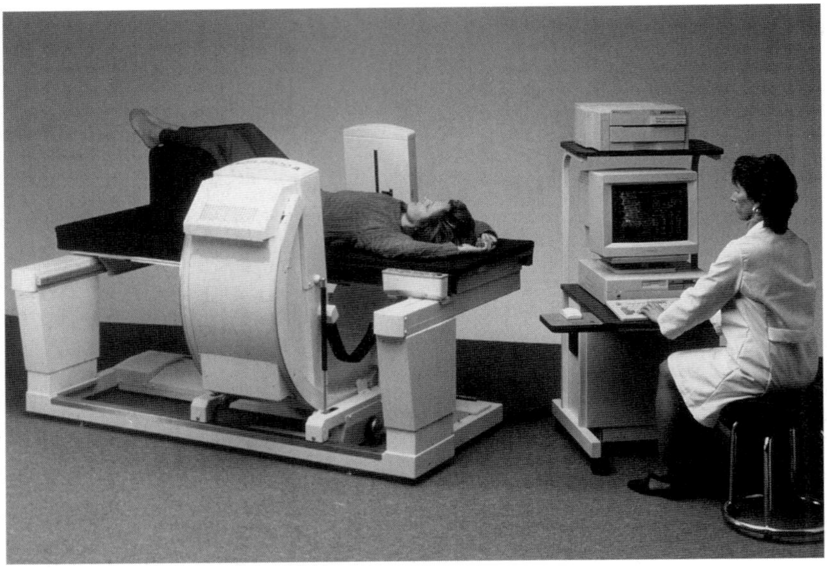

Figure 20.9. The single-energy mode uses a 0.5-mm wide collimator slit and takes 10 seconds to acquire a scan from L4 to T4. The fast and array dual-energy modes both use a 1-mm collimator and scans take 5 and 10 min-utes respectively. The high-definition mode uses a 0.5-mm collimator and scans take 10 minutes.

Although scan time for the single-energy mode is short and image definition below the

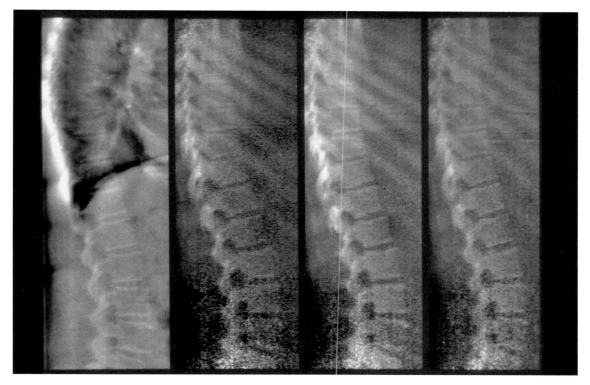

Figure 20.9 MXA images acquired by scanning the same subject (a 60-year-old postmenopausal woman) using each of the four scan modes on the QDR-4500A. From left to right: single-energy mode; dual-energy (DE) fast mode; DE array mode; and DE high-definition mode.

diaphragm is excellent (Figure 20.7A), confusion from soft tissue structures above the diaphragm may make scan analysis difficult, especially for the less experienced operator. These artefacts are absent from the dual-energy images, which often give clearer definition between bone and soft tissue above the diaphragm but may give a poorer image in the lumbar and lower thoracic spine in patients with high soft tissue attenuation.

Rea et al.[47] studied scans of 60 postmenopausal women to make a detailed comparison of the image quality of all four QDR-4500A scan modes. The percentage of vertebrae judged evaluable by vertebral morphometry was plotted as a function of vertebral level from L4 to T4 (Figure 20.10). The high-definition mode performed best with a mean of 11.5/13 (88%) evaluable vertebrae per patient compared with 10.9/13 (84%) for the single-energy mode, 10.7/13 (82%) for the array and 9.4/13 (72%) for the fast dual-energy mode. When both high-definition and single-energy scans were performed and the clearest image used for analysis, there was a mean of 12.2/13 (94%) evaluable vertebrae per patient. The failure to identify and measure every vertebra from L4 to T4 was found to depend principally on the subject's body mass index (BMI = body weight/height^2) (Figure 20.11). The ideal BMI in a healthy subject is 20–25 kg/m^2. However, for obese patients with BMI > 30 the diagnostic

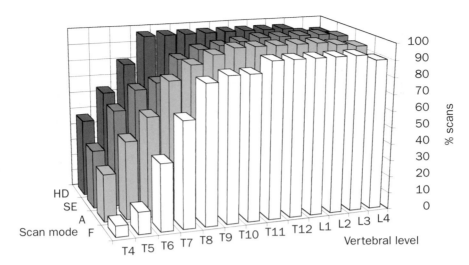

Figure 20.10 Percentage of MXA scans that can be analysed at each vertebral level for the four MXA scan modes on the QDR-4500A. From back to front: HD, high-definition dual-energy (DE) mode; SE, single-energy mode; A, array DE mode; and F, fast DE mode.

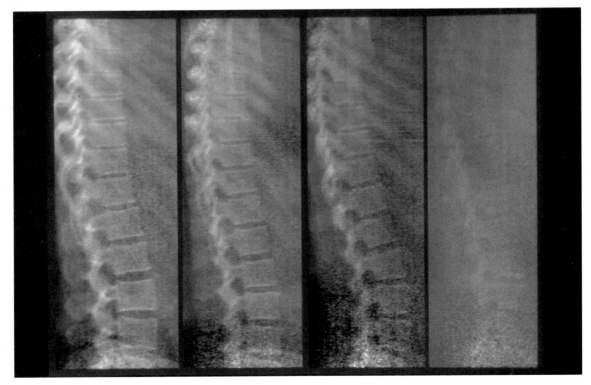

Figure 20.11 MXA images acquired using the dual-energy high-definition scan mode showing the effect of body mass index (BMI) on image quality. From left to right: BMI = 18.0; 25.3; 29.1; and 38.6 kg/m².

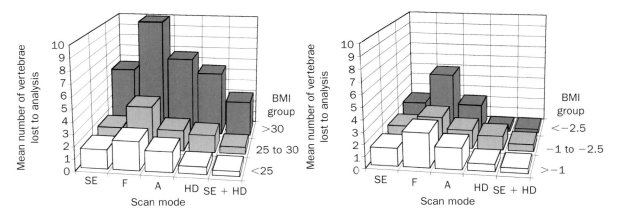

Figure 20.12 Effect of (on the left) body mass index (BMI) and (on the right) bone mineral density (BMD) on the mean number of vertebrae lost to analysis per scan for each scan mode. From left to right: SE: single-energy mode; F: fast dual-energy (DE) mode; A: array DE mode; HD: high-definition DE mode; SE + HD: from assessment of both SE and HD modes. BMI groups: units are kg/m^2; BMD groups: patients grouped by lumbar spine T-scores.

quality of scans deteriorated sharply (Figure 20.12). The effect of lumbar spine BMD was also studied. When subjects were divided into normal, osteopenic and osteoporotic groups by applying the WHO criteria[48] to the patients' lumbar spine T-score values, BMD was found to be a less important factor than BMI in determining the percentage of vertebrae lost to analysis (Figure 20.12). Possibly this is due to the fact that osteoporosis is a systemic disease, and so the BMD of confusing structures such as the ribs and scapulae decrease approximately in proportion to spinal BMD (Figure 20.13). Rea et al. concluded that optimal results are obtained by the acquisition of both single-energy and high-definition dual-energy scans (both scans can be displayed side by side). However, for rapid assessment by an experienced operator, single-energy scans alone offer almost equal utility. Thus, for reasons of speed and patient throughput it is likely that the single-energy mode will be the one most users choose to adopt.

The Hologic QDR-4500A: scan analysis

Vertebral morphometry analysis on the QDR-4500A is performed by the operator placing six points on the vertebra to emulate the conventional radiographic placements (Figure 20.14). Analysis commences at L4 (correct identification of the vertebral level is aided by simultaneous display of the PA centre line scan) and continues up to and including T4 or as many of these vertebrae as can be sufficiently visualized for analysis. The operator first uses a mouse-controlled pointer to identify the anterior inferior corner of each vertebra. The computer software then fits a fourth degree polynomial to these points (Figure 20.15A), after which a level specific co-ordinate system is created for each vertebra (Figure 20.15B) and the computer helps speed the analysis by using a semi-automated knowledge based algorithm to predict the locations of the remaining points.[49] However, it is important that at every stage of the analysis the operator makes adjustments to account for individual variations and deformations. For an experienced operator,

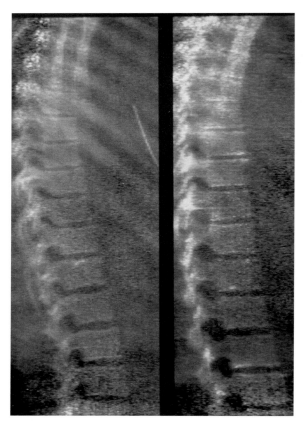

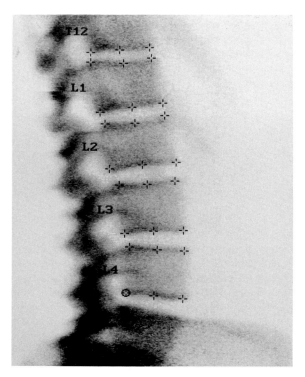

Figure 20.14 Point placement in the lumbar spine on a normal MXA scan.

Figure 20.13 MXA images acquired using the dual-energy high-definition scan mode showing the effect of lumbar spine BMD on image quality. BMD (L1–L4) was: left, 0.689 g/cm^2 (T-score = −3.25); right, 1.034 g/cm^2 (T-score = −0.12).

scan analysis takes approximately 5 minutes. Some guidance on point placement over and above that provided by the QDR-4500 operators' manual is given in the Appendix to this chapter.

After point placement is completed, the anterior, middle and posterior vertebral heights and the anterior and mid-wedge ratios are calculated and displayed by the software (Figure 20.16A and B). The final results (although these latter are not available in the USA) include

interpretations of the data based on the Minne spinal deformity index (SDI) (Figure 20.16C)[27] and the McCloskey algorithm for vertebral deformity (Figure 20.16D).[31] Because T4 is often difficult to measure reliably on DXA images, the Hologic Minne index uses L4 to normalize the vertebral heights. This choice presents a problem if L4 itself is affected by a deformity as in the example shown in Figure 20.16.

The Hologic QDR-4500A: MXA reference data

Currently, the QDR-4500A Minne and McCloskey algorithms use reference data obtained from conventional radiographic morphometry rather than from MXA scans. However, there are strong reasons for thinking that reference data for vertebral morphometry

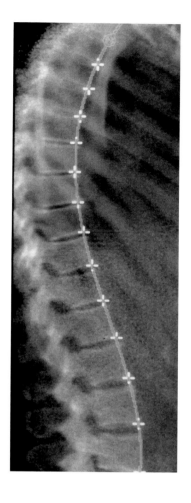

A

B

Figure 20.15 Semi-automated MXA scan analysis algorithm on QDR-4500. (A) Fourth degree polynomial fitted through the anterior–inferior points of L4–T4. (B) Level specific co-ordinate system shown for T10 vertebra: (1) origin of the co-ordinate system is the anterior–inferior point of the vertebra; (2) x-axis is the tangent to the polynomial fit at origin; (3) y-axis is the perpendicular to the x-axis.

are best collected using equipment and methodologies that resemble the clinical application as closely as possible.[50,51]

In the largest MXA reference database published to date, Rea et al. analysed scan data for 1019 white women scanned on QDR-4500A and QDR-2000*plus* systems at three centres in the UK.[50] Although statistically significant differences were found between the data collected at the different centres, different generations of DXA scanner and different scan modes, these differences were small and represented systematic differences of less than 2%. Compared with reference data obtained from spinal radiographs,[27,29] vertebral heights measured by MXA are about 20–25% smaller (Figure 20.17A) because of the elimination of the magnification

error inherent in conventional radiography. However, these differences are almost completely removed when both the MXA and radiography heights are normalized to L3 (Figure 20.17B).

When the vertebral height ratios derived from MXA scans were compared with reference data from radiography,[1,29,31,39] significant differences were seen for the anterior wedge and mid-wedge ratios between the different radiographic studies, as well as between MXA and radiography (Figure 20.18A). However, data for the crush ratio show better agreement between the various studies (Figure 20.18B). It is possible that real population differences could explain some of these results. However, differences in methodology due to different positioning

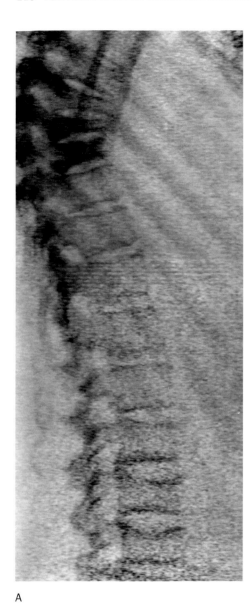

A

	PH (mm)	MH (mm)	AH (mm)	WEDGE	MWEDGE
T4	19.4	18.1	19.6	1.01	0.93
T5	16.9	15.8	16.2	0.96	0.93
T6	14.7	9.4	8.1	0.55	0.64
T7	13.6	7.6	8.1	0.59	0.56
T8	17.5	12.4	11.7	0.67	0.70
T9	22.8	20.4	22.0	0.97	0.90
T10	24.4	21.4	22.6	0.93	0.88
T11	24.6	22.2	25.2	1.03	0.90
T12	26.2	25.5	25.4	0.97	0.98
L1	27.9	26.5	28.1	1.01	0.95
L2	24.7	22.7	24.8	1.00	0.92
L3	23.2	18.7	21.2	0.91	0.80
L4	22.7	17.1	21.2	0.93	0.76

B

Spine Deformity Index (Minne)

	SDI(Ha)	SDI(Hm)	SDI(Hp)	TOTAL
T4	--.--	--.--	--.--	--.--
T5	--.--	--.--	--.--	--.--
T6	0.29	0.02	--.--	0.31
T7	0.31	0.20	0.02	0.54
T8	0.07	--.--	--.--	0.07
T9	--.--	--.--	--.--	--.--
T10	--.--	--.--	--.--	--.--
T11	--.--	--.--	--.--	--.--
T12	--.--	--.--	--.--	--.--
L1	--.--	--.--	--.--	--.--
L2	--.--	--.--	--.--	--.--
L3	--.--	--.--	--.--	--.--
L4	--.--	--.--	--.--	--.--
TOT	0.67	0.22	0.02	0.92

Hologic QDR-4500A (S/N 45008)

C

Vertebral Deformity (McCloskey)

	Ant	Cent	Post	Crush	Total
T4	---	---	---	---	0
T5	---	---	---	---	0
T6	---	---	---	Yes	3
T7	---	---	---	Yes	3
T8	---	---	---	Yes	3
T9	---	---	---	---	0
T10	---	---	---	---	0
T11	---	---	---	---	0
T12	---	---	---	---	0
L1	---	---	---	---	0
L2	---	---	---	---	0
L3	---	---	---	Yes	3
L4	---	---	---	Yes	3
TOT	0	0	0	5	15

D

Figure 20.16 Illustration of the results of a vertebral morphometry scan acquired on a Hologic QDR-4500A. (A) Lateral image of the spine performed in the patient whose radiographs are shown in Figure 20.1; (B) printout of the vertebral height and wedge ratios; (C) interpretation of the data based on the Minne spinal deformity index[27] (note that the Hologic Minne index uses L4 to normalize the vertebral heights and this example illustrates the problems that can arise when the patient has a deformity in L4); and (D) interpretation of the data based on the McCloskey algorithm.[31]

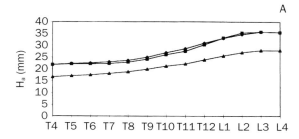
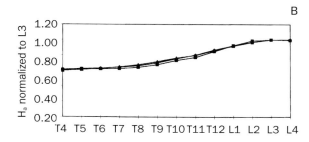

Figure 20.17 Comparison of reference values for mean anterior height (H_a) at each vertebral level derived from MXA[50] (▲), and from conventional radiographic data by Black et al.[29] (■) and Minne et al.[27] (◆). (A) Trimmed H_a values; (B) trimmed H_a values normalized to L3. (Reproduced with permission from Rea et al.[50])

techniques, X-ray parameters and conventions over point placement must also be major factors in the discrepant reference ranges.[51]

Rea's study of MXA reference data also found differences for the population SD values for the height ratios derived from the different studies.[50] Unlike the mean values, the SD figures agreed better between MXA and radiography for the anterior wedge and mid-wedge ratios while agreement was poorer for the posterior height crush ratios (Figure 20.19A and B). While MXA SD figures were comparable with radiography in the lumbar region, the differences tend to increase higher up the thorax. As

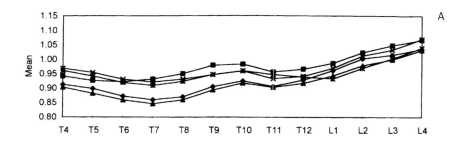

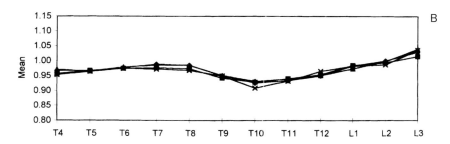

Figure 20.18 Comparison of reference values for mean vertebral height ratios at each vertebral level derived from MXA[50] (■), and from conventional radiographic data by Black et al.[29] (◆), Melton et al.[1] (✕), O'Neill et al.[39] (▲) and McCloskey et al.[31] (✳). (A) Wedge ratio (H_a/H_p) and (B) crush ratio ($H_p(i)/H_p(i-1)$). (Reproduced with permission from Rea et al.[50])

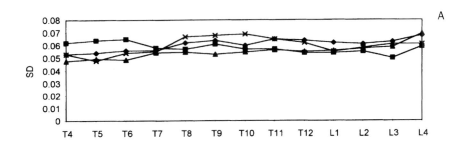

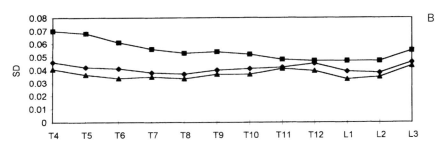

Figure 20.19 Comparison of reference values for the standard deviation (SD) of the vertebral height ratios at each vertebral level derived from MXA[50] (■), and from conventional radiographic data by Black et al.[29] (♦), O'Neill et al.[39] (▲) and McCloskey et al.[31] (✕). (A) Wedge ratio (H_a/H_p); (B) crush ratio ($H_p(i)/H_p(i-1)$). (Reproduced with permission from Rea et al.)

a result of these differences in mean and SD values, threshold values (mean − 3 SD) for identifying vertebral deformities can differ significantly depending on whether reference ranges are derived from MXA or radiographic studies (Figure 20.20A and B).

The Lunar Expert-XL

The Expert-XL (Figure 20.8B) is the first DXA scanner built by Lunar to include a vertebral morphometry capability.[44] The system uses a rotating anode tube and operates at 134 kVp. A PA projection centre line scan is not performed, but instead the operator is left to choose the correct starting point for the lateral scan. The scan itself takes 40 seconds to complete and image quality is comparable to the QDR-4500 single-

energy and high-definition modes (Figure 20.7C).

The scan analysis algorithm on the Lunar Expert is semi-automatic and is similar to one developed previously by Kalender et al.[37] for performing vertebral morphometry studies on QCT scout scans. The operator first places a point within each vertebral body. The algorithm then identifies the end-plates and calculates the horizontal bisecting line through the middle of each vertebra. The anterior, middle and posterior heights are each calculated from the sum of two vertical lines, the first starting from the bisector and cutting the upper end-plate, and the second starting from the bisector and cutting the lower end-plate (Figure 20.21). The position of each vertical line is chosen to maximize the anterior and posterior heights but minimize the middle height. As with the QDR-4500 software, it is important that at the

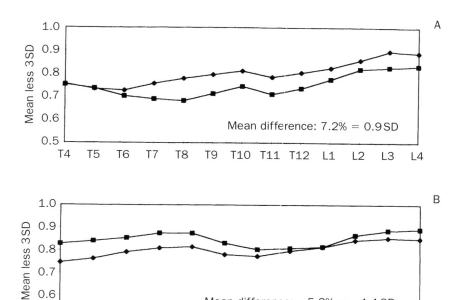

Figure 20.20 Comparison of reference threshold values (mean − 3 SD) for vertebral height ratios to identify deformities at each vertebral level derived from MXA[50] (◆) and from conventional radiographic data[29] (■). (A) Wedge ratio (H_a/H_p); (B) crush ratio ($H_p(i)/H_p(i − 1)$).

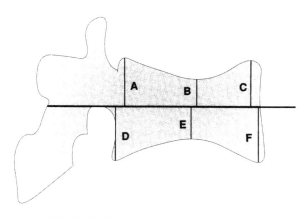

Figure 20.21 Method of point placement on the Lunar Expert-XL. Heights are calculated by summing the distances from points on the vertebral end-plates to a bisecting line.

end of the automatic analysis the operator makes the final adjustments to ensure the optimum point placement. Results are presented as the trend of vertebral heights and Z-scores with vertebral level (Figure 20.22).

PATIENT DOSE FROM DXA VERTEBRAL MORPHOMETRY

Although DXA vertebral morphometry scans do not give the same spatial resolution as lateral radiographs, one advantage of this is the significantly lower radiation dose to the patient. Lewis and Blake published estimates of the effective dose to a patient from vertebral morphometry scans performed on a Hologic

A

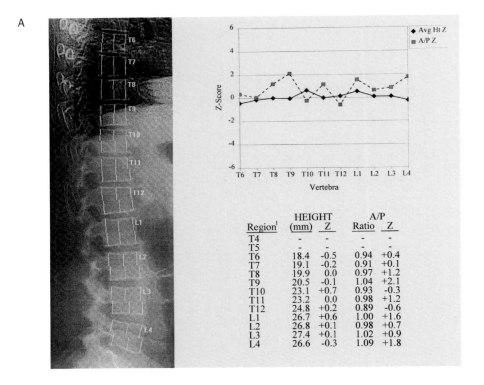

Region[1]	HEIGHT (mm)	Z	A/P Ratio	Z
T4	-	-	-	-
T5	-	-	-	-
T6	18.4	-0.5	0.94	+0.4
T7	19.1	-0.2	0.91	+0.1
T8	19.9	0.0	0.97	+1.2
T9	20.5	-0.1	1.04	+2.1
T10	23.1	+0.7	0.93	-0.3
T11	23.2	0.0	0.98	+1.2
T12	24.8	+0.2	0.89	-0.6
L1	26.7	+0.6	1.00	+1.6
L2	26.8	+0.1	0.98	+0.7
L3	27.4	+0.1	1.02	+0.9
L4	26.6	-0.3	1.09	+1.8

B

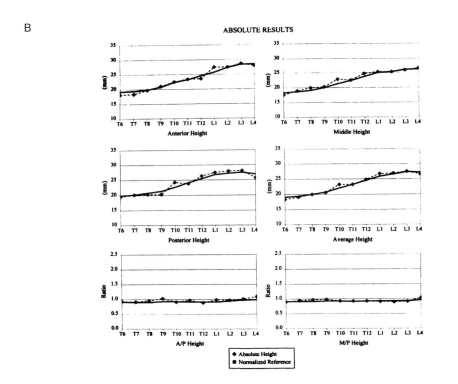

C

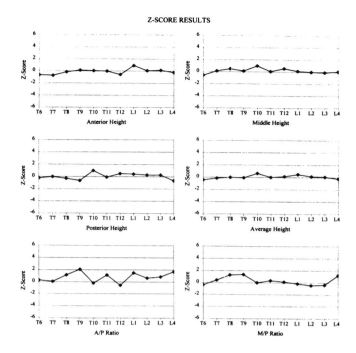

Figure 20.22 Illustration of the results of a vertebral morphometry scan acquired on a Lunar Expert-XL. (A) Lateral image of the spine with vertebral height data; (B) interpretation based on plots of vertebral height against vertebral level; and (C) interpretation based on Z-scores in which the difference of each height measurement from the mean is expressed in units of the population SD.

QDR-2000*plus* system.[52] Their study used organ weighting factors taken from the ICRP Report no. 60[40] and was based on a technique previously developed for calculating patient dose in DXA bone density investigations.[53] They concluded that although the scan length for a vertebral morphometry study is approximately three times greater than a bone density scan of the lumbar spine, patient dose is around 10 times larger (assuming the same collimator, scan speed and tube current) due to the inclusion of the lungs and breasts in the scan field.

Table 20.6 presents equivalent data on patient dose for morphometry scans performed on the QDR-4500A and Expert-XL.[54] Of particular note is that the single-energy mode combines both a fast scan speed and a very low radiation dose to the patient.

ADVANTAGES AND DISADVANTAGES OF DXA SYSTEMS FOR PERFORMING QUANTITATIVE VERTEBRAL MORPHOMETRY

Fan-beam DXA systems with a rotating C-arm have a number of advantages for performing good quality vertebral morphometry studies (Table 20.5). The first of these advantages is that the supine lateral projection ensures that the patient's position is highly standardized and reproducible and no difficulties should occur in patients with normal spinal anatomy. When acquired in combination with a PA projection scan, the operator can check that the patient's spine is straight and identify the correct vertebral level for starting the lateral scan and subsequent analysis. The PA image also enables the lateral scan to track the middle of the spine and

	Table 20.6 Effective dose for vertebral morphometry scans performed on a DXA bone densitometer.[51,53]		
DXA system	Scan mode	PA centre line scan	Lateral morphometry scan
QDR-4500A	Dual-energy fast	4 µSv (30 s)	20 µSv (5 min)
QDR-4500A	Dual-energy medium	10 µSv (90 s)	41 µSv (10 min)
QDR-4500A	Dual-energy hi-res	20 µSv (3 min)	20 µSv (10 min)
QDR-4500A	Single-energy	–	2 µSv (10 s)
Expert-XL	5 mA fast	–	38 µSv (40 s)

Scan times are given in brackets.
Note that QDR-4500A studies require the acquisition of both a PA centre line and a lateral morphometry scan.

maintain a fixed distance between the X-ray tube and the spine. The entire spine is imaged with a single scan, which eliminates the problems of geometrical distortion due to the X-ray cone beam. The final image is stored digitally and point placement may be efficiently performed using semi-automated procedures. Finally, radiation dose is low, making the technique attractive for routine evaluation of patients in the osteoporosis clinic.

Disadvantages of DXA (Table 20.5) include the relatively low resolution that may create difficulties in identification of vertebral contours and allowing for the effects of degenerative changes and scoliosis. Although automated analysis provides efficiency, it may imply a false accuracy so that point placement is too readily accepted by the operator.[43] Finally, exposure factors for DXA scans are not under the control of the operator and therefore difficulties can arise in acquiring usable studies in obese patients.

CONCLUSIONS

Vertebral fractures represent half of all osteoporotic fractures and are an important target for improvements in diagnosis and preventive therapy. Although spinal radiographs are widely performed, they entail a high radiation dose for the patient, and access to vertebral morphometry to supplement the radiologist's interpretation is restricted to a few major centres with the necessary facilities and expertise. In these centres, morphometry is proving a useful tool for epidemiological studies and clinical trials. The development of bone densitometry services has made DXA scanners widely available and the introduction of lateral spinal imaging combining short scan times and user-friendly software for scan analysis offers an exciting opportunity to evaluate the use of vertebral morphometry to improve the assessment and follow-up of patients in the outpatient clinic.

At present, the principal limitation of MXA is the poor definition of the images compared with spinal radiographs. Image resolution is directly associated with radiation dose, and there is a strong case that some of the advantages of low-dose compared with conventional radiography should be traded for an improvement in image quality. A second requirement is to give the operator more control over exposure factors so that clearer images can be obtained in osteoporotic and obese subjects. There is also scope for improvement in the automated software to achieve quicker and more consistent scan analysis. Several studies now underway suggest that the application of sophisticated image processing techniques such as active shape modelling can speed analysis and improve the intra- and interobserver reproducibility of MXA software.[55,56]

APPENDIX: POINT PLACEMENT IN VERTEBRAL MORPHOMETRIC X-RAY ABSORPTIOMETRY

By Jacqueline A Rea

Six points are used to characterize the shape of each vertebral body (Figure 20.A1 (left)), which under normal circumstances is approximately rectangular. The points are placed on the superior–inferior anterior and posterior corners of the vertebral body with a mid-point placed on each of the superior and inferior end-plates that is usually equidistant between the posterior and anterior points.

Inferior–anterior points: each point should be placed at the outer border of the vertebral end-plate at the intersection of the inferior end-plate and the anterior edge of the vertebral body.

Inferior–posterior points: points should be placed at the outer end of the inferior end-plate at the point where it intersects with the posterior edge of the vertebral body.

Superior–anterior points: these points are placed at the outer end of the superior end-plate where it intersects with the anterior edge of the vertebral body.

Superior–posterior points: each point should be placed at the intersection of the superior end-plate and the posterior edge of the vertebral body. There is a small protrusion, known as the uncinate process, at the superior–posterior aspect of some vertebral bodies. This should be excluded in point placement, and superior–posterior points should be placed by projecting the superior end-plate horizontally from the anterior edge straight through the uncinate process and placing the point at the intersection of this line and the posterior edge of the vertebral body.

Mid-points: these points should be placed at the exact middle of the superior and inferior vertebral end-plates, equidistant between the anterior and posterior points. In the case of deformed vertebrae, the mid-points should be placed at the lowest (highest) point of the superior (inferior) end-plate, even if this results in points that are offset from the exact middle of the end-plate (Figure 20.A1 (right)).

Osteophytes: these bony artefacts protruding

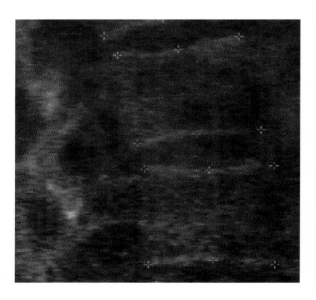 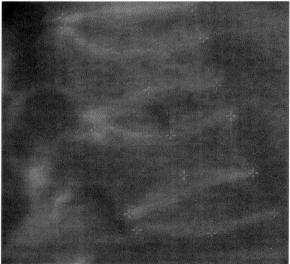

Figure 20.A1 Examples of point placement protocols for normal vertebrae (left) and a subject with mid-wedge deformities (right).

from the corners of some vertebral bodies should be excluded in point placement in a similar way to the uncinate process. For example, if the superior–anterior corner of a vertebral body is affected by an osteophyte, the point should be placed at the intersection of the projected vertical anterior border of the vertebral body and the projected horizontal superior end-plate.

Deformed vertebrae: it is sometimes difficult to place points on deformed vertebrae due to their unusual shape. Point placement should follow the general concepts outlined above for normal vertebrae, but with points placed at the point of maximum height reduction of the vertebral body. More time and care are needed to analyse these vertebrae and the acquisition of both single-energy and high-definition dual-energy MXA scans may improve the visualization of deformed vertebral bodies.

If there seems to be a biconcavity (mid-wedge) deformity of the vertebral end-plates it is important to check that this is not an illusion created by lateral curvature of the spine (scoliosis) as this can result in the imaging of an elliptical projection of the vertebral end-plates. If the PA centre line scan shows a relatively straight spine, then the mid-points should be placed on the interior edge of the end-plates, since it is likely that some sort of deformity is present. However, if the PA scan shows some degree of scoliosis, then the points should be placed in the centre of each elliptical end-plate. Pronounced scoliosis can have a severely detrimental effect on the diagnostic quality of MXA images and scan acquisition, and analysis may not be possible.

It is useful to remember that image contrast and brightness can be adjusted during scan analysis and that it can be helpful to toggle between the standard image of white bone on a black background and the inverted black on white image. These adjustments may help identify the shape of a vertebral body where this is difficult to see because of overlying soft tissue or bony artefacts such as ribs.

During point placement it is important to make use of all the information available, not only from the lateral scan but also the PA centre line scan, and take into consideration the shape, position and size of the vertebral bodies either side of the one in question. This is especially important when analysing vertebrae in the thoracic spine using single-energy scans where soft tissue artefacts may cause problems in accurate point placement.

REFERENCES

1. Melton LJ, Kan SH, Frye MA et al. Epidemiology of vertebral fractures in women. *Am J Epidemiol* (1989) **129:** 1000–11.
2. Cooper C, Campion G, Melton LJ. Hip fractures in the elderly: a world-wide projection. *Osteoporos Int* (1992) **2:** 285–9.
3. Melton LJ, Thamer M, Ray NF et al. Fractures attributable to osteoporosis: report from the National Osteoporosis Foundation. *J Bone Miner Res* (1997) **12:** 16–23.
4. Ray NF, Chan JK, Thamer M et al. Medical expenditures for the treatment of osteoporotic fractures in the United States in 1995: report from the National Osteoporosis Foundation. *J Bone Miner Res* (1997) **12:** 24–35.
5. Cooper C, Atkinson EJ, O'Fallon WM et al. Incidence of clinically diagnosed vertebral fractures: a population based study in Rochester, Minnesota, 1985–1989. *J Bone Miner Res* (1992) **7:** 221–7.
6. Cummings SR, Nevitt MC, Browner WS et al. Risk factors for hip fracture in white women. *N Engl J Med* (1995) **332:** 767–73.
7. Elffors I, Allander E, Kanis JA et al. The variable incidence of hip fracture in Southern Europe: the MEDOS study. *Osteoporos Int* (1994) **4:** 253–63.
8. O'Neill TW, Felsenberg D, Varlow J et al. The prevalence of vertebral deformity in European men and women: the European vertebral osteoporosis study. *J Bone Miner Res* (1996) **11:** 1010–18.
9. Davies KM, Stegman MR, Heaney RP et al. Prevalence and severity of vertebral fracture: the Saunders County bone quality study. *Osteoporos Int* (1996) **6:** 160–5.
10. Melton LJ, O'Fallon WM, Riggs BL. Secular trends in the incidence of hip fractures. *Calcif Tissue Int* (1987) **41:** 57–64.
11. Cooper C, Atkinson EJ, Kotowicz M et al. Secular trends in the incidence of postmenopausal vertebral fractures. *Calcif Tissue Int* (1992) **51:** 100–4.

12. Cummings SR, Black BM, Nevitt MC et al. Bone density at various sites for prediction of hip fractures. *Lancet* (1993) **341:** 72–5.

13. Jergas M, Glüer C-C. Assessment of fracture risk by bone density measurements. *Semin Nucl Med* (1997) **27:** 261–75.

14. Hans D, Dargent-Molina P, Schott AM et al. Ultrasonographic heel measurements to predict hip fracture in elderly women: the EPIDOS prospective study. *Lancet* (1996) **348:** 511–14.

15. Bauer DC, Glüer C-C, Cauley JA et al. Broadband ultrasonic attenuation predicts fractures strongly and independently of densitometry in older women. *Arch Intern Med* (1997) **157:** 629–34.

16. Storm T, Thamsborg G, Steiniche T et al. Effect of intermittent cyclical etidronate therapy on bone mass and fracture rate in women with postmenopausal osteoporosis. *N Engl J Med* (1990) **322:** 1265–71.

17. Liberman UA, Weiss SR, Bröll J et al. Effect of oral alendronate on bone mineral density and the incidence of fractures in postmenopausal osteoporosis. *N Engl J Med* (1995) **333:** 1437–43.

18. Cummings SR, Black DM, Vogt TM. Changes in BMD substantially underestimate the anti-fracture effects of alendronate and other antiresorptive drugs. *J Bone Miner Res* (1996) **11**(suppl 1): S102.

19. Black DM, Cummings SR, Karpf DB et al. Randomised trial of effect of alendronate on risk of fracture in women with existing vertebral fractures. *Lancet* (1996) **348:** 1535–41.

20. Leidig-Bruckner G, Minne HW. The spine deformity index (SDI): a new approach to quantifying vertebral crush fractures in patients with osteoporosis. In: Genant HK, Jergas M, van Kuijk C, eds. *Vertebral fracture in osteoporosis* (University of California Osteoporosis Research Group: San Francisco, 1995), 235–52.

21. Ross PD, Davis JW, Epstein RS et al. Pain and disability associated with new vertebral fractures and other spinal conditions. *J Clin Epidemiol* (1994) **47:** 231–9.

22. Jensen GF, McNair P, Boesen J et al. Validity in diagnosing osteoporosis. *Eur J Radiol* (1984) **4:** 1–3.

23. Deyo RA, McNiesh LM, Cone RO. Observer variability in the interpretation of lumbar spine radiographs. *Arthritis Rheum* (1985) **28:** 1066–70.

24. Barnett E, Nordin BEC. The radiological diagnosis of osteoporosis: a new approach. *Clin Radiol* (1960) **11:** 166–74.

25. Hurxthal LM. Measurement of vertebral heights. *Am J Roentgenol* (1968) **103:** 635–44.

26. Jensen KK, Tougaard L. A simple x-ray method for monitoring progress of osteoporosis. *Lancet* (1981) **ii:** 19–20.

27. Minne HW, Leidig G, Wuster C et al. A newly developed spine deformity index (SDI) to quantitate vertebral crush fractures in patients with osteoporosis. *Bone Miner* (1988) **3:** 335–49.

28. Eastell R, Cedel SL, Wahner HW et al. Classification of vertebral fractures. *J Bone Miner Res* (1991) **6:** 207–15.

29. Black DM, Cummings SR, Stone K et al. A new approach to defining normal vertebral dimensions. *J Bone Miner Res* (1991) **6:** 883–92.

30. Melton LJ, Lane AW, Cooper C et al. Prevalence and incidence of vertebral deformities. *Osteoporos Int* (1993) **3:** 113–19.

31. McCloskey EV, Spector TD, Eyres KS et al. The assessment of vertebral deformity: a method for use in population studies and clinical trials. *Osteoporos Int* (1993) **3:** 138–47.

32. Genant HK, Wu CY, van Kuijk C et al. Vertebral fracture assessment using a semi-quantitative technique. *J Bone Miner Res* (1993) **8:** 1137–48.

33. Genant HK, Jergas M, Palermo L et al. Comparison of semiquantitative visual and quantitative morphometric assessment of prevalent and incident vertebral fractures in osteoporosis. *J Bone Miner Res* (1996) **11:** 984–96.

34. Cummings SR, Melton LJ, Felsenberg D et al. Assessing vertebral fractures. Report of the National Osteoporosis Foundation Working Group on Vertebral Fractures. *J Bone Miner Res* (1995) **10:** 518–23.

35. Jergas M, Valentin RS. Techniques for the assessment of vertebral dimensions in quantitative morphometry. In: Genant HK, Jergas M, van Kuijk C, eds. *Vertebral fracture in osteoporosis* (University of California Osteoporosis Research Group: San Francisco, 1995), 163–88.

36. Banks LM, van Kuijk C, Genant HK. Radiographic technique for assessing osteoporotic vertebral deformity. In: Genant HK, Jergas M, van Kuijk C, eds. *Vertebral fracture in osteoporosis* (University of California Osteoporosis Research Group: San Francisco, 1995), 131–47.

37. Kalender WA, Eidloth H. Determination of geometric parameters and osteoporosis indices for lumbar vertebrae from lateral QCT localizer radiographs. *Osteoporos Int* (1991) **1:** 197.

38. Felsenberg D, Kalender WA. Computer-assisted

morphometry of vertebral fractures. In: Genant HK, Jergas M, van Kuijk C, eds. *Vertebral fracture in osteoporosis* (University of California Osteoporosis Research Group: San Francisco, 1995), 309–17.

39. O'Neill TW, Varlow J, Felsenberg D et al. Variation in vertebral height ratios in population studies. *J Bone Miner Res* (1994) **9:** 1895–907.

40. ICRP. 1990 recommendations of the International Commission on Radiological Protection. Report 60. *Ann ICRP* (1991) **21**(1–3).

41. Shrimpton PC, Wall BF, Jones DG et al. *A national survey of doses to patients undergoing a selection of routine x-ray examinations in English hospitals.* National Radiological Protection Board, NRPB-R200 (HMSO: London, 1986).

42. Steiger P, Cummings SR, Genant HK et al. Morphometric x-ray absorptiometry of the spine: correlation in vivo with morphometric radiography. *Osteoporos Int* (1994) **4:** 238–44.

43. Jergas M, Lang TF, Fuerst T. Morphometric X-ray absorptiometry. In: Genant HK, Jergas M, van Kuijk C, eds. *Vertebral fracture in osteoporosis* (University of California Osteoporosis Research Group: San Francisco, 1995), 331–48.

44. Lang T, Takada M, Gee R et al. A preliminary evaluation of the Lunar Expert-XL for bone densitometry and vertebral morphometry. *J Bone Miner Res* (1997) **12:** 136–43.

45. Slosman DO, Rizzoli R, Donath A et al. Vertebral bone mineral density measured laterally by dual energy x-ray absorptiometry. *Osteoporos Int* (1990) **1:** 23–9.

46. Larnach TA, Boyd SJ, Smart RC et al. Reproducibility of lateral spine scans using dual energy x-ray absorptiometry. *Calcif Tissue Int* (1992) **51:** 255–8.

47. Rea JA, Steiger P, Blake GM et al. Optimizing data acquisition and analysis of morphometric x-ray absorptiometry. *Osteoporos Int* (1998) **8:** 177–83.

48. WHO Technical Report Series 843. Assessment of fracture risk and its applications to screening for postmenopausal osteoporosis (World Health Organization: Geneva, 1994).

49. Steiger P, Weiss H, von Stetten E et al. Automated, knowledge based analysis of morphometric x-ray absorptiometry (MXA) images. *Bone Miner* (1994) **25**(suppl 2): S10.

50. Rea JA, Steiger P, Blake GM et al. Morphometric x-ray absorptiometry: reference data for vertebral dimensions. *J Bone Miner Res* (1998) **13:** 464–74.

51. Mazess R, Barden H, Hanson J. Expert-XL vertebral morphometric normalization. *Osteoporos Int* (1997) **7:** 307.

52. Lewis MK, Blake GM. Patient dose in morphometric x-ray absorptiometry. *Osteoporos Int* (1995) **5:** 281–2.

53. Lewis MK, Blake GM, Fogelman I. Patient dose in dual x-ray absorptiometry. *Osteoporos Int* (1994) **4:** 11–15.

54. Blake GM, Rea JA, Fogelman I. Vertebral morphometry studies using dual-energy X-ray absorptiometry. *Semin Nucl Med* (1997) **27:** 276–90.

55. Smyth PP, Taylor CJ, Adams JE. Automated vertebral morphometry in DXA. *Osteoporos Int* (1997) **7:** 266.

56. Harvey SB, Hukins DW, Hutchison KM et al. Improved vertebral morphometry precision using images from Lunar Expert-XL bone densitometer. *J Bone Miner Res* (1997) **12**(suppl 1): S266.

Index